AF832274

Facial Palsy

Chieh-Han John Tzou
Andrés Rodríguez-Lorenzo
Editors

Facial Palsy

Techniques for Reanimation of the Paralyzed Face

Springer

Editors
Chieh-Han John Tzou
Plastic and Reconstructive Surgery
Hospital of Divine Savior (Krankenhaus Goettlicher Heiland), Sigmund Freud University, TZOU MEDICAL
Vienna
Austria

Andrés Rodríguez-Lorenzo
Department of Plastic and Maxillofacial Surgery and Department of Surgical Sciences
Uppsala University Hospital, Uppsala University
Uppsala
Sweden

ISBN 978-3-030-50783-1 ISBN 978-3-030-50784-8 (eBook)
https://doi.org/10.1007/978-3-030-50784-8

© Springer Nature Switzerland AG 2021
This work is subject to copyright. All rights are reserved by the Publisher, whether the whole or part of the material is concerned, specifically the rights of translation, reprinting, reuse of illustrations, recitation, broadcasting, reproduction on microfilms or in any other physical way, and transmission or information storage and retrieval, electronic adaptation, computer software, or by similar or dissimilar methodology now known or hereafter developed.
The use of general descriptive names, registered names, trademarks, service marks, etc. in this publication does not imply, even in the absence of a specific statement, that such names are exempt from the relevant protective laws and regulations and therefore free for general use.
The publisher, the authors, and the editors are safe to assume that the advice and information in this book are believed to be true and accurate at the date of publication. Neither the publisher nor the authors or the editors give a warranty, expressed or implied, with respect to the material contained herein or for any errors or omissions that may have been made. The publisher remains neutral with regard to jurisdictional claims in published maps and institutional affiliations.

This Springer imprint is published by the registered company Springer Nature Switzerland AG
The registered company address is: Gewerbestrasse 11, 6330 Cham, Switzerland

Preface

> "The facial expressions of human beings fascinate me because they convey both the lowest, most bestial pleasures and the strongest and gentlest emotions of the spirit."—Sir Charles Bells (1774–1842)

Facial paralysis is a devastating condition, which substantially affects a patient's quality of life. The face is one of the most visible parts of the body, and facial expressions are critical in human communication, social interaction, and self-esteem. Injuries to the facial nerve have important functional consequences, such as corneal damage from the impariment of blinking and the derangement of speaking and eating from the loss of oral continence.

Facial paralysis is a fascinating and dynamic field, full of constant innovations, with a vast variety of surgical approaches and techniques. Reanimation of the paralyzed face is considered by many to be one of the most challenging endeavors in reconstructive surgery, as it requires knowledge of multiple complex surgical techniques and disciplines, such as peripheral nerve surgery, microvascular surgery, and aesthetic facial surgery. As reconstructive surgeons with interest in facial palsy, we are passionate and enthusiastic about new technical innovations and surgical approaches to improve the quality of life of patients with paralyzed faces. Success in providing the best clinical outcomes in the rapidly changing field of facial reanimation relies on multidisciplinary collaborations. In this book, we wanted to honor our precious multidisciplinary collaborations and bring up all aspects of therapies by including experts from various disciplines and specialties.

This work, *Facial Palsy: Techniques for Reanimation of the Paralyzed Face,* is a collaborative effort among international experts aiming to provide the most comprehensive and detailed overview of the most pertinent surgical procedures, including a wide spectrum of innovative and cutting-edge approaches and an up-to-date guide to every aspect of reanimating the paralyzed face.

This book is structured in six parts and 38 chapters. The first part focuses on general principles in facial paralysis, including diagnosis, nonsurgical treatments, and documentation of patient outcomes. The second part is related to facial nerve anatomy and reconstruction techniques, including nerve repair, nerve grafts, vascularized nerves, and nerve transfers. The third and fourth parts address the surgical management of long-standing facial palsy, including smile reanimation techniques and rehabilitation of the paretic eye. The fifth part relates to symmetrization of the paralyzed face and ancillary procedures. The sixth and final part focuses on current new frontiers and innovations in reconstructing the paralyzed face.

We are deeply grateful to all authors who devoted an enormous amount of time to this comprehensive coverage of current state-of-the-art knowledge. Your time is a most precious gift—to this book, to the medical society, and to our patients—a gift that can never be returned. Thank you! Moreover, we heartily thank the Springer Nature team—von Behrens Inga, Sasirekka Nijanthan, Martina Himberger, and Daniela Heller—for their continuous professional assistance throughout this project.

Andrés: I would like to dedicate this book to my mentors throughout my career: my first chief and mentor, Dr. Francisco Martelo, for introducing me to plastic surgery; Dr. Pedro Cavadas for showing me what is possible in reconstructive microsurgery; Professor Fu-Chan Wei, for your example of leadership and excellence; and Professor David Chuang, for encouraging me and inspiring me to go into the fascinating field of facial paralysis. I also dedicate this book to my wonderful wife, Debora, and my daughters, Nadia and Olivia, for your endless love, support, and patience. You are the biggest success of my life.

John: I dedicate this book and offer my deepest gratitude to my mentors: Professor Manfred Frey, who introduced me to his beloved field of the reanimation of the paralyzed face; Professor Rafael Leopold Walzer, for showing me amazing and exciting insights in your trick box of plastic and reconstructive microsurgery; Professor Thomas Rath, for globally broadening my view of plastic surgery; Professor Fu-Chan Wei, for your care, leadership, and excellence; and Professor David Chuang, for your amazing inspirations to think outside the box. Moreover, I dedicate this book to my family for your unfailingly support, endless love, and everlasting belief in me.

Last but not least, we would like to express our most sincere gratitude to all patients who have made this book possible by sharing and permitting the publications of photographs related to their treatments. You are a true source of inspiration for all of us.

It is an honor to serve you.

With us, reconstructive surgery has not been a purpose, but a passion.

Uppsala, Sweden — Andrés Rodríguez-Lorenzo
Vienna, Austria — Chieh-Han John Tzou
2020

Contents

About the Editors

Chieh-Han John Tzou completed his medical education and plastic surgery residency at the Medical University of Vienna, Austria, followed by a 1½-year microvascular fellowship at the Chang Gung Memorial University Hospital in Taiwan. Currently, he is the director of the Plastic Reconstructive Surgery Clinic of the Hospital of the Divine Savior and TZOU MEDICAL, Facial Palsy and Lymphedema Center, and is affiliated as an Associate Professor for Plastic and Reconstructive Surgery at the Medical Faculty of the Sigmund Freud University, Vienna, Austria. His focus in clinical work and research is microsurgical and supermicrosurgical reconstruction in facial paralysis, lymphedema, nerve, and tumor patients. He is the co-director of the biennial course "Facial Palsy: A Hands-on Course—www.facialpalsy.eu" in Vienna, Austria.

Andrés Rodríguez-Lorenzo completed his plastic surgery residency and PhD studies at the University Hospital of A Coruña, Spain, followed by a 2-year microvascular fellowship at the Canniesburn Plastic Surgery Unit in Glasgow and the Chang Gung Memorial University Hospital in Taiwan. Currently, he is the Chief and Associate Professor in Plastic Surgery and the program director of the International Fellowship Program in Microsurgery at the Uppsala University Hospital, leading one of the most active microsurgical centers in Scandinavia. His main research focus is head and neck reconstruction, including preclinical studies of face transplantation, virtual planning, and facial paralysis. He is the co-director of the biennial course "Facial Palsy: A Hands-on Course—www.facialpalsy.eu" in Vienna, Austria, and the biannual Scandinavian Facial Nerve Meeting in Uppsala, Sweden.

Part I

Facial Paralysis

1 Facial Paralysis: Etiology, Diagnosis, and Medical Treatment

Lars Jonsson

1.1 The Facial Nerve

The main portion of the facial nerve, cranial nerve VII (CN VII), consists of motor fibers innervating the facial musculature for voluntary and involuntary emotional movements. This is its most important function. The nerve also carries motor fibers to the stapedius, posterior auricular, occipital belly of occipitofrontalis, posterior belly of the digastric and stylohyoid muscles. It also comprises parasympathetic and sensory components that are carried by the intermediate nerve of Wrisberg. The long and inextricable motor pathway of the facial nerve from the cortical region through the brain, brain stem, temporal bone, and parotid gland to the facial muscles makes it susceptible to injury and disease. Depending on the location of injury and origin of disease, facial nerve disorders will present differently in the clinic. Knowledge of nerve anatomy as well as clinical signs of diseases affecting the nerve is thus essential in diagnosing and treating facial nerve dysfunction. This chapter reviews the more common causes of facial paralysis and discusses relevant early medical treatment strategies.

L. Jonsson (✉)
Department of Surgical Sciences,
Otorhinolaryngology and Head and Neck Surgery,
Uppsala University, Uppsala, Sweden

© Springer Nature Switzerland AG 2021
C.-H. J. Tzou, A. Rodríguez-Lorenzo (eds.), *Facial Palsy*,
https://doi.org/10.1007/978-3-030-50784-8_1

1.2 Facial Nerve Pathways

The control of facial muscle movements has a complicated and spread central neural representation. Movements are dually controlled, voluntary and/or involuntary emotional. There are at least five bilateral cortical representations that project to the four paired facial subnuclei in the pons—these subnuclei selectively innervate various facial muscle groups. The primary motor cortex (M1) and the ventral lateral premotor cortex on the lateral side and the supplementary motor region (M2) on the medial aspect of each hemisphere are important for the facial voluntary control. The rostral (M3) and caudal cingulate cortex (M4) on the medial side of the hemispheres receive information from the limbic system and are essential for involuntary emotional facial movements, for overview see Müri [1]. The central innervation of the upper facial muscles is bilateral while the regulation of the lower part of the face mainly is contralateral. One vital clinical sign is therefore the preservation of forehead and eye closure function in a central (contralateral) lesion contrary to the reduced tone and weakness seen in these muscles on the affected side of a peripheral facial lesion (Figs. 1.1 and 1.2). A central (supranuclear) facial injury is often accompanied by tongue weakness and hemiparesis starting with thumb, finger, and hand movements on the ipsilateral side to facial paralysis due to the close relation of these motor centers in

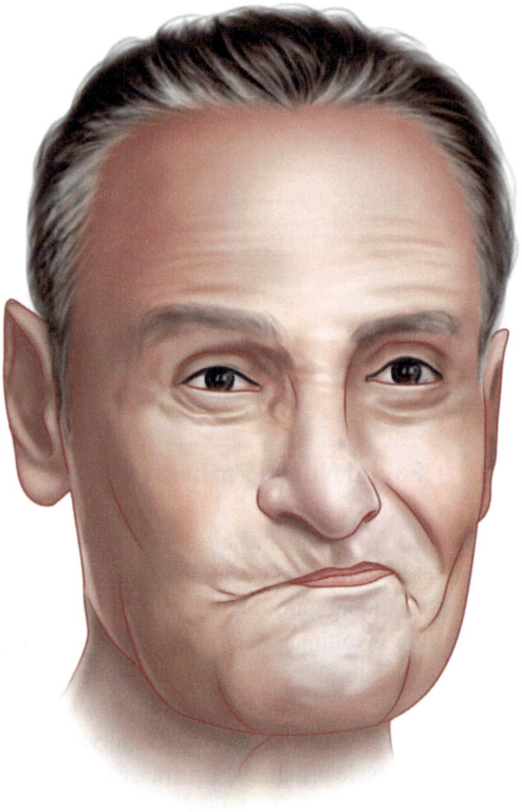

Fig. 1.1 Central facial paralysis on the right side. Central lesion on the left side and contralateral (right) lower facial musculature affected (drooping corner of the mouth and less pronounced nasolabial fold). Upper facial musculature (eye and forehead) unaffected

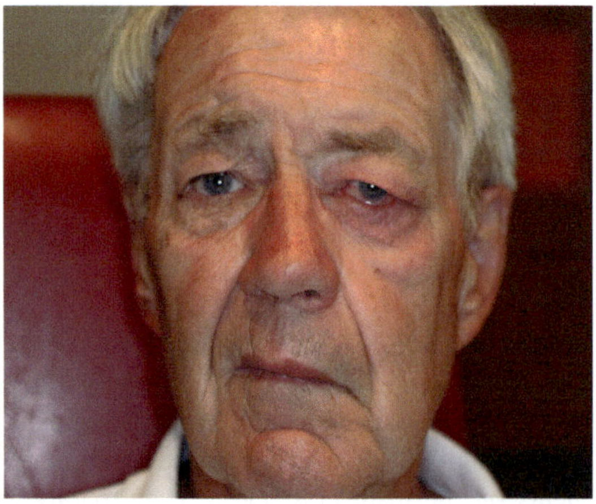

Fig. 1.2 Left-sided peripheral facial paralysis. Ipsilateral lower and upper facial musculature affected with drooping corner of the mouth, less pronounced nasolabial fold, lagophthalmos/wide eye and less pronounced forehead wrinkles. Published with oral and written permission from the patient

the cortex and internal capsule. Signs and appearance of central and peripheral facial palsy (Bell's palsy) are illustrated in Table 1.1. From a clinical viewpoint, the disparity of the central pathways between the voluntary corticofacial projections and involuntary emotional projections explains why emotional responses are intact (except for cases of severe unilateral brain damage) in upper motor neuron (supranuclear) facial paralysis affecting the corticobulbar tract responsible for voluntary facial movements.

A lesion affecting the pontine facial motor nucleus and/or the facial nerve peripheral to the nucleus usually affects both the upper and lower facial muscles. If the peripheral facial palsy originates from a central lesion of the nucleus or fascicle, other signs from nearby structures most often will be present. The palsy is usually accompanied by other nearby neurological signs with gaze palsy/internal strabismus on the side of facial paralysis, plus contralateral hemiparesis, ataxia, and cerebellovestibular signs [2]. Preservation of the forehead, which is a sign of a central (supranuclear) lesion, may, however, appear with a selective lesion in the nucleus as well as intra- or extratemporal portion of the facial nerve.

Before the facial nerve emerges from the pons, fibers loop around the nuclei of CN VI (abducens nerve). The nerve accompanies the CN VIII (vestibulocochlear nerve) in the cisternal and auditory internal meatus pathways. After entering its own bony canal (the fallopian canal in the temporal bone), the nerve makes two bends and divides in labyrinthine, horizontal tympanic, and vertical mastoid segments before leaving the skull base through the stylomastoid foramen. The labyrinthine portion ends at the geniculate ganglion where the nerve makes its first external bend. At this point, the greater petrosal nerve exits with parasympathetic motor fibers to the sphenopalatine ganglion and supply the lacrimal, nasal and palatinal glands. In the horizontal tympanic portion, a second nerve branch exits for the stapedial muscle, which protects the inner ear from loud noise. In the vertical mastoid segment, visceral branches forming the chorda tympany provide submandibular and sublingual gland innervation as well as taste to the anterior two-thirds of the tongue (Fig. 1.3).

Table 1.1 Characteristics of central and peripheral facial palsy (Bell's palsy)

	Central	Peripheral facial palsy
Forehead wrinkle	Normal	Weakened/flaccid
Eye closure	Normal	Lagophthalmos/wide eye
Nasolabial fold/oral commissure	Less pronounced/drooping	Less pronounced/drooping
Onset	Rapid (seconds to minutes)	Hours to 2–3 days
Associated symptoms	Weakness arm/leg, slurred speech, double vision, ataxia vertigo (cerebellovestibular symptoms), problems swallowing	Periauricular and/or neck pain, hyperacusis, taste disturbance, reduced tearing
Age (years)	> 60	20–60

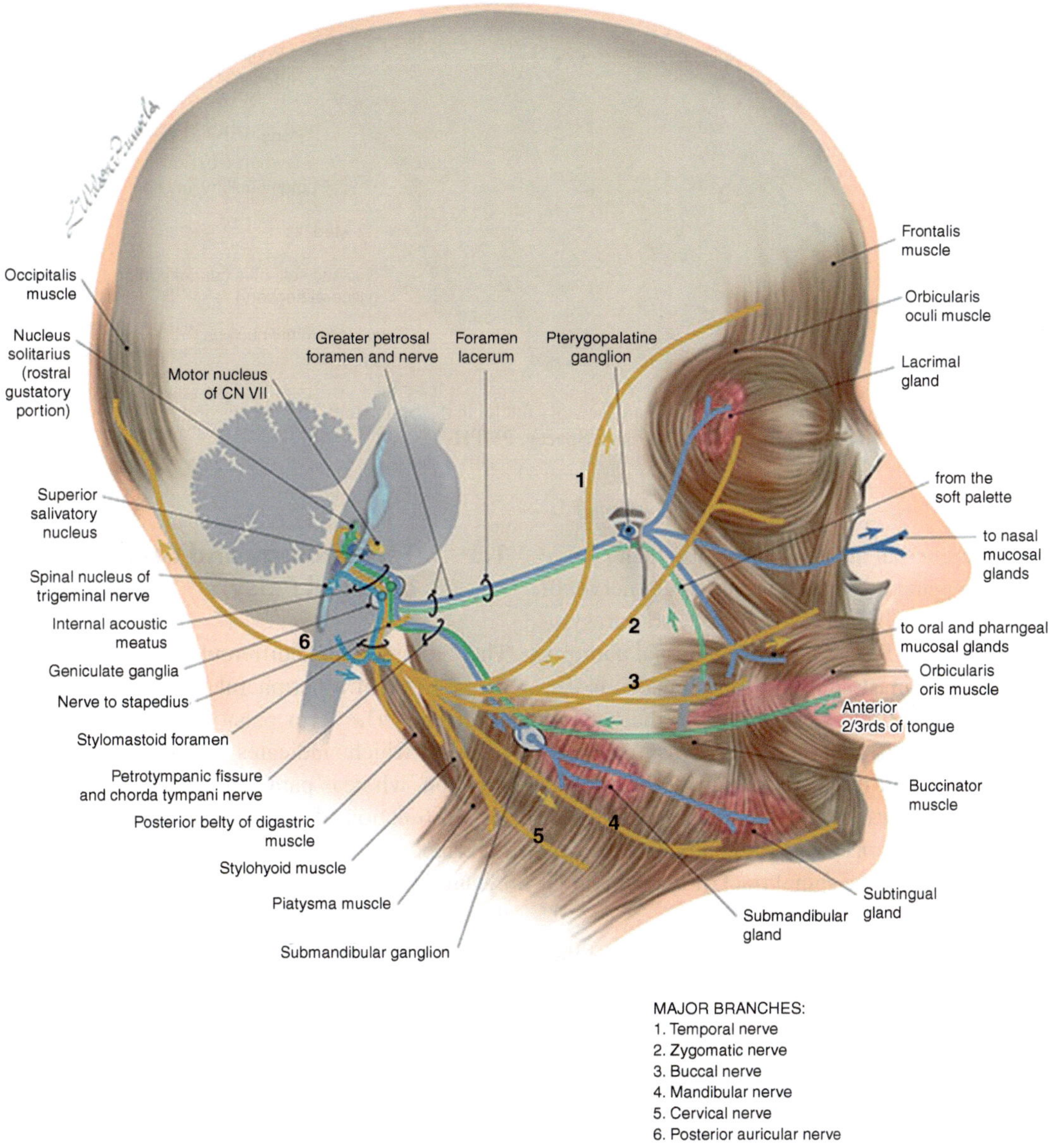

Fig. 1.3 Overview of the facial nerve components (parotid gland removed). (By permission from Cranial Nerves 3rd Ed. © 2010 Wilson-Pauwels, Stewart, Akesson, Spacey, PMPH-USA)

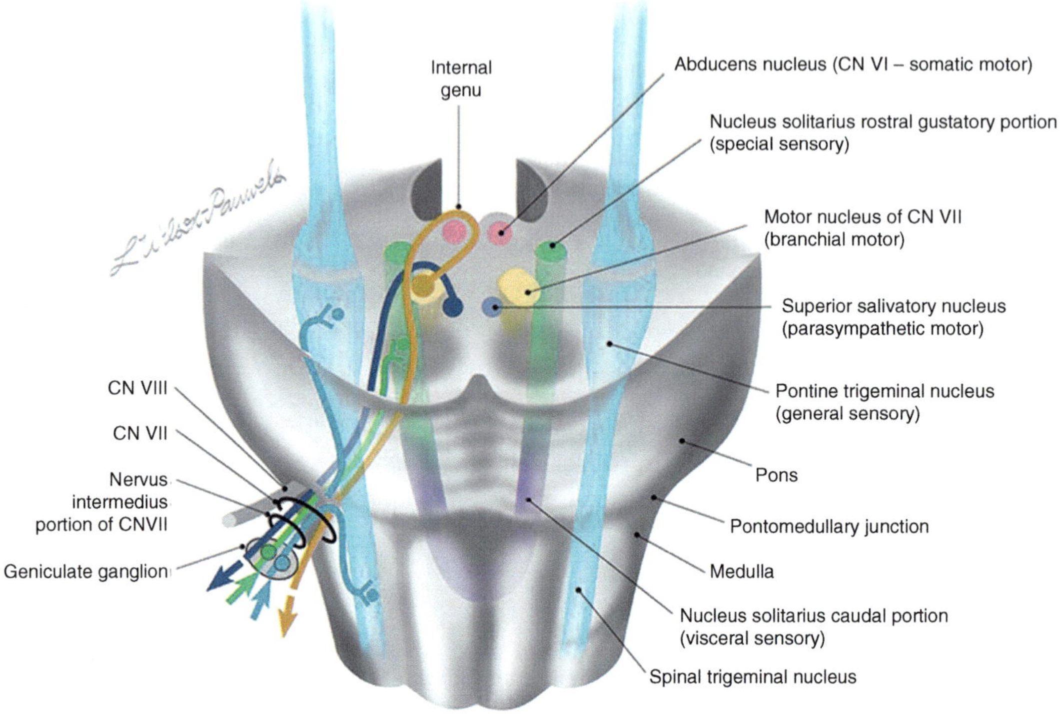

Fig. 1.4 Facial nerve motor, parasympathetic and sensory nuclei in the brain stem. (By permission from Cranial Nerves 3rd Ed. © 2010 Wilson-Pauwels, Stewart, Akesson, Spacey, PMPH-USA)

In the internal auditory canal, the facial nerve is accompanied by the intermediate nerve of Wrisberg, which contains sensory and parasympathetic fibers. Sensation of the external auditory canal, pinna, mastoid, and palate mucosa is carried by afferent fibers, as is taste in the anterior two-thirds of the tongue. The parasympathetic fibers emerge in the superior salivatory nucleus while taste fibers end in the nucleus of tractus solitarius. The sensory afferent fibers terminate in the nucleus of the spinal tract of the trigeminal nerve, CN V (Fig. 1.4).

The facial nerve exits the skull base through the stylomastoid foramen. It gives off the posterior auricular nerve for sensation of the periauricular area before traveling anteriorly through the parotid gland and dividing into five terminal branches that supply the muscles of facial expression; the temporofrontal, zygomatic, buccal, marginal mandibular, and cervical branches.

1.3 Terminology and Grading of Facial Palsy

The literature uses different terms to describe the severity of a peripheral palsy, which can be confusing. The term palsy can be divided into paresis, which indicates some facial muscle function, whereas paralysis indicates a complete loss of function (flaccid face). Palsy may also be described as incomplete or complete, the former meaning still some facial muscle function, while the latter means total loss of function with a flaccid face. The terms incomplete and complete are most often used in the early stage of palsy, but also in the recovery stage of palsy. A better terminology for this would instead be incomplete or complete recovery. In summary, the term palsy respective paralysis is often assimilated with each other in the literature.

Evaluating and describing facial function requires an objective and reliable measurement system that can be used both in the acute stage and to assess the course of recovery over time. Grading facial function is also an instrument for clinical prediction of non-recovery in Bell's palsy [3]. The most widely used systems today are the gross scaled House–Brackmann [4] system and the regional weighted Sunnybrook facial grading systems [5]. Grading scales in facial palsy are described in Chaps. 2, 3.

1.4 Evaluation of Peripheral Facial Palsy

At the initial examination, first determine if the facial weakness is of central or peripheral origin. A central lesion with thrombosis, hemorrhage, tumor, or trauma affecting the voluntary corticofacial projections may cause weakness of the lower contralateral face with flattened nasolabial fold and dropped corner of the mouth. Forehead wrinkle and eye closure is, contrary to a peripheral palsy, intact due to bilateral cortical representation of the upper face. Facial emotional involuntary expressions are not affected. Loss of involuntary emotional facial movements indicates involvement of cingulate corticofacial projections. Acute ischemic cerebral stroke from an arterial obstruction, contrary to the peripheral type, results in an immediate onset of palsy.

1.5 Causes of Peripheral Facial Palsy

A number of diseases are related to/or cause peripheral facial palsy. A lesion that involves the facial nerve in the cerebellopontine angle often affects CN VIII with sensorineural hearing loss, tinnitus, and vertigo. Most common are vestibular schwannomas and meningiomas. Acute idiopathic facial palsy (Bell's palsy), most probably located to the meatal segment and facial hemangiomas, neuromas, acute and chronic (cholesteatomas) ear infection, temporal bone fractures involving the facial canal are other conditions affecting the facial nerve. Topognostic testing may help locate the level of intratemporal lesion. Decreased lacrimation indicates a lesion proximal to the branch of the greater petrosal superficial nerve, hyperacusis, and loss of gustation proximal to the stapedial respective chorda tympani branches.

The proportion of causes of facial nerve disorders varies in the literature. One reason is that referral centers may differ when comparing facial nerve disorders that are examined and treated at the respective institutions. Furthermore, standards for reporting the different causes of facial nerve disorders are lacking. Table 1.2 summarizes the most common main causes of facial disorders from the results of three large studies including 8291 cases. The studies included cases examined in 1963 and 1996 with 3721 cases—3650 patients— [2], 2570 patients seen over 25 years (year of examination not stated) in the study of Peitersen published 2002 [6], and 2000 cases of facial palsy between 2003 and 2013 by Hohman and Hadlock 2014 [7]. The predominating causes are idiopathic facial palsy (53%),

Table 1.2 Proportion (percent) of the main causes of peripheral facial palsy based on three studies including 8291 facial nerve disorders, Schaitkin and colleagues 2000 [2], Peitersen 2002 [6] and Hohman & Hadlock 2014 [7]

Main cause of peripheral facial palsy	Proportion (percent)
Idiopathic including Bell's palsy	53
Trauma (including iatrogenic)	14
Tumor (including benign tumor, malignancy, cholesteatoma and postresection tumor)	9
Herpes zoster oticus	6
Congenital/birth/neonatal	5
Infection (excluding herpes zoster)	4
Stroke, central nervous disease (lesion) and vascular brainstem	2
Facial hyperkinesis/spasm	1
Other—Not classified	6

Reference [2] by permission from Thieme Publishers, New York, United States, reference [6] copyright © Acta Oto-Laryngologica AB (Ltd) by permission Taylor & Francis Ltd., Abingdon, United Kingdom, http://www.tanfonline.com on behalf of Acta Oto-Laryngologica AB (Ltd) and the late author's son Claus Peitersen and reference [7] by permission from the publisher Wiley, United States, © 2013 The American Laryngological, Rhinological and Otological Society, Inc.

trauma (14%), tumor (9%), herpes zoster (6%), congenital palsy (5%), and infection (4%). It should however be noted that the etiological proportions varied between studies. In the study of Peitersen [6], idiopathic palsy had a percentage of 66 compared with 38 percent in the study of Hohman and Hadlock [7]. May reported as many as 849 of 3721 (23%) traumatic cases compared with 95 of 2570 (4%) reported by Peitersen [6].

1.6 Differential Diagnosis of Peripheral Facial Palsy

Lower motor neuron lesion is the most frequent cause of facial nerve disease. The most common clinical sign is ipsilateral facial muscle weakness and, more seldom, stimulation. In rare cases, both sides of the face may be affected [8]. As previously mentioned, the acute idiopathic form of palsy (Bell's palsy) is the commonest type. Nevertheless, a number of differential diagnoses (discussed in Sect. 1.7) have to be excluded when a patient presents with a facial palsy. The comprehensive book on the facial nerve by May and Schaitkin reviews the causes of facial paralysis and classifies them in groups that have since been widely used in the literature [2]. Table 1.3 presents a differential diagnosis of facial palsy and attempts to grade the most common etiological factors with the help of two large studies published during this century, 2500 cases by Peitersen published in 2002 [6] and 2000 cases of facial palsy seen between 2003 and 2013 by Hohman and Hadlock [7].

1.7 Bell's Palsy

Bell's palsy, named after the Scottish surgeon and anatomist Sir Charles Bell, presents as rapid (usually maximal development within 48 h) unilateral weakness or paralysis of the face due to acute dysfunction of the peripheral facial nerve with no readily identifiable cause and some recovery within 3–6 months [9]. Bell's palsy accounts for 50–70% of peripheral facial palsies and the annual incidence is about 30 per 100,000 individuals. There is no difference in gender or side of the face, and no seasonal clustering. Peak incidence is between ages 30 and 60. Diabetes mellitus, hypertension, and pregnancy (third trimester and 2 weeks postpartum) are considered as risk factors. Ipsilateral pain around the ear or in the neck (50–60%), taste disturbance (35%), and/or hyperacusis (30%) are concomitant symptoms.

The rate of misdiagnosis of Bell's palsy by the initial consulting clinician has been reported to be approximately 1% but also as high as 10.8% [10]. Approximately 7% of Bell's palsy patients will have a recurrence—either ipsilateral or contralateral—to previous palsy. Contralateral (alternating) recurrent palsy is usually benign and the need for extended investigation is not so urgent [10]. An ipsilateral (recurrent palsy) recurrence, however, requires a meticulous search for another etiology. Searching for a neoplasm of the facial nerve (schwannoma) or temporal bone and parotid gland is also required. The Melkersson–Rosenthal syndrome with recurrent facial palsy, fissured tongue and periodic lip or facial swelling as well as sarcoidosis is another differential diagnosis to be considered. The diagnosis of Bell's palsy should be reevaluated if there is deviation in history, new or worsening neurologic findings, new symptoms and/or clinical findings or if there are no signs of recovery within 3–4 months [11, 12] (Table 1.4).

The etiology and pathogenic mechanism in Bell's palsy is by definition not known. A possible cause of nerve injury is inflammation of the facial nerve, which might be related to herpes simplex virus type 1 and/or varicella zoster reactivation (zoster sine herpete). The virus theory is supported by the presence of herpes simplex virus type 1 DNA in facial nerve endoneural fluid and/or tissue from posterior auricular muscle in Bell's palsy patients [13]. Edema of the facial nerve within the fallopian canal has been noticed during decompressive surgery for Bell's palsy and the finding of facial nerve contrast enhancement (mainly the meatal/labyrinthine segment) on MRI may be explained by inflammatory damage to the blood-nerve barrier, with increased vascular permeability and/or venous congestion [14].

Table 1.3 Cause of peripheral facial palsy and approximate frequency

Cause of peripheral facial palsy	Approximate frequency Hohman and Hadlock [7]	Approximate frequency Peitersen [6]
Bell's palsy—idiopathic (54%)	761	1701
Neoplastic (10%)	355	105
Acoustic neuroma/vestibular schwannoma[a] (includes neurofibromatosis type 2)		
Head and neck cancer[a]		
Facial nerve tumor		
Parotid tumor lesions (benign and malignant)		
Metastatic carcinoma		
Cholesteatoma		
Leukemia		
Lymphoma		
Meningioma		
Glomus jugulare tumor		
Hemangioblastoma		
Sarcoma		
Anomalous sigmoid sinus		
Carotid artery aneurysm		
Hemangioma of tympanum		
Hidradenoma		
Teratoma		
Histiocytosis		
Fibrous dysplasia		
Temporal bone myeloma		
Carcinomatous encephalitis		
Endolymphatic sac tumors		
Fibrosarcoma		
Ossifying hemangioma		
Granular cell myoblastoma		
Infection (7%)	151	148
Herpes zoster		
Lyme neuroborreliosis		
Acute and chronic otitis/mastoiditis		
HIV		
Mononucleosis		
Poliomyelitis		
Meningitis/encephalitis		
Tuberculosis		
Mumps		
Malignant external otitis		
Chickenpox		
Coxsackie virus		
Influenza		
Acute suppurative parotitis		
Leprosy		
Malaria		
Sinus thrombosis		
Syphilis		
Scleroma		

(continued)

Table 1.3 (continued)

Cause of peripheral facial palsy	Approximate frequency Hohman and Hadlock [7]	Approximate frequency Peitersen [6]
Botulism		
Mucormycosis		
Leptospirosis		
Zika virus		
Acute hemorrhagic conjunctivitis		
Gnathostomiasis		
Mucormycosis		
Cat scratch disease		
Congenital/birth/neonatal age (6%)	99	169
Non-syndromic		
Congenital unilateral lower lip paralysis		
Möbius syndrome		
Forceps delivery		
Myotonic dystrophy		
Trauma (5%)	113	95
Skull base fracture		
Facial soft tissue and bone injuries		
Middle ear injury		
Genetic and metabolic (4%)	82	80
Diabetes		
Pregnancy associated		
Hyper/hypothyroidism		
Hypertension		
Alcoholic neuropathy		
Autoimmune/neurologic/others (3%)	32	124
Melkersson–Rosenthal syndrome		
Sarcoidosis		
Multiple sclerosis		
Collagenosis		
Guillain–Barré syndrome		
Myasthenia gravis		
Amyloidosis		
Hereditary hypertrophic neuropathy (Charcot–Marie–Tooth disease)		
Dejerine–Sottas disease		
Temporal arteritis		
Thrombotic thrombocytopenic purpura (TTP)		
Periarteritis nodosa		
Osteopetrosis		
Osteogenesis imperfecta		
Kawasaki disease		
Iatrogenic (3%) (not including postresection or postradiation acoustic neuroma/head and neck cancer)	143	0
Oral surgery		
Head and neck surgery		
Otologic surgery		
Cosmetic surgery		
Neurosurgery		

Table 1.3 (continued)

Cause of peripheral facial palsy	Approximate frequency Hohman and Hadlock [7]	Approximate frequency Peitersen [6]
Temporal artery biopsy		
Mandibular block anesthesia		
Antitetanus serum		
Rabies vaccination		
Dental		
Sagittal split osteotomy		
Embolization		
Central lesion (2%)	79	34
Central nervous lesion and disease/stroke		
Vascular brainstem lesion/stroke		
Millard–Gubler syndrome (lesion in base of pons with abducens palsy and contralateral hemiplegia)		
Toxicity (0%)	0	0
Thalidomide		
Tetanus		
Diphtheria		
Carbon monoxide		
Lead intoxication		
Ethylene glycol		
Arsenic intoxication		
Alcoholism		
Anticancer drugs		
Not classified (6%)		

Modified after Schaitkin and colleagues 2000 [2]. Approximate frequency according to average numbers given by Peitersen 2002 [6] including 2570 patients and Hohman and Hadlock 2014 [7] including 2000 patients
[a]Includes postresection and postradiation. Reference [2] by permission Thieme Publishers, New York, United States, reference [6] copyright © Acta Oto-Laryngologica AB (Ltd) by permission Taylor & Francis Ltd., Abingdon, United Kingdom, http://www.tanfonline.com on behalf of Acta Oto-Laryngologica AB (Ltd) and the late author's son Claus Peitersen and reference [7] by permission from the publisher Wiley, United States, © 2013 The American Laryngological, Rhinological and Otological Society, Inc.

Table 1.4 History and findings/symptoms that should reevaluate the diagnosis of Bell's palsy

History	Findings/symptoms
Gradual onset of palsy No improvement within 3–4 months Living in a Borrelia-endemic area Risk factors for HIV Facial skin cancer Systemic cancer	Vertigo, hearing loss, tinnitus Bilateral facial palsy Other cranial nerve involvement Febrile illness, fatigue, malaise, radicular pain, and general headache (borreliosis) Limb or bulbar weakness Parotid gland enlargement Otitis media Vesicles in external ear/ear canal, tympanic membrane and/or oropharynx Cervical adenopathy Facial swelling/fissured tongue

Medical treatment of Bell's palsy is based on the theory that inflammation and edema produced by herpes virus of the facial nerve is implicated in its cause. Many trials, limited in size, studying the efficacy of corticosteroids in Bell's palsy had been carried out before two large Class I randomized and placebo-controlled multi-center Bell's palsy trials were published in 2007 and 2008: a Scottish study including 551 patients treated with prednisolone and/or aciclovir [15] and a Scandinavian study including 829 patients treated with prednisolone and/or valaciclovir [16]. In both trials, evidence for the efficacy of oral corticosteroid treatment (compared with no prednisolone) started within 72 h after onset of palsy was demonstrated. In the study of Sullivan and co-workers [15], early treatment with prednisolone 25 mg twice per day for 10 days significantly improved the chances of complete recovery at 3 and 9 months. In the trial of Engström and colleagues [16], patients given prednisolone 60 mg daily for 5 days then tapering to 10 mg daily (total treatment time 10 days) had a significantly shorter time to complete recovery and a significantly higher rate of recovery at 3, 6, and 12 months. With these two Class I studies as base, the guideline development group in the clinical practice guidelines of the American Academy of Otolaryngology—Head and Neck Surgery Foundation published in 2013 recommends a 10-day course of either prednisolone 50 mg for 10 days or prednisolone (the guideline says prednisone) 60 mg for 5 days with a 5-day taper initiated within 72 h of symptom onset [11]. The efficacy of corticosteroids was also stated in the Cochrane Database of Systematic Reviews published in 2016 in which the authors concluded that the available moderate- to high-quality evidence from randomized controlled trials shows significant benefit from treating Bell's palsy with corticosteroids [17]. The benefit of corticosteroid treatment for Bell's palsy after 72 h is less clear since Class I studies with treatment started after this time point are lacking [11]. In his guidelines based on a combination of data and theoretical mechanism of action, Vrabec discusses that the prognosis for those with complete palsy (compared with incomplete) is much poorer, and that treatment is advocated even if presentation is delayed for more than 1 week. After 2 weeks from onset, it is unlikely that any treatment will impact the recovery [18]. With caution regarding side-effects taken into consideration, this reasoning seems logical until further knowledge on the effect of delayed corticosteroid treatment is obtained.

The theory that Bell's palsy is related to a viral herpes infection has led to numerous treatment trials on the effect of antivirals of which aciclovir and valaciclovir are most studied. Including the abovementioned Class I studies [15, 16] both guideline development groups in the clinical practice guidelines of the American Academy of Otolaryngology—Head and Neck Surgery Foundation published in 2013 and the Cochrane Database of Systematic Reviews published in 2015 concluded that antiviral therapy alone in Bell's palsy is no better than placebo with respect to facial recovery [11, 19]. Antiviral treatment in combination with corticosteroids was studied in the two Class I trials by Sullivan and co-workers [15] and Engström and colleagues [16] and the addition of antivirals to corticosteroids was not proven to be of benefit in Bell's palsy. Several Bell's palsy studies of lower methodological class have reported minor improvements in facial nerve recovery with the addition of antivirals to corticosteroids so a small benefit with combination therapy cannot be excluded [11]. The guideline development group in the clinical practice guidelines of the American Academy of Otolaryngology—Head and Neck Surgery Foundation published in 2013 concluded that patients may be offered combination therapy if treated within 72 h of palsy onset, with a large role for shared decision-making. Gagyor and colleagues [19] concluded in the Cochrane Database of Systematic Reviews published in 2015 that low-quality evidence from randomized controlled trials shows a benefit from the combination of antivirals with corticosteroids compared with corticosteroids alone for the treatment of Bell's palsy of various degrees of severity. If the patient is given combination therapy, peroral antiviral valaciclovir 1000 mg 3 times daily for 7 days can be recommended.

In general, mild palsy and signs of improvement within the first 2 weeks indicate a shorter time for recovery. Patients with poor improvement after 8 weeks are at high risk for suffering sequelae. Recovery has generally reached its maximum after 9 or 12 months. In severe cases, synkinesis develops after approximately 3–4 months and may deteriorate up to 12 months after onset of palsy [20]. Recurrent Bell's palsy, on the same or opposite side, occurs in about 7% of cases. About 70% of patients with Bell's palsy recover completely within 6 months without treatment [6]. The remainder will suffer sequelae that consist of residual palsy, contracture, and synkinesis.

Due to inadequate eye closure and/or reduced tearing in most Bell's palsy patients, topical eye care to protect the cornea from dryness and abrasion needs to be initiated as soon as possible: lubricating eye drops at least 6–8 times daily, frequent closure of the upper eye lid with a finger by the patient and tight glasses (sun- or sports glasses) at day time, eye ointment at night, lateral eye lid cross-taping, patching and, in severe cases, a moisture chamber. In case of ocular symptoms such as pain, irritation, or itching, the patient should immediately be referred to an eye specialist. Patients with severe, persistent lagophthalmos also should have an ophthalmologic evaluation [11].

The effect of surgery for treatment of Bell's palsy is dubious and the literature gives no clear recommendations. Since the initial injury is thought to be located in the meatal/labyrinthine portion of the facial nerve only, transmastoid decompression of the facial nerve is insufficient. Middle fossa decompression, including the meatal portion, in patients diagnosed with a severe palsy (House–Brackmann score VI, electroneurography >90% nerve degeneration, and no response on voluntary electromyography) and operated on within 2 weeks after onset was reported to improve outcome compared with corticosteroid treatment only in a case control study by Gantz and colleagues [21]. The Cochrane Database of Systematic Reviews published in 2013 by McAllister and co-workers concluded that only very low quality evidence has emerged from randomized controlled trials and that this is insufficient to decide whether surgical intervention is beneficial or harmful in the management of Bell's palsy [22]. The clinical practice guidelines of the American Academy of Otolaryngology-Head and Neck Surgery Foundation from 2013 state that limited data support surgical decompression of the meatal facial nerve segment in patients with complete palsy and demonstrating severe denervation on electrodiagnostic testing within 2 weeks. It also discussed the substantial costs and rare but serious risks (including seizures, unilateral hearing loss, cerebrospinal fluid leak, and injury to the facial nerve) with this type of surgery. The subject still remains controversial and in their conclusion, the panel could make no recommendation regarding surgical decompression for Bell's palsy [11].

Acupuncture by needle insertion alone or combined with drugs is a treatment modality used for Bell's palsy. The Cochrane Database of Systematic Reviews by Chen and colleagues published in 2010 [23] concluded that the quality of the six included randomized clinical trials was inadequate to allow any conclusion about the efficacy of acupuncture for Bell's palsy. The clinical practice guidelines of the American Academy of Otolaryngology—Head and Neck Surgery Foundation from 2013 summarized that randomized clinical trials do support the use of acupuncture but these trials were downgraded due to poor quality. The panel was unable to determine the ratio of benefit to harm and could make no recommendation regarding acupuncture in Bell's palsy [11]. Li and colleagues, who included 14 randomized controlled trials involving 1541 Bell's palsy individuals in their meta-analysis from 2015, reported that there is insufficient evidence to support the efficacy and safety of acupuncture [24]. To summarize, evidence-based recommendations for acupuncture for Bell's palsy treatment are currently lacking.

Sequelae from severe Bell's palsy are persistent facial muscle weakness, facial muscle contracture, and synkinesis. In the acute stage of severe palsy, the face is flaccid with drooping corner of the mouth, less pronounced nasolabial fold, and a wide eye with lagophthalmos. In the recovery phase starting after 3–6 months, contracture of the facial muscles develops with pulled up corner of the mouth (shortening of lip elevator muscles), deepening of the nasolabial fold, and a smaller eye with contraction of the orbicularis oculi muscle. Synkinesis, which develops 3–6 months after onset of palsy, is an involuntary movement in one region of the face produced during intentional movement in another facial region (Fig. 1.5). The prevailing theory for its mechanism of development is that injured axons undergo aberrant regeneration resulting in innervation of facial muscles other than those originally innervated [25]. Mild synkinesis is present in about 15% and moderate to severe synkinesis in around 7% of Bell's palsy patients 1 year after onset [20]. The most common and troublesome synkinesis affects the muscles of

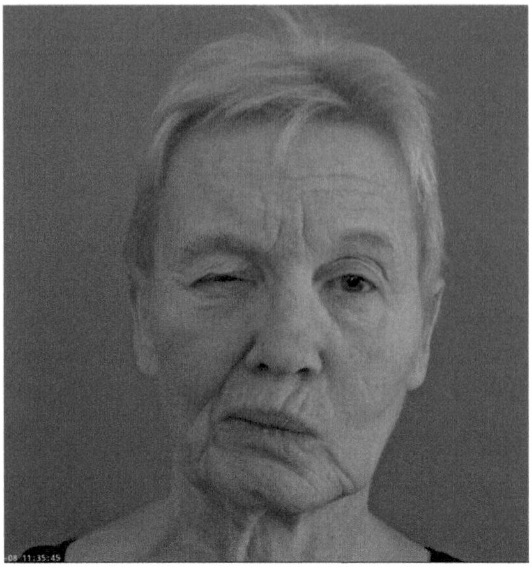

Fig. 1.5 Contracture of the facial muscles with pulled up corner of the mouth, deepening of the nasolabial fold, smaller eye and involuntary facial movements (synkinesis). (Published with oral and written permission from the patient)

the eye and mouth. Rehabilitation and management of synkinesis in facial palsy are discussed in Chaps. 4 and 31, respectively.

1.8 Acquired Peripheral Facial Palsy in Children

Bell's palsy is the leading etiology of acquired acute peripheral facial palsy in children (about 40–50%) but is 2–4 times less frequent than in adults. Its estimated yearly incidence has been reported as about 6 cases per 100,000 in ages 1–15 years, but in a large population-based epidemiologic study it was reported as 18.8 per 100,000 person-years with an increase by age [26]. There are no large randomized controlled Bell's palsy treatment trials on the effect of corticosteroids and/or antivirals in the pediatric population. Etiological factors that can cause peripheral palsy in children resemble those in adults. Infectious causes from otitis media and Lyme disease (especially in borrelia-endemic areas) are more common in children than in adults. Other infectious causes in children (as well as adults, see Table 1.3) are herpes zoster (Ramsay Hunt syndrome), Epstein–Barr virus, cytomegalovirus, adenovirus, rubella, mumps, HIV, Haemophilus influenzae, Mycoplasma pneumoniae, tuberculosis, leprosy, and syphilis. Kawasaki disease (mucocutaneous lymph node syndrome) is a rare acute systemic vasculitic condition that mainly affects children under the age of five and may be accompanied by peripheral facial palsy. The association between severe hypertension and peripheral facial palsy is mainly described in children. Facial palsy can occur in head trauma with fracture of the temporal bone, blunt cheek injury, parotid- and ear surgery, and in vestibular schwannoma surgery for neurofibromatosis type 2. Cholesteatoma of the ear may also cause peripheral facial palsy in children. Tumors and hemopathies as a cause are rhabdomyosarcoma of the temporal bone, Langerhans cell histiocytosis, vestibular and facial schwannoma, parotid tumor, leukemia, and hemophilia. Slow progress (beyond weeks) after onset of palsy or lack of improvement after 3 months suggests a neoplastic or neurological cause. Recurrent facial palsy may relate to Bell's palsy or Melkersson–Rosenthal syndrome (recurrent or persistent orofacial edema, fissured tongue, and relapsing peripheral facial palsy). Alternating recurrent palsy seldom is secondary to causal neoplasm but ipsilateral recurrent palsy needs more comprehensive investigation. Acquired bilateral facial palsy may be due to neurologic disease such as Guillain–Barré syndrome, Lyme borreliosis, most of the other above mentioned viral and bacterial infections (including meningitis), Kawasaki disease, and sarcoidosis.

The role of corticosteroid treatment for Bell's palsy in children is inclusive due to lack of controlled trials. The clinical practice guidelines of the American Academy of Otolaryngology—Head and Neck Surgery Foundation from 2013 note that despite the absence of quality trials supporting corticosteroid use in children, and given the presumed similar disease process and benefit-harm ratio of Bell's palsy in adults and children, corticosteroids may be considered in pediatric patients with a large role for caregiver participation in the decision [11]. Prednisolone may be given in doses of 1 mg/kg (maximum 60 mg/day) per day for 7 days tapered over the following days, started within a week of onset (ideally 72 h) [27]. There is no evidence supporting the use of antiviral therapy alone [11], but addition of antivirals to prednisolone (especially in severe palsy) has been suggested as treatment in children with Bell's palsy. As for adults, it is important to protect the eye to prevent corneal ulcers in children with peripheral facial palsy.

Simultaneous bilateral peripheral facial palsy can be seen in diseases of infectious, neurological, idiopathic, neoplastic or traumatic, autoimmune, iatrogenic, and toxic origin. This is a very uncommon form of palsy and accounts for less than 1% of peripheral facial palsy patients. It requires a careful diagnostic evaluation in order to find the appropriate therapy [2]. The most common causes are Guillain–Barré syndrome, Lyme disease, "bilateral Bell's palsy-herpes simplex type 1," Melkersson–Rosenthal syndrome, sarcoidosis (Heerfordt's syndrome), Epstein–Barr and cytomegalovirus, HIV, meningitis, leukemia, and lymphoma. Trauma with skull base fracture and congenital diplegia seen in Möbius syndrome are other causes for bilateral peripheral facial palsy (Table 1.5).

Table 1.5 Underlying causes of simultaneous bilateral facial palsy

Guillain–Barré syndrome
Borreliosis
Bilateral Bell's palsy
Melkersson–Rosenthal syndrome
Sarcoidosis (Heerfordt's syndrome)
Bacterial meningitis
Epstein–Barr virus
Leukemia
HIV
Lymphoma
Syphilis
Chickenpox
Zika virus
Herpes zoster oticus
Rabies immunization
Granulomatosis with polyangiitis
Botulism
Pontine infarction
Brain stem encephalitis
Kawasaki disease
Amyloidosis
Leptospirosis
Others
Skull base fracture
Mandibular fractures
Congenital diplegia (Möbius syndrome, thalidomide toxicity)
Diabetes mellitus
Myotonic dystrophy
Myasthenia gravis
Bone disorders (sclerosing bone dysplasia, osteogenesis imperfecta, cleidocranial dysostosis)
Acute porphyria
Hypothyroidism
Pregnancy
Benign intracranial hypertension
Bilateral neurofibromas
Prepontine or intrapontine tumor
Charcot–Marie–Tooth syndrome
Bilateral acute or chronic otitis media

1.9 Herpes Zoster Oticus or Ramsay Hunt syndrome

Herpes zoster oticus or Ramsay Hunt syndrome is an acute peripheral facial palsy accompanied by ipsilateral vesicular eruptions in the ear canal, auricle, or mucous membrane of the oropharynx. About 50–75% of patients experience ipsilateral vestibulocochlear symptoms with vertigo and/or sensorineural hearing loss, more severe in the high frequency range. The annual incidence of the disease is about 4 per 100,000 individuals. Herpes zoster oticus is the most common infectious cause of acute peripheral facial palsy in adults and accounts for around 5–10% of peripheral facial palsy cases. Its etiopathology includes the reactivation of latent varicella zoster virus in the geniculate ganglion of the facial nerve. The diagnosis of herpes zoster oticus is mainly clinical via the auricular vesicular herpetic eruptions (Fig. 1.6) that appear in approximately 85% of cases, but in unclear situations, skin/blister analysis by PCR and serologic and/or cerebrospinal examination may add information. Since the palsy may precede vesicular eruptions, herpes

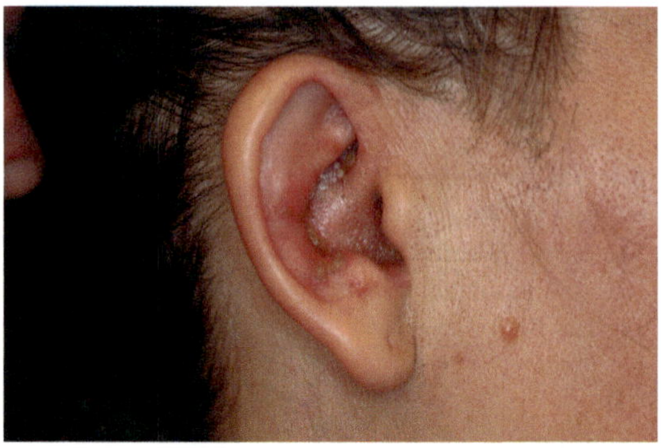

Fig. 1.6 Auricular vesicular herpetic eruptions in a patient with herpes zoster oticus (Ramsay Hunt syndrome). (Published with oral and written permission from the patient)

zoster oticus may be misdiagnosed with Bell's palsy. Even with eruptions present, a Bell's diagnosis with external otitis is sometimes incorrectly made. The facial palsy in herpes zoster oticus may be accompanied by multiple cranial nerve involvement and generally is more severe, which, even with treatment, results in a higher number of patients with sequelae (50%) compared with Bell's palsy. In contrast to Bell's palsy, herpes zoster oticus with facial palsy never occurs simultaneously on both sides and recurrence is extremely rare. Large prospective randomized controlled studies are lacking but the suggested treatment for herpes zoster oticus includes peroral antiviral valaciclovir (500 mg two times daily for 1 week) and peroral corticosteroids in doses as for Bell's palsy. In severe cases, peroral valaciclovir may be replaced with intravenous antivirals. For individuals 60 years or older, vaccinating against varicella zoster virus decreases the risk of herpes zoster.

1.10 Lyme Disease (Neuroborreliosis)

The most common manifestation of Borrelia infection is erythema migrans (25–89%), neuroborreliosis (16–29%), and arthritis (3–41%). Other less common manifestations are acrodermatitis chronica atrophicans, lymphocytoma, and carditis. Lyme neuroborreliosis is caused by a central nervous system infection due to the tick-borne spirochete *Borrelia burgdorferi*. Borrelia may invade the central nervous system directly via tissues, along peripheral nerves or by hematogenous dissemination. Neuroborreliosis is often manifested by cranial nerve engagement. Peripheral facial palsy is the most common neurologic manifestation (approximately 10%) and is often accompanied by radicular pain. Peripheral facial palsy caused by neuroborreliosis is more common in children and increasing risk factors are onset during peak season in an endemic area and a history of an erythema migrans lesion. Patients may have a preceding or concomitant febrile illness, fatigue, malaise, radicular pain, and general headache, in contrast to the more localized periauricular pain that occurs in approximately 50% of Bell's palsy patients. In areas endemic for *Borrelia burgdorferi*, Lyme neuroborreliosis is estimated to cause up to 25% of peripheral facial palsies and should therefore always be considered as a cause of palsy in these regions, especially in bilateral cases and/or if the patient is a child. Borrelia is found in the Northern temperate zone in Europe, Central and North America, and parts of Northern Asia. In peripheral facial palsy cases in endemic areas, serologic testing for immunoglobulin G and M antibodies to *Borrelia burgdorferi* antibodies should be performed in the acute stage and at follow-up within 4–6 weeks. In patients with clinical signs and/or increasing risk factors (especially children) for Borrelia, cerebrospinal examination for mononuclear pleocytosis and Borrelia antibodies should always be considered. Treatment consists of peroral doxycycline 100 mg two times daily for 14 days. Children aged ≥8 years are treated with peroral doxycycline 4 mg/kg once daily for 10 days and children <8 years are given intravenous ceftriaxone 50–100 mg/kg once daily for 10 days. In addition to antibiotics, extra corticosteroid treatment for peripheral facial palsy caused by Borrelia has been advocated, but larger randomized controlled studies to prove this are currently lacking. Findings supporting caution in using corticosteroids in this type of palsy have also been reported.

1.11 Sarcoidosis

Sarcoidosis is a systemic granulomatous disease of unknown etiology but similarities with the two other granulomatous disorders tuberculosis and leprosy have been put forward. It is more common in females than males and peak age is between 20 and 40 years. The most affected organs are the lungs (85%) followed by lymph nodes (65%), liver, skin, and eyes. Radiology and strong clinical evidence of multisystem involvement, together with biopsy findings of non-caseating epitheloid cell granulomas in addition to negative cultures for bacteria, mycobacteria and fungi, support a diagnosis of sarcoidosis.

The central nervous system is involved in sarcoidosis in approximately 10% of cases. The clinical picture involves a peripheral neuropathy or chronic basal meningitis (rarely acute meningitis) with multiple cranial nerves. Peripheral facial palsy, which may be unilateral alternating or recurrent, as well as simultaneous bilateral, is the most common neurological manifestation of sarcoidosis. In Heerfordt's syndrome, which includes peripheral facial palsy, uveitis, enlarged parotid gland, and fever, the underlying disease is sarcoidosis. Radiological diagnosis for sarcoidosis includes chest CT for showing hilar lymphadenopathy and positron emission tomography (PET)/CT/MRI for identifying sites suitable for biopsy and assessing inflammatory active sarcoidosis. Biopsy of lymph node, skin, brain, meninges, or muscle demonstrating non-caseating epitheloid cell granulomas strongly indicates a diagnosis of sarcoidosis. Serum ACE is significantly higher in most (approximately 80%) patients with active sarcoidosis. Serum angiotensin-converting enzyme (ACE) levels are significantly higher in active sarcoidosis patients compared with controls. MRI is a sensitive tool for detecting neurological lesions. Cerebrospinal fluid findings include lymphocytic pleocytosis (which may also be found in borreliosis and viral disease), elevated protein levels and, in some patients, low glucose levels. Cerebrospinal fluid should also be analyzed for ACE levels. Corticosteroids are the first-line medical treatment in neurosarcoidosis. To lower corticosteroid doses, immunosuppressive drugs may be added. Treatment with tumor necrosis factor alfa blockers has also been described.

1.12 Guillain–Barré Syndrome

Guillain–Barré syndrome is an acute to subacute inflammatory polyradiculoneuropathy. It is characterized by the development of bilateral weakness or paralysis, areflexia, paresthesia, pain, and autonomic dysfunction, thus representing a heterogeneous group of immune-mediated neuropathies. In most cases, a demyelinating process with a relatively short recovery period is found, but in its severe form, secondary axonal injury occurs. Severe sequelae from Guillain–Barré syndrome are seen in about 20% of patients. The annual incidence is about 1–2 per 100,000 individuals and its origin is an autoimmune reaction directed against peripheral nerves and nerve roots. An association with vaccines, but also with infection by cytomegalovirus, Epstein–Barr virus, Influenza A virus, *Mycoplasma pneumoniae*, and *Campylobacter jejuni* has been reported. Bilateral facial palsy is common and occurs in about 50% of cases, often with one side affected before the other. Miller Fischer Syndrome, a triad of ataxia, areflexia, and ophthalmoplegia is a variant of Guillain–Barré syndrome that also may occur with facial palsy. Neurophysiological examination shows multifocal demyelination/axonal injury. Cerebrospinal fluid findings with raised protein content and elevated albumin quotient strengthen the diagnosis. Pleocytosis is not prevalent in Guillain–Barré syndrome and if it occurs, Borrelia or HIV infection must be considered. Medical treatment with immunomodulation is performed by plasmapheresis or intravenous immunoglobulin G therapy.

1.13 Melkersson–Rosenthal Syndrome

Melkersson–Rosenthal syndrome is a rare multidisciplinary disease characterized by a triad of symptoms with recurrent orofacial edema (mainly upper lip), facial palsy, and lingua plicata (a deeply fissured tongue). Its annual *incidence* is approximately 0.3 per 100,000 individuals. The cause of the disease is unknown. Typical histology of the orofacial edema shows a non-caseating granulomatous infiltration demonstrating similarities with that of Crohn disease and sarcoidosis. Melkersson–Rosenthal syndrome affects all age groups, but onset is most often seen in young adulthood. The most frequent sign is lingua plicata and the most common initial symptom is edema, which eventually affects most patients and gradually becomes persistent. Facial palsy appears in approximately 30–50% of cases but the complete triad form is only seen in about 20–25%. Onset of palsy is usually associated with ipsilateral orofacial swelling. Relapsing (recurrent or alternating) facial palsy may occur as well as bilateral symptoms (bilateral facial palsy and bilateral orofacial edema). Medical treatment for Melkersson–Rosenthal syndrome is symptomatic. Non-steroid anti-inflammatory drugs and systemic and/or intralesional corticosteroids have remained a mainstay of therapy. Oral antimicrobials have also been reported effective. Other less evaluated treatments include thalidomide, tumor necrosis factor alfa blockers, hydroxychloroquine, methotrexate, dapsone, azathioprine, and mycophenolate mofetil. Plastic surgery of disfiguring refractory orofacial edema may be considered. Total facial nerve decompression has been suggested to prevent further attacks of facial paralysis and its sequelae.

1.14 Ear Infection

The incidence of peripheral facial palsy associated with ear infection, including cholesteatoma, accounts for about 2–3% of all peripheral palsies [2, 6, 7]. Acute otitis media is an infection localized to the mucosa or mucoperiosteum of the middle ear and may be complicated by an acute peripheral facial palsy. Other concomitant complicating symptoms may occur from the inner ear with sensorineural hearing loss and vertigo. A pre-existing dehiscence of the tympanic segment of the fallopian canal is a predisposing factor for facial palsy. Literature shows that the majority of cases are children and that the palsy may be the first sign of acute otitis media with or without mastoiditis. Before antibiotics, otitis media was responsible for a greater proportion of facial palsies. Intravenous antibiotic therapy should be initiated and acute myringotomy drainage with bacterial culture performed. With treatment, the prognosis for facial recovery in general is favorable. Mastoidectomy is performed in cases of complicating acute mastoiditis and/or subperiosteal abscess. In cases of suspected complications (cholesteatoma/bone destruction/sigmoid sinus thrombosis), computed tomography (thin-sliced) is mandatory. Adding corticosteroids to the medical therapy may be considered but convincing reports for their effectiveness are lacking.

Two forms of chronic otitis media associated with peripheral facial palsy are found: chronic suppurative otitis media without cholesteatoma and chronic otitis with cholesteatoma. In contrast to the acute form of otitis media, which mainly affects children, peripheral facial palsy in chronic otitis media mostly affects youths and adults. The palsy in chronic suppurative otitis media with perforation of the tympanic membrane may present as an acute or slowly progressing facial palsy. Prompt treatment with intravenous broad-spectrum antibiotics after bacterial culture from middle ear discharge as well as from blood must be commenced. Computed tomography is needed to evaluate for dehiscence and/or bone destruction within the temporal bone. Pathologic tissue with destruction, progressing disease, and deterioration of facial function demands explorative surgery and facial nerve decompression with elimination of pathological tissue. Cholesteatoma is a non-malignant tumorous process with focal regions of keratinizing squamous epithelium mostly located to the middle ear or mastoid, which may erode surrounding bone. Congenital cholesteatoma occurs in children and acquired cholesteatomas, which are in the majority, are primarily found in adults. Peripheral facial palsy associated with chronic otitis with cholesteatoma needs immediate management in the same manner as for chronic suppurative otitis media. MRI may add further information (cholesteatoma shows characteristic reduced diffusion). Surgery includes facial nerve decompression and removal of cholesteatoma.

1.15 Intratemporal Facial Nerve Trauma

Trauma accounts for about 5% of all peripheral facial palsies. Facial palsy due to intratemporal injury is often associated with external trauma. The most common cause of temporal bone fracture is motor vehicle accidents [7] although seat belts and air bags have reduced these injuries. Computed tomography with thin slices is the radiological method for mapping the extent of injury. It is important to look for cerebrospinal fluid leakage. Temporal bone fracture lines are classically described in relation to the long axis of the petrous pyramid as longitudinal, oblique, and transverse. Transverse fractures account for about 10% of the total but facial palsy is observed in 40–50% of them as opposed to longitudinal fractures (80–90% of total) in which palsy occurs in just 20%. Peripheral facial palsy is twice as common in fractures that cross the otic capsule (also results in sensorineural hearing loss) compared to fractures that do not intersect the capsule. An immediate palsy from head injury will be apparent as soon as the patient is examined in the hospital. Delayed onset of palsy can occur within an interval of 4–5 days. Delayed palsy has a better prognosis than the immediate type and it is generally agreed that delayed palsies should be conservatively treated with corticosteroids as medical treatment. Treatment of immediate palsy depends on the patient's general neurologic condition after the head injury, severity of palsy on electroneuronography as well as computed tomography findings. Surgical exploration of the facial nerve has to be considered in cases with poor prognosis preferably within 2 weeks after onset.

1.16 Extratemporal Facial Nerve Trauma

Injury to the face may wound the facial nerve main trunk or its branches. These injuries account for around 1.5% of peripheral facial palsies. The most common trauma is penetrating, laceration, slash, and facial fracture to the soft tissue. Careful examination of the separate facial nerve branches is important since edema and bruising may mask palsy. Penetrating nerve injuries need prompt exploration and identification of cut nerve branches. Primary nerve repair results in better recovery compared with rerouting or grafting (see Chap. 6).

1.17 Iatrogenic Facial Nerve Trauma

Iatrogenic injury to the facial nerve causes 3% of all peripheral facial palsies. Patients operated for removal of vestibular schwannoma at the cerebellopontine angle comprise one of the largest iatrogenic groups and in larger acoustic neuroma referral centers, these patients account for up to 9% [7]. Facial palsy also occurs after tumor resection alongside any part of the intratemporal or extratemporal facial nerve, including temporal bone tumors, parotid tumors, and head and neck cancer. In tumor surgery, volitional sacrificing of the facial nerve frequently must be performed to obtain radicality. Other causes of iatrogenic injury to the facial nerve are mastoid surgery, middle ear surgery, oral surgery, cosmetic surgery (face lift), neurosurgery, and temporal biopsy surgery [7]. If unexpected facial palsy occurs after surgery and the intactness of the nerve is unclear, facial nerve exploration has to be carried out.

1.18 Tumor

Benign and malignant tumors account for around 5% of peripheral facial palsies [2, 6, 7]. Clinical suspicion of a tumor as cause of peripheral facial palsy is raised with gradual onset, fluctuating or recurrent palsy, hearing loss on the palsy side, and ipsilateral parotid or ear tumor mass. Benign tumors as cause of facial palsy are vestibular schwannoma (often starts with hearing loss) at the cerebellopontine angle and facial neuroma and hemangioma in the intratemporal portion. Malignant tumors in the temporal bone consist of squamous cell carcinomas (primary or metastatic) and basal cell carcinomas. Malignant tumors located in the region of the parotid gland as cause of palsy are mucoepidermoid carcinomas, adenoid cystic carcinomas, adenocarcinomas, and squamous cell carcinomas. Tumor resection (in some cases also reconstructive surgery) and reanimation surgery followed by oncological treatment is the option for these malignant tumors.

1.19 Peripheral Facial Palsy in Newborn, Congenital Facial Palsy

The incidence of peripheral facial palsy at birth, so-called congenital facial palsy, is between 1 and 2 per 1000 newborns. The palsy is categorized as traumatic or developmental and distinguishing between the two is important since prognosis and therapy differ. The spontaneous recovery rate in congenital traumatic palsy is approximately 90%, while developmental facial palsy in general will not improve. The most common cause of unilateral congenital palsy is birth-related trauma. Primipara, birth weight more than 3500 g, prolonged labor, and forceps delivery are risk factors for trauma. Signs of birth-related injury include face or skull lacerations or hematomas as well as mastoid hematomas and hemotympanum. Other anomalies, bilateral palsy or cranial deficits indicate developmental background. Except for history and clinical findings, early-stage computed tomography and/or MR imaging may help differentiate traumatic (fracture of the skull base) from developmental palsy (ear anomalies). Furthermore, congenital traumatic palsy, in contrast to developmental palsy, initially shows normal electroneurographic and electromyographic responses at birth. In severe traumatic palsies, which also contrast to developmental palsies, synkinesis will develop after 3–4 months.

The causes of developmental facial palsy may be isolated (non-syndromic) or related to syndromes. Family history of congenital facial palsy indicates a developmental origin. In Möbius syndrome with an incidence of approximately 1 per 50,000 births, bilateral facial nerve palsy and unilateral or bilateral abducens palsy are the most typical features. Other cranial nerves (especially hypoglossal) may also be affected and deformities of the head, trunk (pectoral muscles), and limbs (syndactylism and club foot) may accompany the cranial nerve defects. The pathogenesis of facial palsy in Möbius syndrome is thought to be caused by a nuclear or peripheral lesion. Oculoauriculovertebral syndrome is a spectrum of craniofacial disorders with unilateral abnormalities related to first and second branchial arches. Hypoplasia of the maxilla and mandible, microtia, and abnormally small mouth opening are clinical features of this syndrome. In addition to facial palsy, sensorineural and/or conductive hearing loss is frequent in hemifacial microsmia. Goldenhar syndrome, a variant of oculoauriculovertebral syndrome, also includes cleft palate, vertebral anomalies and epibulbar dermoids, as well as the above mentioned malformations. Symptoms affect both sides of the face in 10–30% of cases, with the right side usually more severely involved. Heart defects, kidney problems as well as central nervous system abnormalities may be present in this syndrome.

Congenital unilateral lower lip palsy, also called asymmetric crying facies, is confined to the lower lip depressor muscles innervated by the mandibular branch of the facial nerve. At rest, the face is symmetric but when crying or laughing drooping of the lower lip towards the unaffected side is seen. Congenital unilateral lower lip palsy is one of the commonest forms of congenital palsies. Sometimes this type may be associated with other malformations of which heart disease is most common. Other grounds or related disorders to congenital facial palsy are CHARGE syndrome (colobomata, heart defects, atresia of choanae, retarded growth, genital hypoplasia, and ear abnormalities), facioscapulohumeral muscular dystrophy, 22q11 deletion syndrome, osteopetrosis (Albers-Schönberg disease), and the use of thalidomide or misoprostol during pregnancy.

Acknowledgement Thomas Berg, MD, PhD, for technical help.

References

1. Müri RM. Cortical control of facial expression. J Comp Neurol. 2016;524:1578–85.
2. Schaitkin BM, May M, Klein SR. Office evaluation of the patient with facial palsy: differential diagnosis and prognosis. In: May M, Schaitkin BM, editors. The facial nerve. New York: Thieme; 2000. p. 179–212.
3. Marsk E, Bylund N, Jonsson L, et al. Prediction of nonrecovery in Bell's palsy using Sunnybrook grading. Laryngoscope. 2012;122:901–6.
4. House JW, Brackmann DE. Facial nerve grading system. Otolaryngol Head Neck Surg. 1985;93:146–7.
5. Ross BG, Fradet G, Nedzelski JM. Development of a sensitive clinical facial grading system. Otolaryngol Head Neck Surg. 1996;114:380–6.
6. Peitersen E. Bell's palsy: the spontaneous course of 2,500 peripheral facial nerve palsies of different etiologies. Acta Otolaryngol Suppl. 2002;(549):4–30.
7. Hohman MH, Hadlock TA. Etiology, diagnosis, and management of facial palsy: 2000 patients at a facial nerve center. Laryngoscope. 2014;124:E283–93.
8. Diamond C, Frew I. Clinical features of facial nerve disorders. In: Diamond C, Frew I, editors. The facial nerve. Oxford: Oxford University Press; 1979. p. 39–58.
9. May M, Hughes GB. Facial nerve disorders: update 1987. Am J Otol. 1987;8:167–80.
10. Eviston TJ, Croxson GR, Kennedy PG, et al. Bell's palsy: aetiology, clinical features and multidisciplinary care. J Neurol Neurosurg Psychiatry. 2015;86:1356–61.
11. Baugh RF, Basura GJ, Ishii LE, et al. Clinical practice guideline: Bell's palsy executive summary. Otolaryngol Head Neck Surg. 2013;149:656–63.
12. Reich SG. Bell's palsy. Continuum (Minneap Minn). 2017;23:447–66.
13. Murakami S, Mizobuchi M, Nakashiro Y, et al. Bell palsy and herpes simplex virus: identification of viral DNA in endoneurial fluid and muscle. Ann Intern Med. 1996;124:27–30.
14. Sartoretti-Schefer S, Wichmann W, Valavanis A. Idiopathic, herpetic, and HIV-associated facial nerve palsies: abnormal MR enhancement patterns. AJNR Am J Neuroradiol. 1994;15:479–85.
15. Sullivan FM, Swan IR, Donnan PT, et al. Early treatment with prednisolone or acyclovir in Bell's palsy. N Engl J Med. 2007;357:1598–607.
16. Engström M, Berg T, Stjernquist-Desatnik A, et al. Prednisolone and valaciclovir in Bell's palsy: a randomised, double-blind, placebo-controlled, multicentre trial. Lancet Neurol. 2008;7:993–1000.
17. Madhok VB, Gagyor I, Daly F, et al. Corticosteroids for Bell's palsy (idiopathic facial paralysis). Cochrane Database Syst Rev. 2016;7:CD001942.
18. Vrabec JT. Medical treatment of Bell palsy. In: Slattery III WH, Azizzadeh B, editors. The facial nerve. New York: Thieme; 2014. p. 81–8.
19. Gagyor I, Madhok VB, Daly F, et al. Antiviral treatment for Bell's palsy (idiopathic facial paralysis). Cochrane Database Syst Rev. 2015;(11):CD001869.
20. Bylund N, Jensson D, Enghag S, et al. Synkinesis in Bell's palsy in a randomised controlled trial. Clin Otolaryngol. 2017;42:673–80.
21. Gantz BJ, Rubinstein JT, Gidley P, et al. Surgical management of Bell's palsy. Laryngoscope. 1999;109:1177–88.
22. McAllister K, Walker D, Donnan PT, et al. Surgical interventions for the early management of Bell's palsy. Cochrane Database Syst Rev. 2013;(10):CD007468.
23. Chen N, Zhou M, He L, et al. Acupuncture for Bell's palsy. Cochrane Database Syst Rev. 2010;(8):CD002914.
24. Li P, Qiu T, Qin C. Efficacy of acupuncture for Bell's palsy: a systematic review and meta-analysis of randomized controlled trials. PLoS One. 2015;10:e0121880.
25. Husseman J, Mehta RP. Management of synkinesis. Facial Plast Surg. 2008;24:242–9.
26. Rowhani-Rahbar A, Baxter R, Rasgon B, et al. Epidemiologic and clinical features of Bell's palsy among children in Northern California. Neuroepidemiology. 2012;38:252–8.
27. Malik V, Joshi V, Green KM, et al. 15 Minute consultation: a structured approach to the management of facial paralysis in a child. Arch Dis Child Educ Pract Ed. 2012;97:82–5.

A Multi-modal Approach to Outcome Tracking in Facial Palsy

2

Joseph R. Dusseldorp, Charles Meares, and Tessa A. Hadlock

Key Points

- Outcome assessment in facial palsy ought to be multi-modal, including patient-reported outcome measures, clinician-graded scoring systems, objective assessment tools, and layperson and spontaneity assessment.
- Patient-reported outcome measures are required to assess the psychosocial impact of facial nerve dysfunction, as experienced by patients.
- Clinician-graded scoring systems and objective assessment tools are needed to rate severity of disease and the effects of interventions. Time and cost constraints are being decreased with automation.
- Layperson assessments have been used to determine impacts of facial palsy on attractiveness, disfigurement, and non-verbal communication.
- A novel approach using machine learning algorithms to assess the emotionality of smiling has been developed and shown to correlate with layperson assessments. A means of objectively quantifying spontaneity of smile has also been developed.

2.1 Introduction

Outcome tracking in facial palsy is critical in order to improve future outcomes. Currently, outcome measurement tools in facial palsy can be classified into patient-reported outcome measures, clinician-graded scoring systems, objective assessment tools, and emerging systems assessing spontaneity and incorporating layperson assessments. The ideal outcome measurement approach must address the complex dysfunction that occurs in facial palsy, by assessing patient-experienced morbidity, and outcomes of interventions from both the patient and clinician perspective. This approach should also make objective measurements and provide a common language for future research [1]. Clearly a panel of outcome measures are required to capture all of these various domains, and such a panel should be sensitive to change, simple, and low cost to encourage widespread implementation [2].

J. R. Dusseldorp (✉)
Department of Otolaryngology/Head and Neck Surgery, Massachusetts Eye and Ear Infirmary and Harvard Medical School, Boston, MA, USA

Department of Plastic and Reconstructive Surgery, Royal Australasian College of Surgeons and University of Sydney, Sydney, NSW, Australia

C. Meares
Department of Plastic and Reconstructive Surgery, Royal Australasian College of Surgeons and University of Sydney, Sydney, NSW, Australia

T. A. Hadlock
Department of Otolaryngology/Head and Neck Surgery, Massachusetts Eye and Ear Infirmary and Harvard Medical School, Boston, MA, USA
e-mail: Tessa_Hadlock@meei.harvard.edu

© Springer Nature Switzerland AG 2021
C.-H. J. Tzou, A. Rodríguez-Lorenzo (eds.), *Facial Palsy*,
https://doi.org/10.1007/978-3-030-50784-8_2

2.2 Patient-Reported Outcome Measures

Patient-reported outcome measures (PROMs) should be utilized to capture the significant psychological and quality of life impacts associated with facial nerve palsy [3–5]. However, a recent survey of clinicians observed that the majority do not employ a PROM in the assessment of facial palsy patients [6]. The Facial Disability Index (FDI) and the Facial Clinimetric Evaluation (FaCE) scale are facial palsy specific surveys that assess the functioning of facial muscles from the patient's perspective and the effect that dysfunction has on patients' quality of life [7, 8]. Both have been validated; however, neither specifically assess the role of synkinesis in the patient's burden of morbidity [9]. To this end, the Synkinesis Assessment Questionnaire (SAQ) can be used as an adjunct or independent PROM tool for assessment of synkinetic impacts on patients' quality of life.

Introduced in 2001, the Facial Clinimetric Evaluation (FaCE) scale aims to measure both facial impairment and quality of life [8]. It has quickly become the most widely used PROM in facial palsy patients [6, 10]. The tool includes Likert-type questions and visual analogue scales covering facial movement, oral movement, lacrimal control, social function, facial comfort, and eye comfort. Scores for these domains are summed to yield the FaCE scale score. This scale ranges from 0 (worst) to 100 (best). The FaCE scale has demonstrated concurrent and convergent validity with the HBGS and is thought to assess psychometric outcomes more completely than other PROMs [9].

The Facial Disability Index (FDI) consists of ten Likert-type questions addressing physical function and social function [7]. The index includes questions covering normal activities of daily living, such as drinking from a cup. The scores are collated giving a score from 0 (worst) to 100 (best). Developed in 1996, the tool has undergone validation testing [7, 9].

The Synkinesis Assessment Questionnaire (SAQ) was developed in 2007 in order to specifically address the deficiency of established PROMs to observe synkinesis-specific issues for patients [11]. The SAQ consists of nine items answered with five Likert-type responses. The answers are summated yielding a range from 0 to 100, higher scores representing worse synkinesis. The SAQ has demonstrated good retest reliability and construct validity [11, 12]. SAQ focuses on patient experience with synkinesis and can be combined as an adjunct with a facial palsy specific PROM.

2.3 Clinician Grading Scoring Systems

Historically, various clinician-graded scoring systems have been advocated with no single scale being universally utilized. Such tools are subjective assessment of facial function and have continually been proposed over the past 50 years [13]. Each tool assesses static and dynamic asymmetry. Only some scales contain regional assessment or determine degree of synkinesis.

The most widely used scale for facial nerve severity assessment is House–Brackmann grading scale (HBGS) [14]. After being adopted by the American Academy of Otolaryngology-Head and Neck Surgery in 1985, it remains the standard in the United States. The HBGS assesses overall facial nerve function using a six-point scale, from normal function to total paralysis. It accounts for secondary defects and synkinesis, can measure large changes over time and has good interobserver and intraobserver reliability [14–22]. HBGS has been modified several times and used to measure outcomes in facial nerve reanimation, though this was not its original purpose [20, 23]. There are no regional subdomain scores in HBGS and so it is insensitive to regional improvements, which limits its utility in outcome measurement [24–27]. However, its simplicity and widespread use have ensured it remains a favored communication tool between clinicians.

The Sunnybrook Facial Grading Scale (SFGS) is a regional-based composite score, assessing facial symmetry at rest, symmetry with voluntary facial movements and synkinesis [26]. It was developed in 1996 in order to address limitations of the HBGS. Calculation of the SFGS is a three-step process: quantify the symmetry of the eye, cheek, and mouth at rest; assess five standard facial movements; and evaluate the face for synkinesis during facial expressions. These component scores are weighted and the composite score is produced on a continuous scale (0–100). Compared to HBGS, SFGS has a greater ability to detect change [28] and has high intraobserver and interobserver reliability irrespective of observer experience [19, 24, 29–31]. The scale is time-consuming to employ and retains an element of subjectivity.

The Sydney facial grading system is similar to the Sunnybrook system, involving a regional assessment of facial movement. Unlike the Sunnybrook scale, the Sydney approach breaks down the facial regions based on branches of the facial nerve and corresponding muscle groups [19]. The Sydney system has strong correlation with the Sunnybrook system [19]; however, it is not widely utilized and lacks proper assessment of intraobserver reliability.

Noting the limitations of the HBGS, the revised Facial Nerve Grading Scale 2.0 (FNGS2.0) was introduced in 2006 [32]. This system assesses four regions of the face based on movement (scored 1–6) and accounts for synkinesis (scored 0–3). The summed score is then converted to a HBGS grade. Studies have shown high correlation between the FNGS2.0 and HBGS with consistently high interobserver reliability [13, 21, 27, 32, 33]. The FNGS2.0 has been shown to better measure synkinesis when compared to the HBGS over time [21].

The Yanagihara scale was introduced in 1976 and was one of the earliest widely accepted outcome measure systems and remains in use in Japan [34]. The Yanagihara method is a regional system that assesses ten facial movements which are graded on a four-point scale. The summed score characterizes the spectrum of facial palsy from normal movement to total paralysis. Facial palsy resolution is defined as a score greater than 36 with no associated synkinesis or facial muscle contraction [34, 35]. The Yanagihara scale provides useful regional information and correlates well with patient self-evaluation [36]. However, the scale is unweighted, potentially resulting in an inability to highlight specific facial movements [18], only captures ocular synkinesis, and has low intraobserver reliability.

The Terzis Facial Grading System (TFGS) observes the cosmetic and functional outcome of facial reanimation with respect to contraction and symmetry [37]. It was developed in 1997 specifically as a grading tool for comparing surgical outcome with pre-operative state. It is easy to implement, offers dynamic movement assessment and evaluates important endpoints: symmetry at rest, and with smiling [38, 39]. Its use has been widespread due to its ease of application [40–45]. Unfortunately, it lacks regional assessment of function, ignores synkinesis and has not been comprehensively validated.

eFACE is a comprehensive application for clinician grading of facial symmetry in unilateral facial palsy [46]. Using a digital interface, the observer scores 15 visual analogue scales with regard to static, dynamic movement and synkinesis. The complete spectrum of possible dysfunction is represented by the sum score of 0–100, with 100 representing normal function. The eFACE application has been demonstrated to be quick, sensitive to change, have high resolution for regional scoring (which have been weighted according to expert consensus [47]), accurately assesses synkinesis and have high inter-, intraobserver and retest reliability [46, 48, 49]. The eFACE application enables a quick assessment of facial palsy outcome in a zonal manner, yet remains a subjective tool.

2.4 Objective Assessment Systems

Objective assessment systems have been developed to evaluate outcomes in a consistent manner [2, 13]. Photography with staged facial movements is the most commonly utilized objective tool by clinicians [6], yet video-based analysis techniques remain poorly integrated into clinical practice as they can be expensive and time-consuming. The increasing utilization of machine learning in medicine has enabled development of efficient, cheap, and objective measurement systems in facial palsy patients [1, 50, 51].

The Facial Assessment by Computer Evaluation (FACE) application is more commonly referred to as the MEEI Facegram. Developed in 2012 and available from the Sir Charles Bell Society website, the MEEI Facegram can assess any frontal view photograph [2]. It is relatively quick and easy to implement as it does not require markers to be placed. Utilizing the average iris diameter of 11.8 mm, measurements of excursion of the eyebrow, palpebral fissure width, excursion of the commissure, and lip measurements are calculated by the user, scaled and converted into a vector.

The application of machine learning to facial palsy photography assessment is represented by the Emotrics objective tool [50]. Developed in 2018 and available as a freeware application, the Emotrics package is a facial landmark algorithm that automatically calculates facial displacements from standard frontal photographs. Smile excursion and symmetry, brow symmetry, and palpebral width are measured. Additionally, the application can also assess differences between two separate images, thus proving useful tool to automatically compare pre- and post-operative phtographs [50].

An innovative videography assessment tool was developed by Frey et al. in 1994 [52]. Utilizing markers attached to facial landmarks and four video cameras in conjunction with a computer, a dynamic 3D video analysis was obtained. The system identified pairs of facial points to compare movement of the brows, eyes, nose, and mouth. Unfortunately, implementing such a system in clinical practice was time-consuming and expensive, preventing its widespread adoption. Subsequent work simplified this method to a single camera, calibration grid and mirror system located behind the patient [53]. Paired with a facial analysis software package, this has resulted in an automatic standardized objective assessment tool that is a sensitive and reliable quantitative facial outcome measurement tool [54].

An alternative 3D videography assessment tool is the FACIAL CLIMA system [55]. Developed in 2008, the system requires reflective markers and three positioned infrared cameras to evaluate facial movements for the patient. The system is capable of calculating distances between landmarks, velocities, and areas for facial palsy analysis [55]. It is easy to use and quick; however, similar to other 3D videography tools, the need for specialized equipment and cost have prevented its widespread adoption.

3D stereophotogrammetry techniques are becoming more commonplace and may ultimately supersede 2D landmark-based assessment [56], though presently these tools are used predominantly in research settings [57]. A major advantage of 2D outcome measurement systems is that imaging is simple to record using standard cameras, large databases currently exist, to which machine learning approaches can be applied [50, 58].

2.5 Emerging Systems

Recent studies have characterized the layperson impression of facial palsy, highlighting the important role of dynamic facial movements, particularly smiling [59–62]. The layperson may be the ideal assessor of a facial palsy outcome as they ultimately decide if patients are able to communicate emotion non-verbally or appear disfigured when attempting to smile [1, 63]. In practice, routine layperson assessments are impractical due to logistical issues and patient confidentiality.

Layperson assessment studies have identified the negative aesthetic consequence of unilateral facial palsy in patients [60, 64]. This is a complex domain for assessment and is potentially best suited to the layperson interpretation [1]. In a layperson comparison of normal subjects and facial palsy patients, significantly lower attractiveness scores were reported for patients with facial paralysis, which was improved by reanimation surgery [60]. In an effort to better assess disfigurement in facial paralysis, over 500 laypersons assessed disfigurement in facial paralysis patients performing standard facial expressions. The layperson's disfigurement rating was significantly correlated with the clinician-graded facial function (eFACE). Additionally, it was noted that patients with worse dynamic subscores were considered more disfigured by laypersons [62].

Facial movements play an integral role in nonverbal communication, which is greatly impaired in facial palsy patients [3, 65, 66]. The layperson assessment is sensitive to these differences. Machine learning tools developed on large databases of facial expressions once validated could potentially serve as a proxy for the layperson assessment, circumventing the issues of privacy and practicality involved with utilizing layperson assessment in practice [1, 51].

Spontaneous smiling is an important outcome of smile reanimation and there are a number of different approaches to its assessment. Though various studies have defined spontaneous smile, currently no standardized assessment tool has been adopted in practice [67–71]. Despite the proposed "Tickle test" to elicit the patient to laugh, many authors make their assessment during a conversation with the patient [69, 70, 72, 73]. Such a process is open to confounding and confirmation bias [1, 74]. A standardized means of eliciting a spontaneous smile is through a standardized series of humorous videoclips. The spontaneous smile assay has been validated to elicit at least one spontaneous smile in over 95% of both normal subjects and facial palsy patients [67]. Quantifying the spontaneous smile outcome following reanimation surgery is extremely difficult and also prone to bias and error when performed by clinicians [74]. Another machine learning program has been developed to assess the emotionality of spontaneous smiling from videoclips of facial palsy patients watching humorous videos [51, 74]. Hopefully, objective tools such as these will lead to improvement of spontaneity outcomes for patients.

2.6 Conclusion

No ideal single tool exists that is appropriate for facial palsy outcome tracking. Clinician grading scoring systems remain widely utilized, particularly for ease of communication. PROMs should be implemented in order to gain an understanding of the impact of interventions on patient-reported quality of life. Objective assessment tools are available and will gain greater adoption in clinical practice as their utility is better understood. Layperson assessments, and automated equivalents, will continue to give valuable insights into interesting subdomains of facial function such as emotionality and spontaneity following reanimation.

In summary, the complete approach to outcome measures in facial palsy (P.A.L.Sy) should include [1]:

- **P**atient-reported outcome measures
- **A**utomated and clinician-graded scoring systems
- **L**ayperson assessment equivalent
- **S**pontaneous smile anal**y**sis

Disclosure Statement Dr. Hadlock, Dr. Dusseldorp, and Dr. Meares have nothing to disclose. No funding was received for this article.

References

1. Dusseldorp JR, van Veen MM, Mohan S, Hadlock TA. Outcome tracking in facial palsy. Otolaryngol Clin N Am. 2018;51(6):1033–50. https://doi.org/10.1016/j.otc.2018.07.003.
2. Hadlock TA, Urban LS. Toward a universal, automated facial measurement tool in facial reanimation. Arch Facial Plast Surg. 2012;14(4):277–82. https://doi.org/10.1001/archfacial.2012.111.
3. Coulson SE, O'dwyer NJ, Adams RD, Croxson GR. Expression of emotion and quality of life after facial nerve paralysis. Otol Neurotol. 2004;25(6):1014–9. https://doi.org/10.1097/00129492-200411000-00026.
4. Kleiss IJ, Beurskens CHG, Stalmeier PFM, Ingels KJAO, Marres HAM. Quality of life assessment in facial palsy: validation of the Dutch Facial Clinimetric Evaluation Scale. Eur Arch Otorhinolaryngol. 2015;272(8):2055–61. https://doi.org/10.1007/s00405-015-3508-x.
5. Lindsay RW, Bhama P, Hadlock TA. Quality-of-life improvement after free gracilis muscle transfer for smile restoration in patients with facial paralysis. JAMA Facial Plast Surg. 2014;16(6):419. https://doi.org/10.1001/jamafacial.2014.679.
6. Fattah AY, Gavilan J, Hadlock TA, et al. Survey of methods of facial palsy documentation in use by members of the Sir Charles Bell Society. Laryngoscope. 2014;124(10):2247–51. https://doi.org/10.1002/lary.24636.

7. VanSwearingen JM, Brach JS. The Facial Disability Index: reliability and validity of a disability assessment instrument for disorders of the facial neuromuscular system. Phys Ther. 1996;76(12):1288–98; discussion 1298–300. http://www.ncbi.nlm.nih.gov/pubmed/8959998.
8. Kahn JB, Gliklich RE, Boyev KP, Stewart MG, Metson RB, McKenna MJ. Validation of a patient-graded instrument for facial nerve paralysis: the FaCE scale. Laryngoscope. 2001;111(3):387–98. https://doi.org/10.1097/00005537-200103000-00005.
9. Ho AL, Scott AM, Klassen AF, Cano SJ, Pusic AL, Van Laeken N. Measuring quality of life and patient satisfaction in facial paralysis patients: a systematic review of patient-reported outcome measures. Plast Reconstr Surg. 2012;130(1):91–9. https://doi.org/10.1097/PRS.0b013e318254b08d.
10. Luijmes RE, Pouwels S, Beurskens CHG, Kleiss IJ, Siemann I, Ingels KJAO. Quality of life before and after different treatment modalities in peripheral facial palsy: a systematic review. Laryngoscope. 2017;127(5):1044–51. https://doi.org/10.1002/lary.26356.
11. Mehta RP, WernickRobinson M, Hadlock TA. Validation of the Synkinesis Assessment Questionnaire. Laryngoscope. 2007;117(5):923–6. https://doi.org/10.1097/MLG.0b013e3180412460.
12. Rhee JS, McMullin BT. Outcome measures in facial plastic surgery: patient-reported and clinical efficacy measures. Arch Facial Plast Surg. 2008;10(3):194–207. https://doi.org/10.1001/archfaci.10.3.194.
13. Fattah AY, Gurusinghe ADR, Gavilan J, et al. Facial nerve grading instruments: systematic review of the literature and suggestion for uniformity. Plast Reconstr Surg. 2015;135(2):569–79. https://doi.org/10.1097/PRS.0000000000000905.
14. House JW, Brackmann DE. Facial nerve grading system. Otolaryngol Head Neck Surg. 1985;93(2):146–7. https://doi.org/10.1177/019459988509300202.
15. Burres S, Fisch U. The comparison of facial grading systems. Arch Otolaryngol Head Neck Surg. 1986;112(7):755–8.
16. Lewis BI, Adour KK. An analysis of the Adour-Swanson and House-Brackmann grading systems for facial nerve recovery. Eur Arch Otorhinolaryngol. 1995; 252(5):265–9. https://doi.org/10.1007/BF00185387.
17. Saito H. A simple objective evaluation and grading for facial paralysis outcomes. Acta Otolaryngol. 2012;132(1):101–5. https://doi.org/10.3109/00016489.2011.626793.
18. Berg T, Jonsson L, Engström M. Agreement between the Sunnybrook, House-Brackmann, and Yanagihara facial nerve grading systems in Bell's palsy. Otol Neurotol. 2004;25(6):1020–6. https://doi.org/10.1097/00129492-200411000-00027.
19. Coulson SE, Croxson GR, Adams RD, O'Dwyer NJ. Reliability of the "Sydney," "Sunnybrook," and "House Brackmann" facial grading systems to assess voluntary movement and synkinesis after facial nerve paralysis. Otolaryngol Head Neck Surg. 2005;132(4):543–9. https://doi.org/10.1016/j.otohns.2005.01.027.
20. Reitzen SD, Babb JS, Lalwani AK. Significance and reliability of the House-Brackmann grading system for regional facial nerve function. Otolaryngol Head Neck Surg. 2009;140(2):154–8. https://doi.org/10.1016/j.otohns.2008.11.021.
21. Lee HY, Moon SP, Byun JY, Chung JH, Na SY, Yeo SG. Agreement between the facial nerve grading system 2.0 and the House-Brackmann grading system in patients with Bell palsy. Clin Exp Otorhinolaryngol. 2013;6(3):135–9. https://doi.org/10.3342/ceo.2013.6.3.135.
22. Smith IM, Murray JAM, Cull RE, Slattery J. A comparison of facial grading systems. Clin Otolaryngol Allied Sci. 1992;17(4):303–7. https://doi.org/10.1111/j.1365-2273.1992.tb01001.x.
23. Lazarini P, Mitre E, Takatu E, Tidei R. Graphic-visual adaptation of House-Brackmann facial nerve grading for peripheral facial palsy. Clin Otolaryngol. 2006;31(3):192–7. https://doi.org/10.1111/j.1749-4486.2006.01197.x.
24. Kanerva M, Poussa T, Pitkäranta A. Sunnybrook and House-Brackmann Facial Grading Systems: intrarater repeatability and interrater agreement. Otolaryngol Head Neck Surg. 2006;135(6):865–71. https://doi.org/10.1016/j.otohns.2006.05.748.
25. Croxson G, May M, Mester SJ. Grading facial nerve function: House-Brackmann versus Burres-Fisch methods. Am J Otol. 1990;11(4):240–6.
26. Ross BG, Fradet G, Nedzelski JM. Development of a sensitive clinical facial grading system. Otolaryngol Head Neck Surg. 1996;114(3):380–6. https://doi.org/10.1016/S0194-5998(96)70206-1.
27. Henstrom DK, Skilbeck CJ, Weinberg J, Knox C, Cheney ML, Hadlock TA. Good correlation between original and modified House Brackmann facial grading systems. Laryngoscope. 2011;121(1):47–50. https://doi.org/10.1002/lary.21163.
28. Kanerva M, Jonsson L, Berg T, et al. Sunnybrook and House-Brackmann systems in 5397 facial gradings. Otolaryngol Head Neck Surg. 2011;144(4):570–4. https://doi.org/10.1177/0194599810397497.
29. Ahrens A, Skarada D, Wallace M, Cheung JY, Neely JG. Rapid simultaneous comparison system for subjective grading scales grading scales for facial paralysis. Am J Otol. 1999;20(5):667–71.
30. Kayhan FT, Zurakowski D, Rauch SD. Toronto facial grading system: interobserver reliability. Otolaryngol Head Neck Surg. 2000;122(2):212–5. https://doi.org/10.1016/S0194-5998(00)70241-5.
31. Hu WL, Ross B, Nedzelski J. Reliability of the Sunnybrook Facial Grading System by novice users. J Otolaryngol. 2001;30(4):208–11.
32. Vrabec JT, Backous DD, Djalilian HR, et al. Facial Nerve Grading System 2.0. Otolaryngol Head Neck Surg. 2009;140(4):445–50. https://doi.org/10.1016/j.otohns.2008.12.031.
33. Lee LN, Susarla SM, Hohman MH, Henstrom DK, Cheney ML, Hadlock TA. A comparison of facial nerve

grading systems. Ann Plast Surg. 2013;70(3):313–6. https://doi.org/10.1097/SAP.0b013e31826acb2c.
34. Yanagihara N. Grading of facial nerve palsy. In: Fisch U, editor. Facial nerve surgery, proceedings: third international symposium on facial nerve surgery. Birmingham, AL: Aesculapius Publishing; 1977. p. 533–5.
35. Hato N, Fujiwara T, Gyo K, Yanagihara N. Yanagihara facial nerve grading system as a prognostic tool in Bell's palsy. Otol Neurotol. 2014;35(9):1669–72. https://doi.org/10.1097/MAO.0000000000000468.
36. Ikeda M, Nakazato H, Hiroshige K, Abiko Y, Sugiura M. To what extent do evaluations of facial paralysis by physicians coincide with self-evaluations by patients: comparison of the Yanagihara method, the House-Brackmann method, and self-evaluation by patients. Otol Neurotol. 2003;24(2):334–8.
37. Terzis JK, Noah ME. Analysis of 100 cases of free-muscle transplantation for facial paralysis. Plast Reconstr Surg. 1997;99(7):1905–21.
38. Biglioli F, Frigerio A, Rabbiosi D, Brusati R. Single-stage facial reanimation in the surgical treatment of unilateral established facial paralysis. Plast Reconstr Surg. 2009;124(1):124–33. https://doi.org/10.1097/PRS.0b013e3181aa0e2b.
39. Brichacek M, Sultan B, Boahene KD, Ishii L, Byrne PJ. Objective outcomes of minimally invasive temporalis tendon transfer for prolonged complete facial paralysis. Plast Surg (Oakville, Ont). 2017;25(3):200–10. https://doi.org/10.1177/2292550317728033.
40. Balaji S. Temporalis pull-through vs fascia lata augmentation in facial reanimation for facial paralysis. Ann Maxillofac Surg. 2016;6(2):267. https://doi.org/10.4103/2231-0746.200323.
41. Allevi F, Motta G, Colombo V, Biglioli F. Double-bellied latissimus dorsi free flap to correct full dental smile palsy. BMJ Case Rep. 2015;2015. https://doi.org/10.1136/bcr-2015-210436.
42. Ahuja R, Chatterjee P, Gupta R, Gupta G, Shrivastava P. A new paradigm in facial reanimation for long-standing palsies? Indian J Plast Surg. 2015;48(1):30. https://doi.org/10.4103/0970-0358.155265.
43. Gordin E, Lee TS, Ducic Y, Arnaoutakis D. Facial nerve trauma: evaluation and considerations in management. Craniomaxillofac Trauma Reconstr. 2015;8(1):1–13. https://doi.org/10.1055/s-0034-1372522.
44. Leckenby J, Grobbelaar A. Smile restoration for permanent facial paralysis. Arch Plast Surg. 2013;40(5):633–8. https://doi.org/10.5999/aps.2013.40.5.633.
45. Labbè D, Bussu F, Iodice A. A comprehensive approach to long-standing facial paralysis based on lengthening temporalis myoplasty. Acta Otorhinolaryngol Ital. 2012;32(3):145–53.
46. Banks CA, Bhama PK, Park J, Hadlock CR, Hadlock TA. Clinician-graded electronic facial paralysis assessment. Plast Reconstr Surg. 2015;136(2):223e–30e. https://doi.org/10.1097/PRS.0000000000001447.
47. Banks CA, Jowett N, Hadlock CR, Hadlock TA. Weighting of facial grading variables to disfigurement in facial palsy. JAMA Facial Plast Surg. 2016;18(4):292–8. https://doi.org/10.1001/jamafacial.2016.0226.
48. Banks CA, Jowett N, Hadlock TA. Test-retest reliability and agreement between in-person and video assessment of facial mimetic function using the eFACE facial grading system. JAMA Facial Plast Surg. 2017;19(3):206–11. https://doi.org/10.1001/jamafacial.2016.1620.
49. Banks CA, Jowett N, Azizzadeh B, et al. Worldwide testing of the eFACE facial nerve clinician-graded scale. Plast Reconstr Surg. 2017;139(2):491e–8e. https://doi.org/10.1097/PRS.0000000000002954.
50. Guarin DL, Dusseldorp J, Hadlock TA, Jowett N. A machine learning approach for automated facial measurements in facial palsy. JAMA Facial Plast Surg. 2018;20(4):335–7. https://doi.org/10.1001/jamafacial.2018.0030.
51. Dusseldorp JR, Guarin DL, van Veen MM, Jowett N, Hadlock TA. In the eye of the beholder: changes in perceived emotion expression after smile reanimation. Plast Reconstr Surg. 2019;144(2):457–71. https://doi.org/10.1097/PRS.0000000000005865.
52. Frey M, Jenny A, Giovanoli P, Stüssi E. Development of a new documentation system for facial movements as a basis for the international registry for neuromuscular reconstruction in the face. Plast Reconstr Surg. 1994;93(7):1334–49. https://doi.org/10.1097/00006534-199406000-00002.
53. Frey M, Giovanoli P, Gerber H, Slameczka M, Stüssi E. Three-dimensional video analysis of facial movements: a new method to assess the quantity and quality of the smile. Plast Reconstr Surg. 1999;104(7):2032–9. https://doi.org/10.1097/00006534-199912000-00013.
54. Tzou C-HJ, Pona I, Placheta E, et al. Evolution of the 3-dimensional video system for facial motion analysis: ten years' experiences and recent developments. Ann Plast Surg. 2012;69(2):173–85. https://doi.org/10.1097/SAP.0b013e3182223d96.
55. Hontanilla B, Aubá C. Automatic three-dimensional quantitative analysis for evaluation of facial movement. J Plast Reconstr Aesthetic Surg. 2008;61(1):18–30. https://doi.org/10.1016/j.bjps.2007.03.037.
56. Verhoeven T, Xi T, Schreurs R, Berge S, Maal T. Quantification of facial asymmetry: a comparative study of landmark-based and surface-based registrations. J Craniomaxillofac Surg. 2016;44(9):1131–6. https://doi.org/10.1016/j.jcms.2016.07.017.
57. Codari M, Pucciarelli V, Stangoni F, et al. Facial thirds–based evaluation of facial asymmetry using stereophotogrammetric devices: application to facial palsy subjects. J Craniomaxillofac Surg. 2017;45(1):76–81. https://doi.org/10.1016/j.jcms.2016.11.003.
58. McDuff D, El Kaliouby R, Senechal T, Amr M, Cohn JF, Picard R. Affectiva-MIT facial expression dataset (AM-FED): naturalistic and spontaneous facial expressions collected "in-the-wild". In: IEEE Computer Society conference on computer vision and pattern recognition workshops; 2013. p. 881–8. https://doi.org/10.1109/CVPRW.2013.130.

59. Su P, Ishii LE, Joseph A, et al. Societal value of surgery for facial reanimation. JAMA Facial Plast Surg. 2016;21287(2):139–46. https://doi.org/10.1001/jamafacial.2016.1419.
60. Ishii L, Godoy A, Encarnacion CO, Byrne PJ, Boahene KDO, Ishii M. Not just another face in the crowd: society's perceptions of facial paralysis. Laryngoscope. 2012;122(3):533–8. https://doi.org/10.1002/lary.22481.
61. Dey JK, Ishii LE, Byrne PJ, Boahene KDO, Ishii M. Seeing is believing: objectively evaluating the impact of facial reanimation surgery on social perception. Laryngoscope. 2014;124(11):2489–97. https://doi.org/10.1002/lary.24801.
62. Lyford-Pike S, Helwig NE, Sohre NE, Guy SJHT, Lyford-Pike S, Helwig NE, Sohre NE, Guy SJ, Hadlock TA. Predicting perceived disfigurement from facial function in patients with unilateral paralysis. Plast Reconstr Surg. 2018;142(5):722e–8e. https://doi.org/10.1097/PRS.0000000000004851.
63. Hadlock T. Standard outcome measures in facial paralysis getting on the same page. JAMA Facial Plast Surg. 2016;18(2):85–6. https://doi.org/10.1001/jamafacial.2015.2095.
64. Dey JK, Ishii M, Boahene KDO, Byrne PJ, Ishii LE. Changing perception: facial reanimation surgery improves attractiveness and decreases negative facial perception. Laryngoscope. 2014;124(1):84–90. https://doi.org/10.1002/lary.24262.
65. Surakka V, Hietanen JK. Facial and emotional reactions to Duchenne and non-Duchenne smiles. Int J Psychophysiol. 1998;29(1):23–33. https://doi.org/10.1016/S0167-8760(97)00088-3.
66. Hall JA, Carter JD, Horgan TG. Gender differences in nonverbal communication of emotion. In: Gender and emotion: social psychological perspectives; 2000. p. 97–117. https://doi.org/10.1017/CBO9780511628191.006.
67. Iacolucci CM, Banks C, Jowett N, et al. Development and validation of a spontaneous smile assay. JAMA Facial Plast Surg. 2015;17(3):191–6. https://doi.org/10.1001/jamafacial.2015.0083.
68. Buendia J, Loayza FR, Luis EO, Celorrio M, Pastor MA, Hontanilla B. Functional and anatomical basis for brain plasticity in facial palsy rehabilitation using the masseteric nerve. J Plast Reconstr Aesthetic Surg. 2016;69(3):417–26. https://doi.org/10.1016/j.bjps.2015.10.033.
69. Biglioli F, Bayoudh W, Colombo V, Pedrazzoli M, Rabbiosi D. [Double innervation (facial/masseter) on the gracilis flap, in the middle face reanimation in the management of facial paralysis: a new concept]. Ann Chir Plast Esthet. 2013;58(2):89–95. https://doi.org/10.1016/j.anplas.2012.12.001.
70. Cardenas-Mejia A, Covarrubias-Ramirez JV, Bello-Margolis A, Rozen S. Double innervated free functional muscle transfer for facial reanimation. J Plast Surg Hand Surg. 2015;49(3):183–8. https://doi.org/10.3109/2000656X.2014.988218.
71. Watanabe Y, Akizuki T, Ozawa T, Yoshimura K, Agawa K, Ota T. Dual innervation method using one-stage reconstruction with free latissimus dorsi muscle transfer for re-animation of established facial paralysis: simultaneous reinnervation of the ipsilateral masseter motor nerve and the contralateral facial nerve to im. J Plast Reconstr Aesthet Surg. 2009;62(12):1589–97. https://doi.org/10.1016/j.bjps.2008.07.025.
72. Chuang DCC, Lu JCY, Anesti K. One-stage procedure using spinal accessory nerve (XI)-innervated free muscle for facial paralysis reconstruction. Plast Reconstr Surg. 2013;132(1):117e–29e. https://doi.org/10.1097/PRS.0b013e318290f8cd.
73. Sforza C, Frigerio A, Mapelli A, et al. Double-powered free gracilis muscle transfer for smile reanimation: a longitudinal optoelectronic study. J Plast Reconstr Aesthetic Surg. 2015;68(7):930–9. https://doi.org/10.1016/j.bjps.2015.03.029.
74. Dusseldorp JR, Van Veen MM, Guarin DL, Quatela O, Jowett N, Hadlock TA. Spontaneity assessment in dually innervated gracilis smile reanimation surgery. JAMA Facial Plast Surg. 2019;21(6):551–7. https://doi.org/10.1001/jamafacial.2019.1090.

3 Documentation and Imaging in Facial Palsy

Tsz Yin Voravitvet, Chrisovalantis Lakhiani, and Tommy Nai-Jen Chang

3.1 Documentation in Facial Palsy

3.1.1 Overview

The facial palsy patient poses a unique problem to reconstructive surgeons. The myriad etiologies, symptoms on presentation, and clinical course pose a substantial sum of variables that affect reconstructive planning. Thus, standardized and detailed documentation are of paramount importance for assessing the need for reconstruction, surgical planning, and tracking outcomes. To date, while no universally standardized method of facial palsy documentation exists, substantive methods incorporate the factors of disease etiology, degree of facial nerve involvement, presence of synkinesis, and progression of symptoms. As such, photo-videographic evidence are supplementary but necessary for a complete clinical record and communication between practitioners.

Current systems can be classified into measures of impairment, or quality of life. With regard to the former, the most commonly used scales today are the House–Brackmann Facial Nerve Grading System and the Sunnybrook Facial Grading System. The House–Brackmann Facial Nerve Grading System was developed in 1985 by otolaryngologists Drs. John House and Derald Brackmann [1]. It is divided into 6 categories or grades, with Grade 1 being normal and Grade 6 being total paralysis. This scale benefits from its ease of use and rapid application. However, it suffers from the limitations of not individually reporting facial zones (facial nerve branch injury) and limited reporting of synkinesis. In contrast, the Sunnybrook Facial Grading System (developed by Dr. Julian Nedzelski at Sunnybrook Hospital in Toronto in 1994) scores discrete facial zones both at rest and with voluntary contraction. A patient receives points for the degree of normal resting tone or movement. The degree of synkinesis is then measured at the forehead, eye, and mouth and subtracted from the total score. A maximum total score of 100 is normal in this system. The Sunnybrook Facial Grading System benefits from its versatility by examining the patient at rest and with voluntary movement, inclusion of synkinesis in the final scoring, and division of mimetic measurements into zones of facial nerve injury.

Contrastingly, the Facial Clinimetric Evaluation (FaCE) Scale was developed at the Baylor College of Medicine in 2001 as a patient-graded instrument for evaluating quality of life in the facial palsy patient [2]. This study has been well-validated and corroborated compared to the Facial Disability Index and Medical Out-

T. Y. Voravitvet
Department of Surgery, Lerdsin Hospital, College of Medicine, Rangsit University, Bangkok, Thailand

C. Lakhiani (✉) · T. N.-J. Chang
Department of Plastic and Reconstructive Surgery, Chang Gung Memorial Hospital, Taoyuan, Taiwan

© Springer Nature Switzerland AG 2021
C.-H. J. Tzou, A. Rodríguez-Lorenzo (eds.), *Facial Palsy*,
https://doi.org/10.1007/978-3-030-50784-8_3

comes Study Short Form 36 (SF-36) Questionnaire and quality of life index. It requires the patient to self-report their degree of synkinesis, discomfort, quality of life in daily activity, and social interference.

At the Chang Gung Memorial Hospital, Linkou Medical Center in Taiwan, a novel facial palsy documentation system is employed that was designed by Dr. David Chwei-Chin Chuang. Unlike the previous systems mentioned, this documentation method aims to be comprehensive, including information on etiology, history, presentation, palsy of the unique branches of the facial nerve, as well as appearance at rest and with mimetic contraction (Fig. 3.1). The vertical column is for the documentation of intended movements, whereas synkinetic movements would be documented in the horizontal row. This system is employed at the initial visit; however, the other validated scoring systems are used as well for tracking outcomes (Fig. 3.2). For the purposes of this chapter, we shall be discussing the method employed at our institution, as well as the resources utilized for assessing, scoring, and tracking our outcomes. These include photo-videographic recordings, which we shall discuss in the following section.

3.1.2 Patient Assessment

As with any disease presentation, it is imperative to begin with a thorough history and physical examination. For the facial palsy patient, relevant historical data include the onset and timing of symptoms, supposed etiology (infectious, traumatic, iatrogenic, or congenital), laterality, subjective visual impairment, and progression of the disease. In the case of iatrogenic or infectious etiology, it is imperative to ensure that no further treatments will be required, or that the disease has stabilized. Relevant data collection includes previous operative records and the current disease status documentation, especially in some patients who have received prior reconstructive, ablative, or cosmetic procedures.

Name: Gender: Chart No: Left / Right side Birth date(Age): Address:
M F Tel:
Cause of facial nerve palsy: Date of Palsy:
Date of First Visit:
Present Illness
Past History:
Family history:
Physical Examination
At Rest
: symmetry vs. asymmetry (mild, moderate, severe)
(tension or hypertonicity at paretic side, oculofacial synkinesis, deep nasolabial fold, hypertrophy of corrugator, lower lip retraction, chain dimples, neck bands, others__________________)
Bell's phenomenon present (yes / no) Blink (yes / no)

At Dynamic movement

Synkinesis / No Synkinesis	Eye (narrowing)	Upper lip (contracture)	Lower lip (contracture)	Chain (dimpling)	Plastysma (neck bands)	Face asymmetry (mild, moderate, severe)
Forehead raise ☐ Palsy ☐ Weak ☐ Non-palsy						
Eye closure : lagophthalmos ( ) mm						
Smile : visible tooth (0 1 2 3 4 >4)						
Lower lip pull-down ☐ Palsy ☐ Weak ☐ Non-palsy						
Whistling ☐ Palsy ☐ Weak ☐ Non-palsy						

Fig. 3.1 Facial paralysis special chart in Chang Gung Memorial Hospital, Linkou Medical Cener, designed by Professor David Chwei-Chin Chuang

Fig. 3.2 Facial paralysis special chart for follow-up

Facial Nerve Evaluation				
House-Brackmann scale: I II III IV V VI				
Before treatment				
After treatment :	1st year	2nd year	3rd year	longer postop
Chuang's smile score system: 0 1 2 3 4				
Before treatment				
After treatment :	1st year	2nd year	3rd year	longer postop
Chuang's smile cortical adaptation staging system: I II III IV V				
Before treatment				
After treatment :	1st year	2nd year	3rd year	longer postop
Terzis and Noah Aesthetic and Functional Grading System: 1 2 3 4 5				
Before treatment				
After treatment :	1st year	2nd year	3rd year	longer postop

Prior to beginning the physical examination, one must ask for and take into account any previous facial palsy history (i.e., on the contralateral side), related syndrome, or prominent facial asymmetry from any other cause. The physical examination begins with the patient at rest. It is essential to look for facial asymmetry, co-contracture, tension or hypertonicity at paretic side, oculofacial synkinesis, deep nasolabial fold, hypertrophy of corrugator, lower lip retraction, chin dimples, and any neck band. The presence or absence of the Bell's phenomenon must also be separately addressed. Examination with dynamic movement then proceeds with documentation of the following functions, which correspond to the facial nerve branches:

- Forehead raise
- Eye closure
- Smile
- Lower lip pulling down
- Whistling

When asking the patient to activate the function of each facial nerve branch, one must also be searching for the presence of any synkinesis or co-contracture.

Finally, patient follow-up outcomes are recorded using House–Brackmann Scale [1], Chuang's Smile Score System [3], Chuang's Smile Cortical Adaptation Staging System [4] (Table 3.1), and Terzis and Noah Aesthetic and Functional Grading System [5].

Table 3.1 Chuang's Smile Score System

Score	Visible teeth	Contracture	Synkinesis
0	None or minimal central incisor	–0.5	–0.5
1	Full or near-full central incisor	–0.5	–0.5
2	Full central incisor and part of lateral incisor	–0.5	–0.5
3	Full central incisor, lateral incisor, and canine	–0.5	–0.5
4	Full central incisor, lateral incisor, canine, and premolar or more	–0.5	–0.5

3.2 Imaging in Facial Palsy Overview

Photography and to some extent videography have become indispensable components of the reconstructive surgeon's documentation protocol. These tools serve not only to assist in tracking a patient's clinical course, but also to allow for operative planning, transmission of information, and afford some degree of medico-legal protection. With regard to the latter, it is important to note that informed consent should always be obtained for the procurement and use of patient photographs and recordings.

For the facial palsy patient, photo-videography takes on the added role of serving to objectively measure outcomes. While there have been several systems for analysis proposed, there is not yet a single universally adopted standard for photo-videographic analysis of the facial palsy patient. Some may prefer to take measurement from still photographs [6], while others may employ standardized scales, such as the Scaled Measure of Improvement in Lip Excursion system [7]. At the Chang Gung Memorial Hospital, our most used photographic grading system is the Chuang's Smile Excursion Score [3] due to its simplicity and reproducibility (Table 3.1). This score is graded from 0 to 4 and focuses on smile evaluation only. A score of 0 will have no or minimal central incisor show, whereas a score of 4 will have full central and lateral incisors, canine, and the first premolar. From this, 0.5 is subtracted if either contracture of synkinesis is present. The limitation of this grading system, however, is that it focuses only on smile correction as it was developed to track outcomes following reconstruction of buccal branch injuries.

While we will here describe the methods of photo-videographic assessment employed at our institution, the primary factors of importance are standardization, repeatability, and clarity.

3.2.1 Composition and Positioning

Several resources have been developed with regard to photographic standards in plastic surgery [8–10]. These include avoidance of shadow, maintaining consistent and unobtrusive lighting, use of a neutral, solid-color background, and a same photographer using a high-quality camera in order to get the consistent quality photos and videos (Fig. 3.3). As a general rule, facial photographs are recommended to be taken with a fixed-focal length lens to maintain consistency. Modern digital single lens reflex (D-SLR) cameras afford the ability to easily change aperture, shutter speed, and exposure to achieve a high-quality picture in most office lighting conditions. A 5-megapixel or more camera is also generally considered sufficient for medical photography. If possible, a tripod should be routinely employed to minimize blur. When possible, photographs should be taken by the same individual. A variety of commercially available software programs are now available for digitally cataloguing all photographs and recordings.

The protocol at our institution involves a standardized photograph and video recording at the pre-operative and each subsequent post-operative visit. A tripod is always used, and photographs are taken at 2 m from the patient. The camera lens is set at the height of the nasal tip. Adjustments are made to set the inter-canthal line parallel to the horizontal axis of the photograph. For the full-face anteroposterior view, the superior border of the head is framed by a small amount of background (about 10% of the vertical height of the image). The inferior border of the image stops near the level of the suprasternal notch. Thus, we are able to capture an image from frontalis muscle function, orbicularis oculi closure, smile, and mentum, to the platysma. Photographs are then taken at rest, and with voluntary contraction.

Our procedure for capturing dynamic movements is as follows:

1. Frontal Branch: Patients are asked to elevate the forehead and create forehead wrinkles in order to evaluate frontalis muscle function. (Occasionally, this is difficult to observe and palpation of the forehead may be required to substantiate this finding.)
2. Zygomatic Branch: It is imperative to observe for and document lid position first at rest. Subsequently, the patient is asked to close their eyes to examine for paralytic lagophthalmos. In the older patient, this finding may be further compromised by dermatochalasis. Video recordings are also taken at this stage to document lid lag and any concomitant synkinesis.
3. Buccal Branch: The patient is asked to smile at a "mild" ("smile with ease"), "moderate," and "full" ("smile with maximum effort") dentured smile [11]. The patients are asked to pronounce the letter "E" as in "cheese" to facilitate smile performance and expose the teeth. Video documentation is used primarily for confirmation of the measurements made from photographs. In patients with missing

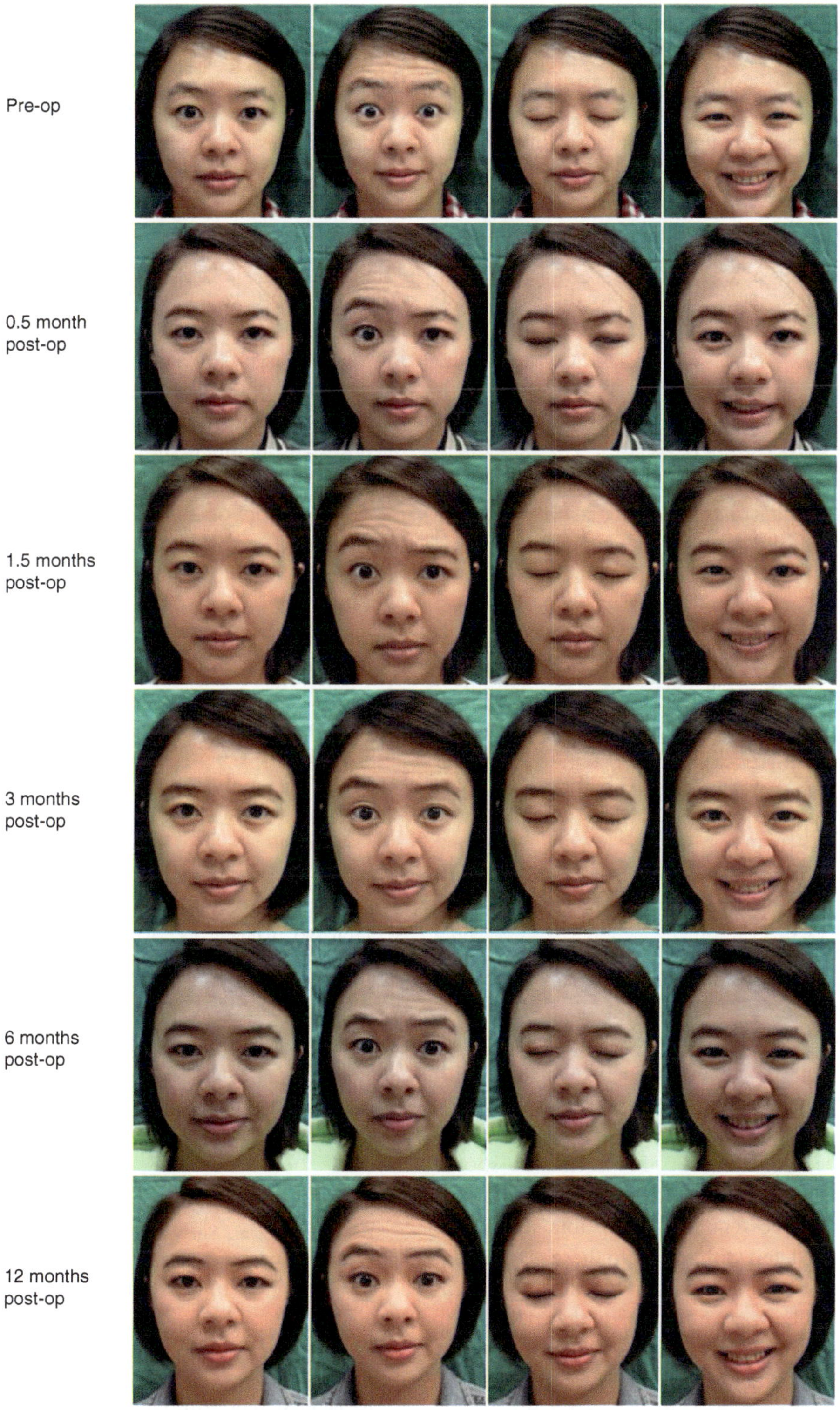

Fig. 3.3 A case demonstration to show a 30-year-old female who suffered from a left facial nerve schwannoma and underwent resection under the microscope. After the surgery, she developed a left sided neuropraxia. This improved over time. A single photographer (Dr. Tommy Nai-Jen Chang) using the same camera can get very consistent high-quality serial photos to identify changes in facial expression

teeth or malocclusion, the scoring is based on the predicted neutral dental position [12].
4. Marginal Mandibular Branch: The isolated marginal mandibular nerve palsy can be checked by asking the patients to evert the lower lip. During the resting stage, the symmetry of the lip needs to be observed. If there is a palsy, the lip will deviate to the contralateral (healthy) side.
5. Cervical Branch: Patients are here asked to contract the neck muscles as in shaving.

3.2.2 Post-paralytic Facial Synkinesis (PPFS)

Other important parameters that need to be observed are the presence of co-contracture and synkinesis [10]. Facial synkinesis is an unwanted facial movement observed in a particular facial region accompanying a voluntary wanted one, usually caused by aberrant reinnervation among facial nerve fibers following nerve injury [11]. In the past, many physicians did not pay much attention to documenting the synkinesis status of the patient and overlooked this condition of facial paralysis. However, we now know the importance of this pathologic movement and the sequelae of this condition.

Facial synkinesis may occur not only during facial expression, but also at rest (i.e., the intermittent blinking reflex causes intermittent cheek muscle twitching). Long-term unresolved synkinesis may result in permanent contracture, such as hypertrophy of the corrugator muscles, deepened nasolabial folds, lower lip retraction, chin skin dimples, and neck bands [12]. As such, the photo documentation of this condition should be taken both at rest and dynamic movement. However, video recordings are able to provide much more detail with regard to these involuntary movements. It is important in these video recordings to use the standard AP view described, with exposure of the platysma in its entirety.

Following reconstruction, there is further benefit of video recording through offering the patient a record of how to perform induction exercises. Consistent recording throughout the follow-up period is able to track the stages of cortical adaptation to various nerve transfer techniques [4].

3.3 Conclusion

Although there is no standard uniform grading system used at the moment, many reliable grading systems exist to aid the surgeon in assessing and following the patient. Photo-videographic data has become an indispensable tool for the purposes of documentation and planning. While it remains up to the surgeon to determine which methods suit his or her practice best, it remains important to employ consistent and thorough documentation for the purposes of reconstructive planning, tracking a clinical course, and measuring outcomes.

References

1. House JW, Brackmann DE. Facial nerve grading system. Otolaryngol Head Neck Surg. 1985;93(2):146–7.
2. Kahn JB, et al. Validation of a patient-graded instrument for facial nerve paralysis: the FaCE scale. Laryngoscope. 2001;111(3):387–98.
3. Tzou CH, Chuang DC, Chen HH. Facial paralysis grading system: a new and simple smile excursion score for evaluating facial reanimation surgery. Ann Plast Surg. 2015;74(2):210–3.
4. Tzou CH, Chuang DC, Chen HY. Cortical adaptation staging system: a new and simple staging for result evaluation of functioning free-muscle transplantation for facial reanimation. Ann Plast Surg. 2014;73(1):50–3.
5. Terzis JK, Noah ME. Analysis of 100 cases of free-muscle transplantation for facial paralysis. Plast Reconstr Surg. 1997;99(7):1905–21.
6. Fattah AY, et al. Survey of methods of facial palsy documentation in use by members of the Sir Charles Bell Society. Laryngoscope. 2014;124(10):2247–51.
7. Bray D, et al. Assessing outcomes in facial reanimation: evaluation and validation of the SMILE system for measuring lip excursion during smiling. Arch Facial Plast Surg. 2010;12(5):352–4.

8. DiBernardo BE, et al. Photographic standards in plastic surgery. Plast Reconstr Surg. 1998;102(2): 559–68.
9. Galdino GM, Vogel JE, Vander Kolk CA. Standardizing digital photography: it's not all in the eye of the beholder. Plast Reconstr Surg. 2001;108(5): 1334–44.
10. Gurtner GC, Neligan PC. Plastic surgery E-book, vol. 1. Principles. Elsevier Health Sciences; 2017.
11. Beurskens CH, Oosterhof J, Nijhuis-van der Sanden MW. Frequency and location of synkineses in patients with peripheral facial nerve paresis. Otol Neurotol. 2010;31(4):671–5.
12. Chuang DC, Chang TN, Lu JC. Postparalysis facial synkinesis: clinical classification and surgical strategies. Plast Reconstr Surg Glob Open. 2015;3(3):e320.

Pre- and Post-op Rehabilitation in Facial Palsy Patients

4

Othmar Schuhfried

Key Points

- The optimal functional recovery is the central aim of the rehabilitation in facial paralysis.
- The therapeutic strategies include facial exercise therapy of the mimic muscles, electromyography-biofeedback, electrotherapy, massage, lymphatic drainage, and botulinum toxin injections.
- Methods of the clinical evaluation and follow-up assessments should be sensitive to changes with rehabilitation interventions.

Therapeutic options used in the rehabilitation in patients with facial dysfunctions include facial exercise therapy (physiotherapy, mirror therapy), electromyography (EMG)-biofeedback, electrotherapy, massage, lymphatic drainage, and botulinum toxin injections. Although each modality has its indication, the facial exercise therapy is the basic intervention. The therapeutic strategy is based on the severity and course of the disease.

O. Schuhfried (✉)
Department of Physical Medicine, Rehabilitation and Occupational Medicine, Medical University of Vienna, Vienna, Austria
e-mail: othmar.schuhfried@meduniwien.ac.at

© Springer Nature Switzerland AG 2021
C.-H. J. Tzou, A. Rodríguez-Lorenzo (eds.), *Facial Palsy*,
https://doi.org/10.1007/978-3-030-50784-8_4

4.1 Facial Nerve Grading Instruments

Approximately every month the clinical assessment should be repeated to assess possible improvement. Muscle strength of the mimic muscle, static and dynamic facial asymmetry, and the presence of spasm and synkinesis should be evaluated. Synkinesis is the involuntary contraction of muscles that accompanies voluntary contraction of other muscles. For example when the patient smiles the eyelid closes on the affected side (synkinesis in the oculi and orbicularis oris muscle). In a large longitudinal multicenter study, synkinesis frequency was 21.3% at 12 months and synkinesis deteriorates between 6 and 12 months [1]. The loss of facial symmetry and ability to smile and abnormal movement pattern create cosmetic and social problems. Therefore the evaluation of the quality of life and impairment in social interaction is important [2].

4.2 House–Brackmann Score

The most popular method for assessing the severity of facial paralysis is the grading system according to House–Brackmann [3]. It analyzes the symmetry, global mobility, stiffness, and synkinesis of the face. This scale ranges from 1 (normal) to 6 (severe dysfunction) and is therefore a rather rough scale that might be unable to detect subtle changes.

4.3 Sunnybrook Score

This grading system measures three components of facial asymmetry: resting asymmetry, symmetry of the voluntary movement, and synkinesis [4, 5]. A score of 100 points is related to normal facial symmetry. This score is sensitive to changes with rehabilitation interventions. Each component of this grading system is sensitive to change and individually contributes to a change in the composite score [5]. The Sunnybrook composite score at 1 month is a good predictor for synkinesis [1].

4.4 Chuang's Smile Excursion Score

The smile excursion score assigns a score from 0 to 4 to characterize patient's smile based on the number of maxillary teeth exposed [6]. It is a simple, quick, and reliable system in evaluating smile before and after reanimation of the paralyzed face (Fig. 4.1).

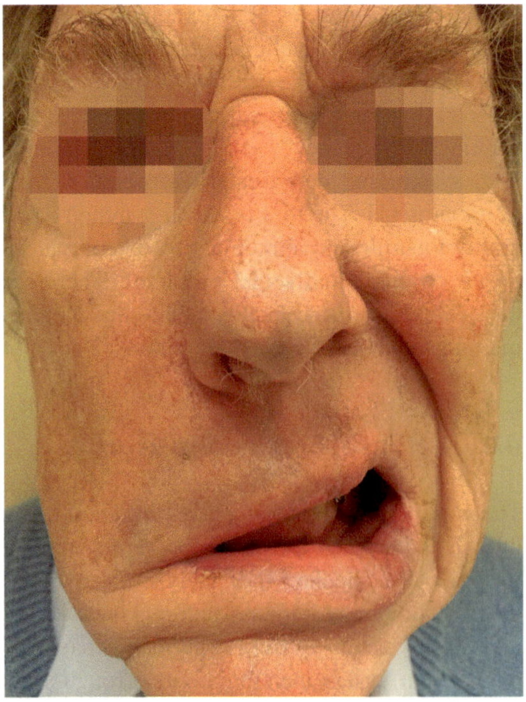

Fig. 4.1 Patient rated with 0 applying the Chuang's smile excursion score. The smiling patient has no maxillary teeth visible on the paralyzed side of the face

Furthermore it is useful to perform an electrophysiological assessment to evaluate the severity of the facial nerve lesion and prognose the time needed for recovery and the quality of recovery.

4.5 Exercise Therapy

Facial exercise therapy can improve functionality of the mimic muscle and therefore should always be included in the rehabilitation process. Facial exercises of the mimic muscles are the basic intervention and try to preserve muscular tone and activity, trophism, facial symmetry and to avoid abnormal movement pattern. Facial exercise therapy is effective for facial palsy for the outcome functionality [7].

Facial exercise therapy should be performed by a specially trained facial physiotherapist or speech therapist. Facial exercise therapy must be adapted to the extent of the lesion, the present facial activity, or any abnormal patterns of movement. Frequent repetitions and frequent daily sessions (individualized home program) are necessary. Repetition improves motor relearning. Based on the clinical evaluation, the facial exercises can be divided into four categories [8, 9]: Initiation, Facilitation, Movement Control, Relaxation.

Initiation treatment category: If there are a moderate to severe facial asymmetry at rest, no visible muscle activity, and a flaccid mimic musculature, the patients are placed in the initiation treatment category. Soft tissue mobilization and superficial massage are indicated. Active assisted range of motion exercises and small range movement exercises are performed. Mass movements and overpowering by the muscle function of the uninvolved side of the face should be avoided (Fig. 4.2).

Facilitation treatment category: If there are a mild to moderate facial asymmetry at rest, an initiate facial movement, and no synkinesis, the patients are placed in the facilitation treatment category. Patients are instructed in individualized soft tissue stretching and mobilization. Active and resistive exercise to increase facial movement excursion are appropriate. Awareness

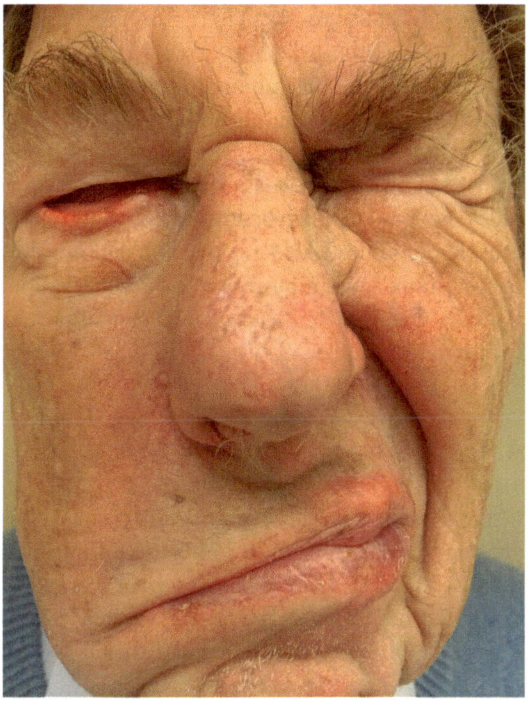

Fig. 4.2 Patient with a severe asymmetry of voluntary movement and overpowered muscle function of the uninvolved side of the face. The loss of facial symmetry and ability to smile creates cosmetic and social problems

of signs of abnormal movement patterns (synkinesis) and avoidance of mass movement is important. Emphasis is on slow, small movements to gain symmetry. Mirror (visual) feedback or EMG-biofeedback can be used to learn adequate movements and to suppress abnormal muscle activity. Mirror mimic exercises and EMG-biofeedback could achieve the awareness, involvement, and engagement of patients in the recovery process.

Movement control category: If there are a mild to moderate facial asymmetry at rest and an initiate facial movement but synkinesis has developed, the patients are placed in the movement control category. Patients are instructed in soft tissue massage of the facial muscles and relaxation techniques. The patients are guided in relearning isolate muscle contractions and to reduce muscle activity of abnormal patterns of movement. Producing desired facial movements without an accompanying synkinetic movement is the aim. Small range movement patterns are recommended. The emphasis is on controlling synkinesis. Mirror feedback and EMG-biofeedback can be used to develop selective muscle control and decrease synkinesis [10].

Relaxation Category: If there are severe muscular hypertonicity and synkinesis, the patients are placed in the relaxation category. The primary treatment for problems of facial twitches and spasm are relaxation exercises, such as modifications of the standard relaxation exercises originally described by Jacobson and small rhythmic, alternating movements to relax muscles. Techniques to inhibit muscle activation include sustained stretching and cross-friction massage to reduce passive tissue restrictions. EMG-biofeedback is helpful to control the muscle relaxation.

After supervised facial exercise therapy every patient is given a homework brochure to perform daily facial mimic exercises autonomously. A study showed that supervised exercises provided by a therapist are equally effective than facial exercises performed autonomously at home in terms of facial paresis recovery rate [11].

4.6 Electromyography-Biofeedback (EMG-Biofeedback)

In order to improve the perception of the correct movement sequences, an electromyography (EMG)-biofeedback apparatus can be used. Here the muscle activity is derived via EMG surface electrodes and visualized on an associated computer screen. This facilitates the relearning of correct movements [12]. Whereas early efforts focus on global animation of the paralyzed face, as the problem of synkinesis is recognized, this technique is successfully directed to minimizing synkinetic motion. EMG-biofeedback electrodes can be placed simultaneously in muscles innervated by different nerve branches to look for co-contraction and synkinesis [13]: frontalis muscle (temporal branch), orbicularis oculi muscle (zygomatic branch), zygomatic muscles (zygomatic branch), orbicularis oris muscle (buccal branch). The patient gets a feedback by a graph on the monitor or a sound when he contracts the target muscle while simultaneously relaxing the synkinetic muscle. Therefore EMG-biofeedback helps the patient to perform selective muscle control and to decrease synkinesis. It is an objective means of measuring movements and outcome. Home-units can be used to perform EMG-biofeedback daily [13].

4.7 Electrical Stimulation

If the facial paresis is not spontaneously declining within 6 weeks, an electrostimulation of the mimic muscles can be started. If there is no electrophysiological sign of denervation and the reason of the facial palsy is neuropraxia, electrical stimulation with short impulses with a duration between 0.1 ms and 1 ms can be used. If there are electrophysiological signs of severe or complete denervation, triangular pulses (disturbances of accommodation of the denervated muscles) with a pulse duration of 100–200 ms are required for this purpose. The stimulation should be performed for 5–10 min each muscle three sessions a week [14]. The current intensity should be as low as possible to initiate a twitch of the stimulated mimic muscle. After ten therapy sessions, the stimulation should be paused for 1 month. If there is still no regeneration, a new electrotherapy session can be added. The electrical stimulation should not be used once contracture or synkinesis occurs [14]. The conclusion of a recent systematic review is that there is no evidence to support the use of electrical stimulation during the acute phase of recovery after Bell's palsy and there is low-level evidence for patients with chronic symptoms [15].

After a muscular gracilis transplantation, the stimulation of the muscle transplant starts 6 weeks after surgery. This is done daily for 5–10 min until an arbitrary activity occurs (usually 4–8 months after surgery). Then the electrical stimulation is ended and the focus is on active mimic exercises.

4.8 Massage

The aim of facial massage is to relax hypertonic muscles and to initiate mimic activity. External and intraoral facial massage are a useful supplement [16]. Soft tissue massage with small amplitude movements has been shown to promote muscle blood flow and keep the skin and muscles in optimum condition prior to reinnervation. Patients can also be instructed to perform self-massage techniques.

4.9 Manual Lymphatic Drainage

Manual lymphatic drainage maneuvers are considered to exert force on the interstitial fluids and thereby shifting them towards collaterals and/or normally functioning lymphatic vessels. These manipulations therefore not only soften tissues directly, but possibly also remove excessive local fluid. Lymphatic drainage can be used in the acute stage of an idiopathic facial nerve palsy, with the idea that it supports the reduction of the nerve's swelling [16]. The manual lymphatic drainage also has a relaxing effect and the cutaneous stimulus has an initiating effect. The manual lymphatic drainage can be recommended as a supportive method in the conservative therapy of idiopathic facial paralysis.

4.10 Botulinum Toxin

In the case of synkinesis, facial hyperkinesis, and imbalance, the application of the neurotoxin botulinum toxin A can be considered [17]. Botulinum toxin injections are a minimally invasive, well-tolerated technique that causes temporary paralysis of hyperkinetic musculature. Nevertheless, side effects like induced lagophthalmos and keratitis, excessive facial weakness, and mild difficulty in talking, eating, or drinking are described [18]. The precise area or point and depth of injection are important. Before the injection of botulinum toxin, the patients should participate in a facial muscle retraining program for a minimum of 16 weeks [9]. After application of botulinum toxin, facial exercise training is crucial for a successful outcome. In the use of botulinum toxin in the management of facial paralysis, regular follow-ups and careful documentation should be undertaken.

The effect of complementary interventions such as acupuncture is dependent on the experience of the therapist. Positive therapeutic effects of acupuncture were described in the treatment of Bell's palsy [19].

4.11 Postoperative Facial Rehabilitation

The postoperative rehabilitation interventions must always be agreed with the surgeon and his guidelines and prescriptions must be followed. Also, the individually healing and recovery process must be taken into account.

4.11.1 Rehabilitation After Temporalis and Masseter Muscle Transposition

In the case of both temporalis and masseter muscle transposition, the innervation of the muscle depends on a nerve other than the facial nerve. Since the temporalis and masseter muscles are chewing muscles, the patients are instructed to bite while they smile. If no movement is visible, the patients are assigned to the initiation category. If movement is possible in the muscle, the patients are assigned to the facilitation category. Treatment includes teaching the patient how to exercise the transpositioned muscle while monitoring for synkinetic movement. EMG-biofeedback can be used for facilitation of the desired movement. Patience and effort are required to overcome the difficulty dissociating and reassociating the function of chewing and smiling or chewing and closing the eye [20]. After months of training, motivated patients will undergo cerebral adaption and can learn to smile without clenching their teeth.

4.11.2 Rehabilitation After Labbé Technique

The rehabilitation should start 3 weeks after surgery to prevent local adhesions. This begins with deep but soft massages of the tendon insertion into the commissure [21]. Furthermore, gentle exercises start and the symmetry of the face and smile, lip movement, swallowing, and articulation are practiced. Using a mirror or EMG-biofeedback desirable movements are learned and unwanted movements are avoided. A smile is achieved by the movement of the lower jaw with consecutive contraction of the temporalis muscle. Over the time patients have to learn how to contract the muscle and lift the corner of the mouth without clenching the teeth using brain plasticity capacities. A standardized protocol was developed by Lambert-Prou to achieve step by step a functional change of the temporal muscle to perform a spontaneous smile [22].

4.11.3 Rehabilitation After Nerve Transfers and Cross-Facial Nerve Grafting

The rehabilitation is similar to the facial motor rehabilitation for nonsurgical patients. If there are no visible muscle activities, patients are assigned to the initiation category. With little movements, the patients are assigned to the facilitation category. The most desirable result would be the complete return of the smile function and facial symmetry.

4.11.4 Rehabilitation After Free Gracilis Muscle Transfer for Reconstruction of the Smile in Irreversible Facial Palsy

In case of free gracilis muscle transfer, the transplanted muscle is completely separated from its original source of innervation, which is a branch of the obturator nerve, and acquires a new source of innervation through the cross-face nerve graft, that is, through the contralateral healthy facial nerve. Thus, the muscle transplant undergoes a process of complete denervation and reinnervation until clinically evident and electrophysiologically measureable function can be registered [23]. After the surgery, special attention should be paid to reduce postoperative edema by soft tissue mobilization. Normally, clinically visible muscle function is not achieved before 6 months postoperatively. Patients undergoing free muscle transplantations for reconstruction of the smile are provided 6 weeks postoperatively with an electrical stimulation device and are instructed to stimulate the muscle transplant twice daily for approximately 10 min [16, 23]. The aim of this treatment is to facilitate motor re-education and prevent atrophy of the muscle transplant. If no motion is visible, patients are classified into the initiation category. If movements of the muscular graft are present, they are classified into the facilitation category. Practicing small movements is important and special lip exercises are performed.

References

1. Bylund N, Jensson D, Enghag S, Berg T, Marsk E, Hultcrantz M, Hadziosmanovic N, Rodriguez-Lorenzo A, Jonsson L. Synkinesis in Bell's palsy in a randomized controlled trial. Clin Otolaryngol. 2017;42:673–80.
2. Györi E, Przestrzelski C, Pona I, Hagmann M, Rath T, Radtke C, Tzou CJ. Quality of life and functional assessment of facial palsy patients: a questionnaire study. Int J Surg. 2018;55:92–7.
3. House JW, Brackmann DE. Facial nerve grading system. Otolaryngol Head Neck Surg. 1985;93(2):146–7.
4. Ross GB, Fradet G, Nedzelski JM. Development of a sensitive clinical facial grading system. Otolaryngol Head Neck Surg. 1996;114:380–6.
5. Fattah AY, Gurusinghe ADR, Gavilan J, Hadlock TA, Marcus JR, Marres H, Nduka CC, Slattery WH, Snyder-Warwick AK. Facial nerve grading instruments: systematic review of the literature and suggestion for uniformity. Plast Reconstr Surg. 2015;135:569–79.
6. Tzou CHJ, Chuang DCC, Chen HH. Facial paralysis grading system. A new and simple smile excursion score for evaluating facial reanimation surgery. Ann Plast Surg. 2015;74:210–3.
7. Pereira LM, Obara K, Dias JM, Menacho MO, Lavado EL, Cardoso JR. Facial exercise therapy for facial palsy: systematic review and meta-analysis. Clin Rehabil. 2011;25(7):649–58.
8. Van Swearingen JM. Facial rehabilitation: a neuromuscular reeducation, patient-centered approach. Facial Plastic Surg. 2008;24(2):250–9.
9. Lindsay RW, Robinson M, Hadlock TA. Comprehensive facial rehabiliation improves function in people with facial paralysis. Phys Ther. 2010;90:391–7.
10. Cronin GW, Steenerson RL. The effectiveness of neuromuscular facial retraining combined with electromyography in facial paralysis rehabilitation. Otolaryngol Head Neck Surg. 2003;128:534–8.
11. Infante-Cossio P, Prats-Golczer VE, Lopez-Martos R, Montes-Latorre E, Exposito-Tirado JA, Gonzalez-Cardero E. Effectiveness of facial exercise therapy for facial nerve dysfunction after superficial parotidectomy: a randomized controlled trial. Clin Rehabil. 2016;30(11):1097–107.
12. Toffola ED, Tinell C, Lozza A, Bejor M, Pavese C, Agosti ID, Petrucci L. Choosing the best rehabilitation treatment for Bell's palsy. Eur J Phys Med Rehabil Med. 2012;48:635–42.
13. Volk FG, Finkensieper M, Guntinas-Lichius O. EMG biofeedback training at home for patient with chronic facial palsy and defective healing. Laryng Rhino Otol. 2014;93:15–24.
14. Shafshak TS. The treatment of facial palsy from the point of view of physical and rehabilitation medicine. Eura Medicophys. 2006;42:41–7.
15. Fargher KA, Coulson SE. Effectiveness of electrical stimulation for rehabilitation of facial nerve paralysis. Phys Ther Rev. 2017;22:169–76.
16. Paternostro-Sluga T, Herceg M, Frey M. Conservative treatment and rehabilitation in peripheral facial palsy. Handchir Mikrochir Plast Chir. 2010;42:109–14.
17. Cabin JA, Massry GG, Azizzadeh B. Botulinum toxin in the management of facial paralysis. Curr Opin Otolarynol Head Neck Surg. 2015;23:272–80.
18. Cooper L, Lui M, Nduka C. Botulinum toxin treatment for facial palsy: a systematic review. J Plast Recontr Aesthet Surg. 2017;70:833–41.
19. Xu S, Huang B, Zhang C, Du P, Yuan Q, Bi G, Zhang G, Xie m LX, Huang G, Wang W. Effectiveness of strengthened stimulation during acupuncture for the treatment of Bell's palsy. A randomised controlled trial. CMAJ. 2013;185:473–9.
20. Michaelidou M, Tzou CHJ, Gerber H, Stüssi E, Mittlböck M, Frey M. The combination of muscle transpositions and static procedures for reconstruction in the paralyzed face of the patient with limited life

expectancy or who is not a candidate for free muscle transfer. Plast Reconstr Surg. 2009;123:121–9.
21. Guarreschi P, Labbe D. Lengthening temporalis myoplasty: a surgical tool for dynamic labial commisuure reanimation. Facial Plast Surg. 2015;31(2): 123–7.
22. Lambert-Prou MP. The temporal smile. Speech therapy for facial palsy patients after temporal lengthening myoplasty. Rev Stomatol Chir Maxillofac. 2003;104(5):274–80.
23. Michaelidou M, Herceg M, Schuhfried O, Tzou CHJ, Pona I, Hold A, Mittlböck M, Paternostro-Sluga T, Frey M. Correlation of functional recovery with the course of electrophysiological parameters after free muscle transfer for reconstruction of the smile in irreversible facial palsy. Muscle Nerve. 2011;44:741–8.

5 Electrophysiology in Facial Paralysis

Othmar Schuhfried

Key Points

- For the electrophysiological evaluation in facial paralysis, the most important methods are nerve conduction studies and the needle electromyography
- The aim is the verification of a peripheral lesion and determination of its extent
- The electrophysiological examination provides a decision support for therapeutic interventions

The electrophysiological evaluation of the facial nerve with nerve conduction studies (NCS) or needle electromyography (EMG) can be performed to answer the following questions [1, 2]:

1. Is the lesion peripheral?
2. Severity of the lesion and what is the underlying pathology: neurapraxia, axonotmesis, neurotmesis?
3. Is there a chance for recovery?
4. Is a surgical intervention necessary (electrophysiological measures are one of the criterions for decision-making besides time of onset of the lesion, physical examination, underlying pathology…)?

To evaluate the proximal segments of the facial nerve, blink reflex studies can be helpful.

5.1 Nerve Conduction Studies (NCS)

The maximum motor evoked action potential or the so-called compound muscle action potential (CMAP) is derived by surface electrodes from the mimic muscles after supramaximal transcutaneous stimulation of the facial nerve. The main trunk of the facial nerve can be stimulated either below the ear anterior to the mastoid, where it exits the stylomastoid foramen, or directly anterior to the tragus. Selective branches of the facial nerve can be stimulated more distally.

5.1.1 Recording

Any of the following muscles can be used for recording: the frontalis, nasalis, orbicularis oculi, orbicularis oris, or mentalis (Fig. 5.1). The reference electrode can be placed over the same muscle on the contralateral side of the face.

Avoiding interference with masseter CMAP is important (Fig. 5.2).

O. Schuhfried (✉)
Department of Physical Medicine, Rehabilitation and Occupational Medicine, Medical University of Vienna, Vienna, Austria
e-mail: othmar.schuhfried@meduniwien.ac.at

© Springer Nature Switzerland AG 2021
C.-H. J. Tzou, A. Rodríguez-Lorenzo (eds.), *Facial Palsy*,
https://doi.org/10.1007/978-3-030-50784-8_5

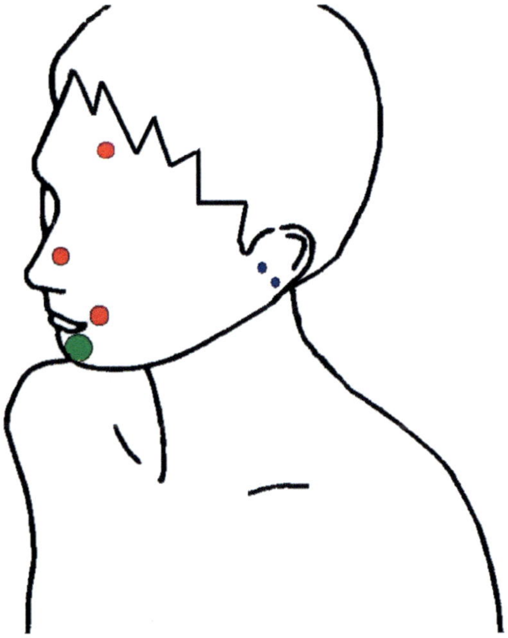

Fig. 5.1 Electrode configuration for nerve conduction studies: stimulation (blue electrodes) directly anterior to the tragus; recording from the frontalis muscle, nasalis muscle, and orbicularis oris muscle with adhesive electrodes (red). The reference electrode is placed over the contralateral muscle. A ground electrode (green) is placed over the forehead, chin, or arm

5.1.2 Parameter

Compound muscle action potential (CMAP): The amplitude is proportional to the number of intact motor axons [1–4].

The latency: reflects conduction time along the fastest conducting fibers of the distal segment of the facial nerve.

CMAPs vary substantially from one patient to the other [5, 6]. Therefore the CMAPs of the affected side are compared with the healthy side. The following is postulated in this regard: the greater the nerve damage, the lower is the CMAP on the affected side compared to the healthy side. Severe degeneration of the nerve is suspected when the CMAP potential on the affected side is more than 90% lower than that on the healthy side (Fig. 5.3). In severe cases, there may be a complete loss of nerve stimulability as an expression of complete degeneration. A definite determination of nerve degeneration can be demonstrated not earlier than 10–14 days after the onset of nerve damage because a Wallerian degeneration takes that long to reach the mimic muscles [1, 2].

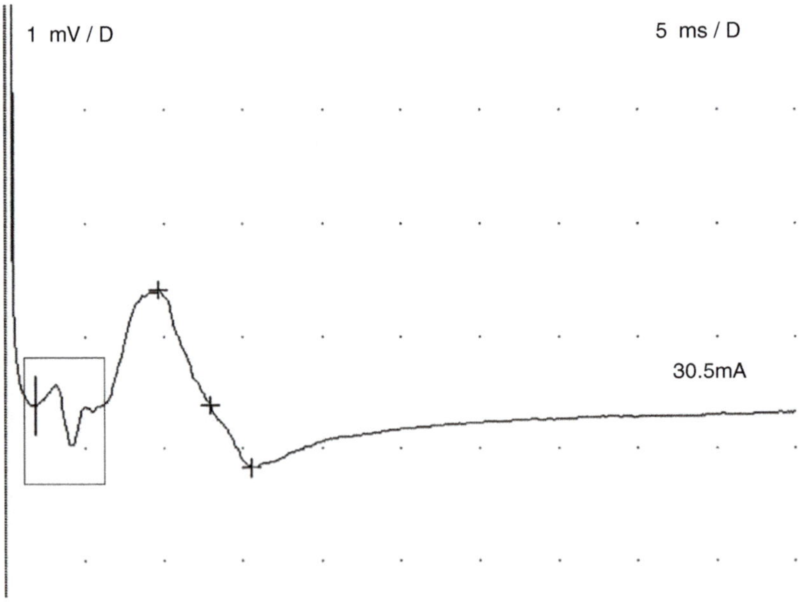

Fig. 5.2 Compound muscle action potential (CMAP) of the orbicularis oris muscle and interference (marked with the rectangle) with a masseter potential (small potential recorded before the origin CMAP of the mimetic muscle with a latency less than 2 ms)

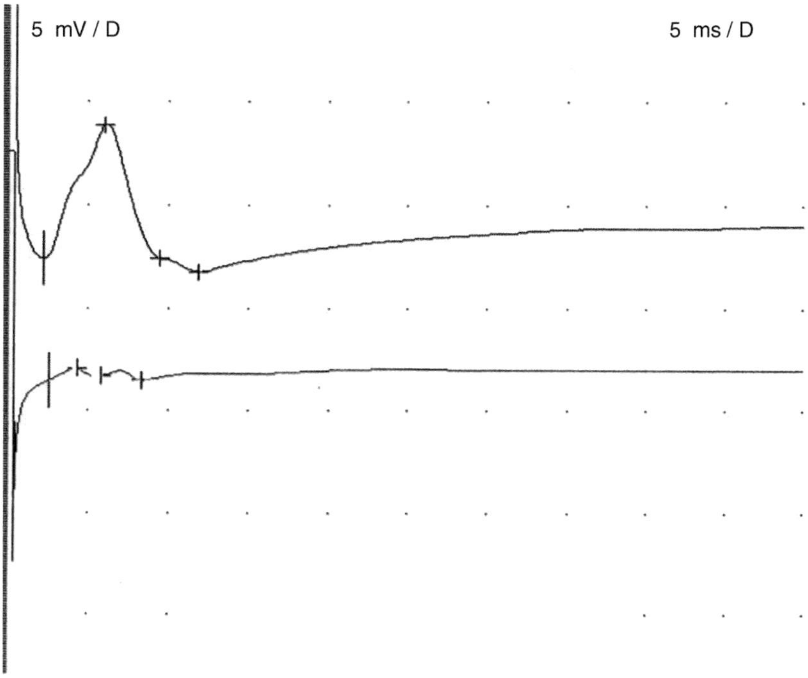

Fig. 5.3 Side to side comparison of the compound muscle action potential (CMAP) of the orbicularis oris muscle showing severe nerve degeneration

Since the lesion site is usually proximal of the stimulation site, a reduction of the CMAP potential may be regarded as an expression of Wallerian degeneration. The degree of axonal loss has direct implication for the prognosis and the time required for recovery. The more the CMAP decrease, the slower the recovery will be. A distinct amplitude decrease and even the lack of the same (0–10% of the contralateral side) point to heavy nerve damage and an incomplete clinical recovery [1].

For example, in the case with percentage degeneration of 50% compared to the not involved side but clinically complete palsy, we can draw that this facial paralysis may result partially from conduction block and the prognosis might be good.

Serial NCS are recommended to predict the status of neural degeneration and the prognosis of the facial palsy. Due to the large intersubject and also intrasubject variability of the results (e.g., in healthy subjects of 22% of the CMAP of the nasal muscle) [6] and the fact that the late term results do not correlate well with clinical symptoms [7], NCS are only partly suitable for the purpose of monitoring.

In patients with hemifacial spasm, a response can be seen also in the muscle that is not directly innervated by the stimulated nerve branch. During stimulation of the zygomatic branch and recording from the orbicularis oculi muscle and simultaneously from the mental muscle, a potential can be recorded in both muscles (delayed response also in the mentalis muscle that is normally not innervated by the zygomatic branch) because of ephaptic spread and transmission.

5.2 Electromyography (EMG)

A procedure to demonstrate an axonal lesion of the facial nerve is the needle EMG of the mimic muscles. The crucial target muscles can be investigated: frontalis muscle (temporal branch), orbicularis oculi muscle (zygomatic branch), orbicularis oris muscle, nasalis muscle (buccal branch), mentalis muscle, depressor anguli oris muscle (marginal mandibular branch). Electrical activity of each muscle is recorded at rest and during volitional movement [1, 2, 8].

When the muscle is at rest, abnormal resting potentials so called pathological spontaneous activity (positive sharp waves and fibrillations) are typical electromyographic signs of axonal damage and concomitant muscle denervation. Such pathological spontaneous activity does not occur in the presence of neurapraxia, but does occur in cases of acute axonal damage to the nerve. This sign of denervation does not appear earlier than 10–14 days after injury [8, 9]. In the mimic muscles, the assessment of pathological spontaneous activity can be difficult. Because of the usually small motor units, the narrow motor unit action potentials (MUAP) often look like fibrillations. In addition, for many patients it is not possible to completely relax these muscles.

The next step is to investigate the volitional activity of the mimic muscles. The configuration, duration, and amplitude of the recorded MUAPs are investigated by this procedure. The normal MUAPs of the mimetic muscles are smaller and shorter than those in the limb muscles (Fig. 5.4). Any MUAP with more than four phases is considered polyphasic and might herald nerve regeneration. Additionally, the density of the interference pattern is evaluated during maximal volitional activity.

Needle EMG may also be helpful to answer the question of the optimal therapy option in facial neuropathy. When needle EMG reveals volitional activity, the nerve lesion is incomplete and at least a few axons are intact. Furthermore

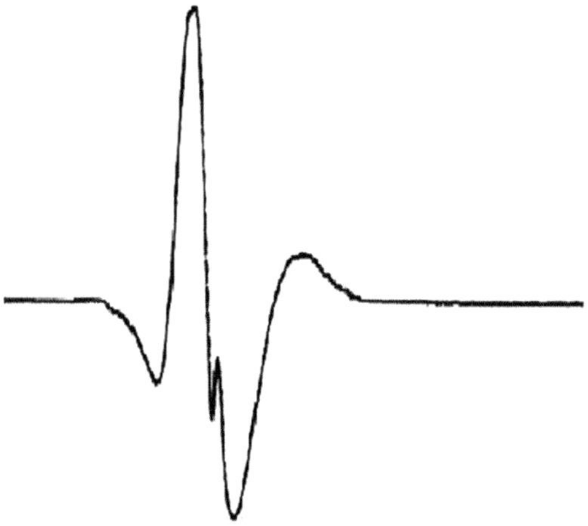

Fig. 5.4 Electromyography: volitional motor unit action potential (MUAP) of the orbicularis oris muscle while the patient is pursing his lips

electrodes can be placed simultaneously in muscles innervated by different nerve branches to look for co-contraction and synkinesis.

EMG can be used to monitor patients after nerve reconstruction. Signs of regeneration are frequently seen on needle EMG before the patient shows any clinical signs of recovery. Processes of reinnervation can be detected earlier by electrophysiological analysis than by clinical analysis. Depending on the type of nerve reconstruction, reinnervation potentials can be found in the mimic muscles about 4–6 months after the nerve reconstruction procedure.

The findings of a low CMAP amplitude in NCS and pathological spontaneous activity (fibrillation potentials, positive sharp waves) with poor or no recruitment of normal configurated MUAPs in EMG are all consistent with an acute peripheral lesion.

5.3 Blink Reflex Studies

The blink reflex measures the entire reflex arc between trigeminal and facial nerves including proximal segments of the facial nerve [1, 2]. Neuropathies or compressive lesion of the facial or trigeminal nerve may be detected, as well as brainstem lesions.

In electrophysiological examination, the blink reflex is triggered by electrical stimulation of the supraorbital nerve. The stimulus response is registered simultaneously from both orbicularis oculi muscles. Afferent impulses are shifted by an oligosynaptic pathway to the ipsilateral facial nerve nucleus, whose stimulation causes an early and exclusively ipsilateral reflex component (R1) in the orbicularis oculi muscle after a latency of about 10 ms. The afferent impulses also descend to the caudal medulla oblongata. Ascending from this site and connected polysynaptically, these impulses reach both nuclei of the facial nerve so that the delayed stimulus response (R2) is registered bilaterally with a latency of about 30 ms. In view of the rapid habituation of the R2 response, a sequence of irregular low-frequency stimuli (below 0.5 Hz) is advisable. Only the R2 component is seen on the contralateral side. The maximal difference in R2 latencies between the two sides is 5 ms. In cases of mild paresis, the sole pathological finding may be a reduction in the amplitude of the stimulus responses on the affected side. In cases of a more pronounced peripheral lesion, the amplitude of both blink reflex responses (R1 and R2) is either reduced and has a prolonged latency or is entirely absent at the affected side. In a central lesion, the first component (R1) is normal in terms of latency and amplitude.

The diagnostic value of the blink reflex lies in the fact that the facial nerve can be stimulated proximal to the site of the lesion through a reflex arc. The blink reflex can be used in chronic facial palsy to look for evidence of aberrant reinnervation: stimulating the supraorbital nerve and simultaneously recording from the orbicularis oculi and oris muscle.

5.4 Magnetic Stimulation

The facial nerve can be stimulated intracranially by magnetic stimulation. The absence of impulse conduction may be indicative of complete neurapraxia or an interruption of axonal continuity. The results of magnetic stimulation are highly variable and its prognostic value is poor. Therefore, this procedure is not used for routine diagnostic investigation.

5.5 Outcome Indicators

Good prognosis: normal NCS after 10–14 days, late onset of Wallerian degeneration, no pathological spontaneous activity in EMG after 14–21 days, volitional EMG-activity, normal interference pattern, improving of volitional EMG-activity. Blink Reflex: R1 delayed or normal, reappearance of blink reflex within 2 weeks.

Poor prognosis: early onset of Wallerian degeneration, progressive decay of NCS-amplitude (CMAP) ≥90% reduction in comparison to the contralateral side, pathological spontaneous activity on EMG after 10–21 days, no volitional EMG. Blink Reflex: R1 absent.

References

1. Mannarelli G, Griffin GR, Kileny P, Edwards B. Electrophysiological measures in facial paresis and paralysis. Operat Tech Otolaryngol Head Neck Surg. 2012;23:236–47.
2. Josep V-S´. Electrodiagnostic studies of the facial nerve in peripheral facial palsy and hemifacial spasm. Muscle Nerve. 2007;36:14–20.
3. Byun H, Cho YS, Jang JY, Chung KW, Hwang S, Chung WH, Hong SH. Value of electroneurography as a prognostic indicator for recovery in acute severe inflammatory facial paralysis: a prospective study of Bell's Palsy and Ramsay Hunt Syndrome. Laryngoscope. 2013;123:2526–32.
4. Mamoli B. Zur Prognoseerstellung peripherer Fazialisparesen unter besonderer Berücksichtigung der Elektroneurographie. Wien Klin Wochenschrift. 1976;53:3–28.
5. Kim SH, Ryu EW, Yang CW, Yeo SG, Park MS, Byun JY. The prognostic value of electroneurography of Bell's palsy at the orbicularis oculi versus nasolabial fold. Laryngoscope. 2016;126:1644–8.
6. Neuwirth-Riedl K, Burian M, Nekahm D, Gstöttner W. Optimizing of electromyography of the facial nerve. J Otorhinolaryngol Relat Spec. 1990;52(6):360–7.
7. Arslan HH, Satar B, Yildizoglu U, Edizer DT, Akgun H. Validity of late-term electroneurography in Bell's palsy. Otol Neurotol. 2014;35(4):656–61.
8. Sittel C, Stennert E. Prognostic value of electromyography in acute peripheral facial palsy. Otol Neurotol. 2001;22:100–4.
9. Grosheva M, Wittekindt C, Guntinas-Lichius O. Prognostic value of electroneurography and electromyography in facial palsy. Laryngoscope. 2008;118:394–7.

Part II

Facial Nerve Reconstruction

6 Principles of Facial Nerve Reconstruction

Andrés Rodríguez-Lorenzo
and Chieh-Han John Tzou

Key Points

- Facial nerve reconstruction requires the viability of distal facial nerve branches, mimetic muscles, and motor end/plates.
- There are six types of facial nerve injuries: Nerve Injuries Type III or above will develop some degree of sequelae if not treated, from facial synkinesias, facial muscle weakness, or muscle contracture.
- The methods of facial nerve reconstruction include nerve decompression, direct nerve repair, interposition of nerve graft, nerve transfers, direct muscle neurotization, and end-to-side nerve repair.
- Timing of reconstruction is critical for optimization of outcomes, early intervention has in general yielded to better outcomes.
- The authors present a classification of Levels of Facial Nerve Injury in relation to the Method of Reconstruction in three levels: Level 1 or Central Nerve System or Intratemporal Nerve Injuries With Not Available Facial Nerve Stump, Level 2 or Intratemporal or Extratemporal Intraparotid Nerve Injuries with Available Facial Nerve Stump, and Level 3 or Extratemporal Extraparotid or Distal Nerve Injuries.

6.1 Introduction

Dysfunction of the facial nerve can occur after nerve insult due to trauma, cancer, or infection among others. It can be a result of an injury located at any level of the course of the nerve from its origin at the central nerve system until it reaches the neuromuscular junction at the mimetic muscles level. Due to its relatively superficial course, the facial nerve is one of the cranial nerves more sensitive to injuries in trauma or oncological resection in the head and neck area. The probability of its recovery depends on several factors such as level, severity, or time of the nerve injury.

Facial nerve reconstruction is defined as the group of surgical procedures that aim to restore the main facial nerve function by reinnervation of the mimetic muscles. Facial nerve reconstruction procedures therefore are indicated in stages of facial nerve injuries where the mimetic muscles are still not atrophied or absent, in oppose to long-standing or congenital facial paralysis, and have as requirement the viability of the motor

A. Rodríguez-Lorenzo (✉)
Department of Plastic and Maxillofacial Surgery, Uppsala University Hospital, Uppsala, Sweden

Department of Surgical Sciences, Uppsala University, Uppsala, Sweden
e-mail: andres.rodriguez.lorenzo@surgsci.uu.se

C.-H. J. Tzou
Plastic and Reconstructive Surgery, Hospital of Divine Savior (Krankenhaus Goettlicher Heiland), Sigmund Freud University, TZOU MEDICAL, Vienna, Austria
e-mail: science@tzoumedical.com, science@tzou.at

© Springer Nature Switzerland AG 2021
C.-H. J. Tzou, A. Rodríguez-Lorenzo (eds.), *Facial Palsy*,
https://doi.org/10.1007/978-3-030-50784-8_6

endplates and mimetic muscles thus allowing for possible reinnervation.

In this chapter, the authors describe the principles of facial nerve reconstruction and the authors' strategy and preferences in different levels of injury.

6.2 Types of Facial Nerve Injuries

The prognosis of a facial nerve injury depends on the severity of the injury, among other factors. The classification of peripheral nerve injuries was described by Seddon [1] and Sunderland [2] in which the degree of nerve injury is associated to the integrity of the axons, its covering of myelin, and the different connective tissue layers of the nerve (epineurium, perineurium, and endoneurium) as displayed in Table 6.1.

If there is only a physiological block in nerve conduction, the degree of injury is called neuropraxia (Seddon) or Type I by Sunderland Classification. It is usually caused by nerve compression and full recovery should be expected. There is no Tinel sign in neuropraxia as there is no nerve degeneration or regeneration. If the nerve injury leads to axonal disruption, it causes distal nerve degeneration (Wallerian degeneration) and the proximal end of the nerve tries to heal by a process named nerve regeneration which translates clinically with the presence of Tinel sign. This level of injury is called axonotmesis in Seddon classification and correlates with the Sunderland Types depending on which connective tissue layer of the nerve is affected: in type II only the axons are disrupted, in type III the endoneurium is affected, and in type IV both endoneurium and the perineurium are affected, being a nerve fascicle disruption. In type II injuries, spontaneous recovery is possible as the axons will grow 1 mm/day through intact distal nerve fibers, and in type III injuries, there is axonal sprouting; however, the loss of endoneurium and the presence of intraneural scar create aberrant reinnervation where the axonal sprouting follows the "wrong" distal nerve channels and potentially creating facial synkinesias. Finally, when the nerve is totally transected including the outer connective tissue layer (epineurium), it is called neurotmesis (Seddon) or type V. In both type IV and V injuries, functional recovery is not possible without facial nerve reconstruction. Mackinnon et al. [3] described type VI nerve injuries, where a combination of types II and IV of injury are encountered.

In facial nerve injuries type III or higher, it is unlikely full clinical recovery of the facial nerve function, with clinical sequelae in the form of synkinesias due to aberrant reinnervation, muscle contracture or muscle weakness in form of incomplete or complete facial paralysis, therefore facial nerve reconstruction techniques may be indicated.

6.3 Methods of Facial Nerve Reconstruction

The reconstruction of the facial nerve includes a number of different surgical methods that aim for restoration of the facial nerve function, which involves guiding axons toward target organ (mimetic muscle) or removing scar tissue that

Table 6.1 Types of nerve injuries

Type of injury					
Seddon	Sunderland	Nerve structure damage	Physiological nerve changes	Tinel sign	Prognosis without intervention
Neuropraxia	**I**	Myelin sheath	Conduction block	No	Complete recovery
Axonotmesis	**II**	Myelin sheath + Axon	Wallerian degeneration	Yes	
Neurotmesis	**III**	Myelin sheath + Axon + Endoneurium			Incomplete recovery with facial synkinesias
	IV	Myelin sheath + Axon + Endoneurium + Perineurium			Facial paralysis
	V	Myelin sheath + Axon + Endoneurium + Perineurium + Epineurium			Facial paralysis

obstructs axons growing. Return of nerve function depends on several factors including the gap size between transected nerve segments and the type and condition of the organs being reinnervated [4].

Facial nerve reconstruction techniques use microsurgical magnification and instrumentation for exploration and repair of the facial nerve. The selection of the surgical method depends on several factors including the type and time of injury, nerve gap, level of injury, or surgeon preference. Facial nerve reconstruction includes the following methods that can be used as single procedure or in combination (Fig. 6.1): neurolysis or nerve decompression, direct nerve repair, interposition nerve graft, direct muscle neurotization, end-to-side and nerve transfers.

(a) ***External Neurolysis or Nerve Decompression.*** In situation of compression of the facial nerve, usually within the temporal bone, nerve decompression by releasing the nerve from surrounding tight tissue allows to restore nerve conduction and function. The surgical decompression of intratemporal facial nerve compression is usually performed through a middle cranial fossa and transmastoid or translabyrinthine approaches based on hearing status. Despite there is no general consensus of the indication, some authors indicate facial nerve decompression in patient with complete acute facial paralysis (House–Brackmann 6), greater than 90% nerve degeneration, and absent electromyog-

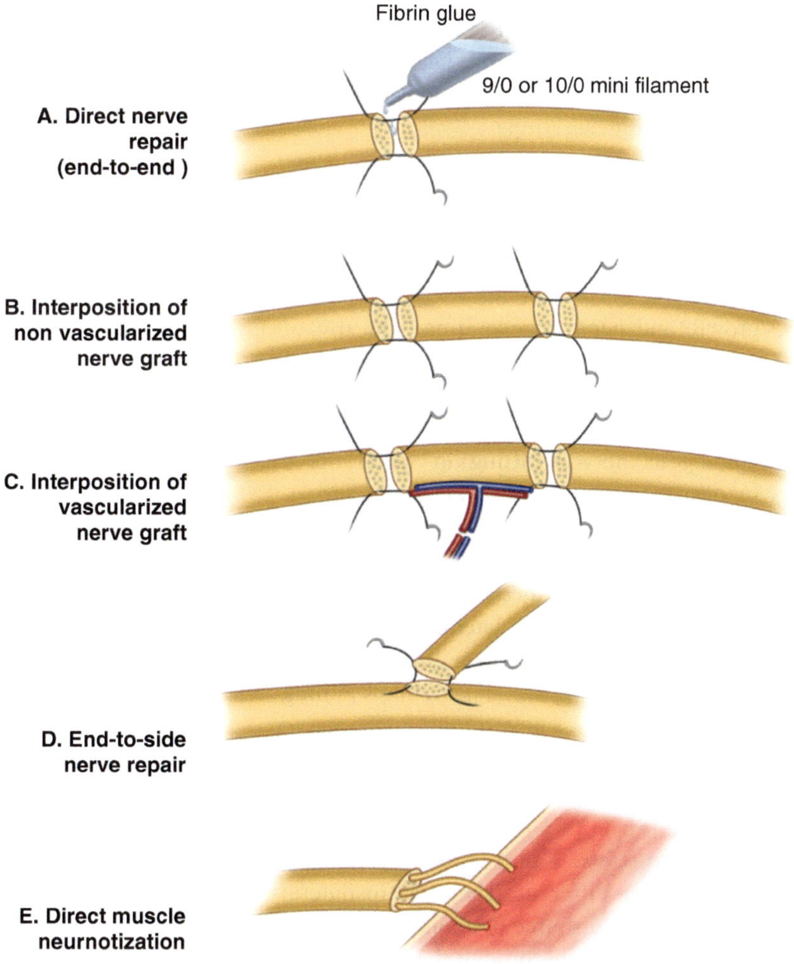

Fig. 6.1 Surgical methods for nerve reconstruction including direct nerve repair, interposition of nonvascularized and vascularized nerve grafts, end-to-side repair, and direct muscle neurotization

raphy activity in patients with temporal bone fractures or in Bell's Palsy [5].

(b) ***Direct Nerve Repair.*** Direct coaptation of the transected ends is the method of choice in facial nerve injuries when possible. Direct nerve repair is performed using microsutures (epineural or fascicular, 9/0 or 10/0 monofilament), fibrin glue, or both allowing for nerve continuity and appropriate alignment of fascicles [4]. The nerve regeneration through the distal end of the repair occurs at an average pace of 1 mm/day, depending on several factors that can influence the rate and quality of recovery [6]. One of the requisites to be able to do a successful direct nerve repair is the presence of healthy nerve stumps that allows for a tension-free nerve repair, therefore in case of a portion of the nerve is destroyed it is advisable to perform other techniques such as nerve graft interposition, nerve transfers, or end-to-side repair to provide more reliable nerve regeneration.

(c) ***Nerve Graft Interposition***. When there is not possible to do tension-free anastomosis due to the presence of a gap in the facial nerve, interposition of nerve grafts is necessary to bridge the nerve gap allowing for axonal growth and nerve regeneration. The use of autologous nerve grafts is the standard of care in reconstruction of nerve gaps [7], and the most commonly used donor nerves for autologous nerve grafting in facial nerve reconstruction are the sural and great auricular nerves. In case of long nerve gaps, composite defects of nerve and soft tissue, or the presence of scarring bed, vascularized nerve grafts such as the vastus lateralis motor nerve or the lateral femoral cutaneous nerve have been used as interposition nerve flaps aiming to enhance the vascular supply of the nerve graft and increase nerve regeneration potential in combination with soft tissue reconstruction [8].

(d) ***Nerve Transfers***. Nerve transfers uses of a donor nerve different from the ipsilateral facial nerve as a source of axons to innervate the mimetic muscle through the distal facial nerve, term that is also known as neurotization. They are indicated when long segments of the facial nerve are irreversibly damaged, there is a lack of proximal facial nerve stump or in central nerve facial paralysis in the presence of intact distal facial nerve branches and viable mimetic muscles. Common clinical scenarios include ablative oncology or trauma involving the brainstem and skull base [9, 10].

The most commonly used donor nerves in nerve transfers are the contralateral facial nerve, the masseter branch of the trigeminal nerve and the hypoglossal nerve, and less frequently the spinal accessory nerve and phrenic nerves (Fig. 6.2). In case of selecting a donor nerve different of the facial nerve, spontaneous smile is only achieved in a group of patients, mostly described when using the masseter nerve transfer, therefore it is important an structured postoperative physiotherapy regime to increase the rate of central relearning that allows effortless smile. In addition, there is a risk of facial synkinesias associated with the activation of the original function of the donor nerve (biting when using the masseter, tongue movement with the hypoglossal nerve or shoulder elevation with the spinal accessory nerve for example), therefore efforts have been made to study the most optimal donor nerve in facial reanimation that allows for easy central relearning and less involuntary facial movements [11, 12]. The nerve transfers can be performed by direct repair, using an interposition nerve graft or in an end-to-side manner; however, the main advantages of using non-facial nerve as donors in nerve transfers is that is possible direct nerve coaptation close to the target muscle allowing a more effective facial reanimation and stronger smile excursion as they provide higher axon counts in comparison with cross-facial nerve grafts.

(e) ***Direct Muscle Neurotization***. When the distal branch of the facial nerve is not present or avulsed but the muscle is still viable, it is possible to implant the nerve

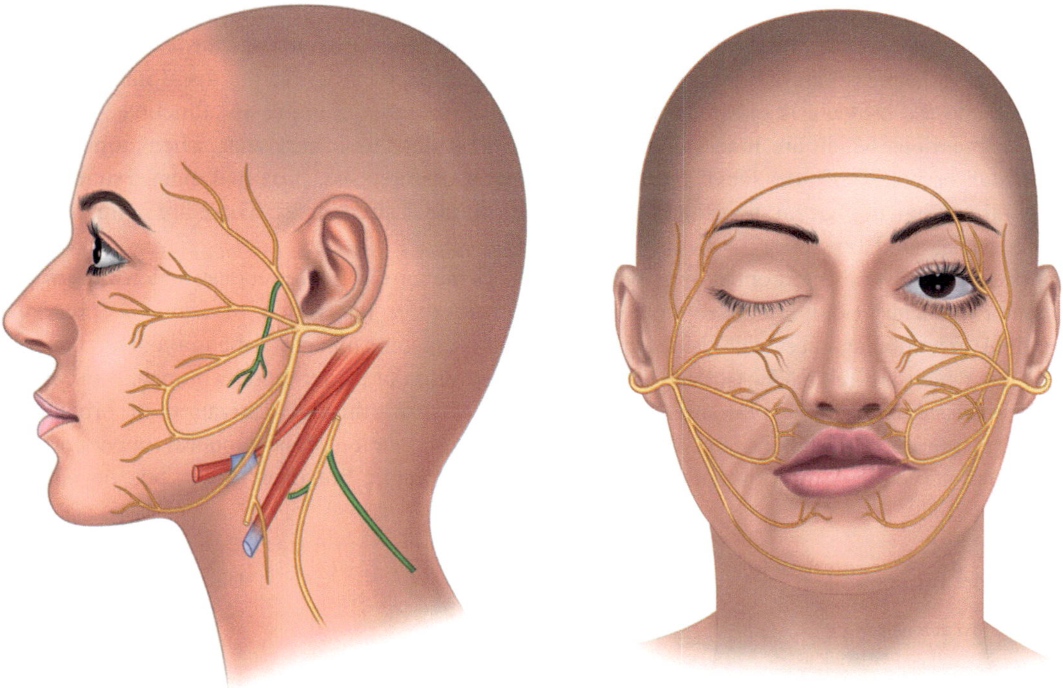

Fig. 6.2 Nerve transfers to the facial nerve. On the left, non-facial donor nerves in green including the masseter, hypoglossal, and spinal accessory nerves as the most commonly used nerve. On the right, nerve transfers using the contralateral facial nerve where different several nerve grafts can be used to target eye closure, smile reanimation, and lower lip depressors using end-to-end repair or end-to-side repair

into the substance of the muscle allowing for muscle contraction, procedure named as direct muscle neurotization. Direct muscle neurotization was pioneered by Terzis et al. [13, 14] using it in mostly pediatric facial paralysis for both eye and lower lip reanimation. In this technique the distal end of a cross-face nerve graft is destined to neurotize a muscle and it is split into two to three fascicles, each one is implanted through a separate incision in the epimysium.

(f) ***End-to-Side repair***. End-to-side repair allows axonal sprouting in the distal nerve segment from a proximal donor nerve with the advantage of decreasing the donor site morbidity from the donor nerve that may be indicated in cases of not useable proximal facial nerve stump or in combination with other nerve reconstruction methods, usually in combination with an interposition nerve graft. The coaptation between the recipient and the donor nerves may be made directly onto the epineurial sheath or through an epineurial window [15].

6.4 The Distal Target in Facial Nerve Reconstruction: Innervation of Mimetic Muscles

The facial nerve is a mixed nerve that has motor fibers allowing facial expressions, sensory fibers that conduct taste sensations from the anterior two-thirds of the tongue, and parasympathetic fibers that are responsible for increasing the saliva flow by innervation of the sublingual and submandibular glands, lacrimal production by innervation of the lacrimal gland, innervation of the nasal mucosa, and participation as the efferent limb in the corneal reflex.

The main goal though in facial nerve reconstruction is to reinnervate the mimetic muscles to restore facial expressions. There are 21 paired muscles and the orbicularis oris responsible for facial expressions which are innervated through the distal branches of the facial nerve [16]: temporal, zygomatic, buccal, marginal mandibular, cervical, and posterior auricular. These branches have several interconnections with the neighbor branches (with the exception of the marginal mandibular, cervical, and posterior auricular which are relatively isolated from the others) and subdivide in several small branches that innervate every facial muscle. When planning facial nerve reconstruction both anatomical reconstruction (direct facial nerve repair or nerve graft) or functional (nerve transfers) is critical to have an appreciation of the distal innervation of facial musculature and its functions in facial expressions, to ensure that when doing nerve reconstruction the proximal nerve stump will reach the desired target. These are represented in Fig. 6.3.

If the aim of nerve reconstruction is ***eyebrow reanimation*** (activation of frontalis, procerus, and corrugator muscles), the main distal target is innervation of the temporalis branches; in case of ***eye closure*** (through activation of orbicularis oculi) innervation of the temporal (upper portion) and zygomatic branches (lower portion) should

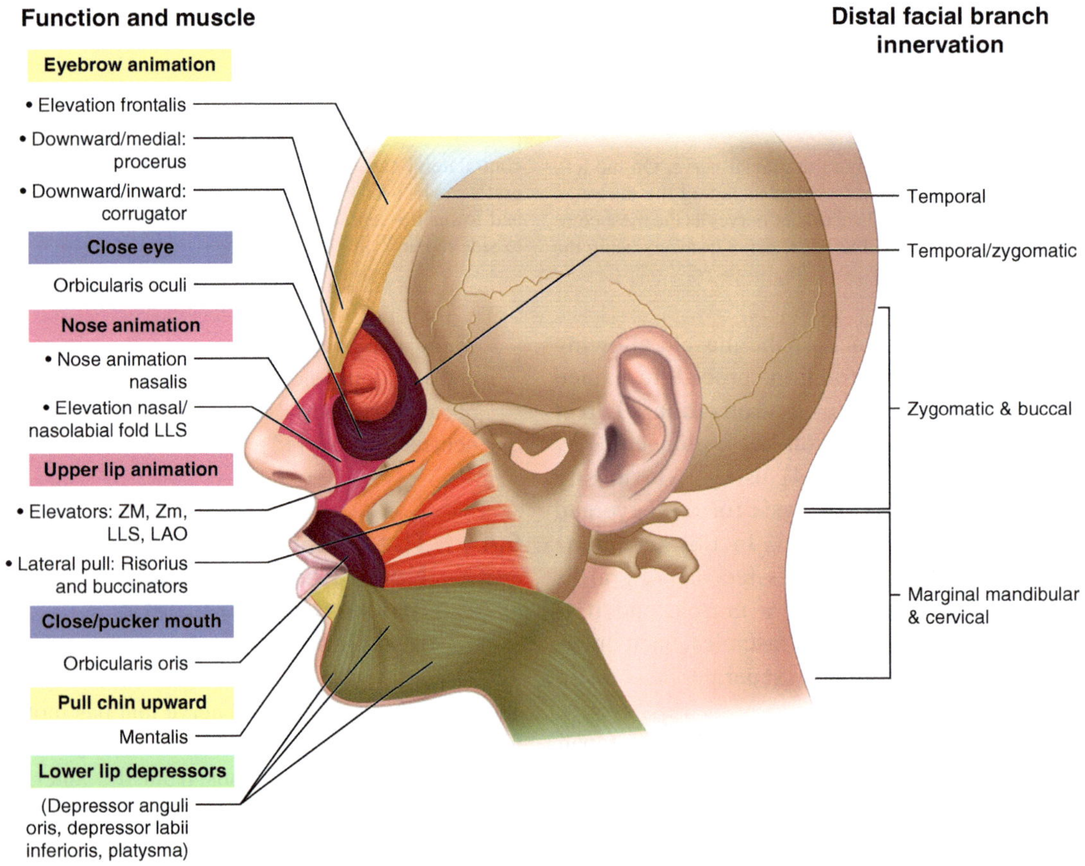

Fig 6.3 Representation of function of mimetic muscles and its innervation which are the selective targets for neurotization

be performed; ***nose animation*** (activation of nasalis and Levator Labii Superioris Alaeque Nasi) is achieved through innervation of mostly zygomatic but also buccal braches; ***upper lip animation*** (elevators: ZM, Zm, LLS, LAO and lateral pull: risorius and buccinators) is achieved through innervation of zygomatic and buccal branches; ***lower lip animation*** (upper pull of chin: mentalis and lower lip depressor DAO, DLI, platysma) is innervated by the marginal mandibular and cervical branches.

Identification of the distal facial nerve branches and its function can be done by anatomical identification during nerve exploration and facilitated with the aid of an intraoperative nerve stimulator in traumatic cases within 72 h (before Wallerian degeneration), in oncological cases where the facial nerve is resected, and in cases of incomplete facial paralysis. In the ideal situation, all mimetic muscles of the facial nerve can be recovered after facial nerve repair; however, there are several situations where there is a need for prioritization of functions to be recovered by facial nerve reconstruction such as eye closure and smile reanimation over forehead and lower lip, in case of suboptimal conditions for nerve regeneration (aged patients, long nerve gaps, scarring bed, concomitant soft tissue and bone defects, etc.).

6.5 Timing of Facial Nerve Reconstruction

The decision of the timing for surgical exploration and facial nerve reconstruction depends on the clinical scenario as the most important factor in determining the optimal dynamic facial palsy reconstruction to perform is to know the viability of existing facial mimetic muscles and motor endplates, thus allowing for possible reinnervation. Increased denervation time and advancing patient age both negatively affect nerve regeneration and may lead to inferior outcomes of reinnervation procedures [10].

6.5.1 Timing or Nerve Reconstruction in Open Facial Nerve Injuries with Facial Nerve Deficits or Oncological Resections Including the Facial Nerve

The indication of early intervention and facial nerve exploration is obvious when there is a clear injury of the facial nerve in traumatic cases (i.e., a facial laceration with loss of one or several functions of the mimetic muscles) or in oncological cases where ablation of the facial nerve is planned as part of the oncological resection. In these scenarios, acute exploration and reconstruction of the facial nerve yield to the best results and ideally should be done within 72 h. During that time period the section of the axon distal to the site of injury tends to remain electrically excitable before Wallerian degeneration is completed, allowing for better topographic identification of the distal nerve branches. In addition, early exploration of the facial nerve allows for more likely direct nerve repair as there is less retraction of the transected ends and easier mobilization due to the lack of scarring.

6.5.2 Timing for Nerve Reconstruction in Acquired Facial Paralysis with Unknown Facial Nerve Status

Patients with acquired paralysis who have undergone serial clinical and/or electrophysiologic testing that has failed to show any functional recovery by 6 months can be considered for a reinnervation procedure before complete muscle and motor endplate atrophy. To aid with decision-making, electrophysiologic testing can be helpful to determine the predicting functional recovery [17] and the viability of distal motor endplates. In case of intracranial tumor resection, such as acoustic neuroma, it is important the intraoperative information of the status of the facial nerve provided by the surgeon to estimate the potential for recovery. Depending on the age of the patient and the type of procedure intended, reinnervation can be successful up to 12–18 months after denervation. Traditionally 2 years has been the limit for indication of facial nerve reconstruction; however, there is no defined cutoff limit for denervation time that is universally applicable [10].

6.6 Classification of Levels of Facial Nerve Injuries in Relation to Facial Reconstruction Method

Insults to the facial nerve can occur along its entire anatomical course from the cerebral cortex to the innervation of the mimetic muscles. The facial nerve originates within the pons in the facial nucleus entering the temporal bone through the internal auditory meatus [18]. The *intratemporal portion of the facial nerve* divides in four segments: meatal, labyrinthine, tympanic, and mastoid. The labyrinthine segment extends from the internal auditory meatus to the geniculate ganglion, where the cell bodies of special visceral afferent neurons carrying taste from the anterior two-thirds of the tongue are located. It is at the geniculate where the nervus intermedius joins the facial nerve proper, and the greater superficial petrosal and lesser petrosal nerves exit the facial nerve. The tympanic segment of the nerve extends posteriorly from the geniculate ganglion to the second genu, where the facial nerve turns inferiorly, transitioning to the vertical or mastoid segment giving off the stapedius nerve and the chorda tympani. The facial nerve exits the temporal bone through the stylomastoid foramen, yielding the *extratemporal portion of the nerve*, runs within the parotid gland and then innervates all muscles of facial expression.

To optimize the clinical outcomes, it is paramount in the selection the adequate method of reconstruction of the facial nerve, taking in consideration the level of injury. Herein, the authors classified the injuries to the facial nerve in three levels in relation to their nerve reconstruction methods of choice or strategies (Fig. 6.4): **Level 1** or Central Nerve System or Intratemporal Nerve Injuries With Not Available Facial Nerve Stump; **Level 2** or Intratemporal Nerve Injuries Extratemporal Intraparotid Injuries with Available Facial Nerve Stump; and **Level 3** or Extratemporal Extraparotid or Distal Nerve Injuries (Table 6.2). This classification serves as a reference to the authors to indicate the method of reconstruction; however, this needs to be individualized to patient's needs.

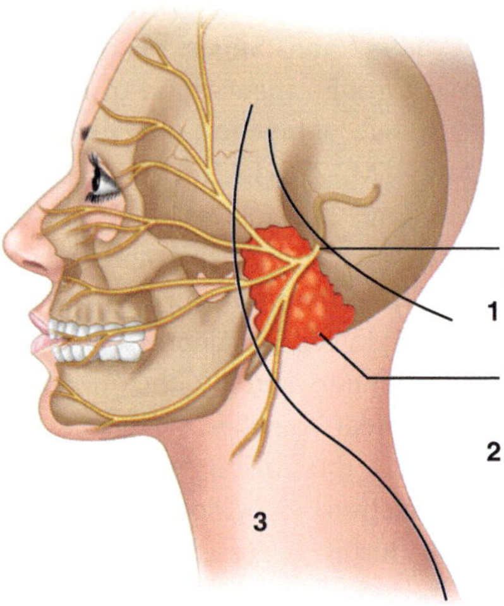

Fig. 6.4 Illustration of classification of levels of facial nerve injury in relation of nerve reconstruction method. **Level 1** or central nerve system or intratemporal nerve injuries with no available facial nerve stump; **Level 2** or intratemporal nerve injuries extratemporal intraparotid injuries with available facial nerve stump; **Level 3** or extratemporal extraparotid or distal nerve injuries

6.6.1 Level 1: Central Nerve System or Intratemporal Nerve Injuries with Not Available Facial Nerve Stump

Common clinical scenarios of this level of injury include patients with complete facial paralysis after ablative oncology or trauma involving the brainstem and skull base. The ipsilateral facial nerve is not usable, therefore the donor nerves for neurotization available are the contralateral facial nerves and/or ipsilateral non-facial cranial nerves (typically the masseter, hypoglossal, and spinal

Table 6.2 Classification of levels of injury to the facial nerve in relation to facial nerve reconstruction method

Level	Description	Source of proximal donor axons for neurotization	Most common etiology of facial nerve injury	Typical clinical and intraoperative findings	Method of choice of facial nerve reconstruction	Donor nerve and recipient target
1	**Central nerve system or intratemporal nerve injuries *with not* available facial nerve stump**	Contralateral facial nerve Non-facial cranial nerves[a]	Brainstem tumors Skull base fractures	Complete facial palsy (exploration of facial nerve is usually not performed)	Combination of nerve transfers with cross-face nerve graft	*Masseter nerve* to the upper trunk of the facial nerve for eye and smile reanimation and *contralateral platysma motor nerve with a nerve graft or mini-hypoglossal transfer* to the marginal mandibular branch for lower lip reanimation
2	**Intratemporal and extratemporal intraparotid nerve injuries *with* available facial nerve stump**	Ipsilateral facial nerve Contralateral facial nerve Non-facial cranial nerves	Oncological resection including parotid or/and lateral temporal bone	Complete facial palsy ± Long nerve gaps ± Soft tissue defect ± Aged patients ± Pre- or postop radiotherapy	Dual innervation of the face by nerve transfers and ipsilateral facial nerve	*Masseter nerve* to the buccal and zygomatic branches for smile, nose and lower orbicularis oris reinnervation *and ipsilateral facial nerve with nerve graft* to the upper zygomatic and temporal branches for eye and forehead reanimation. Lower lip reanimation can be performed with mini-hypoglossal transfer to the marginal mandibular branch
3	**Extratemporal extraparotid or distal nerve injuries**	Ipsilateral facial nerve Contralateral facial nerve Non-facial cranial nerves	Facial trauma or selective oncological procedures (i.e., neck biopsy, submandibular gland, skin cancer excision)	Incomplete facial palsy ± Selective injuries to distal nerve branches	Anatomical reconstruction: Direct nerve repair of nerve grafts or intrafacial nerve transfer in absent proximal stump of the branch of the facial nerve	Ipsilateral facial nerve branches and transected distal nerve

[a]Function of other cranial nerves needs to be evaluated to confirm its functionality

accessory nerves). Clinical exploration or electrophysiological studies of the viability of other cranial nerves are necessary to confirm its usability in nerve transfers.

There are different combinations of neurotizations that can be used; the authors approach is to use the masseter nerve to the upper facial nerve to achieve both eye closure and smile/orbicularis oris reanimation and the contralateral platysma motor nerve or the mini-hypoglossal nerve transfer (end to side or with jump graft) to innervate the marginal mandibular branch for lower lip reinnervation. The synkinesias in eye closure using the masseter nerve are usually discrete.

6.6.2 Clinical Example

A 24-year-old female with neurofibromatosis type 2 with complete left facial paralysis after resection of a left vestibular schwannoma (Fig. 6.5) who received facial nerve reconstruction 3 months after initial tumor resection with masseter nerve transfer to the upper facial nerve and the contralateral platysma motor nerve with a nerve graft to the marginal mandibular nerve (Fig. 6.6). One year post op showing excellent facial reanimation with discrete oro-ocular synkinesias (Fig. 6.7).

6.6.3 Level 2: Intratemporal and Extratemporal Intraparotid Nerve Injuries with Available Facial Nerve Stump

Common clinical scenarios in this level of injury include oncological resection of tumors that require parotidectomy and/or lateral temporal bone resection and often associated with other soft tissue defects (skin och volume defect in the neck), long nerve gaps, the need of adjuvant radiotherapy and mostly likely in aged patients [19]. All these factors affect negatively nerve regeneration, therefore the strategy of facial nerve reconstruction needs to aim for providing high number of axons to the distal facial nerve branches to be able to reanimate the face. Traditionally approaches have used only interpositional nerve grafts between the facial nerve stump and the distal facial nerve branches; however, due to the poor conditions for nerve regeneration, the outcomes have not been consis-

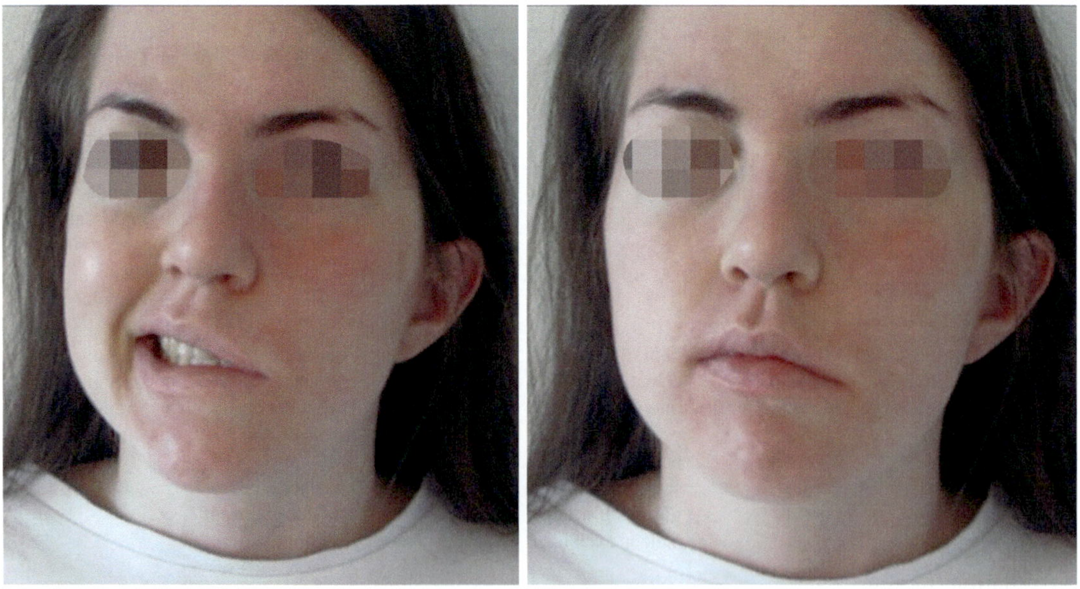

Fig. 6.5 Clinical example of Level 1 Facial Nerve Injury. Twenty-year-old female with complete left facial paralysis after resection of an intracranial vestibular schwannoma

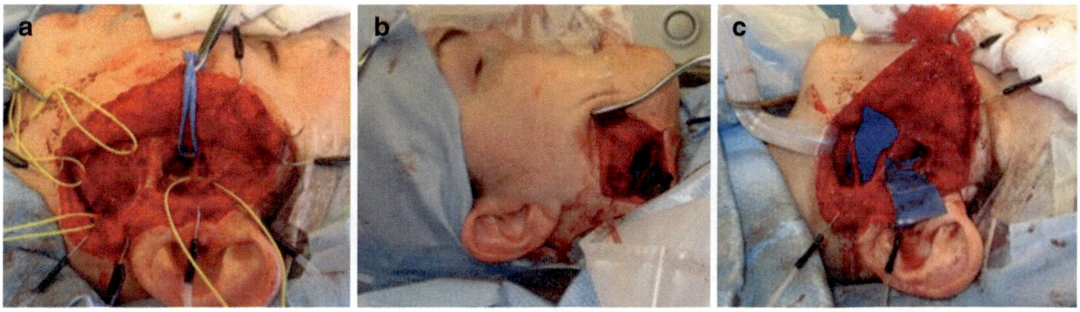

Fig. 6.6 Intraoperative photo of facial nerve reconstruction. (**a**) Exposure of facial nerve branches (yellow vessel loop) and masseter nerve (blue vessel loop). (**b**) Contralateral dissection of platysma motor nerve. (**c**) Nerve coaptation of the masseter nerve with the upper trunk of the facial nerve and contralateral platysma motor nerve with a cross-face nerve graft to the marginal mandibular nerve

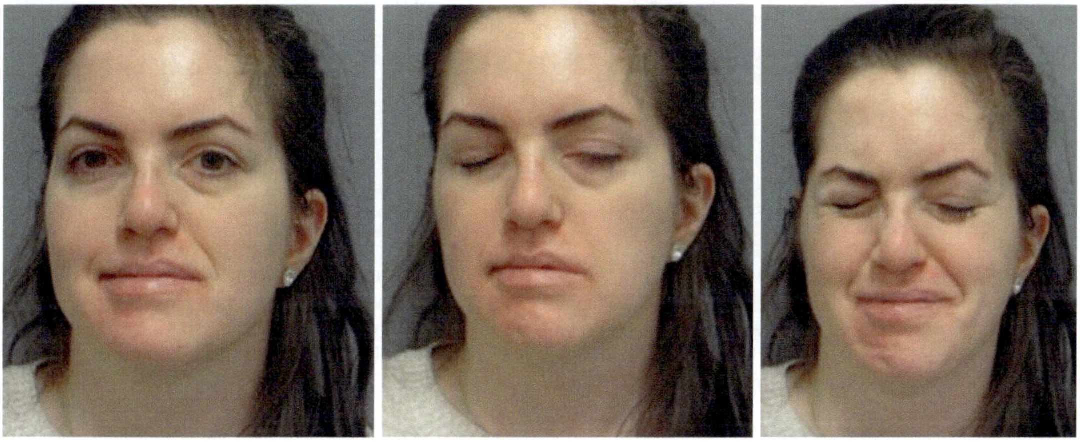

Fig. 6.7 One-year follow-up showing good facial symmetry and facial reanimation. Oro-ocular synkinesias are only evident with maximal eye closure

tently satisfactory and are in our opinion indicated only in short nerve gaps (less than 5 cm) in this level of injury. These factors make that our approach to this level of injury is to maximize the number of axons that reanimate the mimic muscles by using a combination of nerve grafting of the facial nerve with nerve transfers aiming to restore the function of selective distal targets (eye closure and midface reanimation as priorities and forehead and lower lip as secondary targets).

Our method of choice is what we call "dual innervation of the facial nerve" to maximize the number of axons to every target, with prioritization of eye closure, smile reanimation, ad nose reanimation by innervating the nose and oral complex with the masseter nerve and using the facial nerve stump with a nerve graft for eye closure and forehead reanimation. The lower lip depressors are set as a secondary goal and could be addressed by hypoglossal nerve transfer end to side or with jump graft or can be addressed later with ancillary procedures or myomectomy.

6.6.4 Clinical Example

A 37-year-old man with parotid metastasis of a teratocarcinoma needed parotidectomy with facial nerve resection, mastoidectomy, and radical neck dissection. The defect was reconstructed immediately using a fasciocutaneous ALT flap, and facial nerve reconstruction was performed with a dual innervation, using the masseter nerve transfer for midface reanimation and facial nerve stump with

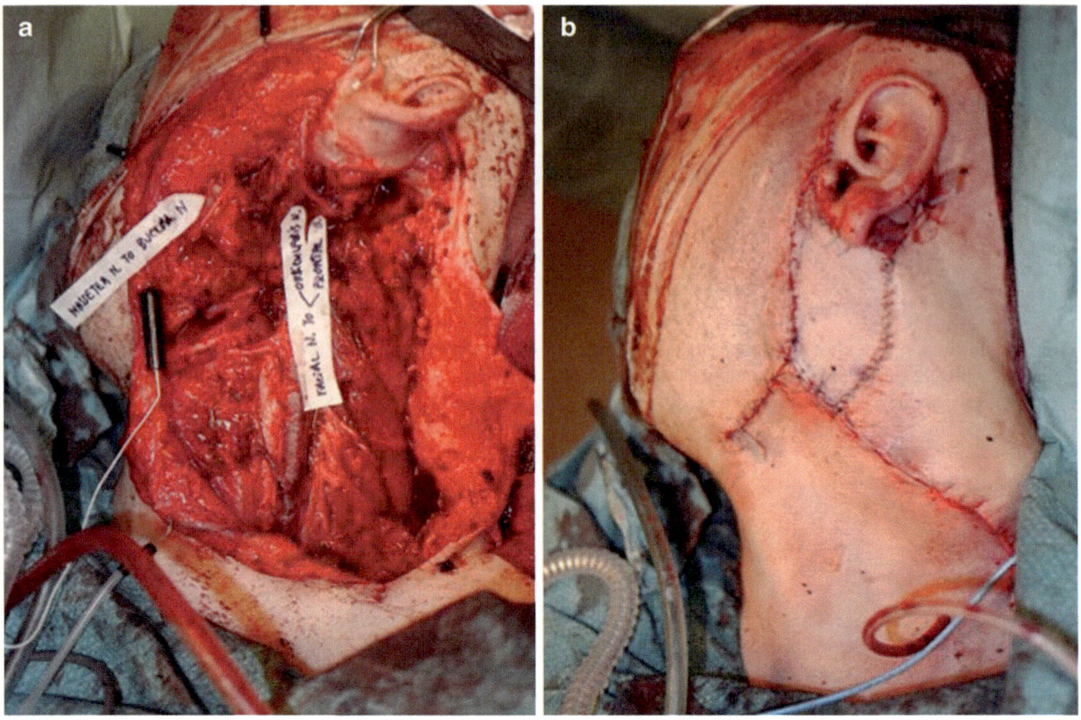

Fig. 6.8 Clinical example of Level 2 Facial Nerve Injury. Thirty-seven-year-old male with complete left facial paralysis after resection of an advanced teratocarcinoma with metastasis in the parotid. (**a**) Photo after parotidectomy, radial neck dissection, and mastoidectomy. Facial nerve reconstruction is performed with dual innervation by using the masseter nerve to midface reinnervation and facial nerve stump with nerve graft to the periocular muscles (**b**). Final closure with a free ALT flap

a nerve graft for eye reanimation (Fig. 6.8). One-year follow-up the patient showed good symmetry at rest and excellent facial reanimation with effortless smile being able to smile with an open mouth (Fig. 6.9). Note that the lower lip was not reanimated or the forehead as priority was given to the perioral and periocular muscles.

6.6.5 Level 3: Extratemporal Extraparotid or Distal Nerve Injuries

Common clinical scenarios seen in this level are facial trauma including branches of the facial nerve of selective oncological procedures that require soft tissue excision that may involve the facial nerve. Therefore, only partial facial palsy may be encountered and only selected branches are affected. Our method of choice in this injuries is anatomical reconstruction of the continuity of the facial nerve branches by direct repair or interposition of nerve grafts. In case of avulsion or absence of the proximal stump of one of the branches, intrafacial nerve transfers can be ***Extratemporal Extraparotid or Distal Nerve Injuries*** performed by using expendandable neighbor branches for neurotization such as the cervical branch to the marginal mandibular branch.

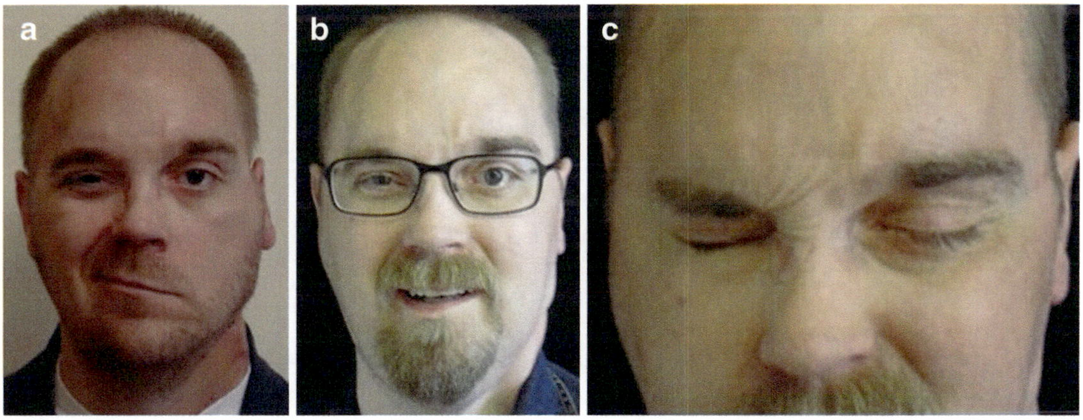

Fig. 6.9 Clinical photos of the patient. (**a**) One week postoperative after tumor resection and reconstruction showing complete facial paralysis. (**b**) Effortless smile with open byte 1 year postop. (**c**) Eye closure 1 year postoperative

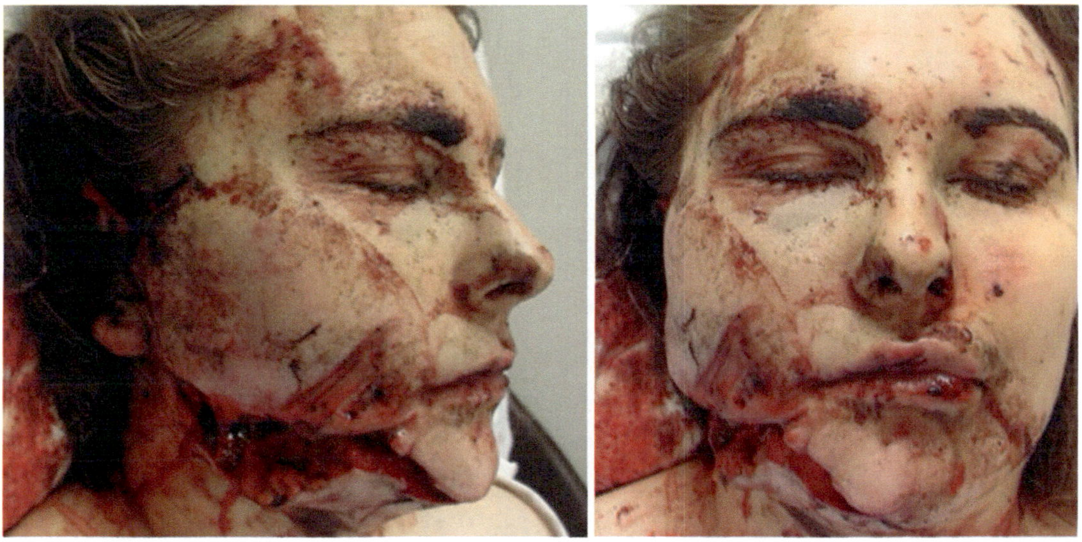

Fig. 6.10 Clinical example of Level 3 Facial Nerve Injury. Twenty-year-old female with incomplete right facial paralysis affection the buccal and marginal mandibular branches after a traffic accident with a penetrated injury with a truck window in the right cheek

6.6.6 Clinical Example

A 20-year-old female with incomplete right facial paralysis affection the buccal and marginal mandibular branches after a traffic accident with a penetrated injury with a truck window in the right ***Extratemporal Extraparotid or Distal Nerve Injuries***cheek (Fig. 6.10). Acute repair within 24 hours was performed with repair of the buccal and marginal mandibular branches (Fig. 6.11). Follow-up after 18 months year showing full recovery of both orbicularis oris function and marginal mandibular branch (Fig. 6.12).

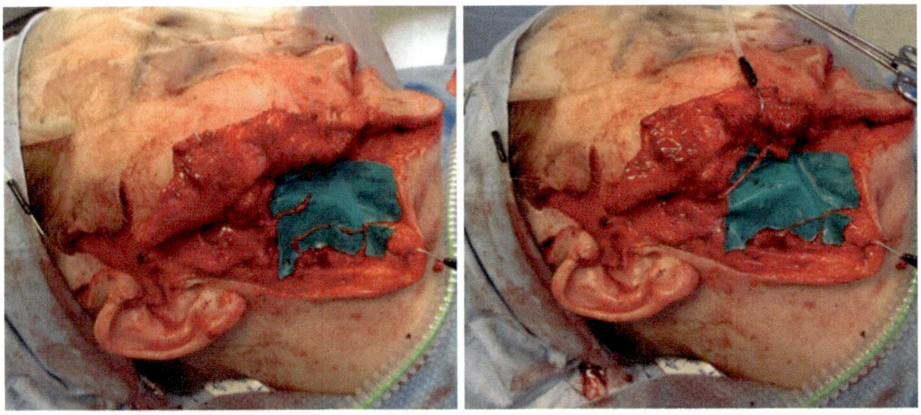

Fig. 6.11 Intraoperative photos of direct nerve repair of both buccal and marginal mandibular nerve branches

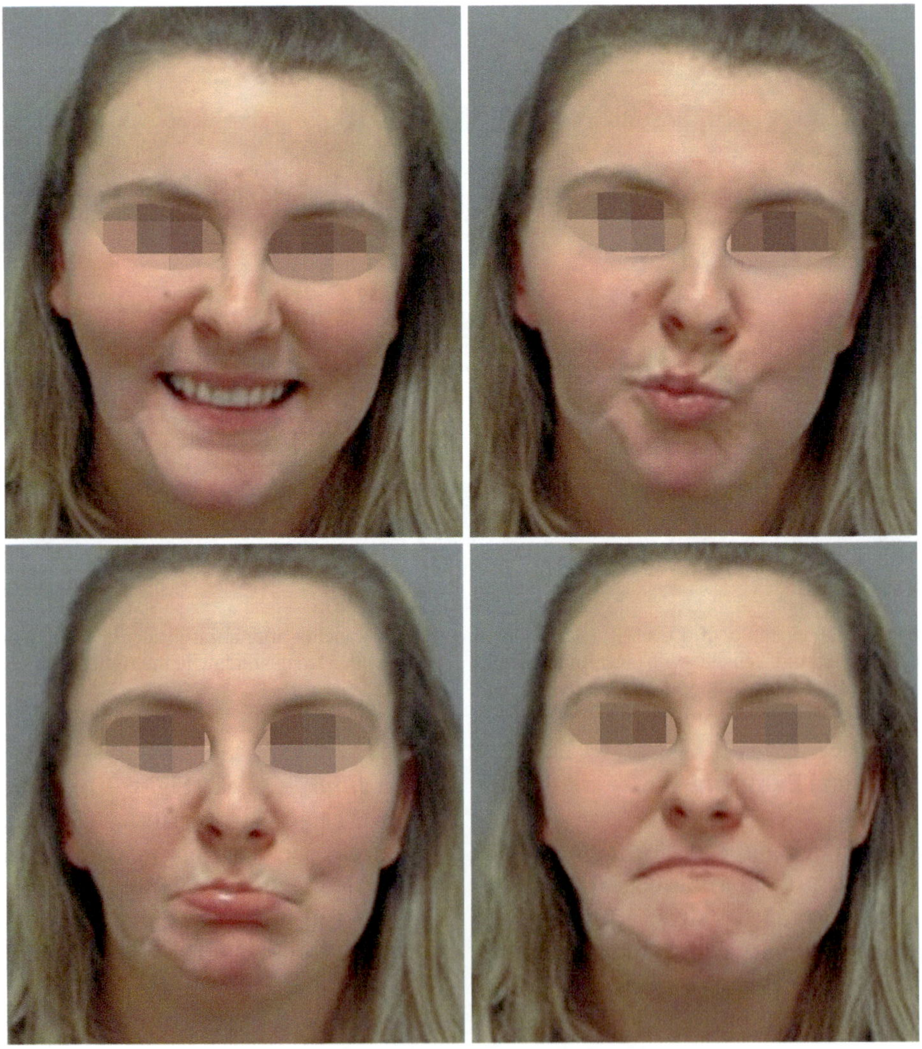

Fig. 6.12 Follow-up at 18 months postoperative showing full recovery of both orbicularis oris function and lower lip depressors

References

1. Seddon H. Three types of nerve injury. Brain. 1943;6:237–88.
2. Sunderland S. A classification of peripheral nerve injuries producing loss of function. Brain. 1951;74:491–516.
3. Mackinnon S, Dellon A. Diagnosis of nerve injury. In: Surgery of the peripheral nerve. New York: Thieme Medical Publishers; 1988. p. 74–9.
4. Kadakia S, Helman S, Saman M, Cooch N, Wood-Smith D. Concepts in neural coaptation: using the facial nerve as a paradigm in understanding principles surrounding nerve injury and repair. J Craniofac Surg. 2015;26(4):1304–9.
5. Sun DQ, Andresen NS, Gantz BJ. Surgical management of acute facial palsy. Otolaryngol Clin N Am. 2018;51(6):1077–92.
6. Walter M. Facial nerve regeneration, growth factors, and return of the mimetic, symmetrical smile. Facial Plast Surg. 1993;9:69–73.
7. Bascom D, Schaitkin B, May M, et al. Facial nerve repair: a retrospective review. Facial Plast Surg. 2000;16:309–13.
8. Kimata Y, Sakuraba M, Hishinuma S, Ebihara S, Hayashi R, Asakage T. Free vascularized nerve grafting for immediate facial nerve reconstruction. Laryngoscope. 2005;115(2):331–6.
9. Klebuc M, Shenaq SM. Donor nerve selection in facial reanimation surgery. Semin Plast Surg. 2004;18:53–60.
10. Garcia RM, Hadlock TA, Klebuc MJ, Simpson RL, Zenn MR, Marcus JR. Contemporary solutions for the treatment of facial nerve paralysis. Plast Reconstr Surg. 2015;135(6):1025e–46e.
11. Schaverien M, Moran G, Stewart K, Addison P. Activation of the masseter muscle during normal smile production and the implications for dynamic reanimation surgery for facial paralysis. J Plast Reconstr Aesthet Surg. 2011;64:1585–8.
12. Jensson D, Enghag S, Bylund N, Jonsson L, Wikström J, Grindlund M, Flink R, Rodriguez-Lorenzo A. Cranial nerve coactivation and implication for nerve transfers to the facial nerve. Plast Reconstr Surg. 2018;141(4):582e–5e.
13. Terzis JK, Karypidis D. Outcomes of direct muscle neurotization in pediatric patients with facial paralysis. Plast Reconstr Surg. 2009;124:1486.
14. Terzis JK, Tzafetta K. Outcomes of mini-hypoglossal nerve transfer and direct muscle neurotization for restoration of lower lip function in facial palsy. Plast Reconstr Surg. 2009;124(6):1891–904.
15. Konofaos P, Bassilios Habre S, Wallace RD. End-to-side nerve repair: current concepts and future perspectives. Ann Plast Surg. 2018;81(6):736–40.
16. Schaitkin B, Eisenman D. Anatomy of facial muscles. In: May M, Schaitkin B, editors. The facial nerve. 2nd ed. New York: Thieme Medical Publishers; 2000.
17. Sittel C, Stennert E. Prognostic value of electromyography in acute peripheral facial nerve palsy. Otol Neurotol. 2001;22:100–4.
18. May M. Anatomy for the clinician. In: May M, Schaitkin B, editors. The facial nerve. New York: Thieme Medical Publishers; 2000. p. 19–56.
19. Cristóbal L, Linder S, Lopez B, Mani M, Rodríguez-Lorenzo A. Free anterolateral thigh flap and masseter nerve transfer for reconstruction of extensive periauricular defects: surgical technique and clinical outcomes. Microsurgery. 2017;37(6):479–86.

Anatomy of the Facial Nerve

7

U. M. Heber and W. J. Weninger

Abbreviations

acf Anterior cranial fossa
an Great auricular nerve
ba Basilar artery
ca Internal carotid artery
cfd Cervicofacial division
ch Cerebellar hemisphere
cn2 Optic nerve
cn3 Oculomotor nerve
cn6 Abducent nerve
cn7 Facial nerve
cn8 Vestibulocochlear nerve
eam Opening of external acoustic meatus
ejv External jugular vein
fa Facial artery
fv Facial vein
iam Ostium of internal acoustic meatus
in Infundibulum
jf Jugular foramen
la Labyrinthine artery
mcf Middle cranial fossa
me Transition zone of medulla spinalis to medulla oblongata
mm Masseter muscle
mp Mastoid process
ob Olfactory bulb
of Oval foramen
p Petrous part of temporal bone
pa Parotid gland
pcf Posterior cranial fossa
pl Platysma muscle
po Pons
rm Retromandibular vein
s Sella turcica
smf Stylomastoid foramen
sp Styloid process
sta Superficial temporal artery
tfa Transverse facial artery
tl Temporal lobe
va Vertebral artery
zm Zygomaticus major muscle

This chapter will briefly recapitulate the anatomy of the facial nerve. As the facial nerve emerges from cranial nerve (CN)7 as its motoric portion the first part will focus on the anatomical course and diverse targets of CN7. The second part of this chapter contains a detailed description of the facial nerve regarding intracerebral, intracranial, and extracranial anatomical and topological characteristics, and also functional aspects.

U. M. Heber (✉) · W. J. Weninger
Division of Anatomy, MIC & CMI, Medical University of Vienna, Vienna, Austria
e-mail: ulrike.heber@meduniwien.ac.at; Wolfgang.Weninger@meduniwien.ac.at

© Springer Nature Switzerland AG 2021
C.-H. J. Tzou, A. Rodríguez-Lorenzo (eds.), *Facial Palsy*,
https://doi.org/10.1007/978-3-030-50784-8_7

7.1 Cranial Nerve (CN)7

Traditionally cranial nerve (CN)7 is referred to as facial nerve. Together with CN8 it leaves the brain at the cerebellopontine angle (Fig. 7.1) and travels through the subarachnoid space towards the posterior surface of the petrous part of the temporal bone. Here the nerves are joined by the labyrinthine artery and together they enter the internal acoustic opening. On their way through the internal auditory (acoustic) meatus CN7 separates and enters the facial (Fallopian) canal (Fig. 7.2a, b).

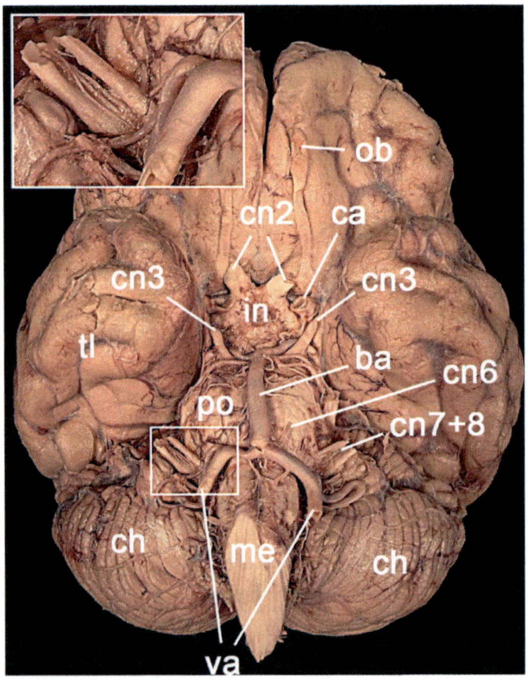

Fig. 7.1 Facial, intermediate, and vestibulocochlear nerve (cn7 + 8) near base of the brain. Inlay shows magnification of right cerebellopontine angle. *tl* temporal lobe, *po* pons, *me* transition zone of medulla spinalis to medulla oblongata, *ch* cerebellar hemisphere, *in* infundibulum, *va* vertebral artery, *ba* basilar artery, *ca* internal carotid artery, *ob* olfactory bulb, *cn2* optic nerve, *cn3* oculomotor nerve, *cn6* abducent nerve, *cn7 + 8* facial and vestibulocochlear nerve

The fallopian canal and the nerve inside have three segments: The first (labyrinthine segment) is very short and oriented fronto-laterally, the second (tympanic segment) is oriented occipito-laterally, and the third (mastoid segment) descends until the canal terminates at the stylomastoid foramen (Fig. 7.2c, d). The nerve leaves the canal through this opening. At the transition of the labyrinthine to the tympanic segments the canal and CN7 form an acute curve, the (second) geniculum, which contains the genicular ganglion with sensory nerve bodies.

While running inside the facial canal, various branches leave CN7. The greater petrosal nerve branches off where the nerve forms the geniculum. The chorda tympani, the stapedial nerve, and a branch joining the auricular branch of the vagus nerve (Arnold's nerve) leave the mastoid segment [1].

7.1.1 Targets of CN7

The branches of CN7 innervate the derivatives of the material derived from the mesenchyme of the second pharyngeal (branchial) arch. They comprise general and special sensory, parasympathetic, and motoric fibers or combinations. Motor targets are the stapedius muscle, mimic, auricular, and posterior suprahyoid muscles. Parasympathetic targets are the lacrimal gland, two salivary glands (sublingual and submandibular), and small glands and the mucosa of the palatine and nasopharynx. General sensory targets are small areas at and near the auricle and the external acoustic meatus. Special sensory targets are taste buds in the anterior two-thirds of the tongue and scattered buds on the hard and soft palate.

Between the cerebellopontine angle and the Fallopian canal, the sensory and parasympathetic fibers run together and form the nervus intermedius (intermediate nerve of Wrisberg), which is

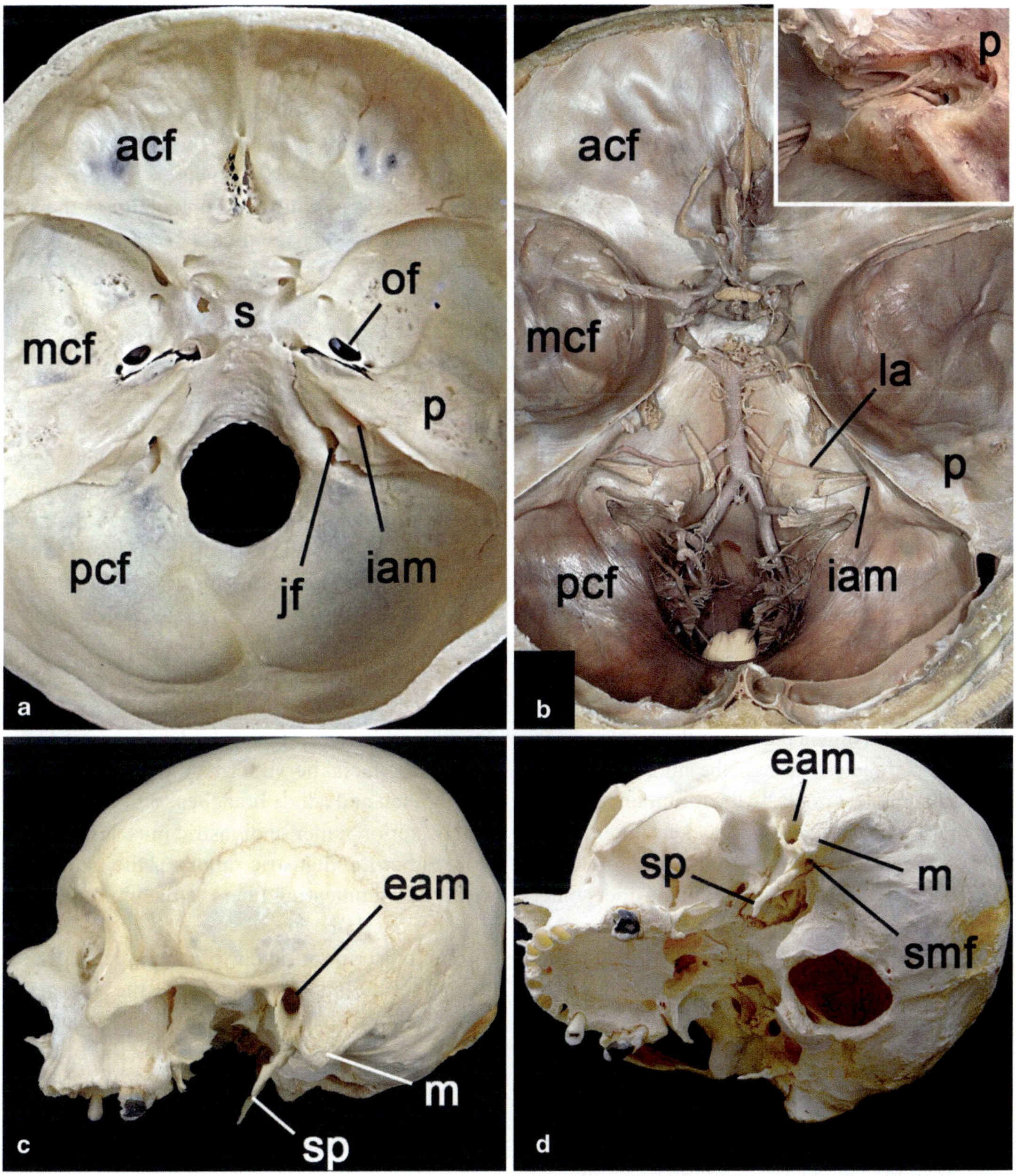

Fig. 7.2 Key features along the passage of facial nerve through cranium. (**a**, **b**) Features of internal skull base without (**a**) and in association with dura mater, nerves, and brain arteries (**b**). The roof of the internal acoustic meatus and the labyrinthine segment of the facial canal are removed in the inlay. (**c**, **d**). Topology of the stylomastoid foramen. *acf* anterior cranial fossa, *mcf* middle cranial fossa, *pcf* posterior cranial fossa, *s* sella turcica, *p* petrous part of temporal bone, *of* oval foramen, *jf* jugular foramen, *iam* ostium of internal acoustic meatus, *la* labyrinthine artery, *eam* opening of external acoustic meatus, *sp* styloid process, *m* mastoid process, *smf* stylomastoid foramen

part of CN7, but separated from its motoric portion. At the level of the geniculum of CN7, the perikaryon of the sensory neurons form the geniculate ganglion.

7.2 Facial Nerve: Motoric Portion of CN7

In addition to its use for describing CN7, the term facial nerve is used for referring to the (branchial) motor portion of CN7 only. This chapter will make use of this definition and focus on the description of the motoric portion of CN7.

7.2.1 Intracerebral Segment

The motor nuclei of the facial nerve are located in the ventral rhombencephalon near the midline. They receive excitatory fibers from neurons sitting in the motor cortices, which are mainly the precentral gyri of the frontal telencephalic lobe. Their axons travel via the internal capsule and the cerebral peduncles towards the nuclei as part of the corticonuclear tracts. In the rhombencephalon, the majority of the corticonuclear fibers cross sides and enter the contralateral motor nucleus of the facial nerve. A smaller amount of fibers enters the ipsilateral nucleus.

The fibers from the contralateral primary motor cortex form synapses with neurons targeting all muscles innervated by the facial nerve. The smaller amount of corticonuclear fibers that do not cross sides and enter the ipsilateral nucleus solely terminate at neurons targeting muscles of the upper face. Hence, the neurons of the motor nucleus of the facial nerve sending fibers towards the muscles of the upper face, including the orbicularis oculi muscle, can be activated by the contralateral and the ipsilateral primary motor cortex. The rest of the neurons and thus all other facial muscles can only be activated by the contralateral primary motor cortex.

The axons leave the nucleus of the facial nerve medially and ascend towards the floor of the fourth ventricle. They circumvent the nucleus of the sixth cranial nerve dorsally, thereby elevating the rhomboid fossa to form the facial colliculus. Then the fibers descend towards the cerebellopontine angle passing ventromedially to the spinal nucleus of the trigeminal nerve.

7.2.2 Intracranial Segment

After leaving the brain the motor fibers run as part of CN7, but separated from the sensory and parasympathetic fibers of the intermediate nerve towards the fallopian canal (see above). Fibers innervating the stapedius muscle leave the mastoid segment and the rest of the motoric fibers then pass through the stylomastoid foramen.

7.2.3 Extracranial Segment

Positioned between the styloid and mastoid processes, the facial nerve forms the posterior auricular branch and sends branches to the stylohyoid and posterior venter of digastric muscles. In addition, either the digastric ramus or the main stem sends communicating fibers to the glossopharyngeal nerve (Haller ansa).

The posterior auricular branch ascends dorsal to the auricle and connects with the vagus, the posterior branch of the great auricular and the lesser occipital nerve. It innervates the occipital belly of the epicranius muscle and, together with the temporal branch of the facial nerve (see 7.2.5) the auricular muscles.

7.2.4 Parotid Plexus

After submitting these branches, the stem of the facial nerve enters the tissues of the parotid gland. It comprises up to 4.000 nerve fibers and bifurcates into a temporofacial and a cervicofacial division [2]. The temporofacial division is joined by a branch of the auriculotemporal nerve, which provides parasympathetic and sympathetic secretory fibers for the innervation of the parotid gland. The secretory fibers use the branches of the facial nerve to distribute in the parotid gland. The perikarya of the parasympathetic fibers are located in the otic ganglion and can be activated by fibers originating from perikarya in the inferior salivatory nucleus and travel to the ganglion via the glossopharyngeal, tympanic, and finally lesser petrosal nerve (Jacobson anastomosis). The sympathetic fibers originate from perikarya in the superior cervical ganglion.

Still inside the parotid gland the temporofacial and cervicofacial divisions form five large branches: the temporal, zygomatic, buccal, mandibular, and cervical branch. The temporal and zygomatic branches derive from the temporofacial division, the mandibular and cervical branch from the cervicotemporal division. The buccal branch leaves either the one or the other, or in a small proportion of individuals has two roots, one from each division. The course of these branches can be classified using various classification schemes [3]. In principle, the branches either simply form sub-branches that spread to reach their targets, or they exchange fibers in a simple or rather complex way, thereby forming a plexus inbetween the superficial and profound parts of the gland.

Either way, the branches leave the gland at its superior, anterior, and inferior borders to enter the more superficial layers of the face. As the branches emerge from the gland, especially the temporal branch has already formed up to five and the zygomatic branch up to three sub-branches. The buccal branch stays a single nerve strand in approximately half of the population, while in the rest it has ramified into two or three sub-branches. The mandibular (in more than 80%) and cervical branch (in more than 90%) usually leave the parotid gland as single nerve strands [4, 5] (Fig. 7.3).

7.2.5 Innervation of Facial Muscles

In the face, the branches continue relatively straight towards the muscles. The mandibular branch usually runs inferior to the mandible [6]. All branches have complex variable topologic relations to anatomic structures such as the facial and transverse facial artery and vein, the parotid duct (Stensen duct), or the tissue compartments of the face [7]. Despite of these variations, several authors successfully defined landmarks for targeting nerve branches through the intact skin or for identifying skin regions and strata which are free of larger nerve branches [8–10].

Anatomical textbooks and studies differ slightly in their descriptions of the facial muscle innervation. This is mainly due to a high degree of individual variation in the topology, branching pattern, and communications between facial nerve branches (Fig. 7.4). According to Gray's textbook of human anatomy, the cervical branch innervates the platysma, the mandibular branch the risorius and muscles of the lower lip and chin. The buccal branch supplies the muscles of the cheek and upper lip and small nasal muscles, the zygomatic branch the orbicularis oculi muscle. The temporal branch innervates the anterior and superior auricular muscles, the frontal belly of the occipitofrontal muscle, and supraorbital muscles [11]. Yet details regarding facial muscle innervation are under heavy dispute [12, 13].

Near their targets the facial nerve branches ramify extensively before and while entering the muscles. Especially these small rami exchange fibers with the branches of the trigeminal nerve and it is hypothesized that those fibers might conduct proprioceptive information. The cervical branch often directly communicates with large branches of the transverse cervical nerve,

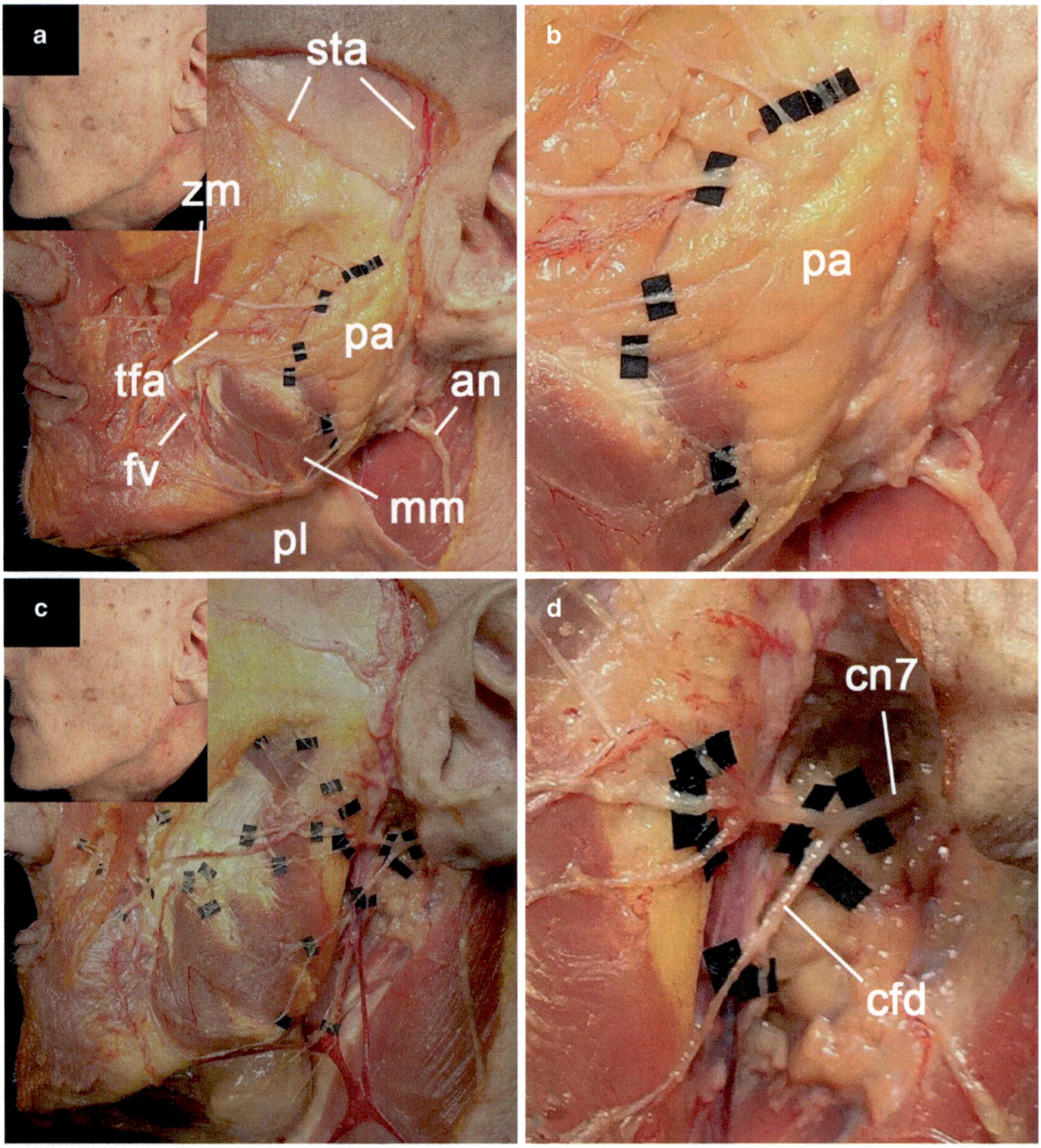

Fig. 7.3 Ramification of the facial nerve (cn7). (**a**, **b**) Branches of CN7 leaving the borders of the parotid gland (pa). (**c**, **d**) Ramification of the stem of the facial nerve immediately distal to the stylomastoid foramen. Note the bifurcation into temporofacial and cervicofacial (cfd) division. *sta* superficial temporal artery, *zm* zygomaticus major muscle, *pa* parotid gland, *tfa* transverse facial artery, *fv* facial vein, *pl* platysma muscle, *mm* masseter muscle, *an* great auricular nerve, *cfd* cervicofacial division, *cn7* facial nerve

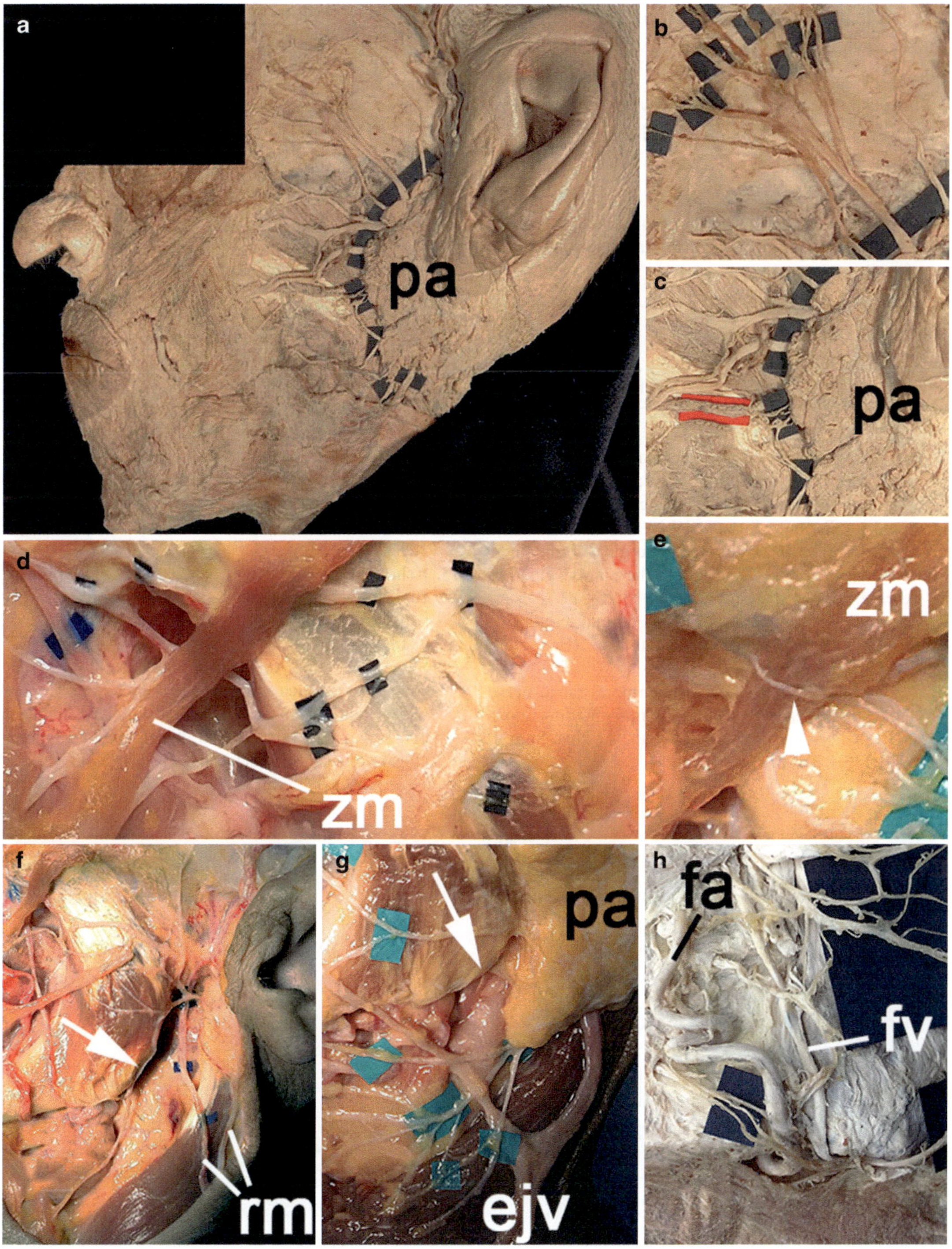

Fig. 7.4 Variations in the topology of the branches of the facial nerve (CN7). (**a**, **b**) Overview (**a**) and detailed (**b**) ramification of branches after exiting the parotid gland. Note the extensive ramification of temporal nerve branches before entering target muscles (**b**). (**c**–**e**) Zygomatic branches can cross the parotid duct (red background, **c**), form a plexus in the masseteric region (**d**) and run underneath (**d**) or around (arrowhead, **e**) the zygomaticus major muscle (zm). (**f**, **e**). The cervicofacial division can either ramify inside the parotid gland (**d**) or later in its course around the mandibular angle (arrow, **f**). The mandibular branch usually runs inferior to the mandible (**f**), and further crosses the facial artery and vein (**h**). The cervical branch can cross the external jugular vein and if so, can run above or underneath it (**g**). *pa* parotid gland, *zm* zygomaticus major muscle, *rm* retromandibular vein, *ejv* external jugular vein, *fa* facial artery, *fv* facial vein

a sensible nerve originating from the second and third cervical nerves, but also with the glossopharyngeal nerve. In general, many constant and inconstant connections between facial nerve branches and cranial and spinal nerves are described [14].

Acknowledgements We would like to thank S. Meng and B. Maurer-Gesek for their support in image creation.

References

1. Eshraghi AA, Buchman CA, Telischi FF. Sensory auricular branch of the facial nerve. Otol Neurotol. 2002;23(3):393–6.
2. Hembd A, et al. Facial nerve axonal analysis and anatomical localization in donor nerve: optimizing axonal load for cross-facial nerve grafting in facial reanimation. Plast Reconstr Surg. 2017;139(1):177–83.
3. Gataa IS, Faris BJ. Patterns and surgical significance of facial nerve branching within the parotid gland in 43 cases. Oral Maxillofac Surg. 2016;20(2):161–5.
4. Martinez Pascual P, et al. Extracranial course of the facial nerve revisited. Anat Rec (Hoboken). 2019;302(4):599–608.
5. Farahvash MR, et al. The extratemporal facial nerve and its branches: analysis of 42 hemifacial dissections in fresh Persian (Iranian) cadavers. Aesthet Surg J. 2013;33(2):201–8.
6. Yang HM, et al. Revisiting the topographic anatomy of the marginal mandibular branch of facial nerve relating to the surgical approach. Aesthet Surg J. 2016;36(9):977–82.
7. Lee JY, et al. Topographic relationships between the transverse facial artery, branches of the facial nerve, and the parotid duct in the lateral midface in a Korean population. Ann Plast Surg. 2014;73(3):321–4.
8. Dorafshar AH, et al. Surface anatomy of the middle division of the facial nerve: Zuker's point. Plast Reconstr Surg. 2013;131(2):253–7.
9. de Bonnecaze G, et al. The frontal branch of the facial nerve: can we define a safety zone? Surg Radiol Anat. 2015;37(5):499–506.
10. Roostaeian J, Rohrich RJ, Stuzin JM. Anatomical considerations to prevent facial nerve injury. Plast Reconstr Surg. 2015;135(5):1318–27.
11. Williams P, Warwick R, Dyson M, Bannister L. Gray's anatomy international student edition. Edinburgh: Churchill Livingstone; 1989. p. 859–1244.
12. Raslan A, et al. High variability of facial muscle innervation by facial nerve branches: a prospective electrostimulation study. Laryngoscope. 2017;127(6):1288–95.
13. Kehrer A, et al. The nerve supply of zygomaticus major: variability and distinguishing zygomatic from buccal facial nerve branches. Clin Anat. 2018;31(4):560–5.
14. Shoja MM, et al. Anastomoses between lower cranial and upper cervical nerves: a comprehensive review with potential significance during skull base and neck operations, part I: trigeminal, facial, and vestibulocochlear nerves. Clin Anat. 2014;27(1):118–30.

8 Nerve Transfers to the Facial Nerve

Andreas E. Krag and Shai M. Rozen

Key Points

- Nerve transfers to the facial nerve are indicated in acute and subacute facial paralysis patients where the proximal facial nerve stump cannot be found or when repair via direct coaptation or nerve grafting is not feasible.
- The distal facial nerve branches and the facial mimetic muscles must be intact for successful nerve transfer.
- Cross-facial nerve grafting as sole reinnervation procedure is not reliable and should likely be performed concomitantly with a nerve transfer on the paralyzed side.
- Nerve transfers will likely work if performed up to 18 months after facial nerve injury, but preliminary data suggest that earlier nerve transfers may provide better excursion.
- Dual innervation via combining masseteric to facial nerve transfer and cross-facial nerve grafts may provide rapid reinnervation and strong excursion from the masseteric nerve for voluntary movements, and possibly improved synchronous motions after reinnervation by the cross-facial nerve grafts occurs.

A. E. Krag · S. M. Rozen (✉)
Department of Plastic Surgery, The University of Texas Southwestern Medical Center, Dallas, TX, USA
e-mail: shai.rozen@utsouthwestern.edu

8.1 Background

To obtain optimal outcomes in facial paralysis patients, the goals should be achieving spontaneity, synchrony, and sufficient excursion. Currently, no single donor nerve can obtain these results consistently in all scenarios of facial paralysis, but for spontaneity to occur the optimal donor nerve is the facial nerve. Hence, it is preferable to use the ipsilateral facial nerve axons, either via direct repair or short nerve grafting, to obtain optimal results, if the recipient mimetic muscles are salvageable and a proximal facial nerve is available. When this is not possible, yet the mimetic muscles are still amenable to reinnervation, then nerve transfers are indicated using a non-facial cranial nerve as the donor nerve.

8.2 Patient Presentation

Patients with acute or subacute facial paralysis, defined as patients in whom their facial mimetic muscles are salvageable, should be considered for nerve transfers to the facial nerve if facial nerve repair, via direct coaptation or via nerve grafting, is not possible.

Patients may present with either complete or incomplete facial paralysis or may present preoperatively in a multi-specialty clinic with varying degrees of facial nerve function, in which case, mimetic function may be salvaged with nerve

© Springer Nature Switzerland AG 2021
C.-H. J. Tzou, A. Rodríguez-Lorenzo (eds.), *Facial Palsy*,
https://doi.org/10.1007/978-3-030-50784-8_8

grafts, nerve transfers, or a combination, concomitantly with tumor resection in a multidisciplinary operation [1].

The underlying pathologies are varied. These may include malignant or benign cerebellopontine angle tumors such as acoustic neuromas, schwannomas, and neurofibromas, malignant or benign parotid gland tumors, or malignant skin tumors; infections including viral and bacterial; traumas including more proximal temporal bone fractures or more distal facial lacerations; iatrogenic injuries during surgeries of the skull base or face; or poor recovery from Bell's palsy.

A detailed patient history should be obtained including etiology, duration of facial paralysis, and previous surgeries in the brain, head, and neck region. The patient must be asked about the rate of deterioration of facial nerve function and any preceding symptoms. Physical examination must include a full cranial nerve examination including any remaining facial nerve function and function of any possible donor nerves, as well as an assessment of the facial musculature. Electroneurography and electromyography may be used in cases of unclear examinations but are not commonly contributory or used. Fibrillations on needle electromyography of the mimetic muscles indicate viable facial musculature despite denervation which can be salvaged by nerve transfer. A silent signal on needle electromyography suggests that the mimetic muscles are atrophic and salvage by nerve transfer is less likely [2].

8.3 Nerve Transfers: Goals, Indications, and Rationale

8.3.1 Goals

The goal of nerve transfers is salvage of the facial mimetic musculature by reinnervation from a non-facial donor motor nerve, thereby preventing mimetic muscle atrophy and fibrosis. The primary realistic objective is to restore voluntary motions, yet achieving spontaneity is more elusive. Certain reports claim that spontaneity can be achieved in some patients when innervating with a non-facial nerve, but this cannot be obtained with consistency. The second goal is to restore facial symmetry in repose. Nerve transfers in general do not provide tone. It is for this reason that additional static support is usually added, and sometimes additional cross-facial nerve grafts are deployed in hope of obtaining or adding some tone and possibly increase synchroneity. Although nerve transfers are more commonly discussed in the setting of the midface, nerve transfers can also be effective if performed in a timely manner in innervating other facial regions such as the periorbital area assisting in voluntary closure of the eye, or the lower lip to improve oral competence. These subjects will be discussed in detail below.

8.3.2 Indications

Nerve transfers to the facial nerve are indicated in acute or subacute facial paralysis patients when the proximal facial nerve stump is not readily available for repair, either via direct coaptation or via nerve grafting, yet the distal facial nerve branches and mimetic muscles are intact. Also, salvageability of mimetic musculature is a prerequisite for a successful nerve transfer and mainly depends on the duration of paralysis. Although the exact denervation duration after which the mimetic muscles are likely not salvageable is not known, most would consider this period not beyond 18 months although some reports describe salvage even at 24 months. Degree of denervation (complete versus incomplete) may play a role in the length of this window of opportunity, but preliminary research suggests that earlier intervention yields improved results [3].

Hence, nerve transfers to the facial nerve will unlikely succeed in congenital complete facial paralysis patients without facial neuromuscular units, e.g., Möbius syndrome, as well as patients with longstanding denervation and facial muscle atrophy regardless of underlying pathology. These conditions should be treated by transfer of a new neuromuscular unit to the face with either a free functional muscle transplant or muscle transfer.

8.3.3 Rationale

The rationale behind nerve transfer is restoration of motor neuron stimuli to the facial nerve branches from another cranial nerve, which partially takes over the function of the proximal facial nerve. Motor axons from the donor nerve regenerate through facial nerve branches and reinnervate the facial mimetic muscles. The donor nerve is transferred to the facial nerve preferably by direct coaptation or through interposition nerve grafts. A non-facial cranial nerve is always used as the motor donor nerve in nerve transfers. The masseteric branch of the trigeminal nerve is likely the most commonly used donor nerve for nerve transfers because of minimal donor-site morbidity and rapid reinnervation. The spinal accessory nerve and the hypoglossal nerve have also been described for this purpose [4].

Several rules hold true to the success of any nerve coaptation or repair: a tension free coaptation, appropriate trimming of the nerve edges, and repair outside the zone of injury. Yet, several additional tenets are important in nerve transfers.

First, there must be a functional donor nerve. Although not common, some patients with cancer or congenital facial paralysis may have more than one cranial nerve involved. Therefore, all patients need a thorough yet simple cranial nerve examination demonstrating active target muscles of the future donor nerve. As an example, preoperative palpation of masseter muscle motion when the patient is asked to bite down is sufficient to assure an intact masseteric nerve.

Second, is assuring the integrity of the recipient facial nerve from the point of coaptation to the target mimetic muscles as well as verifying that recipient muscles are undamaged. In multilevel injuries or large tumor resections, this is key. If either the recipient nerve is discontinuous, or the target muscle is damaged, a nerve transfer will fail.

Third, as a continuation to the second point, is the duration of paralysis. Although the exact duration of paralysis unto which the mimetic musculature cannot be reinnervated is unknown, it is generally thought that beyond 18 months of denervation the muscles are less likely to recover. In fact, many authors, including the senior author, think that earlier nerve transfers yield better results and would generally prefer to perform nerve transfers prior to 1-year duration of paralysis [3].

8.3.4 Advantages of Nerve Transfers

Axonal load: As mentioned previously, nerve transfers are mainly used to salvage and utilize the patient's own paralyzed muscles when ipsilateral facial nerve options are unavailable. In the mid-seventies, original work by Scaramella and others attempted to use cross-facial nerve grafts to directly neurotize the paralyzed mimetic muscles [5]. These techniques have generally been aborted in their original form since the number of axons reaching the paralyzed muscle were small and could not provide sufficient neurotization, in addition to the fact that often axons would arrive too late to the muscle after it had atrophied. Future modifications added nerve transfers concomitantly with cross-facial nerve grafts, a technique commonly termed "babysitting," although the main source of reinnervation would be from the nerve transfer. In other words, nerve transfers have the advantages of high axonal loads and short distances for axonal regeneration, hence the high reliability and strong muscle excursions they provide [2].

Rapid innervation: Due to the short distances of reinnervation from an ipsilateral nerve transfer, the duration of paralysis may be shortened. This allows treating patients who presented late, with facial paralysis durations of up to 12–18 months, with a chance for muscle salvage otherwise not possible due to significantly longer denervation times if cross-facial nerve grafts were used. First motions are expected to be observed 2–6 months after masseteric to facial nerve transfer [4, 6, 7].

Ability to reinnervate several mimetic muscles: Although simultaneous innervation of several muscles may seem an adverse outcome, when those muscles are even partially synergistic, this may be advantageous. Such is the case, when the donor nerve is coapted proximal to the division of branches that innervate the orbicularis oculi muscle as well as the zygomaticus muscle complex. In theory, this creates a mild oral-ocular synkinesis, but in reality, it creates a more natural smile with mild palpebral closure when the patient smiles. An additional advantage is protection of the cornea due to the ability to voluntarily close the eyelids. Also, there have been several descriptions of using different nerve transfers to separately innervate different regions of the face.

Reliability: Due to the high axonal loads, short distance to reinnervation, and the need for only one nerve coaptation, nerve transfers are highly reliable in providing motion to the mimetic muscles.

8.3.5 Disadvantages of Nerve Transfers

Inadvertent motion: Because the donor nerve used in nerve transfers was originally used by nature to perform another activity, when that activity is performed, the patients will inadvertently perform the new motion it is intended to perform. For example, if the masseteric nerve was used for smile reanimation, the patient will smile to some degree when chewing. Despite this, most patients report improvement in eating and would likely tolerate this at the gain of a voluntary smile [8]. Donor-site morbidity following masseteric to facial nerve transfer is low and mastication does not seem to be impaired postoperatively [4, 7].

Lack of tone: Nerve transfers provide strong voluntary muscle excursion but are less effective in restoring resting tone and symmetry. It is the senior author's experience that reinnervation from the contralateral facial nerve is necessary for improvement of facial tone.

Lack of spontaneity: A spontaneous smile means an emotional smile that is produced without thinking nor is it voluntary. It is evoked by emotions. Regardless of which donor nerve is used, one must remember that the donor nerves are not programmed nor have cortical representation in the brain to move the mimetic muscles. Therefore, some degree of retraining is necessary. Although some authors argue that spontaneity is possible through cerebral plasticity, it is likely less common on a consistent basis than previously described [6, 9].

Lack of synchrony: Synchrony means that both sides of the face move at the same time. Although some patients are so well-versed at using their donor nerve and can smile in near synchrony, this occurs more commonly when patients perform a voluntary smile rather than a spontaneous smile, and even then, perfect synchrony is rare.

8.4 Masseteric to Facial Nerve Transfer

The mandibular nerve is the third and largest division of the trigeminal nerve, which provides sensory innervation to the lower third of the facial skin and motor innervation to the muscles of mastication. The masseteric nerve is a pure motor branch from the mandibular nerve innervating the masseter muscle.

To access the masseteric nerve, a preauricular incision is made on the paralyzed side of the face which is extended inferiorly and posteriorly to the mandibular angle. Skin and subcutaneous tissue is incised with monopolar cautery to the sub-superficial musculoaponeurotic system plane, where the cheek flap is raised over the parotid-masseteric fascia. Dissection of the masseteric nerve begins at the center of a triangle between three anatomical landmarks: the coronoid process anteriorly, the mandibular condyle posteriorly, and the mandibular notch caudally (Fig. 8.1). Dissection is performed through the parotid gland with particular care to preserve the facial nerve branches, regardless of degree of paralysis. Once the masseter muscle fibers are encountered, they are carefully split in the area of the mandibular notch. Meticulous hemostasis with bipolar or micro clips should always be performed. The descending branch of the masseteric nerve is encountered between the middle

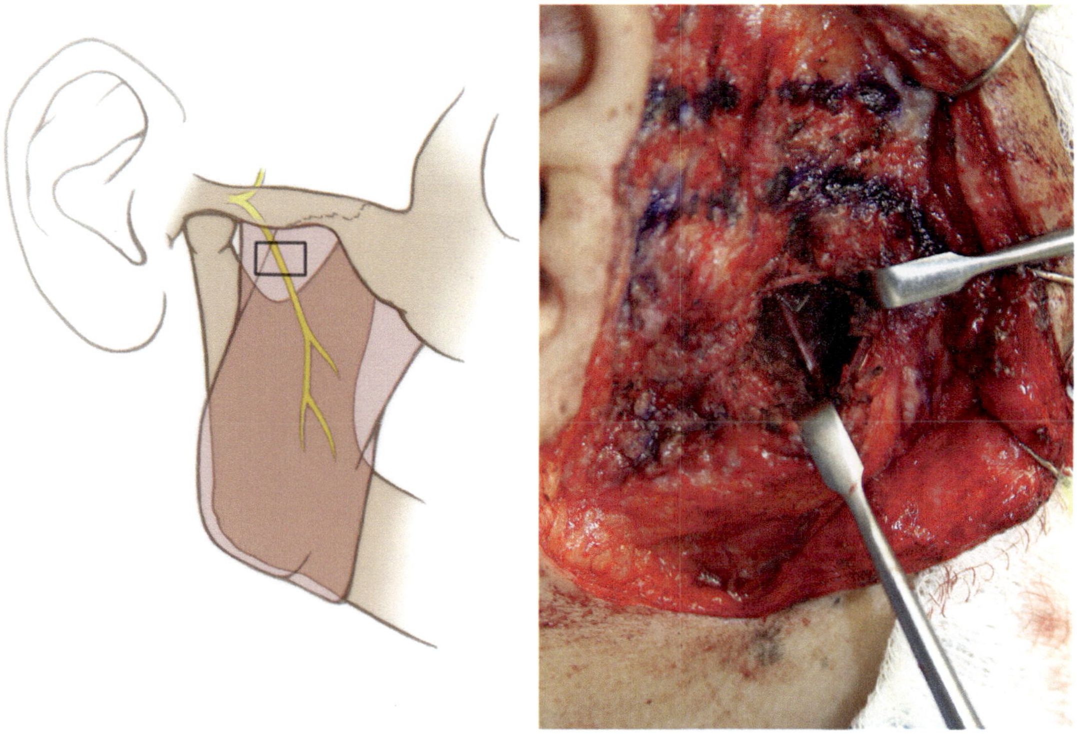

Fig. 8.1 Dissection of the masseteric nerve. Left: the three anatomical landmarks for identifying the masseteric nerve: the coronoid process anteriorly, the mandibular condyle posteriorly, and the mandibular notch caudally. Right: intraoperative photo of the dissected masseteric nerve. (© Shai M. Rozen, MD)

and deep masseter heads. The masseteric nerve is dissected in a direction towards the modiolus for about 2.0 cm, where it is transected before branching and then transposed to the surface of the parotid. A nerve length of 13–14 mm should be expected. For a successful nerve transfer without tension on coaptation or the need for a nerve graft, additional parotid tissue is usually removed to allow comfortable coaptation with either a branch of the facial nerve or the trunk depending on indication [10].

Anatomical placement of the masseteric to facial nerve transfer is performed by coaptation to the facial nerve main trunk in patients with no proximal facial nerve continuity, or to selective zygomatic or buccal facial nerve branches in patients with facial nerve continuity in order to potentially preserve the proximal axonal input which provides facial tone (Fig. 8.2). In this selective coaptation, a recipient branch for the nerve transfer innervating both the zygomaticus major muscle and orbicularis oculi muscle should be chosen as this will provide voluntary smile and eye closure. The masseteric and recipient facial nerve branch is coapted end-to-end with 10-0 interrupted nylon sutures in the epineurium and reinforced with tissue glue based on surgeon preference [11].

8.5 Cross-Facial Nerve Grafting

Cross-facial nerve grafting is an established technique which has the objective of restoring both voluntary and involuntary activation of paralyzed facial muscles. An electric nerve stimulator is used for identification of facial nerve branches. Selection of donor facial nerve branches on the nonparalyzed side is guided by the principles of "specificity and redundancy." "Specificity" entails identifying nerve branches innervating the orbicularis oculi for eye closure and blink,

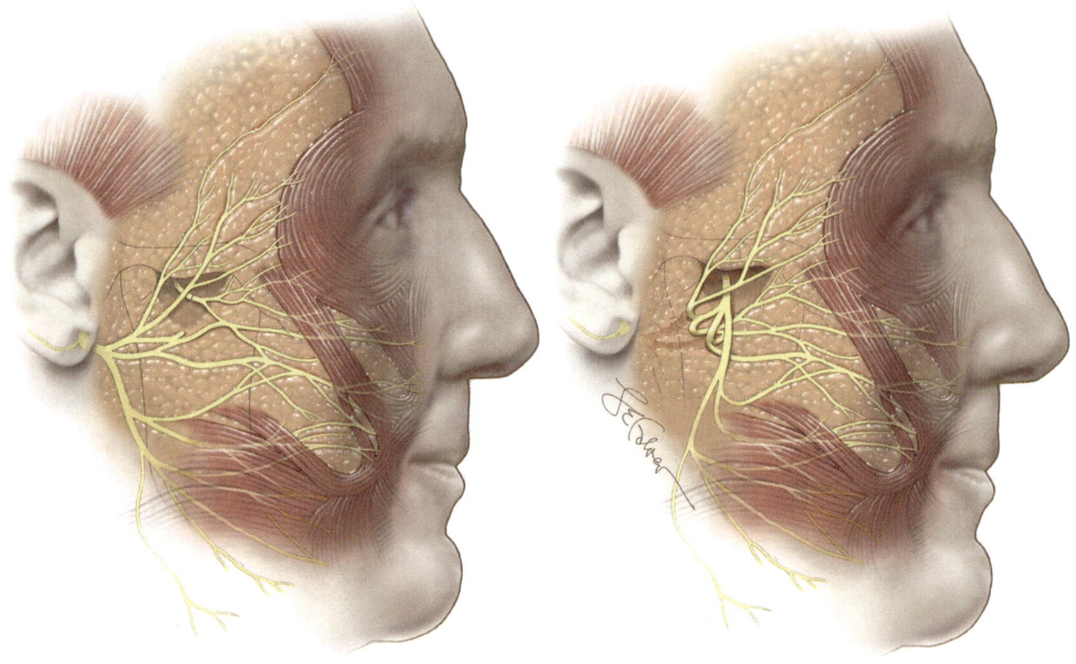

Fig. 8.2 Anatomical placement of the masseteric to facial nerve transfer. Left: selective masseteric nerve coaptation to a zygomatic facial nerve branch. Right: truncal masseteric coaptation to the main facial nerve trunk. (© Shai M. Rozen, MD)

and nerve branches in the midface innervating the zygomaticus major for the smile. Facial nerve branches performing activities other than these intended motions, such as those innervating the risorius muscle, should not be chosen as donor nerves for the smile. "Redundancy" entails that two nerve branches performing a similar activity be identified before sacrificing one of these branches to minimize donor-site morbidity of the nonparalyzed hemiface. Correspondingly, recipient facial nerve branches for coaptation on the paralyzed side should be chosen carefully. In the less common scenario in which cross-facial nerve grafting is performed simultaneously with a tumor resection, stimulation of corresponding branches may be performed. Much more commonly, the recipient facial nerve branches are non-stimulatable, and proper anatomical mapping of the facial nerve branches should be performed [1].

The main disadvantages with cross-facial nerve grafting is the long distance for axonal regeneration, which translates into lengthy denervation of the target facial musculature and a significant decrease in axonal numbers that reach the mimetic muscles. The resulting low axonal load from the cross-facial nerve grafts might result in weak muscle activation or no activation at all. For these reasons, cross-facial nerve grafting alone is not recommended. To overcome this issue, the so-called "babysitter" procedure was introduced. As originally described, a direct hypoglossal to facial nerve coaptation was performed concomitantly with the first stage of cross-facial nerve grafting. The hypoglossal nerve provided fast reinnervation and stimulation of facial mimetic muscles until axons had regenerated though the cross-facial nerve grafts [2]. The hypoglossal nerve is rarely used any more, but based on similar principles it has been replaced by the masseteric nerve as donor nerve. Also, most authors would perform this in one setting. Earlier attempts to cut the transferred donor nerve and then directly coapt the cross-facial nerve grafts were aborted since the patients were re-paralyzed, and regained little motion, which strengthens the notion that the transferred donor nerve overtakes the majority of mimetic muscle motor control, rather than the cross-facial nerve grafts.

8.6 Dual Innervation

As described in the previous sections, nerve transfers to the facial nerve are effective in producing voluntary motion in different portions of the face with good excursion symmetry compared with the nonparalyzed side. However, reinnervation from a non-facial motor donor nerve does not restore spontaneous facial expressions, and facial tone may be weak compared with the paralyzed side.

The aim of dual innervation is to obtain the advantages of both worlds: fast and strong reinnervation stemming from the nerve transfer, combined with cross-facial nerve grafts, coapted either end-to-end or end-to-side with specific paralyzed branches, to hopefully provide increased tone, synchroneity, and perhaps even some spontaneity. Although the idea is warranted, strong data supporting this idea has yet to be published, but from the senior author's experience it likely deserves merit. In cases of nerve transfers, as opposed to dual innervation of a muscle transplant which the senior author prefers performing in two stages, masseteric to facial nerve transfer and cross-facial nerve grafting is performed in the same procedure, where two cross-facial nerve grafts are inserted, one for the periorbital area and one for the smile. The selection of cross-facial nerve graft donors should follow the principles of "specificity and redundancy" as described in the previous section (Fig. 8.3). Following the dual innervation procedure, first voluntary motions are observed after 2–6 months by reinnervation from the masseteric nerve. As for the effect of the cross-facial nerve graft, the improved tone and possibly improved synchroneity likely start taking effect 1 year after the surgery when axonal regrowth has reached its target muscles (Fig. 8.4). In the senior author's opinion, improvements are seen over several years with increasing tone and synchroneity, but this has yet to be demonstrated with good methodology (Fig. 8.5) [1, 6, 12].

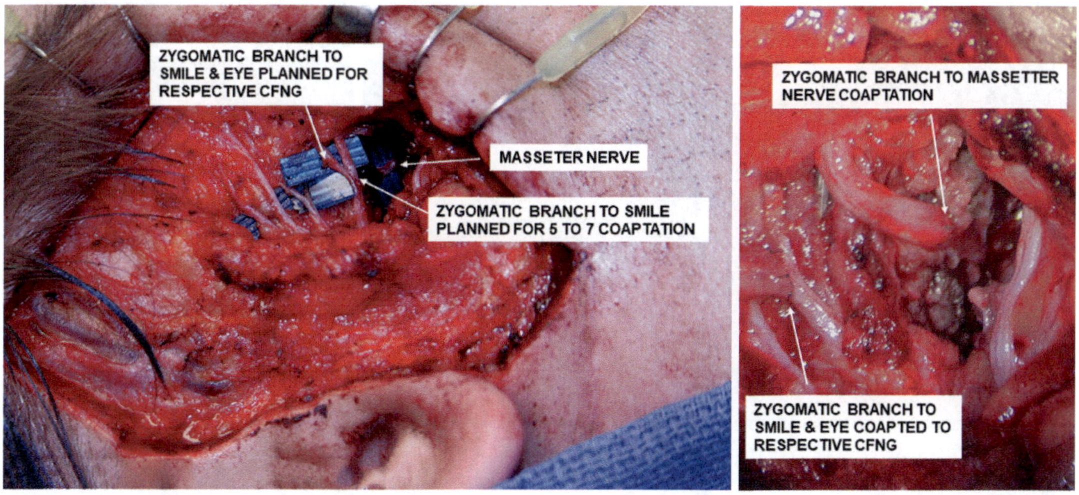

Fig. 8.3 Intraoperative photos of a selective masseteric nerve coaptation to a zygomatic facial nerve branch with concomitant cross-facial nerve grafting. Left: dissection of recipient facial nerve branches on the paralyzed side prior to cross-facial nerve grafting and masseteric to facial nerve transfer. Right: after selective end-to-end masseteric to facial nerve transfer and end-to-side cross-facial nerve graft coaptations. (Courtesy of Shai M. Rozen, MD)

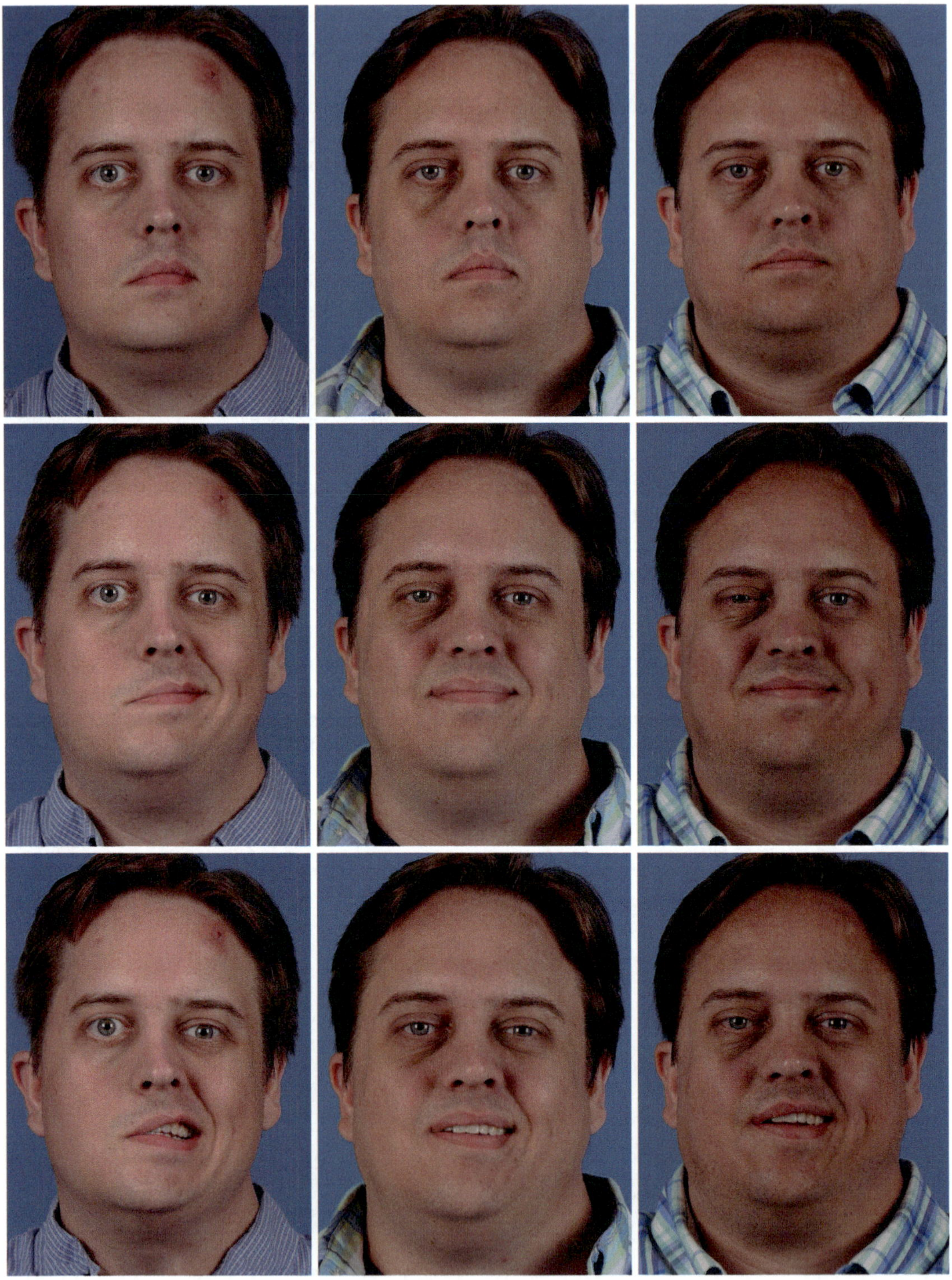

Fig. 8.4 Thirty-five-year-old male who presented with complete right sided facial paralysis after acoustic neuroma resection with intratemporal nerve grafting to the facial nerve. The patient underwent selective masseteric to facial nerve transfer and two cross-facial nerve grafts, one to the midface and the other to the periorbita on the right side 75 days after acoustic neuroma resection. Right upper eyelid gold weight insertion and right lower eyelid canthoplasty were performed 12 months after the nerve transfer procedure. Left column: Patient before nerve transfer and cross-facial nerve grafting. Center column: Patient 12 months after nerve transfer and cross-facial nerve grafting. Right column: Patient 23 months after nerve transfer and cross-facial nerve grafting. (Courtesy of Shai M. Rozen, MD)

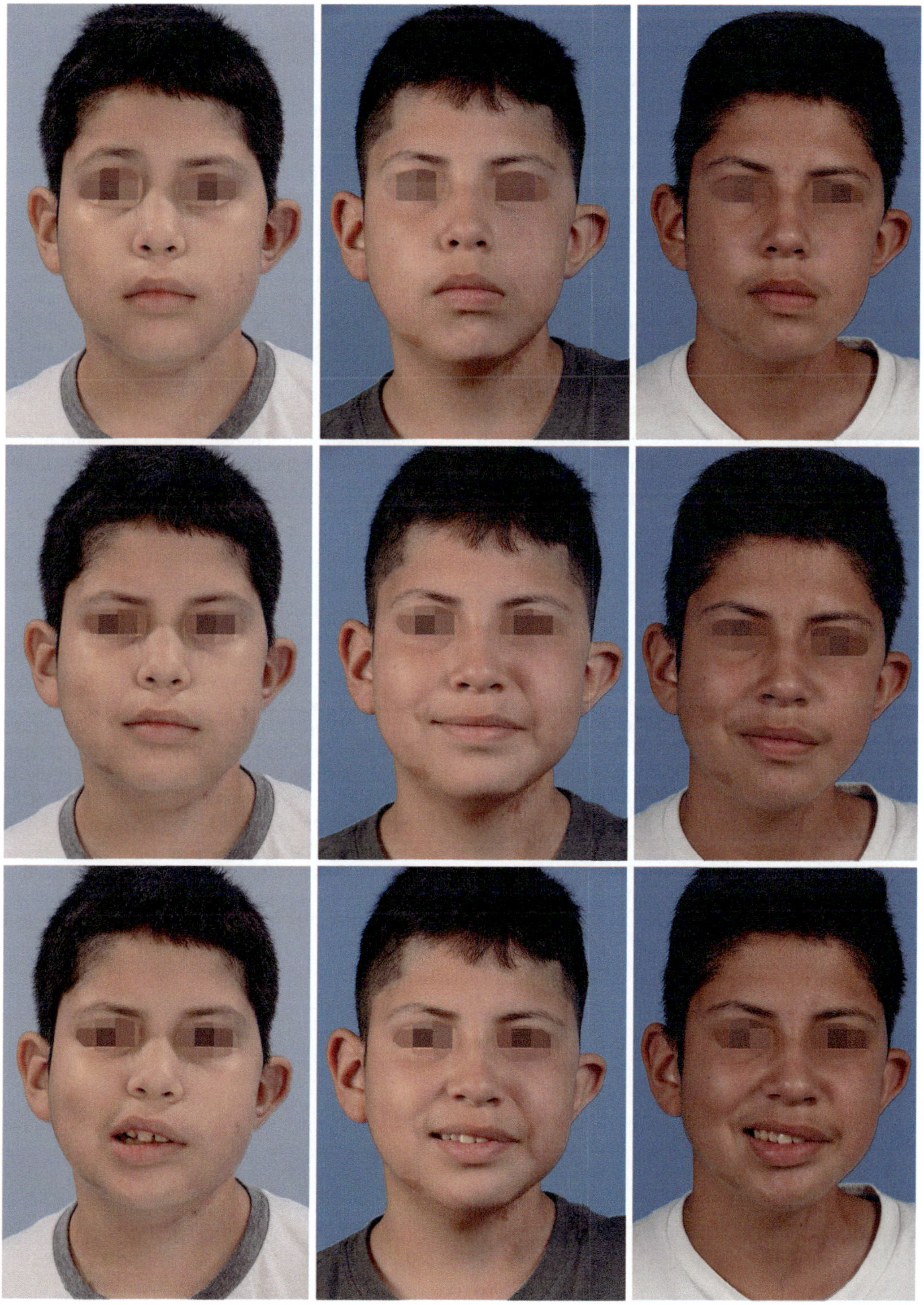

Fig. 8.5 Eleven-year-old male who underwent left total parotidectomy including proximal facial nerve resection and neck dissection due to mucoepidermoid carcinoma of the parotid gland. He underwent immediate reconstruction with masseteric to facial nerve transfer coapted to the facial nerve main trunk and two cross-facial nerve grafts coapted end-to-side to a distal facial nerve branch to the periorbital area and the midface. Reconstruction was immediately followed by radiation treatment. The left column: Patient 3 weeks after nerve transfer and cross-facial nerve grafting. The center column: Patient 18 months after nerve transfer and cross-facial nerve grafting. Right column: 36 months after nerve transfer and cross-facial nerve grafting. (Courtesy of Shai M. Rozen, MD)

8.7 Summary

Nerve transfers to the facial nerve reinnervate and salvage the facial mimetic musculature when performed up to 18 months after onset of facial paralysis, but earlier intervention may improve results. The masseteric nerve is the preferred donor nerve as it provides rapid reinnervation and restores voluntary smile excursion with minimal donor-site morbidity. However, masseteric to facial nerve transfer cannot be expected to restore facial tone, synchroneity, and spontaneity. Hence, dual innervation utilizing cross-facial nerve grafting as an adjunct to masseteric to facial nerve transfer in a single stage procedure should be considered for optimal outcomes. Future research and development in nerve transfer procedures should focus on specific reinnervation in all segments of the face.

References

1. Rozen SM. Facial reanimation: basic surgical tools and creation of an effective toolbox for treating patients with facial paralysis: part B. Nerve transfer combined with cross-facial nerve grafting in the acute facial palsy patient. Plast Reconstr Surg. 2017;139(3):725–7.
2. Terzis JK, Tzafetta K. The "babysitter" procedure: minihypoglossal to facial nerve transfer and cross-facial nerve grafting. Plast Reconstr Surg. 2009;123(3):865–76.
3. Zhang S, Hembd A, Ching CW, Tolley P, Rozen SM. Early masseter to facial nerve transfer may improve smile excursion in facial paralysis. Plast Reconstr Surg Glob Open. 2018;6(11):e2023.
4. Hontanilla B, Marre D. Comparison of hemihypoglossal nerve versus masseteric nerve transpositions in the rehabilitation of short-term facial paralysis using the Facial Clima evaluating system. Plast Reconstr Surg. 2012;130(5):662e–72e.
5. Scaramella LF. Anastomosis between the two facial nerves. Laryngoscope. 1975;85(8):1359–66.
6. Biglioli F, et al. Masseteric-facial nerve neurorrhaphy: results of a case series. J Neurosurg. 2017;126(1):312–8.
7. Hontanilla B, Marre D, Cabello A. Masseteric nerve for reanimation of the smile in short-term facial paralysis. Br J Oral Maxillofac Surg. 2014;52(2):118–23.
8. Rozen S, Harrison B. Involuntary movement during mastication in patients with long-term facial paralysis reanimated with a partial gracilis free neuromuscular flap innervated by the masseteric nerve. Plast Reconstr Surg. 2013;132(1):110e–6e.
9. Manktelow RT, Tomat LR, Zuker RM, Chang M. Smile reconstruction in adults with free muscle transfer innervated by the masseter motor nerve: effectiveness and cerebral adaptation. Plast Reconstr Surg. 2006;118(4):885–99.
10. Cheng A, Audolfsson T, Rodriguez-Lorenzo A, Wong C, Rozen S. A reliable anatomic approach for identification of the masseteric nerve. J Plast Reconstr Aesthet Surg. 2013;66(10):1438–40.
11. Rozen SM, et al. Intracranial facial nerve grafting in the setting of skull base tumors: global and regional facial function analysis and possible implications for facial reanimation surgery. Plast Reconstr Surg. 2016;137(1):267–78.
12. Bianchi B, Ferri A, Ferrari S, Copelli C, Magri A, Ferri T, Sesenna E. Cross-facial nerve graft and masseteric nerve cooptation for one-stage facial reanimation: principles, indications, and surgical procedure. Head Neck. 2014;36(2):235–40.

Vascularized Nerve Grafts in Facial Nerve Reconstruction

9

Eleonora O. F. Dimovska, Jorga Zabojova, and Andrés Rodríguez-Lorenzo

Key Points

- Nerves have predictable patterns of vascular supply.
- Non-vascularized nerve grafts rely on specific features of the graft and favorable conditions in the recipient bed for their survival.
- Vascularized nerve grafts yield superior histologic and functional outcomes to their non-vascularized counterparts, when used in hostile wound beds.
- Superior histologic and functional outcomes can be achieved by using motor nerves to bridge motor nerve gaps, rather than sensory nerves.
- The use of vascularized nerves as a component of chimeric free flaps should be considered in complex facial reconstructions when facial nerve gaps form part of the defect.

9.1 Introduction

Reconstructing a discontinuity in a nerve has several potential surgical solutions. Direct coaptation between the two divided ends is generally preferred, but is not always possible nor is it always able to yield the best outcome. Factors that should be considered when planning a nerve repair relate to the injured nerve itself (location of nerve, length of defect, type of injury, time since denervation), and its host patient (wound bed conditions, age, morbidity, compliance). The clinical circumstances around a nerve defect influence the decision of how to repair, as well as whether to repair at all.

Nerve repair and reconstruction has been studied for over 100 years, and our techniques have evolved in line with the development of a greater understanding of tissue blood supply, nerve anatomy, tissue transfer, and microsurgical techniques. Peripheral nerves and plexus injuries of the limbs have been vastly studied and serve as the basis for our understanding of nerve biology and nerve grafting today [1]. From conventional non-vascularized nerve grafting (NVNG), to pedicled vascularized nerve grafting (pedicled VNG), to free vascularized free nerve grafting (free VNG), the options for nerve reconstruction have evolved with methods to preserve blood supply. The introduction of nerve transfer on a vascular pedicle, technically converting it into a free flap, provides faster nerve regeneration than conventional non-vascularized nerve grafts and is clinically superior in cases where long nerve gaps exist. Ideal options for vascularized nerve transfer (VNG), without added donor morbidity, are limited and a consensus regarding worthy indications is lacking.

E. O. F. Dimovska (✉) · J. Zabojova
A. Rodríguez-Lorenzo
Department of Plastic and Maxillofacial Surgery, Uppsala University Hospital, Uppsala, Sweden
e-mail: andres.rodriguez.lorenzo@surgsci.uu.se, andres.rodriguez.lorenzo@akademiska.se

© Springer Nature Switzerland AG 2021
C.-H. J. Tzou, A. Rodríguez-Lorenzo (eds.), *Facial Palsy*, https://doi.org/10.1007/978-3-030-50784-8_9

Facial nerve defects present a relatively novel but significant indication for the application of free VNG. As one of the longest and more vulnerable of the cranial nerves, the facial nerve is relatively susceptible to damage in its extratemporal course. Facial trauma or, more commonly, deliberate resections in combination with parotidectomies for head and neck cancers leave patients with inevitable functional and aesthetic disfigurement. Oncological clearance is of course of primary concern, but as reconstructive microsurgery is becoming more sophisticated, neither patients nor surgeons willingly accept suboptimal primary reconstructions. Stand-alone nerve defects or those in combination with composite tissue defects have several operative solutions, of which vascularized nerve grafting offers a valuable and effective option to be considered.

9.2 A Historical Overview

Free nerve grafting was trialed as early as in 1870 when Phillipeaux and Vulpian grafted hypoglossal nerve defects with lingual nerve grafts in dogs [2, 3]. These were short defects with unfortunately mostly unsuccessful results. In 1876, Eduard Albert used a human tibial nerve from a freshly amputated leg to reconstruct a 3 cm median nerve defect in a human subject, but was unsuccessful in restoring function and sensibility [3]. Nerve grafting continued to be experimented with during the first and second world war, with varied success. The reason for its occasional failure was presumed to be inadequate blood supply. Experimental work began targeting understanding of nerve biology and to enhance the success rate of nerve grafting. It became clear that the length of defect and diameter of nerve played an important role in the survival of a nerve graft. It was postulated that a thin nerve graft spanning a short defect would survive better due to faster revascularization through the nerve. In 1939, Bunnell and Boyes trialed the concept of cable grafting to improve blood supply to a nerve graft [3]. By using multiple strands of thin nerves grouped together, instead of one large caliber nerve to bridge a nerve gap, they attempted to prevent nerve graft necrosis, but failed. Tension was also realized to be detrimental to blood flow and both Millesi and Terzis performed morphological and electrophysiologic studies in the early 1970s showing how tension in a nerve led to a decrease in blood supply and increase in fibrosis [4]. The progression of improving blood supply to nerve grafts and enabling longer nerve graft reconstructions was undertaken by Strange in 1947. He proposed a pedicled nerve graft; by preserving the blood supply to the nerve through its pedicle, he eliminated the need for vascular support from the wound bed [3]. By using the ulnar nerve as a pedicled vascularized nerve transfer, he managed to bridge a large median nerve gap successfully. Despite this huge breakthrough, there were obvious disadvantages to sacrificing large mixed nerves in the upper limbs. This limited the utility of Strange's technique.

Free vascularized nerve transfers were next in line in the advancement of nerve grafts, and in 1976 Taylor and Ham successfully performed the first autogenous vascularized nerve transplant of a 26 cm vascularized radial nerve graft to a median nerve defect in two patients with Volkmann's ischemic contracture [5]. Furthermore, they demonstrated how a vascularized nerve graft reinnervates at twice the rate to a conventional non-vascularized graft and described vascularization patterns of nerves. Terzis and Breidenbach also performed an extensive anatomical study in 1984 on the vascular supply of possible graftable nerves and proposed donor options most suitable for transplantation based on the dominance of its blood supply [3].

9.3 The Blood Supply of Nerves

In 1977, Lundborg described the blood supply to nerves as extrinsic and intrinsic—two integrated, but yet individually functioning systems [1]. The extrinsic system originates either from axial vessels providing perforators through the epineurium, or small perforating vessels from fascial, musculocutaneous, and periosteal vessels that enter the epineurium directly. Both are considered nutrient vessels to the nerve, but only axial vessels are large and dominant enough to serve as a pedicle on which one may base a potential free vascularized nerve transfer. The intrinsic blood supply consists of epineural, perineural, and endoneural plexuses arranged longitudinally across the nerve. The two systems connect through anastomosing vessels. Sunderland described the blood supply to nerves in 1945 as the *Vasa Nervorum,* but without distinguishing separate systems. Lundborg elaborated on Sunderland's description and showed how the extrinsic and intrinsic systems function independently of each other by performing experimental studies on rat tibial nerves. The intrinsic microcirculation in the nerve remained undisturbed across its entire length after dividing it from its external blood supply. This had huge implications for understanding nerve graft survival. However, the length of nerve capable of surviving a non-vascularized transfer was found to be limited, and later studies showed how an inadequate blood supply produced fibrosis and central necrosis of nerves.

The search for understanding the blood supply to nerves, and how one could transfer them vascularized, continued in 1984 as Terzis and Breidenbach carried out cadaveric dissections of commonly accessible peripheral nerves [3]. They dissected out their blood supply in order to determine the possibility for free vascularized nerve transfer. They dissected out between 20 and 25 samples of 13 different nerves from the upper and lower extremity. Blood supply was classified according to patterns Type I to IV, with a type II (and potentially type III) patterns considered most appropriate for the use in free vascularized nerve transfers (see Fig. 9.1). Type I nerves have no dominant pedicle and receive their blood supply from intrinsic vascular plexuses only, or from extrinsic perforators that enter the epineurium directly without running across the length of the nerve. Vessels available for transfer are thus of

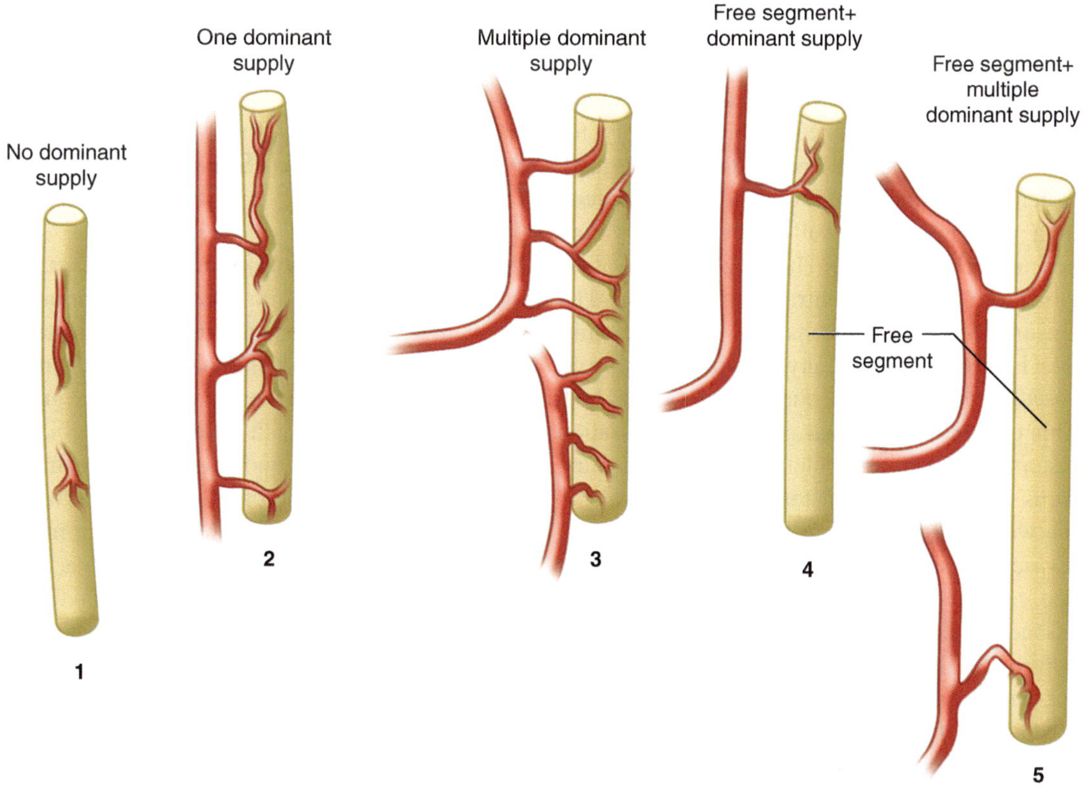

Fig. 9.1 Representation of classification of blood supply to nerves, types I-V [3]

small caliber or non-existent. Type II nerves have one dominant large caliber vessel running across the length of the nerve, supplying its epineurium with perforating vessels along its course. Type III nerves have multiple dominant pedicles. Type IV nerves have one dominant pedicle that supplies only a small portion of the nerve, leaving a larger distal portion unsupplied. Finally, type V nerves have multiple dominant pedicles, but intermittently large segments of the nerve are unsupplied. Nerves found to have a type II blood supply were the posterior cutaneous nerve of the thigh and the intercostal nerve. However, their small vessel size, small nerve diameter, and multiple nerve branching patterns made them unsuitable for most applications.

9.4 Evidence for Vascularized Nerve Grafts

9.4.1 Blood Supply

The evidence for improved functional outcomes with vascularized nerves has historically been contradictory, contributing to its cautious use. However, the significance of blood supply for nerve graft survival has been judiciously argued. A nerve graft transferred to a short nerve defect, in a thin nerve and well vascularized wound bed experiences faster healing and revascularization with less central graft necrosis [1]. Unsurprisingly, the mechanism of nerve graft take is similar to that of any graft take, relying on vascular supply from the surrounding wound bed. This type of conventional graft revascularization occurs mainly by inosculation (vessel sprouting from the graft and anastomosing to vessels in the wound bed), but is facilitated by centripetal revascularization (vessels from the surrounding bed growing into the graft) [6]. Timing is of the essence as these processes need to have started before distal muscle atrophy occurs, in order for successful nerve function to follow. Thus, VNG can offer benefits superior to traditional nerve grafting. The theoretical advantages are improved healing and faster axonal regeneration even in large nerve gaps in the face, thick nerves, and poorly vascularized wound beds.

Vascularized (VNG) and non-vascularized nerve grafts (NVNG) were compared in animal models in the 1980s, and later also examined in human subjects. Although initially little difference was identified between VNG and NVNG under favorable revascularization conditions, Koshima and Harii compared VNG and NVNG in scarred burn wound beds and showed that nerve conduction and axonal regeneration was faster in VNG [1]. Terzis et al. used the same principle and transplanted VNG and NVNG into acutely burnt rat thighs concluding histological superiority in VNG with greater number of axons, more mature myelin sheath, and larger diameter vessels [1]. Evidence also grew for the superiority of VNG in human subjects and in both scarred and normal vascular beds [1]. Rose et al. restored sensibility in scarred fingers by transplanting vascularized peroneal nerve grafts [7]. Doi et al. transplanted 25 cm long vascularized sural nerve grafts to 16 upper extremity defects and proved their survival using a monitoring skin paddle [8].

9.4.2 Motor Versus Sensory Nerve Grafts

With increasing scrutinization of function, an interest has developed in the effect of donor-to-recipient sensory versus motor nerve mismatch. Sensory nerves are commonly transplanted to motor nerve gaps. Peripheral sensory nerve grafts are easily accessible with little donor morbidity. The mismatch in the modality of nerve transplants is however of potential concern. When vascularized motor nerves are used for a motor nerve or mixed nerve defect, the outcomes have been found to be histologically superior to the outcomes seen with sensory nerves, in preclinical studies. Chu et al. performed a recent experimental study on rats comparing motor neuron survival and regeneration after transplanting peripheral sensory nerves and motor nerves in spinal root avulsions in rats [9]. They showed a higher neurotrophic percentage in the motor nerves and more motor neurons regenerating axons into the motor rather than the sensory nerves. Nichols et al. showed robust nerve regeneration and functional recovery in their study on rat tibial nerves when using motor and mixed nerve grafts, where sensory nerve grafts failed [10]. Brenner et al. supported these findings showing in their histological study how sensory nerve grafts impair nerve regeneration when grafted to mixed and motor nerves. Motor nerves clearly showed a higher nerve density and total fiber number with normal muscle mass compared to sensory nerve grafts [11].

9.5 Clinical Applications

9.5.1 The Dilemma

Finding a gold standard in facial nerve reconstruction is a challenge and a standardized reconstructive algorithm taking into account the etiology, degree of nerve defect, and potential associated tissue defect is lacking. Different experiences in both surgical techniques and patient outcomes continue to divide surgeon opinion on the management of facial nerve defects. There are currently no absolute indications for using VNGs options for facial reanimation. However, there are clinical situations where NVNG options could have inadequate regenerative potential and a VNG is technically feasible to attain and a valuable option to consider (Table 9.1).

Table 9.1 Suggested indications for vascularized nerve grafts for the facial nerve

Long nerve gap (>6 cm)
Defects requiring free flap reconstructions
Elderly patient
Poor local vascularity (radiation, prior infection, scarring)
Comorbidity
Smoking
Previously failed non-vascularized nerve graft

9.5.2 Facial Nerve Defects in the Head and Neck Cancer Patient

The ideal patient scenario for any nerve graft candidate would ideally be a young, healthy, non-smoker. The nerve recipient site should be free from radiation, infection, and scarring. The nerve defect should be short and present in a thin nerve. The nerve graft procedure should be performed immediately after resection. These combinations of ideal conditions are seldom met in the oncological setting. Segmental defects in the facial nerve commonly occur deliberately with parotidectomies, in head and neck cancer ablations. A general reconstructive consensus in this specific scenario is currently lacking and management differs widely internationally. Options are many and could include a combination of secondary versus immediate procedures, static methods versus nerve grafts, VNG versus NVNG, pedicled versus free nerve grafts, nerve transfers, stand-alone or combined procedures.

The head and neck cancer group presents the surgeon with several challenges, complicating the decision on how to reconstruct the facial nerve. Patients are often elderly and comorbid with a limited physiological reserve. In the case of comorbid patients, a history of smoking, diabetes, and alcohol are detrimental to healing. Advanced age further decreases nerve regeneration potential, and considering patients' already limited life expectancy, the commitment to a potentially long facial nerve recovery with a graft is often questioned. Ablative procedures leave long nerve gaps and often require radiotherapy, both obstacles to nerve regeneration, healing and good functional outcomes in conventional nerve grafting. It is thus often argued that secondary static procedures provide a faster and more predictable restoration of function than nerve grafts, and should be preferred. Despite achieving immediate symmetry, these procedures unfortunately fail to restore animation and spontaneity of the facial musculature.

Reducing time of denervation is important for success in nerve grafting. Areas with important functional and aesthetic muscular functions, such as the face, benefit from a faster reinnervation with a vascularized nerve graft and immediate post-resective reconstruction. This would reduce nerve ischemia and muscle denervation time, ultimately improving both the potential for and the speed of nerve regeneration. This type of approach to facial nerve reconstruction is of great value in head and neck cancer patients where nerve regeneration potential is often drastically reduced. Using a VNG in these patients can supersede the obstacle of poor regenerative potential due to age, morbidity, long nerve gaps, and radiotherapy. Thus, age should form part of an indication, rather than contra-indication, to vascularized nerve grafting.

9.6 Pedicled Nerve Graft Options

The pedicled nerve graft is one method of reconstructing a nerve defect with a nerve still attached to its blood supply. The first known nerve transposition of this kind was performed by Balance in 1895 when he successfully restored generalized facial nerve palsy in an 11-year-old boy (in whom he by accident severed the facial nerve during a middle ear operation) by transposing the spinal accessory nerve to the facial nerve stump in the middle ear [2]. Results were however suboptimal and morbidity from sacrificing the spinal accessory nerve was significant. Koshima et al. recently described the posterior auricular nerve, transposed to bridge a facial nerve gap after a schwannoma resection, and presented positive results [12]. Nerves from the cervical plexus, such as the lesser occipital nerve and the greater auricular nerve have also been used for pedicled nerve co-aptations, but apart from Koshima's technique, local nerves in the head and neck area are fairly unsuited for complete facial nerve reconstruction. More often, these nerves are used as adjuncts to assist in composite reconstructions, or to restore function in specific single nerve branches only. Also, most tumor-ablative nerve defects are long and more suited to a composite reconstruction. A more appropriate procedure is to aim for a synchronous restoration of both soft tissue integrity, volume and nerve function. Such a holistic reconstruction is gaining more popularity as nerves associated with common free flaps are harvested and used as chimeric flaps to bridge the facial nerve gap in the same sitting as the soft tissue fills in the remaining defect. Occasionally, some pedicled nerve transpositions are used as adjuncts to this technique, in order to improve outcomes. Two nerves commonly used like this today are the hypoglossal and masseter nerve transfers. Their use is described in previous chapters in this book (see Chap. 8).

9.7 Vascularized Nerve Grafts and the ALT Free Flap

The anterolateral thigh (ALT) flap is a well-known workhorse flap for head and neck reconstruction. Donor morbidity is minimal, even in the case of nerve harvest. The ALT carries possibilities to simultaneously harvest the adjacent lateral sensory nerve of the thigh or motor nerve to vastus lateralis as vascularized nerve grafts. The preserved blood supply improves survival despite long nerve gaps, radiotherapy, and patient age (poor regenerative potential). In addition, the ALT can serve as a multifaceted chimeric flap with harvest of skin/fat, muscle, and nerve, sophisticating reconstructive possibilities with improved synchronous reconstruction of skin envelope, volume, and nerve.

Kimata et al. described the concept of immediate post-ablative facial nerve reconstruction in 2005 using four such nerves in ten patients with parotid gland or cutaneous squamous cell tumors (with facial nerve gaps of 5–7 cm) [13]. He used the sural nerve, the deep peroneal nerve, the lateral femoral nerve (LFCN), and the vastus lateralis motor nerve (VLMN) with an ALT free flap. He faced heavy critique with regard to the small cohort and a result of only 6 in 10 patients partly regaining function after a significant post-operative time. It was argued that VNG offered no benefit over conventional NVNG. However, the interest of a synchronous multimodal reconstruction of radical post parotidectomy defects began to grow. Lida et al. published another trial of using the ALT with a LFCN in a 32-year-old man, this time with measurable and acceptable results at 14 months [2]. Kashiwa et al. presented another case in 2010, a 58-year-old man with function visible at 6 months post-operatively [14].

The possibilities of the ALT and combined VNG have in recent years been thoroughly anatomically and clinically studied, and the VLMN has gained popularity over the LFCN. As a motor nerve, it is suggested to propagate stronger facial nerve function than the LFCN, and its branching pattern facilitates anastomosis to several facial nerve branches. Its close proximity to the ALT vascular pedicle makes it ideal for synchronous harvest. The nerve was found to have multiple branches in variable patterns and relations to the pedicle. These branches, although of benefit in multiple facial nerve branch reconstructions, were found to mostly exit at a distal portion, unfavorably related to the ALT dissection and often necessitating a division. In addition, Kuo et al. found that division of several branches of the VLMN in the flap harvest was required in 22% of cases. Surprisingly, limb weakness was not always encountered or was found to improve over time. Initial explanations included redundancy of the nerve supply to the muscle or reinnervation. However, in 2015 Toia et al. expanded on the anatomical understanding of the relation of the VLMN to the vastus lateralis muscle, showing a segmental anatomy of the vastus lateralis muscle composed of three different muscle bellies, each supplied by their own neurovascular pedicle [15]. The superficial partition was found to be supplied by the descending branch of the lateral circumflex artery, the intermediate partition was found to be supplied by the oblique branch of the artery, and the deep partition had perforating branches supplying it from the deep femoral artery. The notion of segmental anatomy of the vastus lateralis was not new, but not previously evaluated in such anatomical precision. This advanced understanding of the anatomical architecture suggested options for selective neuro-muscular harvests with potentially decreased donor morbidity. The most important partitions to preserve were suggested to be the intermediate and deep partitions, due to their insertion into the patella and hence its influence on knee stability. Further to the findings by Toia et al., Agrogiannis et al. presented a cadaveric and radiologic study of the anatomy of the VLMN and found its branches to be arranged in oblique and descending patterns (See Fig. 9.2) [16]. The descending branch runs parallel with

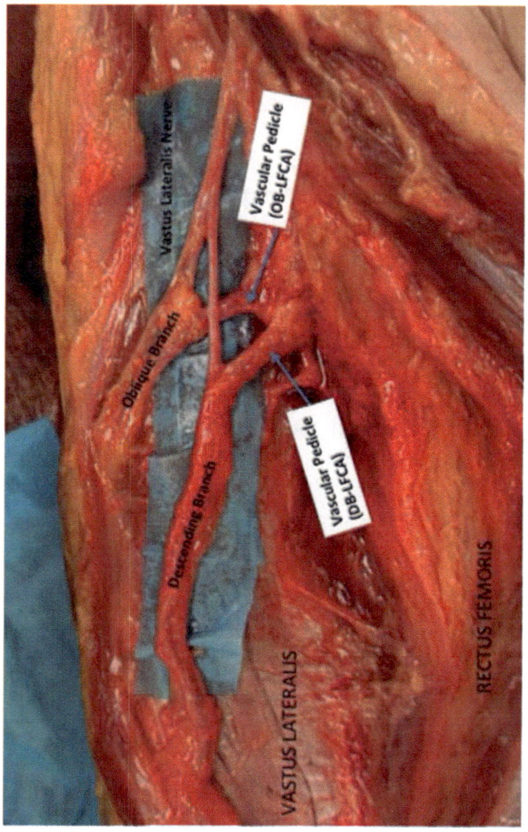

Fig. 9.2 Cadeveric dissection of the VLMN [16]. (*Authors Choice: "The One Stop Shop"*)

(and has a constant blood supply from) the lateral femoral circumflex artery, with the possibility of selectively being harvested without sacrificing the oblique branch. According to Toia et al., the descending branch would correlate with sacrificing the nerve to the superficial partition of the vastus lateralis, thereby achieving a composite free flap harvest with even further precision on decreasing donor morbidity.

In his own practice, the author uses the ALT free flap as a gold standard for composite hemifacial reconstructions and proposes a further modification to the nerve anastomotic techniques. Three cases are presented where the ALT is used as a composite flap with the VLMN coapted to a masseter nerve transfer to maximize reinnervation of the facial nerve. This serves to increase symmetry, but also strength of the smile in all vectors. The nerve anastomosis is performed end-to end—facial nerve branches are anastomosed in a united fashion, in an epineural repair onto the end of the VLMN.

9.8 Clinical Example of a Chimeric Free Flap Reconstruction of Soft Tissue and Facial Nerve

Operative course of a 61-year-old female with a large left sided basal cell carcinoma invading the parotid gland and facial nerve, which required resection.

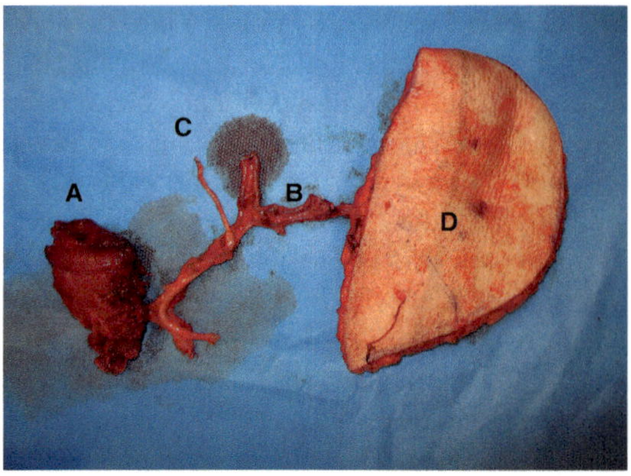

Intra-operative picture of harvested free chimeric anterolateral thigh flap. Vastus lateralis (a), vascular pedicle (b), vastus lateralis motor nerve (c), fasciocutaneous component (d).

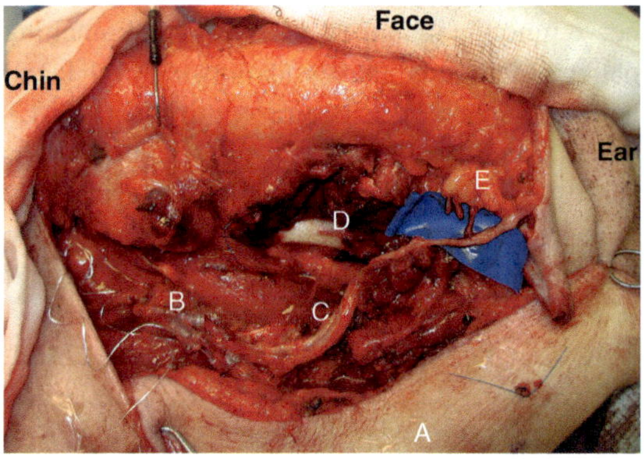

Intra-operative picture of the composite soft tissue and facial nerve reconstruction. The position of the chin, face, and ear are marked for orientation. The fasciocutaneous portion of the chimeric ALT (a) is shown along with the vascular anastomosis (b) and the vastus lateralis motor nerve (VLMN) (c). The masseter nerve (d) will be anastomosed to nerves innervating the smile. The VLMN will serve to bridge the gap between the facial nerve stump and the nerve branches to the orbicularis (e).

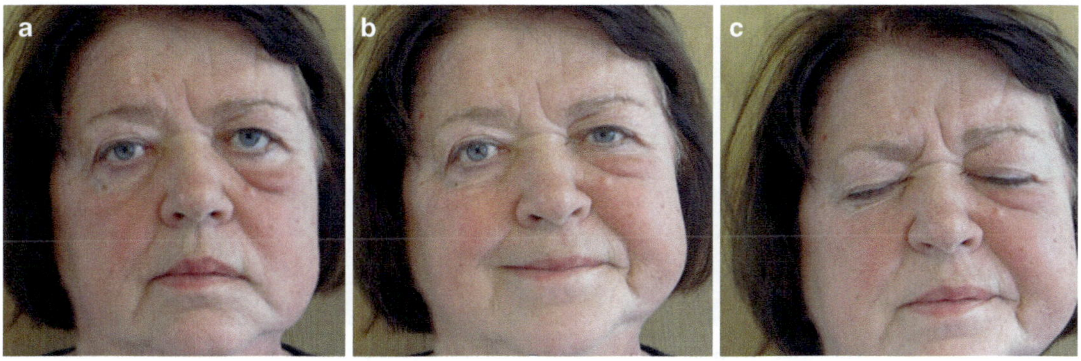

Functional result 1.5 years post-operative of a left sided chimeric free flap reconstruction of soft tissue and facial nerve. The patient has a symmetrical appearance in repose (a), with visible nasolabial fold, demonstrating a good resting tone. During animation, the patient can elevate her left commissure in a smile (b) and has good contraction of her orbicularis oculi (c).

9.9 Clinical Example of Vascularized Nerve Graft to the Marginal Mandibular Nerve

A 57-year-old man with a soft tissue sarcoma in the right jaw angle that underwent tumor resection including soft tissue, part of the mandible and the marginal mandibular branch, with a resulting nerve gap of 7.5 cm (figure a). Nerve reconstruction was performed with a vascularized vastus lateralis motor nerve graft along with a free anterolateral thigh flap. (Figure b, c) Follow-up at 15 months showed good symmetry and function in the lower lip depressors and mentalis (figure d–f).

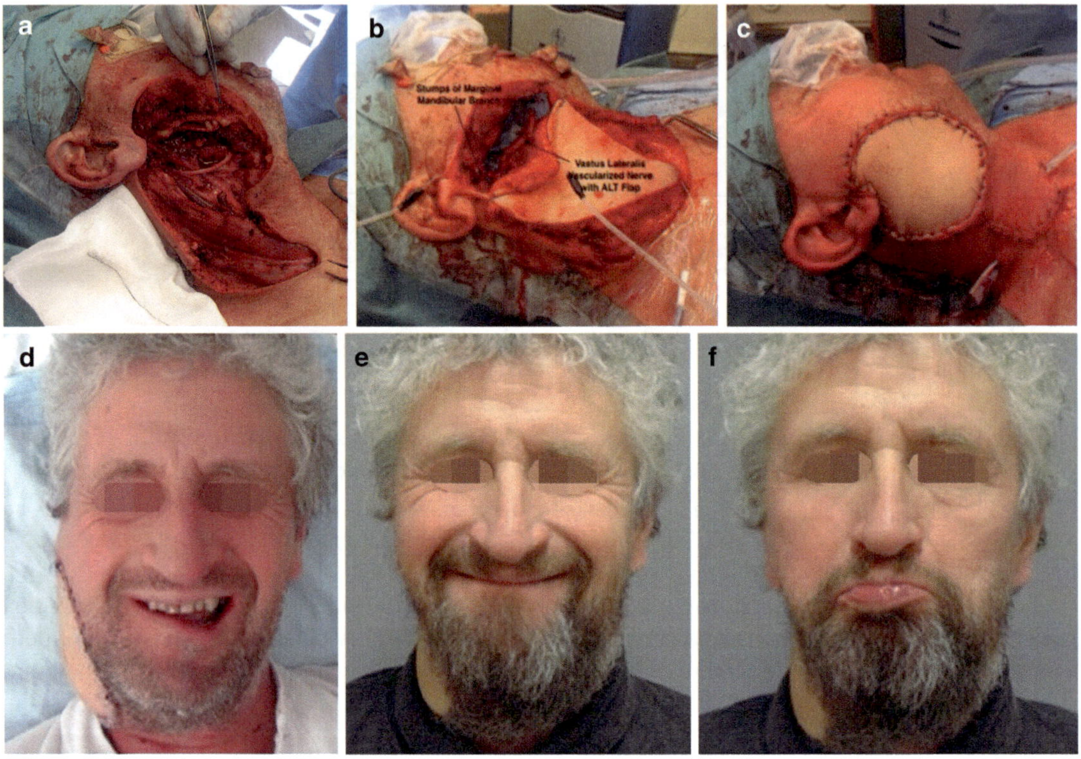

9.10 Conclusion

Nerve grafts (NVNGs) for the reconstruction of the facial nerve are cautiously used due to the increased time of reinnervation and results. Static procedures provide an instant and predictable result but fail to provide movement. A more sophisticated solution, such a vascularized nerve graft (VNG), can serve as an adjunct to the surgical repertoire of reconstructive options.

References

1. Terzis JK, Skoulis T, Soucacos P. Vascularized nerve grafts—a review. Int Angiol. 1995;14(3):264–77.
2. D'Arpa S, Claes KY, Stillaert F, Colebunders B, Monstrey S, Blondeel P. Vascularized nerve "grafts": just a graft or a worthwhile procedure? Plast Aesthetic Res. 2015;2(4):183. http://www.parjournal.net/text.asp?2015/2/4/183/160882.
3. Breidenbach W, Terzis JK. The anatomy of free vascularized nerve grafts. Clin Plast Surg. 1984;11(1):65–71.

4. Terzis J, Faibisoff B, Williams HB. The nerve gap: suture under tension vs. graft. Plast Reconstr Surg. 1975;56:166–70.
5. Taylor GI, Ham FJ. The free vascularized nerve graft. Plast Reconstr Surg. 1976;57:413–26.
6. Terzis JK, Kostopoulos VK. Vascularized ulnar nerve graft: 151 reconstructions for posttraumatic brachial plexus palsy. Plast Reconstr Surg. 2009;123(4):1276–91.
7. Rose E, Kowalski T, Norris M. The reversed venous arterialized nerve graft in digital nerve reconstruction across scarred beds. Plast Reconstr Surg. 1989;83(4):593–604.
8. Doi K, Tamaru K, Sakai K, Kuwata N, Kurafuji Y, Kawai S. A comparison of vascularized and conventional sural nerve grafts. J Hand Surg Am. 1992;17(4):670–6.
9. Wang W, Qi Z, Lin X, Hu Q, Dong J, Zhou L, et al. Neurovascular musculus obliquus internus abdominis flap free transfer for facial reanimation in a single stage. Plast Reconstr Surg. 2002;110:1430–40.
10. Nichols CM, Brenner MJ, Fox IK, Tung TH, Hunter DA, Rickman SR, et al. Effects of motor versus sensory nerve grafts on peripheral nerve regeneration. Exp Neurol. 2004;190(2):347–55. [cited 2018 Aug 20]. https://www.sciencedirect.com/science/article/pii/S0014488604003036?via%3Dihub.
11. Brenner MJ, Hess JR, Myckatyn TM, Hayashi A, Hunter DA, Mackinnon SE. Repair of motor nerve gaps with sensory nerve inhibits regeneration in rats. Laryngoscope. 2006;116(9):1685–92.
12. Koshima I, Nanba Y, Tsutsui T, Takahashi Y, Itoh S. New one-stage nerve pedicle grafting technique using the great auricular nerve for reconstruction of facial nerve defects. J Reconstr Microsurg. 2004;20(5):357–61.
13. Kimata Y, Sakuraba M, Hishinuma S, Ebihara S, Hayashi R, Asakage T. Free vascularized nerve grafting for immediate facial nerve reconstruction. Laryngoscope. 2005;115(2):331–6.
14. Kashiwa K, Kobayashi S, Nasu W, Kuroda T, Higuchi H. Facial nerve reconstruction using a vascularized lateral femoral cutaneous nerve graft based on the superficial circumflex iliac artery system: an application of the inferolateral extension of the groin flap. J Reconstr Microsurg. 2010;26(9):577–82.
15. Toia F, D'Arpa S, Brenner E, Melloni C, Moschella F, Cordova A. Segmental anatomy of the vastus lateralis: guidelines for muscle-sparing flap harvest. Plast Reconstr Surg. 2015;135(1):185e–98e.
16. Agrogiannis N, Rozen S, Reddy G, Audolfsson T, Rodriguez-Lorenzo A. Vastus lateralis vascularized nerve graft in facial nerve reconstruction: an anatomical cadaveric study and clinical implications. Microsurgery. 2015;35:135–9.

10 Non-vascularized Nerve Grafts

Benedikt M. Schwaiger and Chieh-Han John Tzou

10.1 Introduction

All dynamic procedures reconstructive surgery has to offer for the reanimation of the paralyzed face rely either on the restoration or the replacement of nerve and muscle function. Nerve grafts are an important part of the facial reanimation toolkit in situations where tensionless neurorrhaphy is not possible. Nerve grafts are necessary when the goal is to supply innervation—either to the mimic musculature or to muscle transplants, either from the ipsilateral facial nerve, the contralateral facial nerve or from other regional motor nerves. As the facial nerve is relatively small in diameter, thin nerves can be used for grafting. Provided the bed is sufficiently vascularized, which usually is the case in facial nerve reconstruction, the use of non-vascularized grafts is possible. It has been established as a trusted method since Bunnell first reported successful repair of the facial nerve with an interposition graft in 1930 [1]. Today, nerve grafts are commonly used to restore innervation from the facial nerve to the ipsilateral musculature as well as for nerve transfers. Cross-facial nerve grafting from the contralateral, non-paralyzed side takes a special role. Firstly, because it allows the restoration of spontaneous and emotional facial expression [2]. And secondly, the length of the nerve graft poses certain limitations which current research is trying to address. Nerve grafts provide a mechanical scaffolding for regenerating axons to reach the desired target organ. As important as the mechanical guidance offered by endoneurial tubes is, also biochemical effects appear to play a vital role for successful regeneration. Namely Schwann cells are thought to offer trophic support for regenerating axons, increasing the chances for successful reinnervation [3]. However, denervated Schwann cells, such as in nerve grafts and distal nerve stumps, undergo degenerative processes and cannot support nerve regeneration indefinitely [3, 4].

10.2 Donor Nerves

The most commonly harvested nerves for facial reanimation surgery are the sural nerve and the greater auricular nerve. But other alternatives have been described by various authors. Table 10.1

B. M. Schwaiger (✉)
Plastic and Reconstructive Surgery, Department of Surgery, Hospital of the Divine Savior Vienna (Krankenhaus Goettlicher Heiland), Vienna, Austria

C.-H. J. Tzou
Plastic and Reconstructive Surgery, Hospital of Divine Savior (Krankenhaus Goettlicher Heiland), Sigmund Freud University, TZOU MEDICAL, Vienna, Austria

Facial Palsy and Lymphedema Center Vienna, Vienna, Austria
e-mail: science@tzoumedical.com, science@tzou.at

© Springer Nature Switzerland AG 2021
C.-H. J. Tzou, A. Rodríguez-Lorenzo (eds.), *Facial Palsy*,
https://doi.org/10.1007/978-3-030-50784-8_10

Table 10.1 Donor nerves for autologous nerve grafting in facial reanimation

Donor nerve	Harvestable length	Diameter	Morbidity and limitations
Sural nerve	20–60 cm	3.5–3.8 mm	Numbness on the lateral edge of the foot
Greater auricular nerve	5–10 cm		Numbness of the lower third of the ear and angle of the mandible Visible scar on the side of the neck
Lateral antebrachial cutaneous nerve	5–20 cm		Numbness of the lateral forearm Visible scar on the forearm
Medial antebrachial cutaneous nerve	<28 cm	1.5–2 mm	Numbness of the medial arm Visible scar on the forearm
Saphenous nerve			Numbness of the medial calf Variable course, veno-nervous adhesions [5]
Lateral femoral cutaneous nerve			Numbness of the lateral thigh
Superficial radial nerve			Numbness of the back of the hand Visible scar on the forearm

summarizes some of the options mentioned in the literature for autologous nerve grafts.

10.2.1 Sural Nerve

The diameter of the sural nerve matches that of the facial nerve closely. And its exceptional length of up to 60 cm makes it the best option for long or numerous nerve grafts, such as cross-face nerve grafting (CFNG) or reconstruction of the parotid plexus. If necessary, the nerves from both legs can be harvested for multiple cross-face nerve grafts. The regional numbness resulting from nerve harvest is usually well tolerated [6]. Scar formation can be limited with a minimally invasive harvesting technique as described below. Other minimally invasive techniques have been described in the literature, including approaches using balloon dissection or endoscopic instruments [7, 8]. The location of the nerve far from the primary surgical field enables a second surgical team to harvest the nerve during preparation of the nerve stumps by the primary team. If only one nerve is going to be harvested, there is no reason to prefer either side apart from the patient's and surgeon's preference.

10.2.1.1 Surgical Technique for Sural Nerve Harvest

The sural nerve can be located through a small incision posterior to the lateral malleolus. It is found by blunt dissection just below the skin 1–2 cm posterior to the malleolus and runs superficial to the fascia in close vicinity to the small saphenous vein. After dissecting the nerve from the subcutaneous tissue proximally and distally it can be transected sharply and should be marked with a suture. Then a vein stripper is introduced into the incision and over the nerve. With extreme caution the instrument is guided along the expected path of the nerve, between the bellies of the gastrocnemius muscle, and towards the popliteal fossa. If unexpected resistance is encountered along the path of dissection, additional horizontal incisions can be placed while using the head of the vein stripper to protect the nerve. Ultimately, an incision is placed to transect the nerve proximally. The graft is set aside wrapped in sterile gauze moistened with saline solution. Rozen et al. stated that they neurolyze the harvested sural nerve internally to create two full-length cross-face nerve grafts from a single donor nerve [9].

The literature holds differing opinions from various authors, whether sural nerve grafts should be placed keeping their orientation or reversing it [10–16]. The advocates of maintaining the natural orientation theorize that it facilitates axon regeneration while the proponents of reversing the graft fear the loss of regenerating axons through lateral branches of the sural nerve. However, there have been no comparative outcome-based studies that provide sufficient evidence to favor one hypothesis over the other.

10.2.2 Greater Auricular Nerve

The greater auricular nerve is often used as an interposition graft in facial nerve repair or as a jump graft in regional nerve transfer. Its length of less than 10 cm and extensive branching make it unfit for cross-face nerve grafting. The branching pattern, however, has led some authors to advocate its use in replacing the parotid plexus [11, 17]. Access to the nerve is gained through an incision over the sternocleidomastoid muscle, which makes it a favorable option in cases of concomitant neck dissection. The nerve runs deep to the platysma and can best be located at the nerve point of the neck, sometimes referred to as Erb's point, at the posterior border of the sternocleidomastoid muscle. From there it can be dissected cranially along its course towards the ear.

10.2.3 Motor Nerves

Brenner et al. were able to show in an animal model that the histomorphometric markers of regeneration are consistently superior in nerve repair with grafts taken from motor nerves rather than from sensory nerves [18]. Moradzadeh et al. confirmed these findings and furthermore observed that also the functional outcomes as well as the wet muscle mass of the target muscle showed a trend towards better regeneration after nerve repair with motor nerve grafts [19]. Their findings might be able to contribute to an explanation why the outcome of nerve grafting is inferior to direct repair. In humans, however, harvesting motor nerves of adequate length and diameter to fulfill the requirements of facial nerve repair would lead to inacceptable donor site morbidity. In recent years, cadaveric nerve allografts have shown positive results in reconstruction of peripheral nerves. Currently, the use of cadaveric allografts for facial reanimation is still rarely reported and comparative studies of autografts and allografts in humans are not yet available [20, 21].

10.3 Ipsilateral Nerve Repair

Repair of the injured facial nerve is preferably performed by coaptation of the nerve stumps and direct suture. If nerve stumps can be identified but the gap cannot be closed without tension, either because of retraction or because of an extensive defect, interposition grafting allows restoration of the innervation of the mimic muscles. Depending on the etiology, location, and extent of the nerve injury, a number of grafting techniques are at the disposal of the reconstructive surgeon. The choice of nerve graft depends on the length of the defect as well as on concomitant surgeries.

In cases where the facial nerve is thought to be anatomically intact and spontaneous recovery is expected, it is difficult to decide when nerve repair is best planned. It is known that early repair leads to superior results [22, 23]. Therefore, surgeons strive for an early decision but there is a lack of reliable prognostic factors. In case of partial recovery, a functional augmentation as described below may be considered rather than ipsilateral repair risking the partially regained function.

Segmental repair, i.e., grafting to restore individual branches of the facial nerve distal to the parotid plexus generally produces good outcomes with low risk for synkinesia [24]. Injuries involving the main trunk of the facial nerve, however, involve a high risk of aberrant innervation by regenerating axons. It is known for peripheral nerves that the fascicular anatomy can change significantly over short distances within the nerve [25, 26]. In a recent study, we found that the same is true for the extracranial trunk of the facial nerve, suggesting that after resection or debridement of even a short portion of the nerve, fascicles cannot be identified and coapted reliably. Some authors have suggested the use of fascicular repair with perineural sutures rather than epineural sutures; however, there is no conclusive evidence for superiority in facial nerve grafting.

10.4 Cross-Face Nerve Grafts

Since the procedure of supplying paralyzed facial muscles with neural input from the contralateral side of the face was first published in the 1970s by Scaramella and Smith independently, it has become the staple of facial reanimation. During its history, the procedure has been refined and adapted by different surgeons in slightly differing ways, but the basic principle remains the same: Innervation from the contralateral, healthy side is transferred to the paralyzed side of the face via nerve grafts across the midline. On the paralyzed side, the target of innervation can be either the native mimic musculature or free functional muscle transplants. This technique is used in patients who do not have a viable ipsilateral nerve stump. Patients must be willing to undergo the two stages necessary to complete the procedure and further surgeries may be needed nevertheless.

In CFNGs (cross-face nerve grafts), the speed of axon regeneration has been observed to average 1.8 mm per day [27]. Taking into consideration the length of facial nerve grafts, often exceeding 10–15 cm, it is obvious that considerable time will elapse before muscular function can be expected to return. This delay until regenerating axons reach the distal end of the graft must be considered when planning the procedure. If the onset of paralysis is fairly recent or the paralysis is incomplete, the mimic muscles are likely viable for reinnervation from the contralateral side. A cut-off of 6 months has been widely accepted for CFNG as a standalone procedure for complete paralysis [28, 29]. For paralyses of longer duration, so called *babysitter* procedures combining CFNG (for emotional expression) and regional nerve transfers from the ipsilateral hypoglossal or masseteric nerve (for early and powerful motor innervation) are widely used [28, 30]. In doubt, electromyography (EMG) of the target muscles can guide decision-making. Fibrillations on EMG indicate susceptibility of the musculature for reinnervation [31]. After 18 months to 2 years of denervation, facial muscles must be expected to have become atrophied beyond viability for reinnervation. Therefore, in these cases CFNGs can be combined with a free functional muscle transfer to replace muscular function of the midface, the eye, or both [32, 33]. Muscle transplants can also be added in a salvage procedure, when primary cross-face nerve grafting does not produce the desired improvement [32].

CFNG has become widely accepted as the standard for restoration of spontaneous and emotional smile. It is therefore most commonly used in reanimating the corner of the mouth and the nasolabial fold. For reanimation of the forehead, brow, and lower lip, CFNG has not proven as a reliable source of innervation and is usually foregone in favor of other procedures to improve symmetry. For restoration of blink and eye closure, long regeneration periods after CFNG render other procedures more attractive, like temporalis muscle transfer or eyelid loading surgeries. Nevertheless, Terzis et al. have reported good results for eye closure after direct neurotization of the native orbicularis oculi muscle by CFNG as well as with platysma transfer innervated by CFNG [34]. Biglioli et al. similarly reported good results with platysma transplants innervated by CFNG combined with lower eyelid suspension [33]. Frey et al. proposed that a territorially differentiated gracilis muscle transplant innervated by CFNGs to restore smile as well as eye closure is the preferable option in children or in adult patients when temporalis transfer to the eye is not possible [35].

Advanced patient age has been found to correlate with decreased regeneration rates as well as a decreased axon count in potential donor nerves, which could adversely affect functional regeneration [27, 36]. These findings should be taken into consideration when discussing the management with elderly patients.

10.4.1 Timing of Surgery

Cross-face nerve grafting is usually performed in two stages. In the first stage, the donor nerves on the healthy side are identified and long sural nerve grafts are placed through a subcutaneous tunnel created by blunt dissection. A small incision is made in the midline, either intraorally in the upper lip or in the bottom of the nasal cavity, to facilitate the inflection of the tunnel towards the paralyzed side. The graft is placed in overlength and marked by nonabsorbable sutures on the paralyzed side for easier identification during the second stage. The proximal end of the graft is then approximated to a transected donor branch and coapted using 10-0 nonabsorbable epineural sutures.

The second stage can usually be planned around 6–9 months after the first surgery. Axonal outgrowth can be observed by monitoring Tinel's sign. Percussion along the course of the nerve graft will produce a tingling sensation over the frontier of regenerating axons. When sufficient time has elapsed and Tinel's sign has progressed to the distal end of the nerve graft, the graft can be coapted on the paralyzed side. After identification of the nerve graft, the distal neuroma is resected before suturing the CFNG to the recipient nerve. As described above, the CFNG can be anastomosed to facial nerve branches supplying the native facial muscles or to a muscle transplant which is placed at the time of the second stage.

Additional static procedures such as suspensions or eyelid loading can be performed simultaneously with these two surgeries. Subsequent corrective surgeries may become necessary nevertheless after awaiting the functional results of the CFNG procedure.

10.4.2 Donor Branch Selection

To supply innervation to the paralyzed side, branches of the healthy contralateral facial nerve must be identified and transected. A modified preauricular facelift incision is used to elevate the skin and the superficial musculoaponeurotic system on the healthy side. Branches of the facial nerve can be identified at the anterior border of the parotid gland. Zygomatic branches supplying movement to the corner of the mouth and upper lip usually emerge 2 cm below the zygomatic arch, halfway between the tragus and the corner of the mouth. For identification and selection of suitable donor branches, electrical stimulation is used. Therefore, it is important that either no muscle relaxant is used for this procedure or that the effect of the muscle relaxant is antagonized in advance. The goal is to find redundant, but specific branches for the desired function with minimal synkinesis on stimulation. In a cadaveric study, Hembd et al. have shown that all individuals had at least two redundant branches per territory [37]. Intuitively, surgeons might tend towards sacrificing smaller branches for nerve grafting but it has been shown that increased axonal load of donor nerves correlates with better results. Terzis et al. have proposed that an axon count greater than 900 characterizes donor nerve branches with excellent potential for regeneration [38]. Since determining the axon count intraoperatively is not possible, Hembd et al. have sought to provide useful anatomical landmarks for donor nerve selection. They report that a branch with an axonal load greater than 900 can be found in all individuals after short retrograde intraparotid dissection of less than 1 cm [37]. Since they based their findings on examination of cadaveric specimens, nothing is known about the specificity of these branches. Ultimately, electrical nerve stimulation should be used to identify the largest redundant branch which does not produce synkinesis. A diameter greater than 0.6 mm predicts an axonal load of 900 or more in that branch [37]. When selecting a redundant branch as donor for the contralateral side, transient muscle weakness on the healthy side must be expected, but normal amplitudes of facial motions are usually regained [15, 39].

10.4.3 Augmentation of Partial Function

Frey et al. have proposed the use of cross-face-nerve grafting with distal end-to-side neurorrhaphy to "supercharge" residual or partially regenerated innervation in incomplete paralyses [10]. The procedure is characterized by coaptation of the distal end of a CFNG to a facial nerve branch on the paralyzed side through a fenestration in the epineurium without transecting the recipient nerve. Thus, it is expected to upgrade neural input without sacrificing the partial function. In the initial case series, Frey et al. reported increased symmetry of the smile after distal end-to-side neurorrhaphy [10, 40].

10.4.4 Sensory Pathway Protection

A novel approach addressing the issue of exceptionally long grafts in cross-face grafting involves the coaptation of sensory nerves to the nerve graft [41, 42]. The proposed mechanism is that sensory neurons populate the nerve graft and keep the distal denervated graft viable for regeneration of the motor nerve axons [41, 43, 44]. Placheta et al. observed superior outcomes after end-to-side sensory pathway protection of CFNGs in rats [41]. And Catapano et al. reported promising results after end-to-end coaptation of an infraorbital nerve branch to the distal end of a CFNG in five patients [42]. Furthermore, they found no detectable loss of sensory function after sacrificing small branches of the infraorbital nerve. When sensory protection by infraorbital nerve is planned, the CFNG should be tunneled through the upper lip. The infraorbital nerve can be identified and anastomosed to the graft through an intraoral incision above the canine tooth on the paralyzed side.

10.5 Coaptation Techniques

Microsutures using 8-0, 10-0, or even finer sutures have long been the undisputed standard to affix nerve stumps and nerve grafts and continue to be the most prevalent method of coaptation in extracranial facial nerve repair. However, in recent years the use of fibrin tissue adhesives or "fibrin glue" has gained traction, especially in intracranial facial nerve repair. Fibrin tissue adhesive consists of two separate components, fibrinogen and thrombin. The components are combined to mimic a physiological blood clot creating a bond between tissues. Since good comparative studies of different methods of coaptation for facial nerve grafting in humans are not available, the following insights are based on research in animal models.

Early reports in the literature attributed inferior electrophysiologic and histomorphometric outcomes to the use of fibrin glue [45, 46]. Yet more recent research mostly demonstrates equal or superior electrophysiological, histomorphometric, and even functional results after nerve repair and nerve grafting with fibrin glue [47–50]. The risk of dehiscence appears to be equal to that of conventional nonabsorbable sutures in the more recent studies [47, 49, 51]. The coaptation side can be secured by wrapping it in a fascial graft and securing it with additional adhesive. Furthermore, coaptation with fibrin glue is consistently reported to be quicker than microsutures. Whitlock et al. showed that the microsurgical experience of the surgeon greatly influences the outcome of nerve repair with epineural sutures but less so the outcome after coaptation with fibrin glue [51]. Therefore, although microsutures are an excellent option for experienced microsurgeons, the use of fibrin glue may be preferable in novice surgeons or in centers where microsurgical neurorrhaphy is performed infrequently.

Laser welding of coaptation sites has been proposed as another alternative to epineural sutures. Menovsky et al. have reported comparable outcomes after CO_2 laser welding and suturing [49]. The technique they describe still uses sutures to secure the coaptation site, however. Therefore, the advantage is unclear. Evidence for the safety and efficacy of laser welding in facial nerve repair in humans is lacking and does not allow a recommendation.

References

1. May M, Schaitkin BM. History of facial nerve surgery. Facial Plast Surg. 2001;16(4):301–7.
2. Chuang DC-C, Lu JC-Y, Chang TN-J, Laurence VG. Comparison of functional results after cross-face nerve graft-, spinal accessory nerve-, and masseter

nerve-innervated gracilis for facial paralysis reconstruction: the Chang Gung experience. Ann Plast Surg. 2018;81(6S Suppl 1):S21–9.
3. Sulaiman O, Gordon T. Effects of short and long term Schwann cell denervation on peripheral nerve regeneration, myelination, and size. Glia. 2000;32(3):234–46.
4. Sulaiman OAR, Gordon T. Role of chronic Schwann cell denervation in poor functional recovery after nerve injuries and experimental strategies to combat it. Neurosurgery. 2009;65(Suppl 4):105–14.
5. Dayan V, Cura L, Cubas S, Carriquiry G. Surgical anatomy of the saphenous nerve. Ann Thorac Surg. 2008;85(3):896–900.
6. Martins RS, Barbosa RA, Siqueira MG, Soares MS, Heise CO, Foroni L, et al. Morbidity following sural nerve harvesting: a prospective study. Clin Neurol Neurosurg. 2012;114(8):1149–52.
7. Koh KS, Park S. Endoscopic harvest of sural nerve graft with balloon dissection. Plast Reconstr Surg. 1998;101(3):810–2.
8. Oliveira MT, Marttos ACJ, Fallopa F. Endoscopic harvesting of the sural nerve graft: a cadaveric investigation. Orthopedics. 2000;23(11):1189–91.
9. Rozen SM. Facial reanimation: basic surgical tools and creation of an effective toolbox for treating patients with facial paralysis: part B. Nerve transfer combined with cross-facial nerve grafting in the acute facial palsy patient. Plast Reconstr Surg. 2017;139(3):725–7.
10. Frey M, Giovanoli P, Michaelidou M. Functional upgrading of partially recovered facial palsy by cross-face nerve grafting with distal end-to-side neurorrhaphy. Plast Reconstr Surg. 2006;117(2):597–608.
11. Sainsbury D, Borschel G, Zuker R. Surgical reanimation techniques for facial palsy/paralysis. In: Fagan J, editor. Open access atlas of otolaryngology, head & neck operative surgery [Internet]; 2008. p. 1–30. www.entdev.uct.ac.za.
12. Tate JR, Tollefson TT. Advances in facial reanimation. Curr Opin Otolaryngol Head Neck Surg. 2006;14(4):242–8.
13. Celis-Aguilar E, Lassaletta L, Roda JM, Gavilán J. End-to-side interposed donor grafting as a facial nerve reinforcement technique after vestibular schwannoma surgery. Ann Otol Rhinol Laryngol. 2013;122(8):520–3.
14. Nakatsuka H, Takamatsu K, Koshimune M, Imai Y, Enomoto M, Yamano Y. Experimental study of polarity in reversing cable nerve grafts. J Reconstr Microsurg. 2002;18(6):509–15.
15. Anderl H. Cross-face nerve transplantation in facial palsy. Proc R Soc Med. 1976;69(10):781–3.
16. Sahovaler A, Yeh D, Yoo J. Primary facial reanimation in head and neck cancer. Oral Oncol. 2017;74:171–80. https://doi.org/10.1016/j.oraloncology.2017.08.013.
17. Rabie AN, Ibrahim AMS, Kim PS, Medina M, Upton J, Lee BT, et al. Dynamic rehabilitation of facial nerve injury: a review of the literature. J Reconstr Microsurg. 2013;29(5):283–96. http://www.ncbi.nlm.nih.gov/pubmed/23564297.
18. Brenner MJ, Hess JR, Myckatyn TM, Hayashi A, Hunter DA, Mackinnon SE. Repair of motor nerve gaps with sensory nerve inhibits regeneration in rats. Laryngoscope. 2006;116(9):1685–92.
19. Moradzadeh A, Borschel GH, Luciano JP, Elizabeth L, Hayashi A, Hunter DA, et al. The impact of motor and sensory nerve architecture on nerve regeneration. Exp Neurol. 2008;212(2):370–6. https://doi.org/10.1016/j.expneurol.2008.04.012.
20. Carlson TL, Wallace RD, Konofaos P. Cadaveric nerve allograft. Single center's experience in a variety of peripheral nerve injuries. Ann Plast Surg. 2018;80:S328–32. http://insights.ovid.com/crossref?an=00000637-201806006-00003.
21. Gunn S, Cosetti M, Roland JT. Processed allograft: novel use in facial nerve repair after resection of a rare facial nerve paraganglioma. Laryngoscope. 2010;120(Suppl 4):2009.
22. Terzis JK, Konofaos P. Experience with 60 adult patients with facial paralysis secondary to tumor extirpation. Plast Reconstr Surg. 2012;130(1):51–66.
23. Özmen ÖA, Falcioni M, Lauda L, Sanna M. Outcomes of facial nerve grafting in 155 cases: predictive value of history and preoperative function. Otol Neurotol. 2011;32(8):1341–6.
24. Bascom DA, Schaitkin BM, May M, Klein S. Facial nerve repair: a retrospective review. Facial Plast Surg. 2000;16(4):309–13. http://www.ncbi.nlm.nih.gov/pubmed/11460296.
25. Lundborg G. Nerve regeneration and repair: a review. Acta Orthop. 1987;58(2):145–69.
26. Sunderland S. The intraneural topography of the radial, median and ulnar nerves. Brain. 1945;68(4):243–98.
27. Braam MJI, Nicolai JA. Axonal regeneration rate through cross-face nerve grafts. Microsurgery. 1993;14(9):589–91.
28. Terzis JK, Konofaos P. Nerve transfers in facial palsy. Facial Plast Surg. 2008;24(2):177–93.
29. Kim L, Byrne PJ. Controversies in contemporary facial reanimation. Facial Plast Surg Clin North Am. 2016;24(3):275–97. https://doi.org/10.1016/j.fsc.2016.03.016.
30. Terzis JK, Tzafetta K. The "babysitter" procedure: Minihypoglossal to facial nerve transfer and cross-facial nerve grafting. Plast Reconstr Surg. 2009;123(3):865–76.
31. Boahene K. Facial reanimation after acoustic neuroma resection: options and timing of intervention. Facial Plast Surg. 2015;31(2):103–9.
32. Frey M, Michaelidou M, Tzou CH, Hold A, Pona I, Placheta E. [Proven and innovative operative techniques for reanimation of the paralyzed face]. Handchir Mikrochir Plast Chir. 2010;42(2):81–9. http://www.ncbi.nlm.nih.gov/pubmed/20178074.
33. Biglioli F, Zago M, Allevi F, Ciprandi D, Dell'Aversana Orabona G, Pucciarelli V, et al. Reanimation of the paralyzed lids by cross-face nerve graft and platysma transfer. J Craniomaxillofacial Surg. 2018;46(3):398–412. https://doi.org/10.1016/j.jcms.2017.12.022.

34. Terzis JK, Bruno W. Outcomes with eye reanimation microsurgery. Facial Plast Surg. 2002;18(2):101–12.
35. Frey M, Giovanoli P, Tzou CHJ, Kropf N, Friedl S. Dynamic reconstruction of eye closure by muscle transposition or functional muscle transplantation in facial palsy. Plast Reconstr Surg. 2004;114(4):865–75.
36. Hembd A, Nagarkar P, Perez J, Gassman A, Tolley P, Reisch J, et al. Correlation between facial nerve axonal load and age and its relevance to facial reanimation. Plast Reconstr Surg. 2017;139(6):1459–64.
37. Hembd A, Nagarkar PA, Saba S, Wan D, Kutz JW, Isaacson B, et al. Facial nerve axonal analysis and anatomical localization in donor nerve: optimizing axonal load for cross-facial nerve grafting in facial reanimation. Plast Reconstr Surg. 2017;139(1):177–83.
38. Terzis JK, Wang W, Zhao Y. Effect of axonal load on the functional and aesthetic outcomes of the cross-facial nerve graft procedure for facial reanimation. Plast Reconstr Surg. 2009;124(5):1499–512.
39. Cooper TM, McMahon B, Lex C, Lenert JJ, Johnson PC. Cross-facial nerve grafting for facial reanimation: effect on normal hemiface motion. J Reconstr Microsurg. 1996;12(2):99–103. http://www.ncbi.nlm.nih.gov/pubmed/8656408.
40. Fattah A, Borschel GH, Zuker RM. Reconstruction of facial nerve injuries in children. J Craniofac Surg. 2011;22(3):782–8.
41. Placheta E, Wood MD, Lafontaine C, Liu EH, Hendry JM, Angelov DN, et al. Enhancement of facial nerve motoneuron regeneration through cross-face nerve grafts by adding end-to-side sensory axons. Plast Reconstr Surg. 2015;135(2):460–71.
42. Catapano J, Demsey DRB, Ho ES, Zuker RM, Borschel GH. Cross-face nerve grafting with infraorbital nerve pathway protection. Plast Reconstr Surg Glob Open. 2016;4(9):e1037. http://insights.ovid.com/crossref?an=01720096-201609000-00022.
43. Bain JR, Veltri KL, Chamberlain D, Fahnestock M. Improved functional recovery of denervated skeletal muscle after temporary sensory nerve innervation. Neuroscience. 2001;103(2):503–10.
44. Ladak A, Schembri P, Olson J, Udina E, Tyreman N, Gordon T. Side-to-side nerve grafts sustain chronically denervated peripheral nerve pathways during axon regeneration and result in improved functional reinnervation. Neurosurgery. 2011;68(6):1654–65.
45. Moy OJ, Peimer CA, Koniuch MP, Howard C, Zielezny M, Katikaneni PR. Fibrin seal adhesive, versus nonabsorbable microsuture in peripheral nerve repair. J Hand Surg Am. 1988;13(2):273–8. https://doi.org/10.1016/S0363-5023(88)80063-7.
46. Maragh H, Meyer BS, Davenport D, Gould JD, Terzis JK. Morphofunctional evaluation of fibrin glue versus microsuture nerve repairs. J Reconstr Microsurg. 1990;6(4):331–7.
47. Ornelas L, Padilla L, Di Silvio M, Schalch P, Esperante S, Infante PL, et al. Fibrin glue: an alternative technique for nerve coaptation—part I. Wave amplitude, conduction velocity, and plantar-length factors. J Reconstr Microsurg. 2006;22(2):119–22. http://www.ncbi.nlm.nih.gov/pubmed/16456772.
48. Sameem M, Wood TJ, Bain JR. A systematic review on the use of fibrin glue for peripheral nerve repair. Plast Reconstr Surg. 2011;127(6):2381–90.
49. Menovsky T, Beek JF. Laser, fibrin glue, or suture repair of peripheral nerves: a comparative functional, histological, and morphometric study in the rat sciatic nerve. J Neurosurg. 2001;95(4):694–9. http://www.ncbi.nlm.nih.gov/pubmed/11596965.
50. Ramos DS, Bonnard D, Franco-Vidal V, Liguoro D, Darrouzet V. Stitchless fibrin glue-aided facial nerve grafting after cerebellopontine angle schwannoma removal: technique and results in 15 cases. Otol Neurotol. 2015;36(3):498–502.
51. Whitlock EL, Kasukurthi R, Yan Y, Tung TH, Hunter DA, Mackinnon SE. Fibrin glue mitigates the learning curve of microneurosurgical repair. Microsurgery. 2010;30(3):218–22.

11 Avoiding Damage of the Facial Nerve in Parotid Surgery

Stefan Janik and Boban M. Erovic

Key Points

- Temporary and permanent facial palsy occurs in 10–66% to 2.5–8.0% of cases.
- The marginal mandibular branch is at most risk for injury during parotidectomy.
- Risk for facial palsy increases with extend of parotidectomy.
- Be aware of anatomic landmarks during dissection to avoid damage of the facial nerve.
- The posterior belly of digastric muscle, the tragal pointer, and the tympanomastoid suture line represent the three key anatomic landmarks for identification of the extratemporal main trunk of the facial nerve.

11.1 Introduction

Iatrogenic facial nerve injuries account for approximately 7% of facial palsy (FP) [1]. Among them, temporomandibular joint surgeries are the most common procedures associated with facial nerve injuries (2.2%), followed by parotid surgery (1.5%), and tympanomastoidectomy (0.8%) [1]. With regard to parotid surgery, temporary FP occurs in 10–66% of patients after primary parotid surgery, while permanent FP is less common and occurs in 2.5–8.0% of cases [2]. The marginal mandibular branch is at most risk for injury during parotidectomy [2].

11.2 Type of Parotidectomy

Extend of parotidectomy and consequently risk of temporary or permanent FP depend on type of parotidectomy, which are classified into extracapsular dissection (ECD), superficial parotidectomy, and total parotidectomy (see Table 11.1). Moreover, procedures requiring resection or sacrification of the facial nerve due to oncological purpose are classified as radical parotidectomies. In daily clinical practice, the parotid gland is differentiated into a superficial (lateral) and a deep (medial) lobe seperated by the facial nerve.

S. Janik
Department of Otolaryngology, Head and Neck Surgery, Medical University of Vienna, Vienna, Austria
e-mail: stefan.janik@meduniwien.ac.at

B. M. Erovic (✉)
Department of Otolaryngology, Head and Neck Surgery, Medical University of Vienna, Vienna, Austria

Institute of Head and Neck Diseases, Evangelical Hospital Vienna, Vienna, Austria
e-mail: b.erovic@ekhwien.at

© Springer Nature Switzerland AG 2021
C.-H. J. Tzou, A. Rodríguez-Lorenzo (eds.), *Facial Palsy*,
https://doi.org/10.1007/978-3-030-50784-8_11

Table 11.1 Association between type of parotidectomy, extend of surgery, and facial palsy [2–4, 7]

Type of parotidectomy	Identification of the facial nerve	Extend of parotidectomy	Rate of temporary FP (%)	Rate of permanent FP (%)
Extracapsular dissection	–	Part of the superficial lobe	0.0–11.4	1.4–2.2
Superficial parotidectomy	+	Superficial lobe	10.6–20.4	0.6–10.9
Total parotidectomy	+	Superficial and deep lobe of the parotid gland	40.0–60.5	40.0–44.7

FP facial palsy

11.2.1 Extracapsular Dissection

ECD is performed for small and benign tumors of the lateral part of the parotid gland. ECD involves careful dissection of the encapsulated tumor with safety margins under magnified visualization, but without identification of the facial nerve. Principally, ECD should be considered only in solitary, clinically benign tumors, smaller than 4 cm, and located in the superficial lobe of the parotid gland [2].

11.2.2 Superficial Parotidectomy

Superficial parotidectomy is defined as complete removal of the parotid gland superficially (laterally) of the plane of the facial nerve. Subsequently, it is mandatory to identify and dissect the facial nerve and its branches. Superficial parotidectomy is mostly performed for benign parotid tumors. Partial superficial parotidectomy is carried out when particular facial nerve branches and parts of the superficial parotid gland are dissected [2, 3].

11.2.3 Total Parotidectomy

The complete removal of the superficial (lateral) and deep (medial) lobe of the parotid gland is defined as total parotidectomy. In case of tumor infiltration of the facial nerve, it is sometimes necessary to sacrifice branches of the facial nerve, which is classified as radical parotidectomy. Here it is highly recommended to examine proximal and distal margins of the resected nerve by frozen section to exclude perineural invasion and to ensure clear resection margins.

11.3 Pre- and Perioperative Considerations

11.3.1 Facial Nerve Monitoring

Facial nerve monitoring in parotid surgery for benign and malignant diseases reduces the risk of transient postoperative FP as well as the grade of palsy [4]. After the patient is positioned, scrubbed and draped, the facial nerve monitoring is positioned. All electrodes, the nose, and the mouth are covered with an OP-site® foil. At least two electrodes are placed into the orbicularis oris muscle and orbicularis oculi muscle to ensure monitoring of the superior and inferior division of the facial nerve. Frequently, there are additional electrodes available, which are placed into the mentalis and frontalis muscle to monitor all main peripheral branches (temporal, zygomatic, buccal, and marginal branch) of the facial nerve. The green electrode (ground electrode) is placed into the sternocleidomastoid or other muscles providing grounding (Fig. 11.1). For stimulating the facial nerve, a stimulation probe is used.

11.3.2 Surgical Microscope or Surgical Loupes for Parotidectomy?

Whether surgical microscope or surgical loupes are used for parotid surgery and especially for

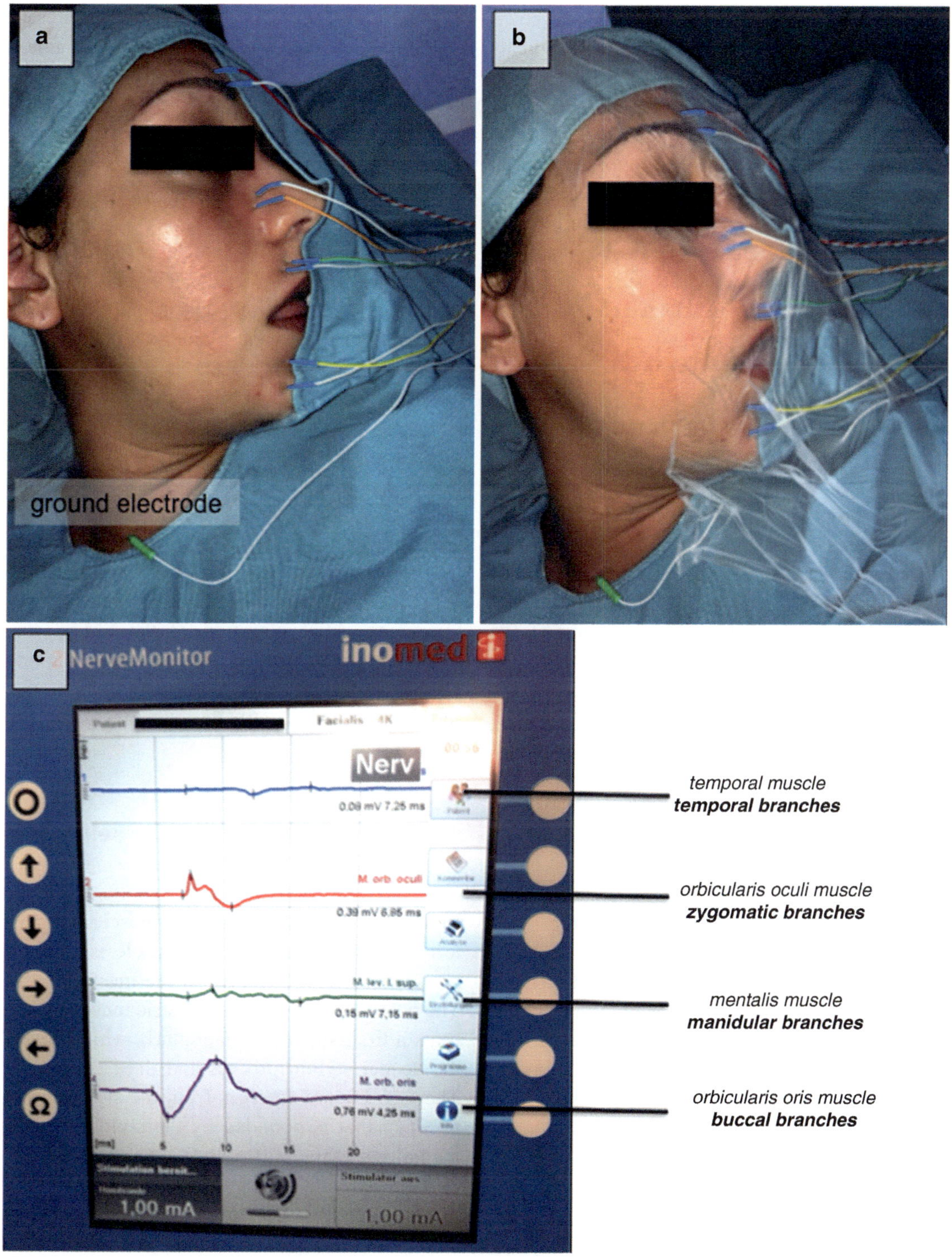

Fig. 11.1 Neuromonitoring. Neuromonitoring of the facial nerve is recommended for all parotid surgeries. Depending on the system, two to four electrodes and one ground electrode are used. Herein the electrodes were placed after the patient was positioned, scrubbed and draped. Electrodes were placed into the temporalis, orbicularis oculi, orbicularis oris, and mentalis muscle, which are supplied by the temporal, zygomatic, buccal, and marginal branch of the facial nerve (**a**). An additional electrode has to be placed as ground electrode into any muscle of the neck. All electrodes, the nose, and the mouth are covered with an OP-site® foil (**b**). All muscles with corresponding branches are monitored separately (**c**)

dissection of facial nerve depends on surgeon's preference. Currently, there exist no data indicating that parotid surgery with surgical microscope is superior regarding complications, FP, and recurrence compared to surgical loupes. Nonetheless, the use of surgical loupes, with less magnification, provides a higher amount of flexibility and are more practicable compared to surgical microscopes. Hence, surgical loupes are most commonly used, while surgical microscopes are applied only in selected cases (e.g. re-anastomosis of facial branches).

11.3.3 Single Shot Antibiotic Treatment

Routine prophylactic antibiotic treatment as a single shot does not provide any significant benefit in preventing postoperative wound infection or function of the facial nerve. Since parotid surgery is principally considered as uncontaminated, the use of antibiotic prophylaxis is not recommended. Due to the fact that the risk for wound infections increases with operation time and extend of surgery, prophylactic perioperative antibiotic treatment is only recommended for patients undergoing parotid gland surgery with resection of adjacent structures and/or neck dissection [5].

11.4 Superficial Parotidectomy

11.4.1 Positioning and Skin Incision

The patient is placed into the supine position with the head turned to the opposite site. Additionally, it may be helpful to slightly overextend the head to improve exposure. The standard incision for parotidectomy is the modified Blair's incision, which is done within a preauricular crease, starting superiorly to the root of the helix, going inferiorly around the lobule of the ear and reaching the tip of mastoid. The incision extends further downwards on the anterior border of the sternocleidomastoid muscle, where it curves gently within a skin crease caudal along the anterior, upper neck.

11.4.2 SMAS Flap

To expose the parotid gland, it is mandatory to dissect skin flaps within the preauricular plain, superficial to the parotid fascia and within the submandibular, cervical plain, superficial to the sternocleidomastoid muscle and platysma. At this point, we are elevating a superficial musculo-aponeurotic system (SMAS) flap. The SMAS represents a natural layer between the skin and the parotid fascia, comprising muscle fibers and connective tissue, which facilitates activity of all facial muscles. Dissection of the SMAS flap provides bulky tissue that can be used to reduce the risk of gustatory sweating, known as Frey Syndrome. After elevation of the SMAS flap superiorly to the parotid fascia, the anterior border of the sternocleidomastoid muscle is dissected inferiorly until its attachment to the mastoid bone.

11.4.3 Landmark I: Posterior Belly of the Digastric Muscle

Below the sternocleidomastoid muscle, the posterior belly of the digastric muscle is exposed proximal to its attachment at the mastoid bone. The posterior belly of the digastric muscle represents a first, superficial landmark, which covers the deeper styloid process and the facial nerve. The facial nerve emerges from the stylomastoid foramen that is bounded by the styloid process medially and the mastoid process of the temporal bone laterally. Therefore, the posterior belly of the digastric muscle indicates the depth at which the facial nerve will be encountered (Drawing I).

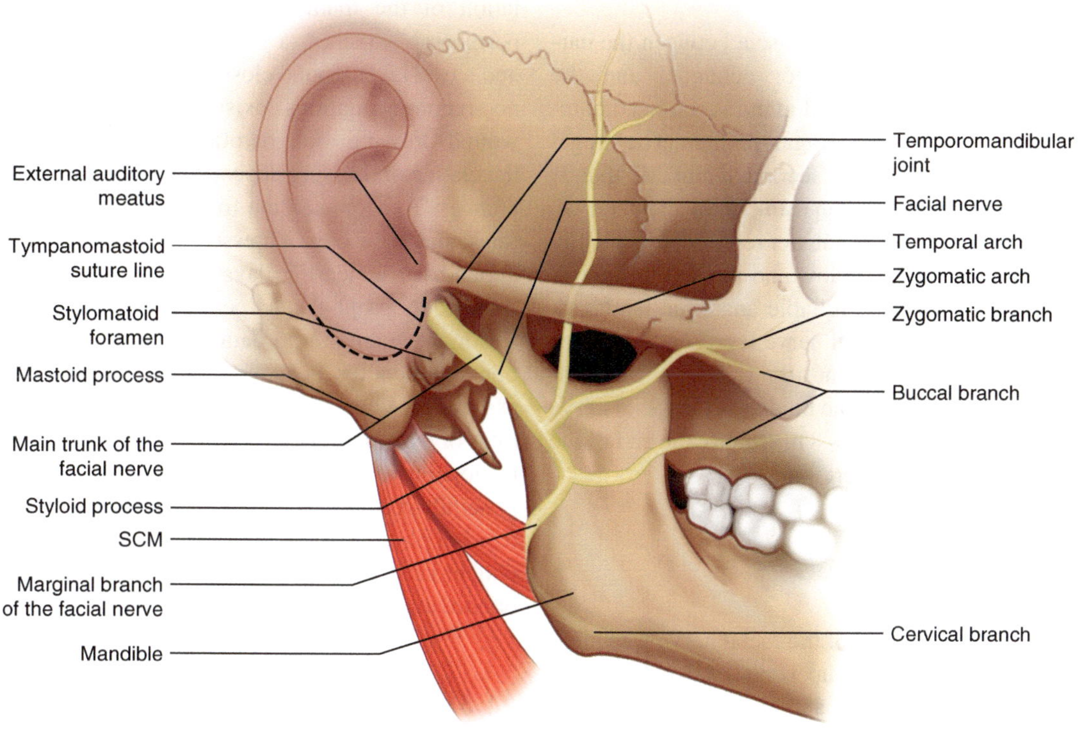

SCM - Sternocleidomastoid muscle

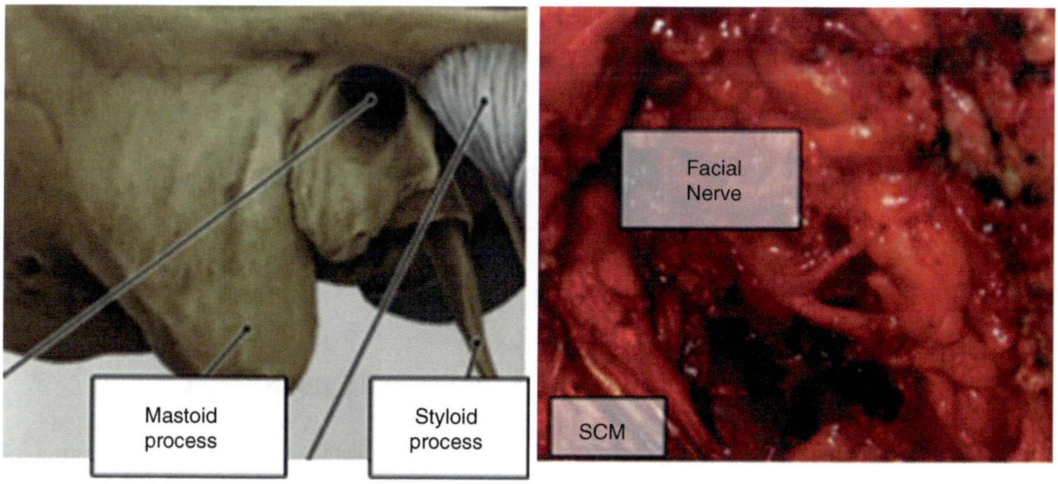

Template for professional Drawing I

11.4.4 Landmark II: Tragal Pointer

After dissecting the tight fascia between the cartilaginous external auditory channel and the parotid gland, the parotid gland is retracted anteriorly to expose the tragal pointer. The tragal pointer represents the second landmark that is used to identify the main trunk of the facial nerve. In particular, the facial nerve can be typically localized 1–1.5 cm below and inferior to the tragal pointer. Another reliable anatomic landmark for detecting the facial nerve represents the tympanomastoid suture line. By following the tympanomastoid suture line medially, the facial nerve can be usually found 6–8 mm along the end of the tympanomastoid suture line.

11.4.5 Dissection

Once the main trunk of the facial nerve was identified, the overlying (superficial) parotid tissue is meticulously tunneled and elevated with the tips of a fine mosquito clamp. The tips of the mosquito clamp should be directed upwards and surgeon should be always aware of the position of the facial nerve. Then the bridge of parotid tissue between the mosquito clamps can be safely divided as the facial nerve typically doesn't pass its plain. There is no significant difference regarding FP comparing cold steel preparation with bipolar dissection technique. The superficial parotid tissue is stepwise elevated, dissected and followed peripherally until the whole superficial parotid gland is removed from the peripheral branches of the facial nerve, which completes a superficial or lateral parotidectomy.

11.4.6 Wound Closure, Dressing, and Postoperative Antibiotic Treatment

Finally, the wound is carefully rinsed with saline and all bleeding sites are coagulated with bipolar electrocautery. After the integrity of the facial nerve has been finally proved by electrical stimulation of the main trunk and occasionally of peripheral branches, a suction drain is inserted, and a two-layer wound closure is done. Currently, no recommendations exist regarding optimal wound dressing after parotidectomy. Therefore, the choice of dressing depends on surgeons' preferences. To avoid seroma formation, salivary fistulas, and sialoceles, a pressure dressing could be applied for at least 3 days with daily changes. Similar to prophylactic perioperative antibiotic treatment, there are no data showing that antibiotic treatment for 5–7 days after parotid surgery is associated with improved outcome and lower rates of wound infections. Therefore, prophylactic postoperative application of antibiotics cannot be generally recommended after parotid surgery, and treating physicians have to decide individually on patient risk factors whether postoperative antibiotic treatment is warranted or not (Fig. 11.2).

11.5 Neck Dissection and Facial Nerve

Neck Dissection (ND) is defined as surgical dissection and removal of neck lymph nodes with adjacent connective tissue. Lymph nodes of the neck are classified into six neck levels. Among them, ND of level I, particularly level Ib, has the highest risk for damage of the marginal mandibular branch of the facial nerve. ND is necessary to evaluate regional neck node involvement of malignant head and neck tumors and parotid malignancies.

11.5.1 Level I: Boundaries

The mandible represents the superior border of the level I, while the anterior belly of the contralateral digastric muscle represents the anterior border and the stylohyoid muscle the posterior border of level I. This triangle can be further divided in level Ia and level Ib. Level Ia (submental triangle) is bounded by the anterior bellies of

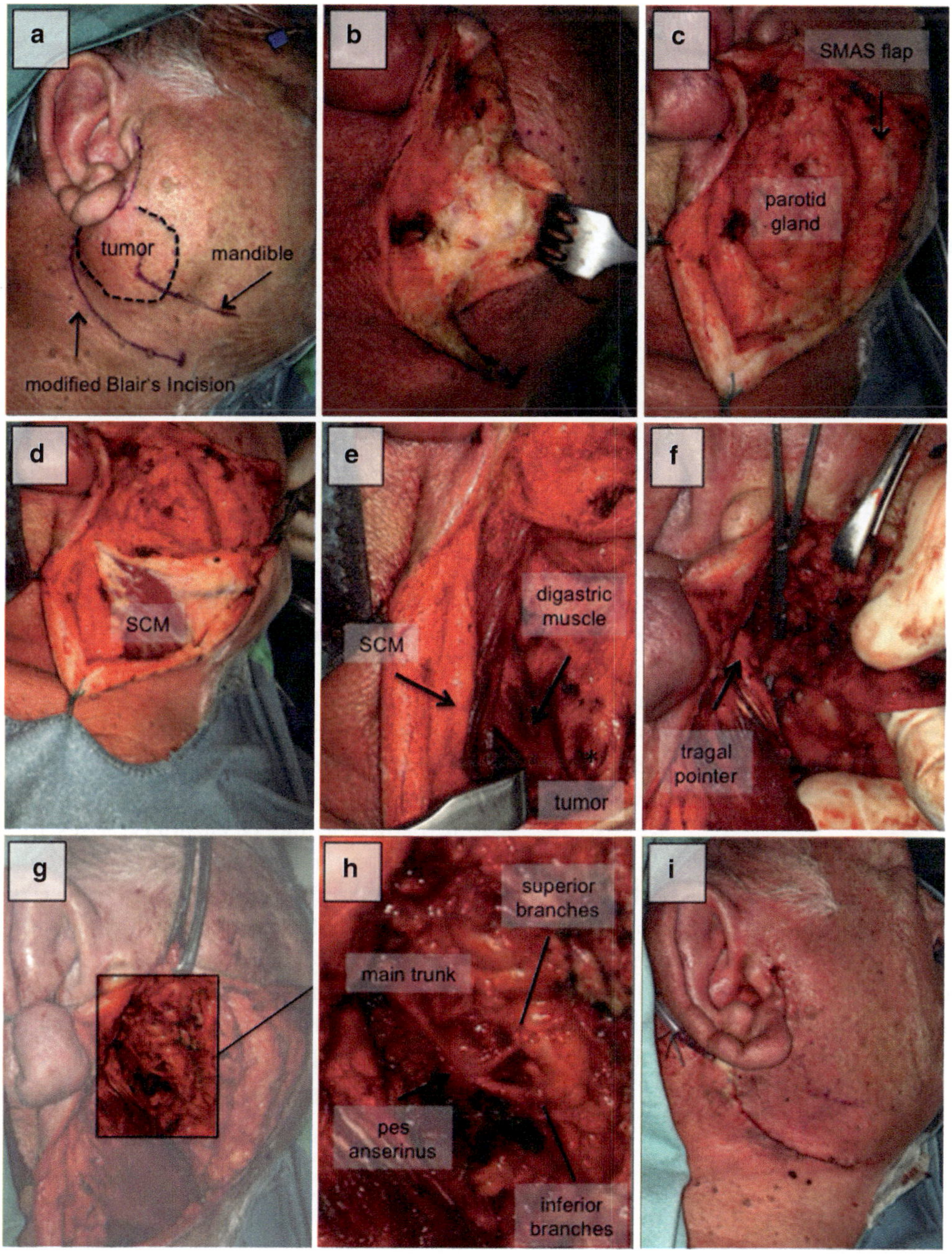

Fig. 11.2 Superficial parotidectomy. Modified Blair's incision, tumor (dotted lines), and mandible are marked (**a**). Skin incision and dissection to expose the fascia of the parotid gland, the sternocleidomastoid muscle (SCM), and the platysma (**b**). Elevation of SMAS (superficial musculoaponeurotic system) flap (**c**) and identification of the anterior border of the SCM (**d**). Retraction of the SCM posteriorly and further dissection to expose the posterior belly of the digastric muscle (Landmark I) proximal to its attachment to the mastoid bone (**e**). Next, the fascia between the cartilaginous external auditory channel and the parotid gland is dissected, and the parotid gland is retracted anteriorly to expose the tragal pointer (**f**). The tragal pointer serves as another landmark (Landmark II) that is most commonly used for identification of the main trunk of the facial nerve, which can be typically found 1–1.5 cm below and inferior to the tragal pointer (**g**). Once the trunk of the facial nerve is identified, dissection proceeds distally until pes anserinus and further branches (**h**) are identified. Superficial parotidectomy is completed after removal of the entire lobe of the parotid gland superficial of the plane of the facial nerve. Finally, suction drain is inserted and a two- to three-layer wound closure is done (**i**). *SMAS flap*

each digastric muscle and the hyoid, while level Ib (submandibular triangle) is anteriorly bounded by the anterior belly of the ipsilateral digastric muscle, posteriorly by the stylohyoid muscle, and superiorly by the mandible.

11.5.2 Risk for Damage of the Marginal Mandibular Branch

The marginal mandibular branch of the facial nerve is of particular risk for damage during parotid and submandibular gland surgery and level Ib ND including removal of the submandibular gland. Temporary and permanent palsy of the marginal mandibular branch are reported in 12.9% and 2.7% of patients after level Ib ND, compared to 33.3% and 11.1% after parotid surgery with level Ib ND, respectively [6]. Although temporary weakness of the marginal mandibular branch is frequently noticed during level Ib ND and parotid surgery, palsy is reversible in the majority of patients over time when the integrity of the facial nerve has been preserved [6].

11.6 Level Ib Neck Dissection

Although palsy of the marginal mandibular branch is temporary in the majority of patients, the treating head and neck surgeon has to know all surgical and anatomical landmarks during level Ib ND to avoid damage of the marginal mandibular branch.

11.6.1 Skin Incision

Skin incision for ND, resection of submandibular gland or the cervical part of the modified Blair's incision for parotidectomy should be placed at least 2 cm (or 1 finger) below the lower border of the mandible.

11.6.2 Elevation of Platysma Flaps

After skin incision, the platysma muscle should be divided horizontally to elevate a superior and an inferior platysma flap. The submandibular gland can be identified directly below the platysma in level Ib.

11.6.3 Identification of the Marginal Mandibular Branch

After exposure of the submandibular gland, all landmarks have to be identified. It has always to be kept in mind that the marginal mandibular branch is crossing superficially the facial artery. In particular, the facial artery arises from the external carotid artery, runs superior to the submandibular gland, and enters the lower border of the mandible, at the mandibular notch. The facial artery enters the mandibular notch 2.5–3 cm ventrally from the mandibular angle. The marginal mandibular branch can be easily identified approximately 1.5 cm superior the mandibular notch, superficial to the facial artery (Fig. 11.3).

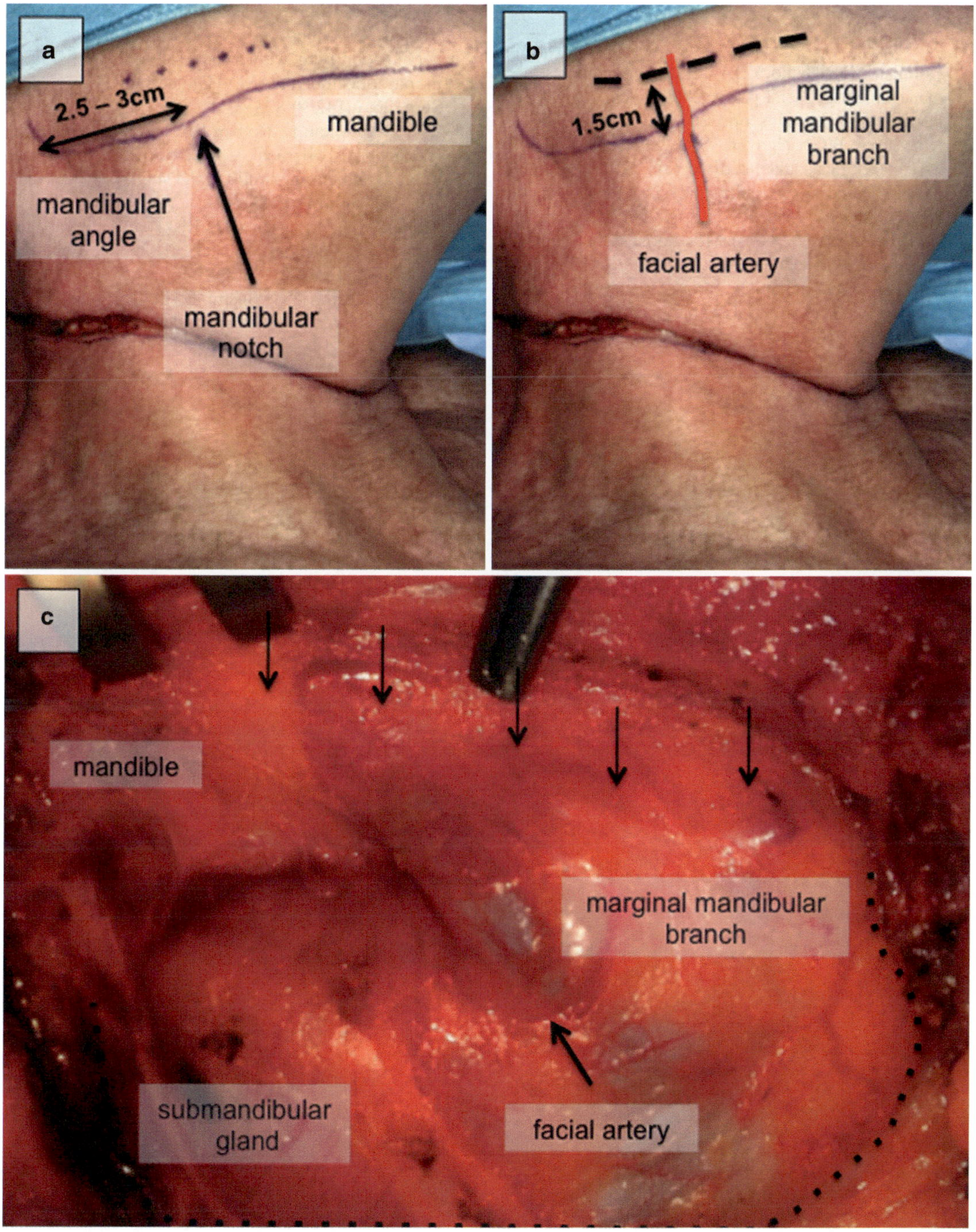

Fig. 11.3 Level Ib neck dissection with special emphasis on the marginal mandibular branch. Skin incision should be done at least 2 cm (1 finger) below the lower border of the mandible. Dotted line indicates marginal mandibular branch and arrow points at marginal notch, 2.5–3 cm ventrally from mandibular angle, where facial artery enters the lower border of the mandible (**a**, **b**). Importantly, marginal mandibular branch runs superficially to facial artery and can be easily identified approximately 1.5 cm superior to the mandibular notch (**b**, **c**). After elevation of platysma flaps, the submandibular gland and the superiorly running facial artery are exposed. Arrows indicate the course of the marginal mandibular branch, which is superior to the facial artery and parallel to the lower border of mandible (**c**)

References

1. Hohman MH, Hadlock TA. Etiology, diagnosis, and management of facial palsy: 2000 patients at a facial nerve center. Laryngoscope. 2014;124(7):E283–93.
2. Albergotti WG, Nguyen SA, Zenk J, Gillespie MB. Extracapsular dissection for benign parotid tumors: a meta-analysis. Laryngoscope. 2012;122(9):1954–60.
3. Kadletz L, Grasl S, Grasl MC, Perisanidis C, Erovic BM. Extracapsular dissection versus superficial parotidectomy in benign parotid gland tumors: the Vienna Medical School experience. Head Neck. 2017;39(2):356–60.
4. Savvas E, Hillmann S, Weiss D, Koopmann M, Rudack C, Alberty J. Association between facial nerve monitoring with postoperative facial paralysis in parotidectomy. JAMA Otolaryngol Head Neck Surg. 2016;142(9):828–33.
5. Shkedy Y, Alkan U, Roman BR, Hilly O, Feinmesser R, Bachar G, Mizrachi A. Role of perioperative antibiotic treatment in parotid gland surgery. Head Neck. 2016;38(Suppl 1):E1876–80.
6. Møller MN, Sørensen CH. Risk of marginal mandibular nerve injury in neck dissection. Eur Arch Otorhinolaryngol. 2012;269(2):601–5.
7. Gaillard C, Périé S, Susini B, St Guily JL. Facial nerve dysfunction after parotidectomy: the role of local factors. Laryngoscope. 2005;115(2):287–91.

12 Avoiding Facial Nerve Injury in Oral and Maxillofacial Surgery

Christos Perisanidis
and Nikolaos Papadogeorgakis

Key Points

- Approaches to the mandible and the temporomandibular joint have the highest incidence of iatrogenic facial nerve injury.
- The buccal branch is at most risk for injury during the retromandibular anteroparotid transmasseteric approach.
- The marginal mandibular branch is at most risk for injury during the retromandibular transparotid approach.
- The submandibular approach and the retromandibular transparotid approach have the highest risk for transient facial nerve injury.
- In-depth understanding and proper dissection of fascial planes in the neck, face, and temporal region is essential to avoid damage of the facial nerve.

12.1 Introduction

Surgical interventions to the mandible and the temporomandibular joint (TMJ) account for up to 40% of iatrogenic facial nerve injuries, followed by oncologic resections in the head and neck region (25%), otologic surgery (17%), and cosmetic surgery (11%) [1]. The TMJ commonly requires surgical exposure for the management of condylar fractures as well as for a plethora of pathologic conditions, including internal derangements of the joint, developmental disorders, ankylosis, and tumors. Over the years, the following surgical approaches to the TMJ and the mandible have been used: retromandibular, preauricular, auricular, endaural, retroauricular, rhytidectomy, periangular, submandibular, and intraoral approach. This chapter will provide an in-depth description of the commonly used retromandibular and preauricular approaches to the TMJ and the associated risks for facial nerve injury.

12.2 Retromandibular Approach to the TMJ

In the literature, the following retromandibular approaches have been described based on route of surgical dissection with regard to the parotid gland and masseter muscle: (1) the anteroparotid transmasseteric approach (dissection proceeds along the anteroinferior border of the parotid and through the masseter muscle), (2) the transparotid approach (dissection enters the parotid). The main advantages of the retromandibular approaches are the reduced distance from the skin incision to the mandibular condyle and the TMJ, adequate exposure of the surgical field, and hidden scars [2].

C. Perisanidis (✉) · N. Papadogeorgakis
Department of Oral and Maxillofacial Surgery, University of Athens, Athens, Greece
e-mail: cperis@dent.uoa.gr

© Springer Nature Switzerland AG 2021
C.-H. J. Tzou, A. Rodríguez-Lorenzo (eds.), *Facial Palsy*,
https://doi.org/10.1007/978-3-030-50784-8_12

12.2.1 Surgical Anatomy

During the anteroparotid transmasseteric approach, the branch of the facial nerve mostly at risk is the buccal branch. The buccal branch emerges from the parotid gland deep to the parotidomasseteric fascia. The nerve runs parallel and inferior to the parotid duct in approximately 75% of cases (Fig. 12.1), while in the remaining 25% the nerve runs parallel and superior to the duct [3]. The buccal branch pierces the parotidomasseteric fascia at the anterior border of the masseter, in vicinity to the masseteric cutaneous ligaments. The clinical consequences of injury to the buccal branch are less severe compared to the marginal mandibular and the frontal branches as there are several communicating branches between the buccal and zygomatic branches of the facial nerve.

During the transparotid approach, the branch of the facial nerve mostly at risk is the marginal mandibular branch. In the literature, several variations of both the path of the marginal mandibular nerve and its position in fascial planes of the face and neck have been described. Within the parotid gland, the marginal mandibular nerve arises most often from the lower (cervicofacial) division of the facial nerve as a single branch. After exiting the parotid gland near its inferior border, the nerve is covered by the parotidomasseteric fascia and courses from posterosuperior to anteroinferior towards the mandibular angle. This trajectory leaves a space between the marginal mandibular branch and the buccal branch, through which the mandible can be safely accessed [4]. Posterior to the facial artery, the marginal mandibular nerve runs 1–2 cm above the lower border of the mandible in 81% of cases, while in the remaining 19% one or more rami of the nerve form a downward arc whose lowest point extends into the neck up to 1.2 cm below the lower border of the mandible. The marginal mandibular branch lies initially within or deep to the investing layer of the deep cervical fascia. Near the mandibular mid-body, the nerve crosses superficial to the facial vessels (Fig. 12.2) and perforates the deep cervical fascia to continue in a plane between the platysma and the deep cervical fascia. Anterior to the facial artery, all of the rami of the marginal mandibular nerve run above the lower border of the mandible [5].

Facial nerve injury can be avoided by: (1) dissecting above the superficial musculoaponeurotic system (SMAS) and platysma, (2) identification of the marginal mandibular branch in the subplatysmal plane, (3) ligation of the facial vessels and dissection in a plane below the deep cervical fascia and deep to the ligated facial vessels (Fig. 12.3a–d).

Throughout the retromandibular approaches, care should be taken to avoid hemorrhage from the retromandibular (posterior facial) vein, which is formed by the superficial temporal vein and the internal maxillary vein at the level of the mandibular condyle. The retromandibular vein runs downward just posterior to the mandibular ramus and crosses the marginal mandibular branch, which runs superficial to the vein in 98% of cases [5].

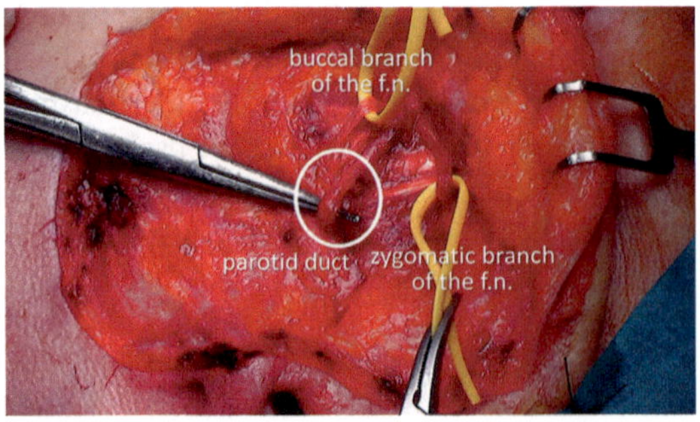

Fig. 12.1 Relation of the buccal branch of the facial nerve to the parotid duct

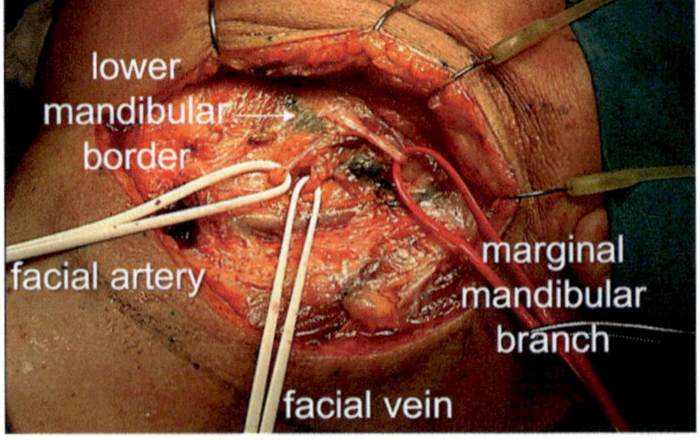

Fig. 12.2 Relation of the marginal mandibular branch of the facial nerve to the facial vessels and the lower border of the mandible

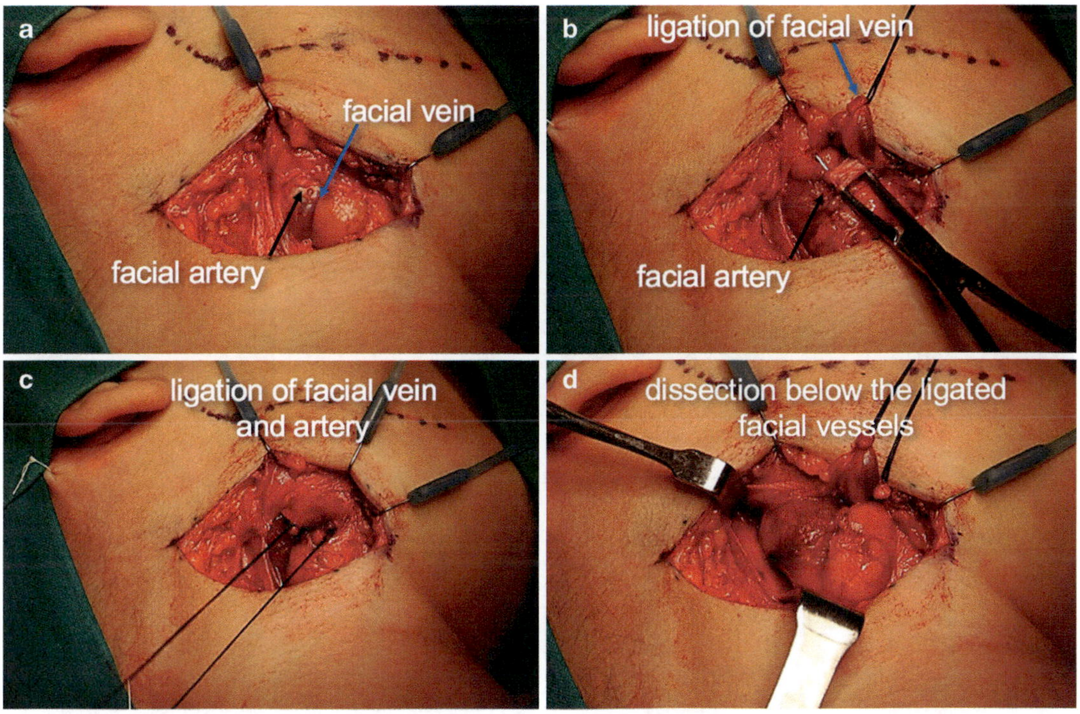

Fig. 12.3 Prevention of marginal mandibular branch injury by ligation of facial vessels. The facial vein and artery are identified through a submandibular incision (**a**). Ligation of facial vein (**b**) and facial artery (**c**). Dissection in a plane below the deep cervical fascia and deep to the ligated facial vessels (**d**)

12.2.2 Retromandibular Anteroparotid Transmasseteric Approach

The skin incision is placed 0.5 cm below the earlobe and approximately 1 cm behind the posterior border of the mandibular ascending ramus (Fig. 12.4b). The incision is carried downwards for 3–3.5 cm and maybe extended preauricular and/or periangular. The depth of incision is the parotidomasseteric plane (Fig. 12.4c) and undermining of subcutaneous tissue with scissors is performed in all directions to allow for better exposure and maximal tissue retraction. Incision of the parotidomasseteric fascia near the anterior-inferior edge of the parotid exposes both the masseter muscle and parotid substance (Fig. 12.4d). Then, the parotid is bluntly pushed upwards while looking on the surface of the masseter muscle for branches of the facial nerve (Fig. 12.4e). The surgical field near the anterior-inferior edge of the parotid gland is usually free of branches of the facial nerve; occasionally the buccal branch can be encountered. The use of a nerve stimulator-locator is recommended in order to reduce the possibility of accidental nerve damage. Then, the masseter is bluntly dissected parallel to its muscle fibers until the mandibular periosteum is reached, which then is sharply incised. A periosteal elevator is used to strip the periosteum and masseter muscle to expose the mandibular angle, ascending ramus, sigmoid notch, coronoid process, and condyle (Fig. 12.4f) [6].

12.2.3 Retromandibular Transparotid Approach

The position and depth of incision is placed as described for the retromandibular anteroparotid transmasseteric approach. The parotidomasseteric fascia is incised at the level of the posterior border of the mandibular ramus and the parotid gland becomes visible. Then, blunt dissection

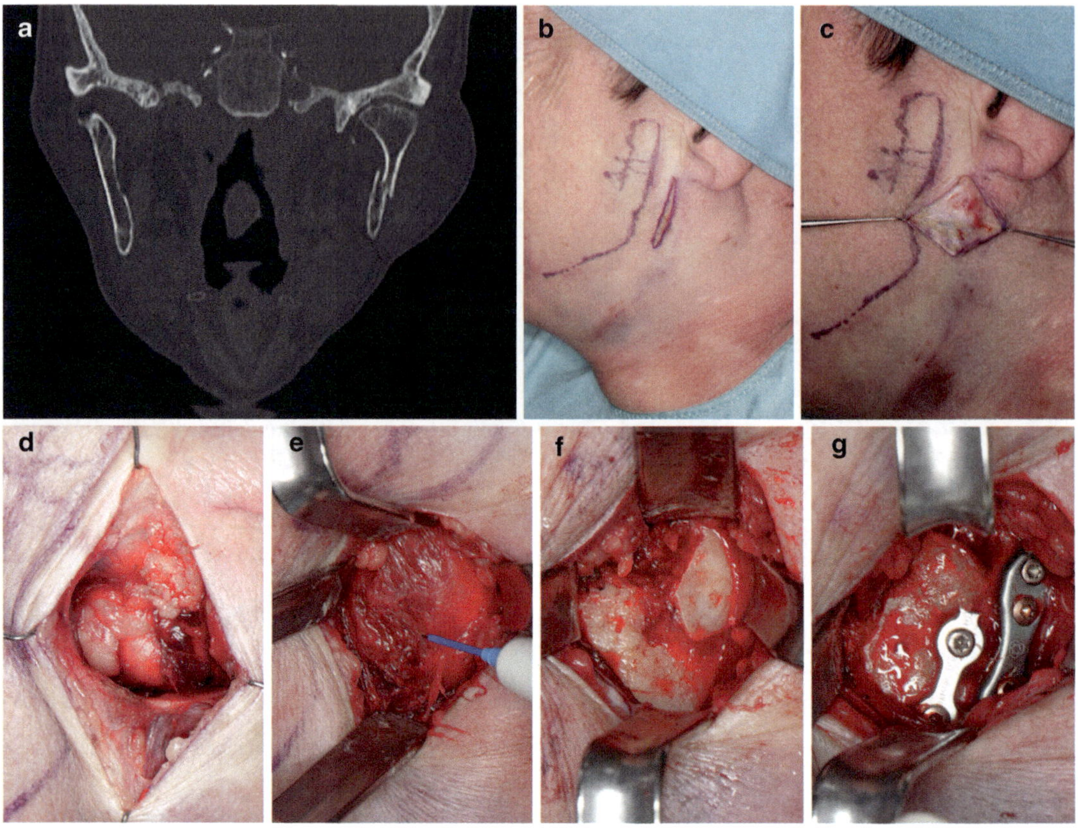

Fig. 12.4 Retromandibular anteroparotid approach for treatment of condylar fracture. The condylar fracture is shown on computed tomography scan (**a**). The skin incision is made right below the earlobe and approximately 1 cm behind the posterior border of the mandible (**b**) to the depth of the parotidomasseteric fascia (**c**). The parotidomasseteric fascia is incised (**d**) and the parotid gland is pushed upwards to expose the masseter muscle while looking for branches of the facial nerve (**e**). The masseter is bluntly dissected and the mandibular periosteum incised to expose the fracture site (**f**). Reposition and osteosynthesis of the condylar fracture with two plates (**g**)

within the parotid parallel to the expected course of the facial nerve branches and towards the periosteum of the posterior border of the mandible is performed. The marginal mandibular branch and/or the retromandibular vein maybe encountered during dissection and should be protected (Fig. 12.5). The pterygomasseteric sling is exposed and sharply divided superiorly, posteriorly, and around the mandibular angle. A periosteal elevator is used to detach the periosteum and the masseter from the mandible and thus expose the condyle and the TMJ.

12.3 Preauricular Approach to the TMJ

The preauricular approach provides direct access to the TMJ and is particularly useful in cases of antero-medially displaced condylar head and condylar neck fractures. Otherwise, exposure of the mandibular ramus is limited and plate fixation technically difficult. In the literature, the following preauricular approaches have been described based on route of surgical dissection: (1) the subfascial approach (dissection deep to the superfi-

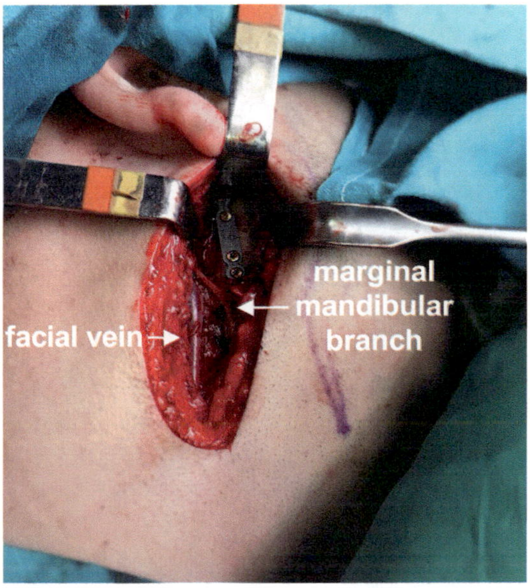

Fig. 12.5 Retromandibular transparotid approach for treatment of condylar fracture. The marginal mandibular branch of the facial nerve crosses above the retromandibular vein in 98% of cases. Reposition and osteosynthesis of the condylar fracture with one plate placed at the posterior edge of the mandibular condyle

cial layer of the deep temporal fascia), (2) the deep subfascial approach (dissection just below the deep layer of the deep temporal fascia). The auricular approach presents a modification of the preauricular approach resulting in better cosmetic outcome.

12.3.1 Surgical Anatomy

During the preauricular approach, the branch of the facial nerve mostly at risk is the frontal (or temporal) branch. In their classic anatomic study, Pitanguy and Ramos described the cutaneous course of the frontal branch on a line extending 0.5 cm below the tragus to a point 1 cm above the lateral edge of the eyebrow (or 1.5 cm lateral to the supraorbital rim) [7]. The frontal branch, which consists of 2–4 nerve branches, emerges from the parotid gland deep to the parotidomasseteric fascia

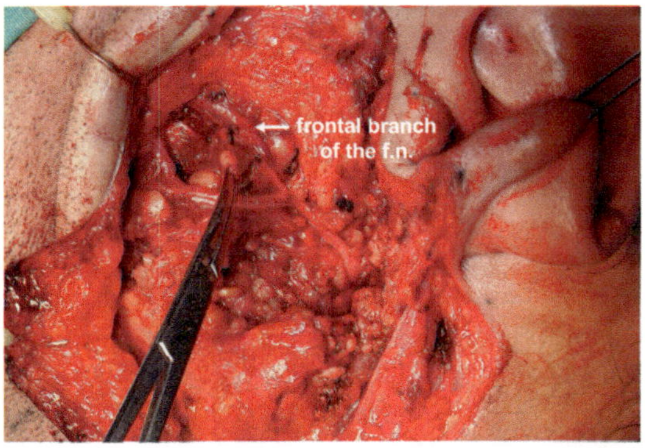

Fig. 12.6 Frontal (or temporal) branch of the facial nerve. The frontal branch of the facial nerve crosses right above the periosteum of the zygomatic arch in a distance of about 20 mm from the bony external auditory canal

lying on the masseter muscle. Then, it crosses the zygomatic arch in a distance of 8–35 mm (average 20 mm) from the anterior-most portion of the bony external auditory canal (Fig. 12.6) [8]. At the level of the zygomatic arch the frontal branch abuts the periosteum and is covered by the parotidotemporal (or innominate) fascia, SMAS, subcutaneous tissue, and skin [9, 10]. At 1 cm above the zygomatic arch, the frontal branch lies just above the deep temporal fascia and is covered by the parotidotemporal fascia, temporoparietal fascia (extension of the SMAS), subcutaneous tissue, and skin. At approximately 2–3 cm above the zygomatic arch, the frontal branch pierces the parotidotemporal fascia and lies just deep to the temporoparietal fascia [9]. In the temporal region, dissection either deep to the superficial layer of the deep temporal fascia or just below the deep layer of the deep temporal fascia will prevent injury to the frontal branch. At the zygomatic arch, the nerve can be protected by incising the periosteum within 8 mm in front of the anterior edge of the bony external auditory canal.

12.3.2 Subfascial Approach

The skin incision is placed in a preauricular natural skin crease from the lobule to the top

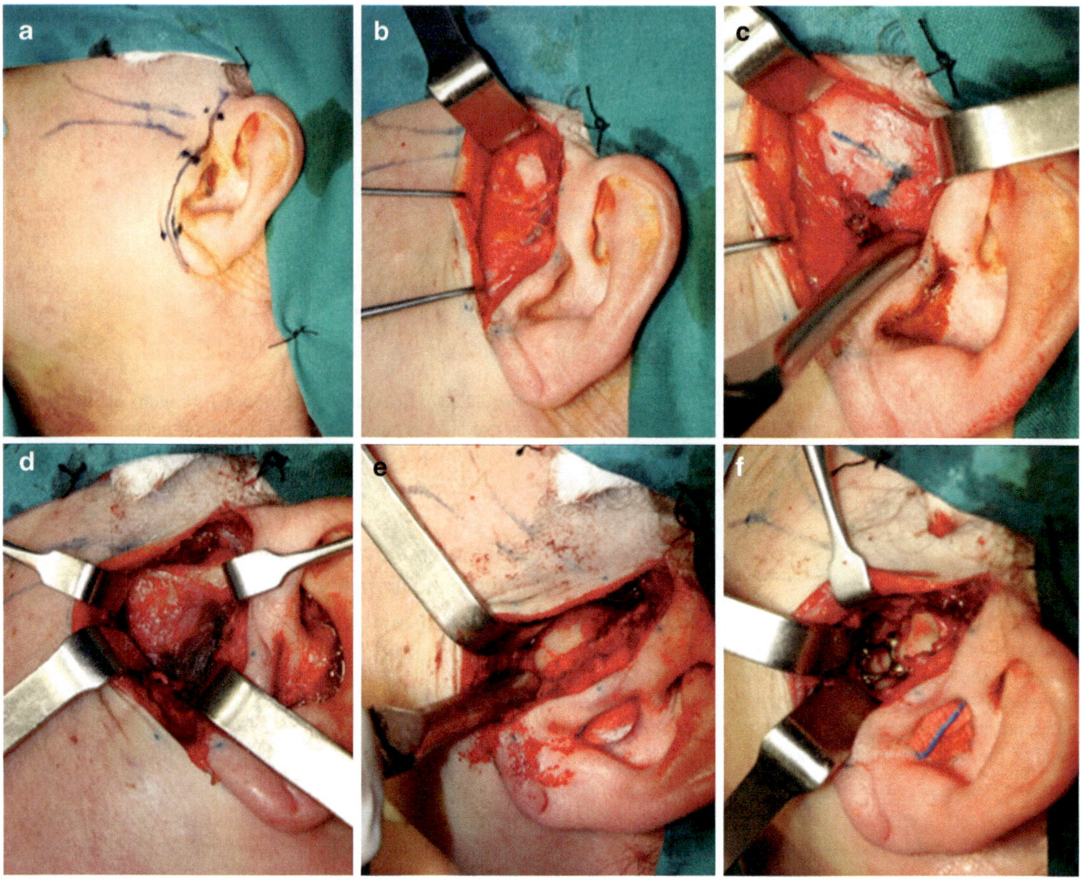

Fig. 12.7 Preauricular subfascial approach for treatment of high condylar neck fracture. The skin incision is designed in a preauricular natural skin crease from the ear lobule to the top of the helix (**a**). Above the zygomatic arch, the incision is made through subcutaneous tissue, the temporoparietal fascia, and the parotidotemporal fascia (**b**) exposing the deep temporal fascia (**c**). The superficial layer of the deep temporal fascia is incised and subperiosteal dissection along the zygomatic arch is performed (**d**). The TMJ and condylar head is exposed (**e**). Reposition and osteosynthesis of the high condylar neck fracture (**f**)

of the helix (Fig. 12.7a) and maybe extended superoanterior in the temporal area (hockey-stick extension). Above the zygomatic arch, the incision goes through subcutaneous tissue, the temporoparietal fascia, and the parotidotemporal fascia (Fig. 12.7b) exposing the well-defined, white superficial layer of the deep temporal fascia (Fig. 12.7c), and a flap is bluntly dissected anteriorly. Below the zygomatic arch, blunt dissection is performed alongside and parallel to the external auditory cartilage to avoid injury to the ear. The superficial layer of the deep temporal fascia is then incised beginning at the root of the zygomatic arch and the incision line continues at 45° in a superoanterior direction. The superficial temporal fat pad enclosed between the superficial and deep layers of the deep temporal fascia is exposed and dissection continues within the fat pad towards the zygomatic arch. The periosteum of the zygomatic arch is incised on its superomedial surface and subperiosteal dissection proceeds anteriorly to the articular eminence (Fig. 12.7d), thus retracting from beneath the flap and protecting the frontal branch of the facial nerve. Then, blunt dissection with scissors and/or periosteal elevators is performed downwards to expose the TMJ capsule, the condylar head, and the condylar neck (Fig. 12.7e).

12.3.3 Deep Subfascial Approach

The deep subfascial approach is a modification of the traditional subfascial approach. In this technique, both the superficial and the deep layer of the deep temporal fascia are incised and the superficial temporal fat pad is dissected. Thus, compared to the traditional technique, the deep subfascial approach provides two additional tissue layers (superficial temporal fat pad and deep layer of the deep temporal fascia) of protection for the frontal branch of the facial nerve.

12.4 Approaches to the TMJ and Risk for Facial Nerve Injury

Approaches to the mandible and the TMJ have the highest incidence of iatrogenic facial nerve injury. Al-Moraissi et al. evaluated in a recent meta-analysis the risk for permanent and transient facial nerve injury based on different surgical approaches to the TMJ [2]. They found that all described surgical approaches to the TMJ have low or no risk for permanent facial nerve injury. The highest risk for permanent damage to the facial nerve was found for the submandibular approach (2.2%) followed by the retromandibular transparotid approach (1.4%), while the retromandibular anteroparotid transmasseteric approach, the preauricular deep subfascial approach, and the intraoral approach showed no risk for permanent facial nerve injury. Similarly, the highest risk for transient facial nerve injury was found for the submandibular approach (15.3%) followed by the retromandibular transparotid approach (14.4%). The retromandibular anteroparotid transmasseteric approach (3.4%) and the intraoral endoscopic-assisted approach (4.2%) showed a relatively low risk for transient damage to the facial nerve.

References

1. Hohman MH, Bhama PK, Hadlock TA. Epidemiology of iatrogenic facial nerve injury: a decade of experience. Laryngoscope. 2014;124:260–5.
2. Al-Moraissi EA, Louvrier A, Colletti G, et al. Does the surgical approach for treating mandibular condylar fractures affect the rate of seventh cranial nerve injuries? A systematic review and meta-analysis based on a new classification for surgical approaches. J Craniomaxillofac Surg. 2018;46:398–412.
3. Pogrel MA, Schmidt B, Ammar A. The relationship of the buccal branch of the facial nerve to the parotid duct. J Oral Maxillofac Surg. 1996;54:71–3.
4. Ellis E III, Zide MF. Surgical approaches to the facial skeleton. 2nd ed. Philadelphia: Lippincott Williams & Wilkins; 2006.
5. Dingman RO, Grabb WC. Surgical anatomy of the mandibular ramus of the facial nerve based on the dissection of 100 facial halves. Plast Reconstr Surg Transplant Bull. 1962;29:266–72.
6. Wilson AW, Ethunandan M, Brennan PA. Transmasseteric antero-parotid approach for open reduction and internal fixation of condylar fractures. Br J Oral Maxillofac Surg. 2005;43:57–60.
7. Pitanguy I, Ramos AS. The frontal branch of the facial nerve: the importance of its variations in face lifting. Plast Reconstr Surg. 1966;38:352–6.
8. Al-Kayat A, Bramley P. A modified pre-auricular approach to the temporomandibular joint and malar arch. Br J Oral Surg. 1979;17:91–103.
9. Agarwal CA, Mendenhall SD III, Foreman KB, Owsley JQ. The course of the frontal branch of the facial nerve in relation to fascial planes: an anatomic study. Plast Reconstr Surg. 2010;125:532–7.
10. Trussler AP, Stephan P, Hatef D, Schaverien M, Meade R, Barton FE. The frontal branch of the facial nerve across the zygomatic arch: anatomical relevance of the high-SMAS technique. Plast Reconstr Surg. 2010;125:1221–9.

Part III

Smile Reanimation in Long Standing Facial Paralysis

13 Principles of Smile Reanimation

Chieh-Han John Tzou
and Andrés Rodríguez-Lorenzo

Key Points

- Smile reanimation is a key goal in the reconstruction of the paralyzed face due to the importance of the smile as one of the main facial expressions.
- Smiling displays joy, but it is also a signaling system that evolved to communicate many kinds of information in ways that vary between cultures and geographic locations.
- The type of smiles can be classified as *Duchenne* versus *non-Duchenne smiles* (depending on if there is co-contraction of the orbicularis oris with the smile or not) and by the *Rubin's classification of smile* (Mona Lisa type, Canine type, and full denture type).
- The vector of pull of the oral commissure from the mimetic muscles, particularly the zygomaticus major, is the main reference for adequate position of the transplanted muscle in facial reanimation.
- Smile reanimation with muscle flaps needs to take into consideration several important factors, such as the selection of the surgical technique (free muscle vs regional muscle), donor muscle, type of neurotizer (facial nerve, nonfacial nerve, or dual innervation), and surgical staging (one versus two stages) and its perioperative management.

13.1 Introduction

13.1.1 History of the Smile

The face is one of the most visible parts of the body, and therefore facial expressions are widely recognized as one of the main tools for communication and social intelligence. Facial expressions allow for nonverbal communication and the expression of emotions that are intrinsic features in the evolution of human behavior and social interaction [1]. Darwin first described the six basic facial expressions (disgust, joy, fear, surprise, anger, sadness), which result from combinations of synchronous movements of different

C.-H. J. Tzou (✉)
Plastic and Reconstructive Surgery, Hospital of Divine Savior (Krankenhaus Goettlicher Heiland), Sigmund Freud University, TZOU MEDICAL, Vienna, Austria

Faculty of Medicine, Sigmund Freud University, Vienna, Austria
e-mail: science@tzoumedical.com

A. Rodríguez-Lorenzo
Department of Plastic and Maxillofacial Surgery, Uppsala University Hospital, Uppsala, Sweden

Department of Surgical Sciences, Uppsala University, Uppsala, Sweden
e-mail: andres.rodriguez.lorenzo@surgsci.uu.se

© Springer Nature Switzerland AG 2021
C.-H. J. Tzou, A. Rodríguez-Lorenzo (eds.), *Facial Palsy*,
https://doi.org/10.1007/978-3-030-50784-8_13

facial mimic muscles [2]. Many variations within these facial expressions are influenced by anatomical differences, demographic differences, and cultural backgrounds [1]. Among all facial expressions, smiling or the display of joy is one of the most relevant ones for social interaction.

Smile reanimation is a key goal in treating the paralyzed face so as to restore one of the main facial expressions and thereby increase the patient's quality of life. In this chapter, we review essential aspects in smiling, including the evolution, sociocultural aspects, and types of smiles, followed by a description of the main factors to be considered in smile reanimation in longstanding facial paralysis.

13.1.2 Evolution of the Human Smile

Facial expressions and the human smile in particular have been studied from the evolutionary point of view as biological adaptations. Facial expressions are socially important signals among most nonhuman primates as well as humans [1]. Primatologist Signe Preuschoft traces the smile back over 30 million years. With clenched teeth and relaxed lips monkeys and apes showed predators that they were harmless and signal submission to more dominant members in their group. Moreover, this open mouth gesture expresses happiness and fun [3], which is so called "fear grin" and conveys a sign of playfulness among barbary macaques [4]. Chimpanzees have been observed to do so to signal both dominant and nonaggressive behavior [5]. Kinesic and psychological studies reveal that a smile can communicate feelings such as contempt, embarrassment, happiness, love, and pride [6]. The "fear grin" smile may have evolved differently among different species. Among humans, it might be a natural evolutionary precursor to the human smile, a "metacommunicative signal of bi-directional affiliative social engagement" [4].

13.1.3 Social and Cultural Aspects of the Smile

The smile is a nonverbal signal of communication, which can be universally associated with emotional experiences of happiness, signaling friendliness, approachability, and cooperativity [5]. It can convey politeness or appeasement and improve interpersonal communication. Numerous studies have shown that smiling individuals were perceived as more attractive, communal, competent [7], approachable [8], friendly, more likable [9], and happier [10]. Moreover, a smile induces a "safe and satisfying interaction" [11], as suggested in the song "When You're Smiling": "When you're smiling, the whole world smiles with you" [12]. There are vast different types of smile with various meanings. A smile can communicate positive emotions, psychological signals, social intentions, or a person's social status [13]. Spontaneous smile is prevalent among apes and humans, whereas social smiling may be unique to humans only. Spontaneous smile is the emotional experience of happiness independent of social context, which may highly correlate with social motivations, such as signaling approachability, cooperativity, friendliness, and politeness to convey appeasement to diffuse social tension. The silent bared-teeth display, e.g., "fear grin," observed in nonhuman primates might be a phylogenetic precursor to the human social smile. It has been observed in dominant chimpanzees toward their subordinates, as a submissive and nonaggressive signal to deflect hostile interactions [5]. In human social contexts, smiling and laughing have different functions in the following order: smiling may be a "pre-laughing device," a common pattern before laughing; smile can also be a response to previous laughter [14]. It is also a signaling system that evolved to communicate various information. One of these is to advertise sexual interest. Research examined gender difference in relative sexual attractiveness of individuals showing expressions of happiness, pride, and shame. Happiness was the most attractive female emotional expression. Female smiles increase physical attractiveness, enhance sex appeal, and are appealing to heterosexual males. In contrast, pride was the most attractive male expression, and one of the least attractive in women to attract heterosexual gender. Shame was attractive for females and males. Younger adult women were mostly enticed by male shame and pride, and less by male happiness or smile [15]. Studies confirmed gender-specific effect of distinct expressions on sexual attractiveness and irrespective of their nationality, women smile more than men [16].

Smiling is a means of communication throughout the world [17]. Spontaneous smile in humans occurs cross-culturally early in infancy and appears more frequent in a population engaged in many face-to-face interactions between caregivers and offspring than in a population in which face-to-face interaction was uncommon [18].

Smiling is perceived commonly as a positive emotion, but for some cultures smile is a negative and unwelcome expression, and may be used to convey confusion or embarrassment [17]. Asian people may smile when they are embarrassed, in emotional pain, or to indicate a friendly greeting; sometimes it is only reserved for close friends and family members. In the blog post "The Cross-Cultural Meanings of a Smile," Shelley Batts reflected smile in North America as a friendly, positive gesture of trust. This gesture is based on historic frontier society in the USA with little official law enforcement, where the first sight communication—"I am a friend"—was important. In more hierarchical cultures, where emotional expressions are less expected, such as Russia or East Asia, the smile is not central to communication. Anecdotal evidence confirms this finding, where smiling at strangers is considered to be unusual and even suspicious behavior [19]: well-known Russian proverb says "Улыбка, без причины - признак дурачины" ("smiling with no reason is a sign of stupidity"), a Korean proverb conveys "He who smiles a lot is not a real man," and a saying in Japanese phrases "when in trouble, get away with a smile." The Norwegian government wittily indicated that Norwegians may assume a smiling stranger as insane [20]. British guidebook informed tourists that smiling at strangers is perceived as a sign of stupidity by Poles [21] and too much smiling can be viewed as a sign of shallowness or dishonesty [22]. Even Darwin [2] wrote about "the large class of idiots who are ... constantly smiling" [20]. Smiling may be seen as a frivolous activity for a government document (e.g., driver's license photo) and might indicate an unserious driver's responsibility of the license holder.

According to Kuba Krys, a Polish psychologist, smiling is not consistently perceived as a sign of intelligence among cultures. Smiling faces are rated significantly *more* intelligent than those of non-smiling people in Germany, Switzerland, Malaysia, China, Austria, Egypt, Philippines, United Kingdom, Denmark, Brazil, Pakistan, Nigeria, Portugal, Nigeria, Australia, Turkey, Georgia, Canada, and Zimbabwe out of 44 studied cultures [20]. But in France, Russia, South Korea, Iran, India, and Japan, smiling faces are considered significantly *less* intelligent. No significant difference in the intelligence ratings of smiling versus non-smiling individuals was found in Taiwan, USA, Ireland, Albania, Kuwait, South Africa, Indonesia, Maldives, Colombia, Norway, Argentina, Italy, Hong Kong, Hungary, Greece, Poland, Mexico, and Israel. The variability of smile perception is neither embedded geographically (e.g., neighboring countries like China and Japan or Germany and France are on different ends of the distributions) nor economically, but is deeply rooted in cultural dimensions [20] (Fig. 13.1).

Countries that rank lower on a cultural phenomenon known as "uncertainty avoidance" tend to have unstable healthcare, court, and political environments. People in those cultures, e.g., Russia, India, and Argentina, view the future as unpredictable and uncontrollable, thus may associate dishonesty with smiling. A smile looks unwise to them or causes them to suspect that the smiling person has done something untrustworthy.

Studies of the complex interactions between cultures and the social perception of nonverbal behavior are only a few [7]. Rychlowska and collaborators (2015) accessed cultural variation of smile that goes beyond East–West cultural comparisons. They pointed out the importance of heterogeneity versus homogeneity of cultures in predicting the "endorsement of smiling."

Three characteristic smile codes (American, Japanese, Polish) have been analyzed and are found to be closely related to cultural norms and values: in the USA, cheerfulness and friendliness; in Japan, social harmony; in Poland, sincer-

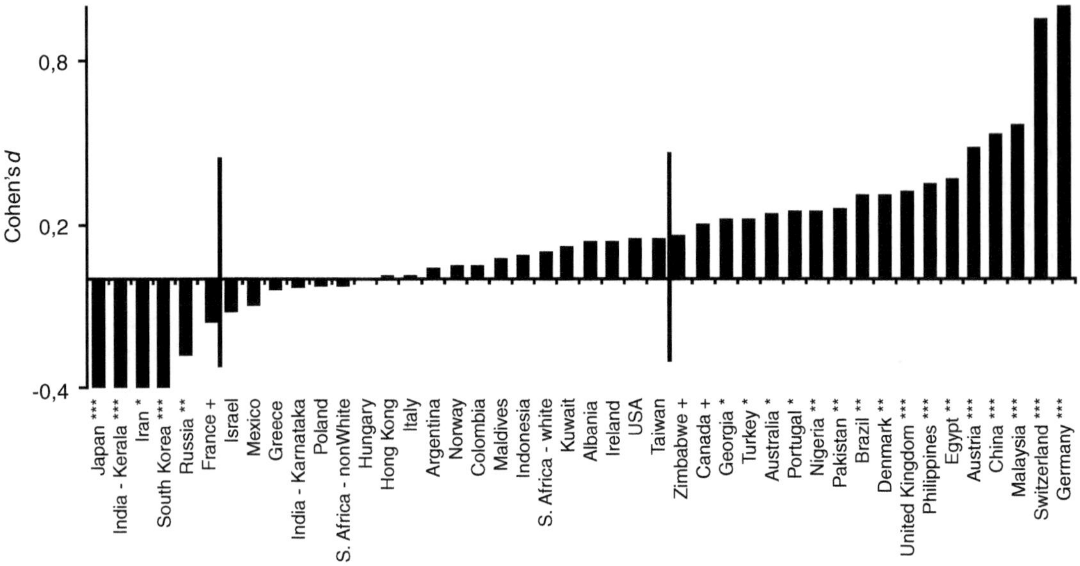

Fig. 13.1 Cohen's *d* for the difference in intelligence ratings of smiling and non-smiling individuals across cultures. Vertical doted lines separate cultures in which smiling individuals are rated as significantly more intelligent (on the right) or significantly less intelligent (on the left) [20]—permission via Open Access under the terms of the Creative Commons Attribution 4.0 International License (http://creativecommons.org/licenses/by/4.0/)

ity. According to Szarota et al. the social act of smiling is related to the given culture and its ideas of "happiness." In the USA, "an ethic of cheerfulness is closely connected to a cultural preoccupation with happiness, construed as an internal attribute to be pursued and attained via personal striving," but Japanese and Polish people understand happiness as ephemeral and temporary [16].

The motivation for smiling differs cross-culturally: Americans usually smile to present themselves as happy and friendly, Japanese smile to look agreeable and self-controlled, and Poles smile to reflect inner feelings and rarely engage in social smiling [23]. Part of this variability is also the beholder's cultural background how smile is perceived among cultures. Americans interpret emoticons by observing expression at the mouth area, seeing ☺ as happy and ☹ as sad, while Japanese find eye expressions, ^_^ as joyful and;_; as tearful. Japanese emphasize the upper half of a face when determining its trustworthiness, but Americans focus more on the lower half [24]. This variation may call into question how true the lower face reflects emotions as Duchenne described that the mouth can be manipulated into a smile more easily than the eyes.

13.1.4 Types of Smile and Anatomical Variations

The smile is a mechanical consequence of an upturn of the commissures of the mouth and is generally associated with joy display, but it also serves as a nonverbal communication tool, as previously described. It is formed primarily by flexing about 42 muscles around the mouth and cheeks [25]. Research has evaluated distinctions among smiles that have led to different classifications of types of smiles.

In 1862, Guillaume-Benjamin Duchenne de Boulogne studied the physiology of facial expressions and evaluated the movement of individual facial muscles with electrodes. He saw the human face as a map, with each muscle representing a "movement of the soul," and classified 53 emotions in terms of muscular action. He classified two distinct types of smiles, a *Duchenne smile* and a *non-Duchenne* smile (Fig. 13.2) [27].

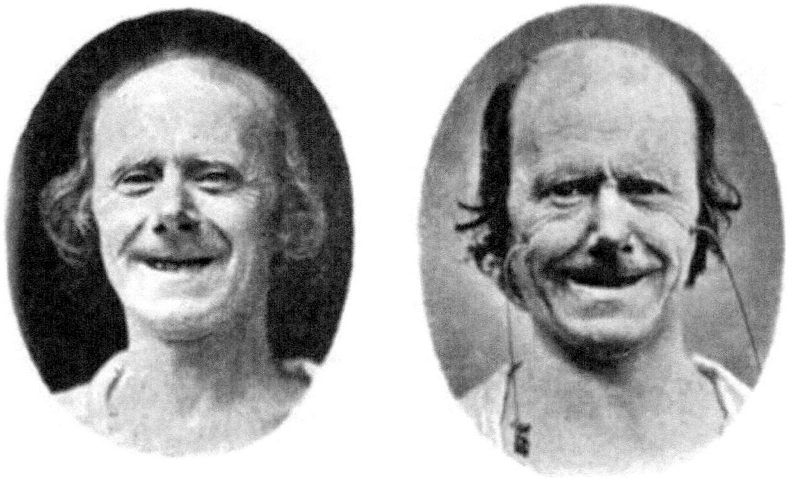

Fig. 13.2 Darwin reported that everyone recognizes the left photo (Duchenne's Plates 32) as happiness, but the right photo (Plate 31), in which there is only zygomaticus major muscle activity without orbicularis oculi muscle, is said not to be a smile of enjoyment—permission from @ Wikicommons cropped from Fig. 13.4, p. 277, from Mécanisme de la Physionomie Humaine [26]

A *Duchenne smile* involves contraction of the zygomatic major muscle and the orbicularis oculi muscle, as Duchenne depicted in his book *Mécanisme de la physionomie humaine* [26]. Duchenne wrote that only the "sweet emotions of the soul" force the orbicularis oculi to contract in a smile, and its inertia in smiling unmasks a false friend. Research suggests that a smile with muscle contraction around the eyes and highly raised cheeks is uniquely associated with positive emotion [28]. A *Duchenne smile* has been described as "smizing" [29] and "smiling with the eyes" [30]. It significantly enhances the perception of advertisements and improves their evaluation [31]. A few people can deliberately initiate a *Duchenne smile* [32]; those with the ability to do so on command are more persuasive in interpersonal interactions [33] and likelier to evoke a positive mood from viewers and trigger affirmative emotional response. However, an exaggerated *Duchenne smile* has been reported to be associated with lying [34].

A *non-Duchenne smile* involves only the zygomatic major muscle without any eye contraction [27]. This mouth-only smile has been called the *Pan Am smile,* named after the former Pan American World Airways, whose flight attendants showed politeness to passengers with a perfunctory smile (Fig. 13.3). Another form of *non-Duchenne smile* is the *Botox smile,* described with the introduction of botulinum toxin treatment in 2002 to paralyze muscles around the eyes and forehead [35]. Genuine smiles may indeed reflect a "sweet soul" and intensity of a true grin can predict marital happiness [36], personal well-being, and even longevity [8, 37, 38]. *Non-Duchenne smile* does not reflect enjoyment, but rather a wide range of emotions, including embarrassment, deceit, and grief. Humanity's simplest expressions are beautifully complex. Frequency and character of smile are influenced by age, gender, culture, and social settings.

In 1974, Leonard Rubin described three basic types of smile: about 59% were the *Mona Lisa smile*, where the mouth corners went up and outward, slightly baring the upper teeth, with the dominant muscle action from the zygomaticus major; about 29% were the *canine smile*, where the canine teeth were exposed, with the dominant muscle action from the levator labii superioris; about 2% were the *full dentured smile*, where the smile showed both upper and lower rows of teeth, with all muscles equally dominant (Fig. 13.4) [25].

The classification of smiles described above is limited to specific cultures [32]. It has been suggested that *smile* may be recognized specifically as a universal display of authenticity in Western culture, whereas judgments of its authenticity go beyond the sender's face to include elements from the perceiver's mind [39].

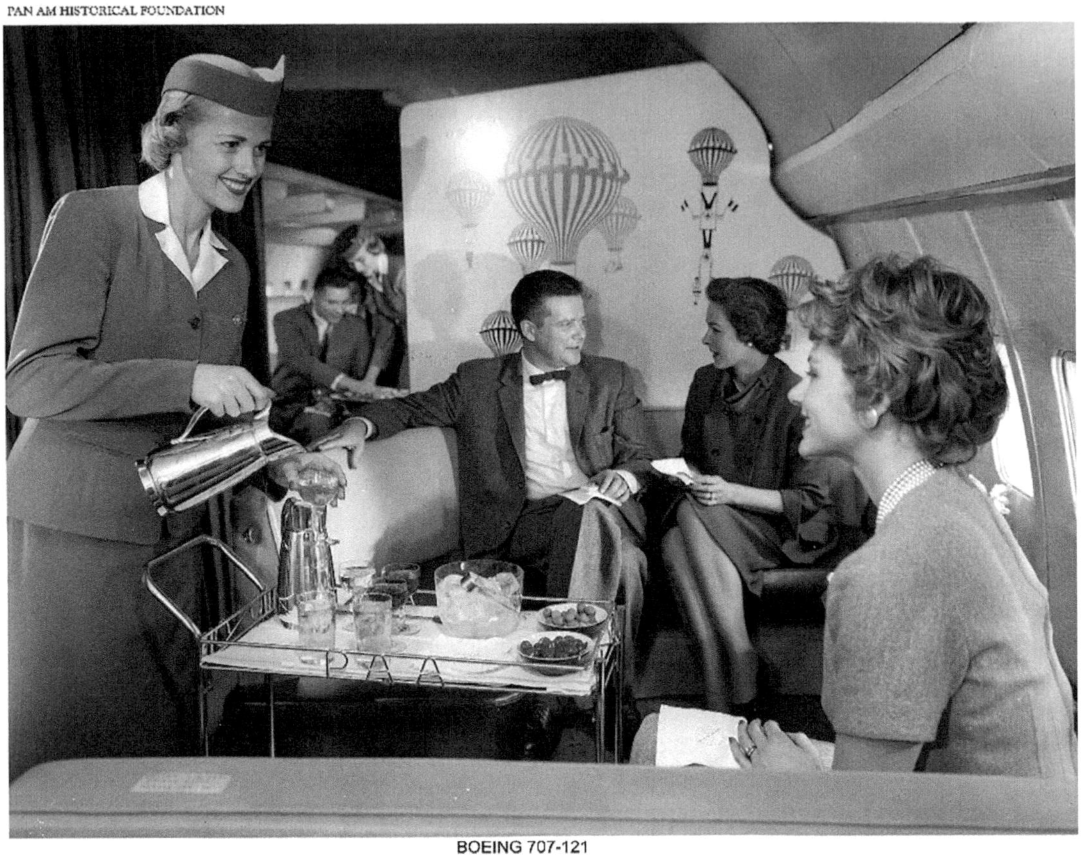

Fig. 13.3 Pan Am flight attendant in 1958. Courtesy of The Pan Am Historical Foundation (www.panam.org), permission granted by Dough Miller

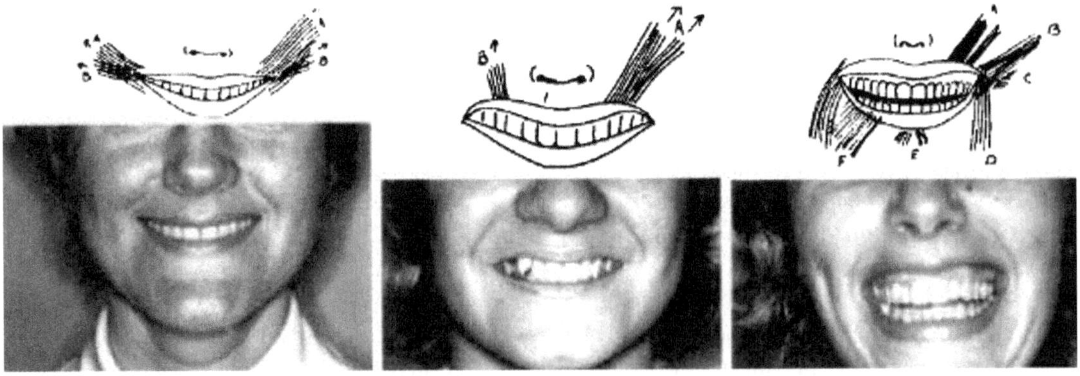

Fig. 13.4 (Left) "Mona Lisa" smile shows dominant activity of zygomatic major muscle; (center) "canine" smile shows dominant levator labii superior muscle contraction; and (right) "full denture" smile shows both muscles equally dominant [25]—permission granted by Wolters Kluwer Health, Inc., Copyright Clearance Center License Number 4880960453860

In 2010, Niedenthal et al. described three types of smiles according to their purpose: *enjoyment*, *affiliative*, and *dominance* smiles [40]. An enjoyment smile can be seen when humans and some primates smile spontaneously during pleasure or success [41]. Affiliative smiles are essential for creating and maintaining social bonds by signaling positive social intentions. Dominance smiles have different physical attributes than those of affiliative and enjoyment smiles: they reflect social status or control and may include conspiratorial, critical, and proud smiles [40].

13.1.5 The Dimple and the Smile

Facial dimples are visible indentations of the epidermis, caused by dermocutaneous insertion of underlying muscle at smile. They supposedly enhance beauty and expression and are much appreciated. Dimples may accentuate the smile, which might in turn increase viewers' perception of attractiveness, sociability, and facial beauty. Moreover they may enhance a smile with more memorable and distinct impressions, and associate it with more cheerfulness. They can be seen on different parts of the body, such as abdomen, back, extremities, and shoulder. A deep dimple on the cheek is usually perceived to be more attractive than a shallow one, but a shallow dimple on the chin can be perceived to be "adorable." Dimples make a smile more prominent and increase the perception of expressions and facial beauty [42]. In many cultures dimples feature prosperous lives. Their presence on the cheek is considered a symbol of good luck in Chinese culture and as a sign of beauty in Arabian culture [43]. Some Chinese women believe that a dimple can bring good fortune to their family. They also believe that a dimple is an important part of a beautiful smiling face. Hence, there is a high demand for dimples surgeries [43].

Dimples are genetically autosomal dominant inherited and occur in both sexes, with no predominance [44–46]. Cheek dimples are believed to occur on chromosome 16, whereas cleft chin dimples occur on chromosome 5 [45]. Single dimple, which occurs on one side of the face only, is rare. Anatomically, formation of dimples may be explained by variations of double or bifid zygomaticus major muscles [47]. Bifid variation of the muscle originates as a single structure from the zygomatic bone and divides with a superior bundle to insert in the typical position above the corner of the mouth and the inferior bundle inserts below the corner of the mouth. In contrast, chin dimples result from an underlying bone defect [48].

13.2 Preoperative Evaluation of the Smile

13.2.1 Mouth Corner Vector for Smile Reanimation

The human smile is an active complex coordinated mimetic function, predominantly with a supero-lateral pull of the mouth corners and elevation of the upper lip, through four main mimetic muscles: zygomaticus major, levator labii superioris, levator labii superioris alaeque nasi muscles, and zygomaticus minor (Fig. 13.5). Knowledge of the mimetic muscles and anatomic variability is key to understanding facial movement, the smile, and consequently the management of long-standing facial nerve palsy [49].

In the following chapters of this section, several authors describe the use of both free muscle and local muscle transfers for smile restoration in long-standing facial paralysis. Many technical and strategic aspects need to be taken into consideration in this surgery, but a factor in achieving the most natural reconstruction is the adequate insetting and location of the muscle transplant that resembles the line of dynamic of mimetic muscles, particularly the zygomatic major muscle. Zabojova et al. studied the angular relations between these mimetic muscles and their anatomical variations to allow for better understanding of the reconstruction needs using muscle transplants for smile reanimation [49]. This anatomic study demonstrated a vertical orientation of the free muscle to reconstruct the zygomaticus

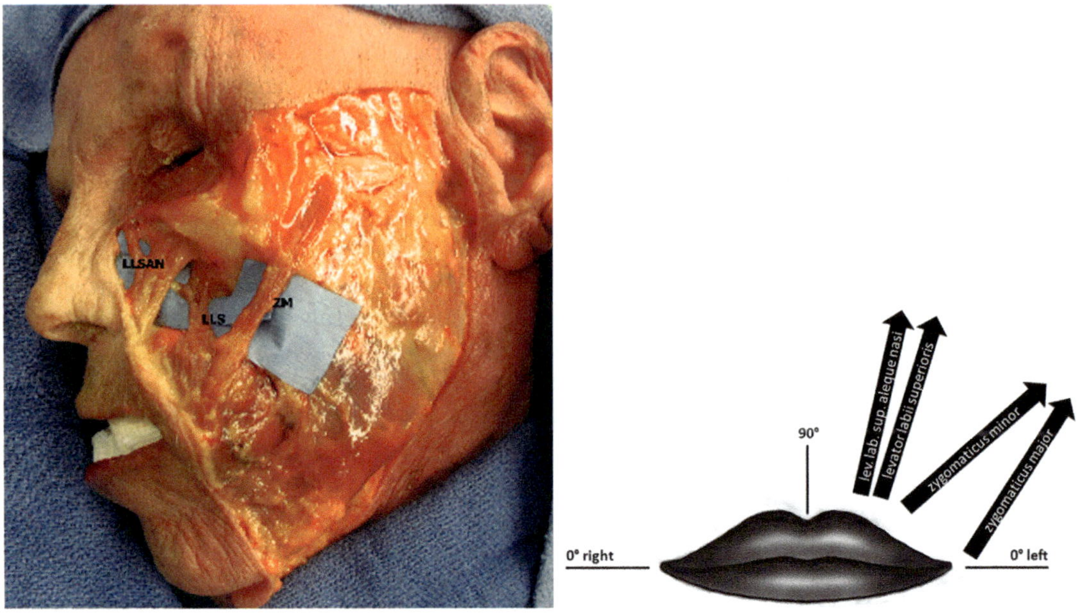

Fig. 13.5 Anatomical photo representing the main mimetic muscles for smiling on the left (LLSAN, LLS, ZM) and its vector of pull in relation to the oral commissure on the left [49]. Used with permission from Wolters Kluwer Health, Inc.: Zabojova, J. Thrikutam, N. Tolley, P. Perez, J. Rozen, S. M. & Rodriguez-Lorenzo, A. (2018). Relational Anatomy of the Mimetic Muscles and Its Implications on Free Functional Muscle Inset in Facial Reanimation. Annals of Plastic Surgery, 81(2), 203–207. https://doi.org/10.1097/SAP.0000000000001507

major muscle angle orientation at least at 55.5° to achieve the best result (Figs. 13.5 and 13.6).

13.2.2 Donor Nerves and Muscles in Smile Reanimation

The gold standard of smile restoration in long-standing facial paralysis is the use of muscle transfers to allow for the dynamic rehabilitation of the smile. There are several considerations when performing muscle transfer for smile reanimation, including the selection of the muscle flap, the selection of the neurotizer, muscle insetting, and the selection of the surgical strategy (one versus two- or three-stage procedures) (Table 13.1).

Free functional muscle transfer has become a common treatment modality for facial reanimation. It can be performed as a one-, two- or three-stage procedure, usually depending of several factors, such as surgeon preference, age, etiology, facial morphology, and patient preference [50, 51]. The two- and three-stage operation using a cross-face nerve graft from the contralateral facial nerve may provide a synchronized, coordinated, and spontaneous emotional expression; however, it has drawbacks, including two surgeries and a long regeneration time. A one-stage procedure using a long nerve pedicle coapted to the contralateral face has also been proposed by several authors, using mostly the latissimus dorsi, allowing for a quicker recovery period and overcoming the potential sequelae involved with nerve harvesting and nerve bridging. There is an increasing trend to use one-stage procedures with a nonfacial nerve as neurotizers, mostly the masseter nerve. Natghian et al. have published a comparative study and metanalysis between both one-stage and two-stage procedures in the literature [51], showing that one-stage procedures using nonfacial nerve neurotizers produce better excursion and symmetry than two-stage procedures, but these comparisons do not include one important variable: the spontaneity of the smile. To overcome this, dual innervation procedures combining the

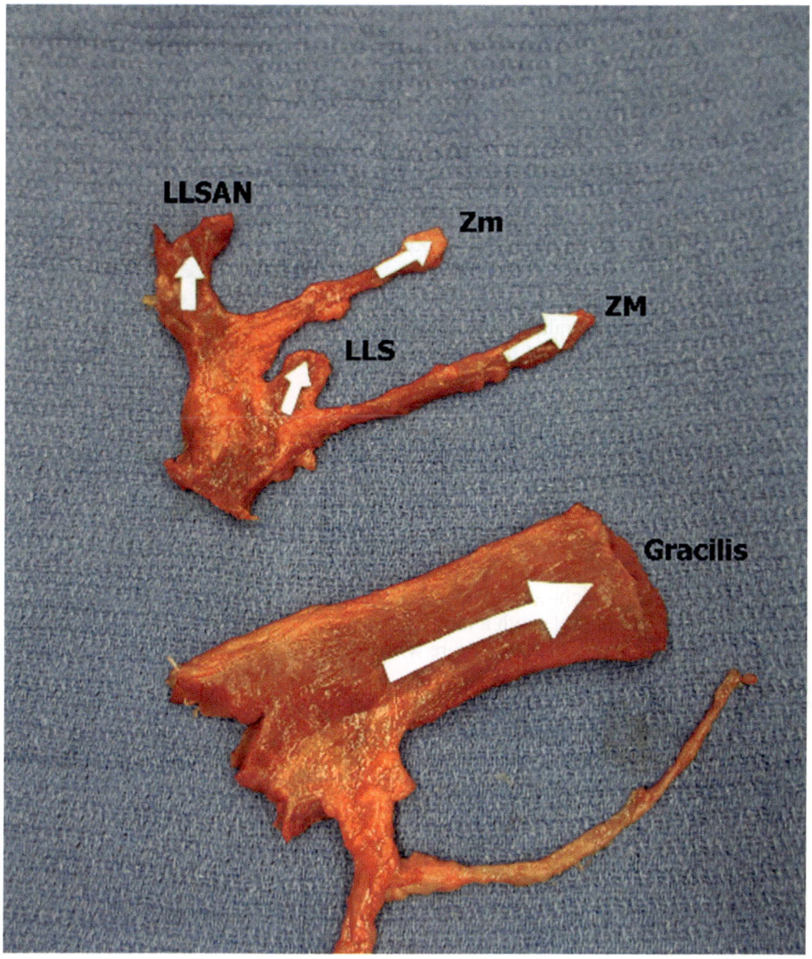

Fig. 13.6 Photograph of the left facial mimic muscles harvested en bloc in relation to a gracilis muscle flap to demonstrate the different vectors of pull. (*ZM* zygomaticus major, *Zm* zygomaticus minor, *LLS* levator labii superioris, and *LLSAN* levator labii superioris alaeque nasi) [49]. Used with permission from Wolters Kluwer Health, Inc.: Zabojova, J. Thrikutam, N. Tolley, P. Perez, J. Rozen, S. M. & Rodriguez-Lorenzo, A. (2018). Relational Anatomy of the Mimetic Muscles and Its Implications on Free Functional Muscle Inset in Facial Reanimation. Annals of Plastic Surgery, 81(2), 203–207. https://doi.org/10.1097/SAP.0000000000001507

power of the masseter nerve and the muscle transfer with the cross-facial nerve grafts for achieving spontaneity have recently been developed. This book reflects the complexity and variety of treatment options in facial reanimation, as described in the following chapters. Each technique and approach has advantages and disadvantages and needs to be individualized to the patient and based on surgeon experience.

13.3 Intraoperative Evaluation of the Smile

Before starting an operation, go through the operation procedure and steps with the operation team (scrub nurse, anesthesiologist, and so forth), especially in cases of cross-face nerve transplantation or facial nerve transfer. Information of nonrelaxation must be passed on to the anesthesiologist to be able to stimulate the facial nerve and to select the best nerve needed. If relaxation was given at intubation, the pharmacokinetics should be kept in mind, as relaxation no longer has any effect on the nerve. Keep the anesthesiologist aware that no relaxation should be given for the rest of the operation in order for the surgeon to stimulate the facial nerve.

The preoperative resting position and smile photographs with and without showing teeth should be printed out. The smile vector of the mouth corner and the movement of the lips should be marked on the photographs to match

Table 13.1 Types and general considerations in smile restoration in long-standing facial paralysis when using free functional muscle transfer (FFMT) and regional muscle transfer (RMT)

Free functional muscle transfer (FFMT)	
(a) Selection of donor muscle	Pectoralis minor Latissimus dorsi Serratus anterior Extensor digitorum brevis Rectus abdominis Gracilis
(b) Selection of donor nerve	Contralateral facial nerve Ipsilateral facial nerve (in partial facial palsy) Masseter nerve Spinal accessory nerve Hypoglossal nerve
(c) Surgical approach	One-stage procedure with FFMT to nonfacial nerve neurotizer One-stage procedure with FFMT to contralateral facial nerve (muscle with a long nerve) two-stage procedure with CFNG and FFMT Dual innervation with CFNG and FFMT to masseter nerve
Regional muscle transfers (RMT)	
(a) Selection of donor muscle	Temporalis muscle Masseter muscle
(b) Type or transposition	Orthodromic: Lengthening myoplasty or elongation with fascial graft Antidromic/reverse

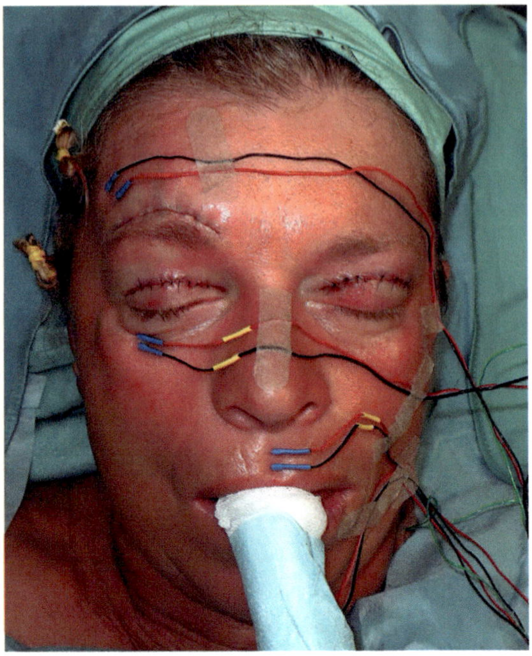

Fig. 13.7 Intraoperative setting of facial nerve neuromonitoring AVALANCHE® SI (Seda S.p.A., Trezzano s/ Naviglio, Milan, Italy)

the best intraoperative stimulation and achieve the most similar smile reconstruction to the healthy side.

Intraoperative stimulation is an important means of finding the most suitable donor facial nerve on the healthy side for a cross-face nerve transplantation. This donor nerve should perform the designated movement of the smile on the paralyzed side.

Static symmetry will be the first goal to achieve during the facial reanimation, so as to support the dynamic reconstruction a static symmetry is a good starting point to build on the dynamic reconstruction. Especially in elder patients, a combination of static and dynamic in the same operation is recommended to achieve the best result [52]. Overcorrection of the paralyzed side must be considered so as to compensate the pull of gravity postoperatively. Gravity will change the position of the corrected eyebrow, eyelids, lips, and mouth corner by at least 1 cm [53–55].

Facial monitoring is a good choice to be used in case of partial facial palsy, where cross-face nerve transplantation is performed. Facial monitoring helps the surgeon locate the facial nerve on the incomplete paralyzed or on the healthy side (Fig. 13.7).

13.4 Postoperative Care of the Smile

Postoperative care is as important as the operation and preoperative evaluation. In the case of a nerve or muscle operation, immobilization of the facial movement is essential to initiate good healing, the dislocation of nerve coaptation and anchoring points of the muscles in the face.

13.4.1 Immediate Postoperative Care

The following food plan is recommended: 3 days of fluid food, followed by 3 days of mushy food and 3 days of soft food. Normal food intake is possible on the tenth day postoperatively.

A bandage around the head (Fig. 13.8) with gauze, cotton, and Peha-haft® (Paul Hartmann GmbH, Vienna, Austria) is important on the one hand to help the patient talk and chew less, and on the other hand to keep the transplanted muscle warm to avoid spasm of the pedicle.

Patients should be instructed to maintain their oral hygiene by gurgling and flushing the mouth with Chlorhexamed FORTE alkoholfrei 0.2% (GlaxoSmithKline Consumer Healthcare GmbH & Co. KG, Munich, Germany) at least three times a day after the meal and if possible in between meals.

Moreover, patients should be advised not to open the mouth and smile well into the immediate postoperative period and during the first 3 weeks. Postoperative swelling will appear immediately and will usually subside after 4–8 weeks. The natural static symmetry will appear within 6–10 months.

13.4.2 Long-Term Postoperative Care

Electrostimulation should be initiated 6 weeks postoperatively, once daily, between 5 and 10 min [56]. The rationale of the 6 weeks waiting time is due to wound tensile strength and muscle-anchoring points. Tensile strength increases linearly slowly for about 2 weeks and then rapidly for 4 weeks. Six weeks postoperatively, the wound has gained about 50% of its ultimate strength and is stable to tolerate moderate forces. In elder patients gains in tensile strength are slower [57] and must be considered before rehabilitation. A standardized evaluation method for assessing the best postoperative physical therapy after neurotized free muscle transplantation to reanimate the paralyzed face uses the following five stages [58]:

Stage I: no movement: electrostimulation, induction exercise, smile exercise.
Stage II: dependent movement: smile exercise.
Stage III: independent movement: spontaneous smile exercise.
Stage IV: spontaneous movement with and without involuntary movement: spontaneous smile exercise.

According to these stages, postoperative physical therapy will be applied as follows.

At stage I, all patients will be advised to enter a rehabilitation program for electrostimulation, smile exercise, and induction exercise of all neurotized free muscle transplantation. Induction exercise is like an internal nerve stimulation and is used to stimulate nerve growth into the muscle and to induce the reinnervated muscle to contract: after XI nerve transfer, shoulder raising or shoulder bending back against resistance; after phrenic or intercostal nerve transfer, running, walking, or climbing hills; after contralateral C7 spinal nerve transfer, donor limb shoulder-grasping exercises with resistance; after masseteric nerve transfer, biting and clenching with the teeth. The patient should be ordered to smile and then, for example, elevate or abduct the shoulder (trigger movement) at the same side as the paralyzed face until movement of FFMT is observed when triggered. These exercises are motor reeducation, which can progressively induce cortical adaptation. The realization of the importance of these exercises is crucial; good results are commonly achieved by psychologically strong and ambitious patients who cooperate well in their rehabilitation programs, whereas poor results are often obtained by lazy or uncooperative patients. When trigger movement can initiate a smile, the next stage of exercise will be initiated.

Stage II: dependent movement becomes more and more dominant during the next 3–6 months postoperatively. Once the triggered FFMT movement becomes dominant, the patient is advised to decrease the trigger movement progressively until it becomes independent—a smile without using the trigger movement.

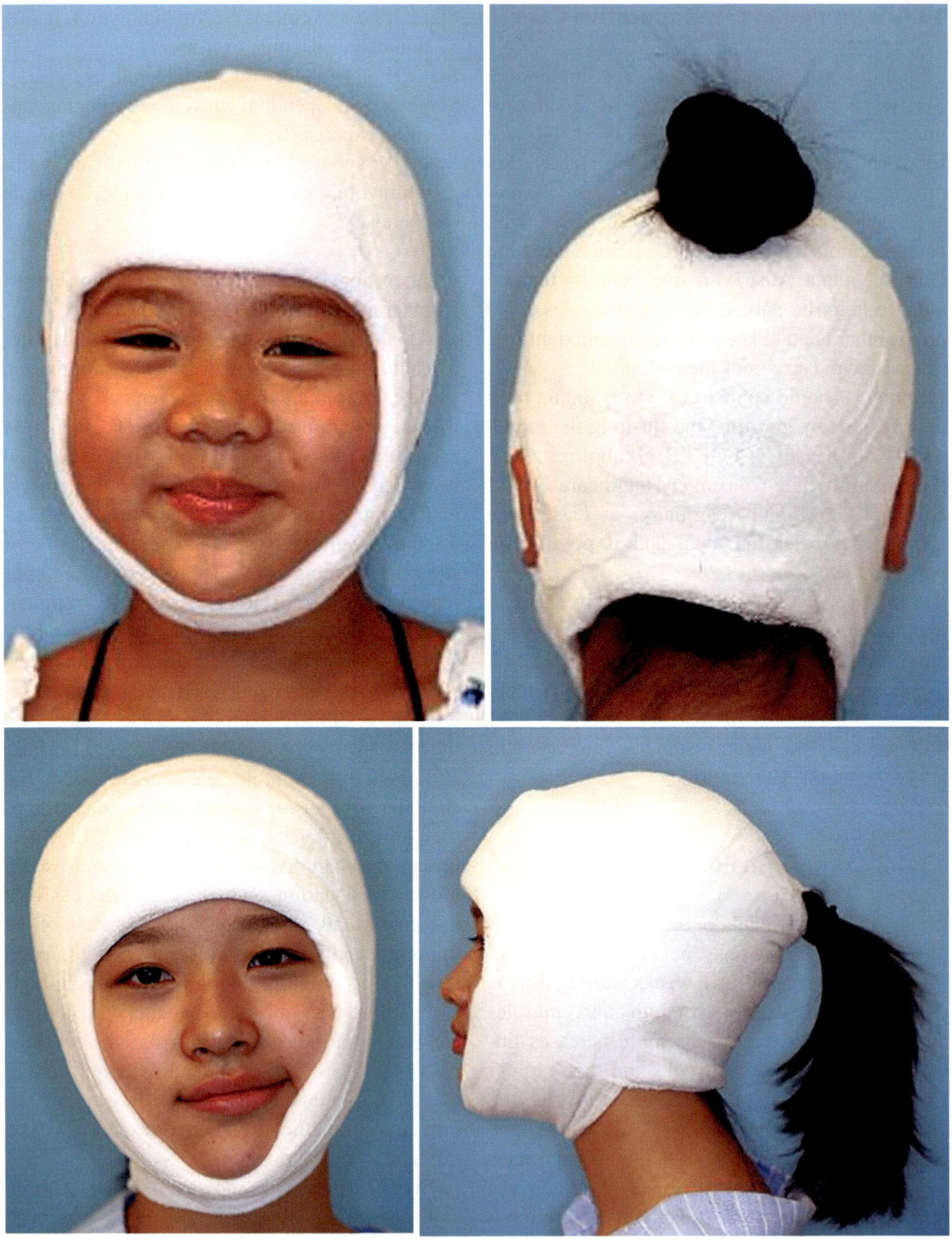

Fig. 13.8 Head bandage, ears can be cut out and spare if there is no wound on that side; for female patients with long hair a high pony tail or dutt/bun would be easy to the postoperative care

Stage III: independent movement usually occurs at 6 months postoperatively. After this period, mirror smile training is started to achieve a spontaneous smile with less or without involuntary movement (stage IV/V). Moreover, the patient should be advised to learn how to control the different degrees of FFMT for small, moderate, and big smiles, also to learn how to adjust the normal side of the face to smile with the FFMT on the paralyzed side to achieve a symmetrical smile. This is called mirror therapy rehabilitation.

For more information, please refer to the chapter "Pre- and Post-Op Rehabilitation in Facial Palsy Patients" by Othmar Schuhfried.

References

1. Schmidt KL, Cohn JF. Human facial expressions as adaptations: evolutionary questions in facial expression research. Am J Phys Anthropol. 2001;Suppl 33:3–24. https://doi.org/10.1002/ajpa.2001.
2. Darwin CR. The expression of the emotions in man and animals. 1st ed. London: John Murray; 1872.
3. Castro É. The neuropsychophysiological construction of the human smile. In: Freitas-Magalhães A, editor. Emotional expression: the brain and the face. Porto, Portugal: Edições Universidade Fernando Pessoa; 2009. p. 2–22.
4. Preuschoft S. "Laughter" and "Smile" in Barbary Macaques (Macaca sylvanus). Ethology. 1992;91(3):220–36. https://doi.org/10.1111/j.1439-0310.1992.tb00864.x.
5. Kraut RE, Johnston RE. Social and emotional messages of smiling: an ethological approach. J Pers Soc Psychol. 1979;37(9):1539–53.
6. Freitas-magalhães A. Emotional expression: the brain and the face. EscrytoslEd. Autor; 2015.
7. Hess U, Beaupré MG, Cheung N. Who to whom and why—cultural differences and similarities in the function of smiles, p. 187–216;2002.
8. Gladstone G, Parker G. When you're smiling does the whole world smile for you? Aust Psychiatry. 2002;10(2):144–6. https://doi.org/10.1046/j.1440-1665.2002.00423.x.
9. Palmer MT, Simmons KB. Communicating intentions through nonverbal behaviors conscious and nonconscious encoding of liking. Hum Commun Res. 1995;22(1):128–60. https://doi.org/10.1111/j.1468-2958.1995.tb00364.x.
10. Otta E, Lira BB, Delevati NM, Cesar OP, Pires CS. The effect of smiling and of head tilting on person perception. J Psychol. 1994;128(3):323–31. https://doi.org/10.1080/00223980.1994.9712736.
11. Miles LK. Who is approachable? J Exp Soc Psychol. 2009;45(1):262–6. https://doi.org/10.1016/j.jesp.2008.08.010.
12. Wikipedia. When you're smiling. 2020. https://en.wikipedia.org/w/index.php?title=When_You%27re_Smiling&oldid=967001376. Accessed 10 July 2020.
13. Matsumoto D, Willingham B. Spontaneous facial expressions of emotion of congenitally and noncongenitally blind individuals. J Pers Soc Psychol. 2009;96(1):1–10. https://doi.org/10.1037/a0014037.
14. Haakana M. Laughter and smiling: notes on co-occurrences. J Pragmat. 2010;42(6):1499–512. https://doi.org/10.1016/j.pragma.2010.01.010.
15. Tracy JL, Beall AT. Happy guys finish last: the impact of emotion expressions on sexual attraction. Emotion. 2011;11(6):1379–87. https://doi.org/10.1037/a0022902.
16. Szarota P. The mystery of the European smile: a comparison based on individual photographs provided by internet users. J Nonverbal Behav. 2010;34(4):249–56. https://doi.org/10.1007/s10919-010-0093-y.
17. Izard CE. The face of emotion. [S.l.]. New York: Appleton; 1971.
18. Woermann V, Holodynski M, Kärtner J, Keller H. A cross-cultural comparison of the development of the social smile: a longitudinal study of maternal and infant imitation in 6- and 12-week-old infants. Infant Behav Dev. 2012;35(3):335–47. https://doi.org/10.1016/j.infbeh.2012.03.002.
19. Levine DR, Adelman MB. Beyond language: cross-cultural communication. Englewood Cliffs, NJ: Prentice Hall Regents; 1993.
20. Krys K, Melanie Vauclair C, Capaldi CA, Lun VM-C, Bond MH, Domínguez-Espinosa A, et al. Be careful where you smile: culture shapes judgments of intelligence and honesty of smiling individuals. J Nonverbal Behav. 2016;40:101–16. https://doi.org/10.1007/s10919-015-0226-4.
21. Bedford, N., et al. "Lonely planet—Destination Poland." Oakland, CA: LPP; 2008.
22. Tidwell C. Non-verbal communication modes. 2018. https://www.andrews.edu/~tidwell/bsad560/NonVerbal.html.
23. Szarota P. Smiling and happiness in cultural perspective. Aust Asian J Cancer. 2011;10(4):277–82.
24. Yuki M, Maddux WW, Masuda T. Are the windows to the soul the same in the East and West? Cultural differences in using the eyes and mouth as cues to recognize emotions in Japan and the United States. J Exp Soc Psychol. 2007;43(2):303–11. https://doi.org/10.1016/j.jesp.2006.02.004.
25. Rubin LR. The anatomy of a smile: its importance in the treatment of facial paralysis. Plast Reconstruct Surg. 1974;53(4):384–7.
26. Duchenne GB. Mécanisme de la physionomie humaine, ou, Analyse électro-physiologique de l'expression des passions, vol. 1. Paris: Jules Renouard, libraire; 1862.
27. Duchenne GB, de Boulogne GBD, Cuthbertson RA, Manstead ASR, Oatley K. The mechanism of human facial expression. Cambridge: Cambridge University Press; 1990.

28. Messinger DS, Fogel A, Dickson KL. All smiles are positive, but some smiles are more positive than others. Dev Psychol. 2001;37(5):642–53. https://doi.org/10.1037/0012-1649.37.5.642.
29. Lefler A. The chicktionary: from A-line to Z-snap, the words every woman should know; 2011.
30. Davis D (2014) How to design a life worth smiling about: developing success in business and in life.
31. Scanlon AE, Polage DC. The strength of a smile: Duchenne smiles improve advertisement and product evaluations. Pac Northw J Undergrad Res Creative Activities. 2011;2(3).
32. Thibault P, Levesque M, Gosselin P, Hess U. The Duchenne marker is not a universal signal of smile authenticity—but it can be learned! Soc Psychol. 2012;43(4):215–21. https://doi.org/10.1027/1864-9335/a000122.
33. Gunnery SD, Hall JA. The Duchenne smile and persuasion. J Nonverbal Behav. 2014;38(2):181–94. https://doi.org/10.1007/s10919-014-0177-1.
34. Marcotte B. Using data science to tell which of these people is lying. 2018. http://www.rochester.edu/newscenter/data-science-facial-expressions-who-if-lying-321252/
35. Leigh A. Charisma: the secrets of making a lasting impression. Pearson Education Limited; 2012.
36. Gottman J, Levenson R, Woodin E. Facial expressions during marital conflict. J Fam Commun. 2001;1(1):37–57. https://doi.org/10.1207/S15327698JFC0101_06.
37. Hacker J, Stanistreet D. Equity in waiting times for two surgical specialties: a case study at a hospital in the North West of England. J Public Health. 2004;26(1):56–60. https://doi.org/10.1093/pubmed/fdh115.
38. Keltner D. Ekman, emotional expression, and the art of empirical epiphany. J Res Pers. 2004;38(1):37–44. https://doi.org/10.1016/j.jrp.2003.09.006.
39. Maringer M, Krumhuber EG, Fischer AH, Niedenthal PM. Beyond smile dynamics: mimicry and beliefs in judgments of smiles. Emotion. 2011;11(1):181–7. https://doi.org/10.1037/a0022596.
40. Niedenthal PM, Mermillod M, Maringer M, Hess U. The simulation of smiles (SIMS) model: embodied simulation and the meaning of facial expression. Behav Brain Sci. 2010;33(6):417–33.; ; discussion 433–480. https://doi.org/10.1017/s0140525x10000865.
41. Ekman P. Lie catching and microexpressions. In: Martin CW, editor. The philosophy of deception. Oxford: Oxford University Press; 2009. p. 118–33.
42. Kumar M, Dey A, Singh D, Sudhakar KN, Mohanty R. Facial dimple creation surgery: a review of literature. Indian J Dent Sci. 2017;9(4):282–6. https://doi.org/10.4103/ijds.ijds_62_17.
43. Bao S, Zhou C, Li S, Zhao M. A new simple technique for making facial dimples. Aesthetic Plast Surg. 2007;31(4):380–3. https://doi.org/10.1007/s00266-006-0191-8.
44. Argamaso RV. Facial dimple: its formation by a simple technique. Plast Reconstr Surg. 1971;48(1):40–3.
45. Omotoso O, Adeniyi P, Medubi L. Prevalence of facial dimples amongst South-western Nigerians: a case study of Ilorin, Kwara State of Nigeria, vol. 6; 2010.
46. Pentzos Daponte A, Vienna A, Brant L, Hauser G. Cheek dimples in Greek children and adolescents, vol. 19;2004.
47. Pessa JE, Zadoo VP, Garza PA, Adrian EK Jr, Dewitt AI, Garza JR. Double or bifid zygomaticus major muscle: anatomy, incidence, and clinical correlation. Clin Anat. 1998;11(5):310–3. https://doi.org/10.1002/(sici)1098-2353(1998)11:5<310::aid--ca3>3.0.co;2-t.
48. Keyhan SO, Khiabani K, Hemmat S. Dimple creation surgery technique: a review of the literature and technique note. J Oral Maxillofac Surg. 2012;70(6):e403–7. https://doi.org/10.1016/j.joms.2012.02.015.
49. Zabojova J, Thrikutam N, Tolley P, Perez J, Rozen SM, Rodriguez-Lorenzo A. Relational anatomy of the mimetic muscles and its implications on free functional muscle inset in facial reanimation. Ann Plast Surg. 2018;81(2):203–7. https://doi.org/10.1097/sap.0000000000001507.
50. Frey M, Giovanoli P. The three-stage concept to optimize the results of microsurgical reanimation of the paralyzed face. Clin Plast Surg. 2002;29(4):461–82.
51. Natghian H, Fransén J, Rozen SM, Rodriguez-Lorenzo A. Qualitative and quantitative analysis of smile excursion in facial reanimation: a systematic review and meta-analysis of 1- versus 2-stage procedures. Plast Reconstr Surg Glob Open. 2017;5(12):e1621. https://doi.org/10.1097/gox.0000000000001621.
52. Kiefer J, Braig D, Thiele JR, Bannasch H, Stark GB, Eisenhardt SU. Comparison of symmetry after smile reconstruction for flaccid facial paralysis with combined fascia lata grafts and functional gracilis transfer for static suspension or gracilis transfer alone. Microsurgery. 2018;38(6):634–42. https://doi.org/10.1002/micr.30324.
53. Abbasi R. Facial reanimation by masseteric muscle-mandibular periosteum transfer. World J Plast Surg. 2013;2(1):44–6.
54. Frey M, Michaelidou M, Tzou C, Pona I, Mittlböck M, Gerber H, Stüssi E. Three-dimensional video analysis of the paralyzed face reanimated by cross-face nerve grafting and free gracilis muscle transplantation: quantification of the functional outcome. Plast Reconstr Surg. 2008;122(6):1709–22.
55. Labbe D, Bussu F, Iodice A. A comprehensive approach to long-standing facial paralysis based on lengthening temporalis myoplasty. Acta Otorhinolaryngol Ital. 2012;32(3):145–53.

56. Paternostro-Sluga T, Herceg M, Frey M. [Conservative treatment and rehabilitation in peripheral facial palsy]. Handchir Mikrochir Plast Chir. 2010;42(2):109–14. https://doi.org/10.1055/s-0029-1243215.
57. Hsu A, Mustoe TA. The principle of wound healing. In: Weinzweig J, editor. Plastic surgery secrets plus e-book. 2nd ed. Philadelphia: Elsevier Health Sciences; 2010. p. 4.
58. Tzou CH, Chuang DC, Chen HY. Cortical adaptation staging system: a new and simple staging for result evaluation of functioning free-muscle transplantation for facial reanimation. Ann Plast Surg. 2014;73(1):50–3.

14 One-Stage Facial Reanimation Using Masseter Nerve Free Flap

D. Braig and Steffen U. Eisenhardt

Key Points

- The masseteric nerve is a branch of the mandibular nerve (V3) and is therefore not compromised in its function in isolated facial palsy. The technique evolved from the treatment of congenital bilateral facial palsy, e.g., Moebius Syndrome, to an increasingly popular alternative to CFNG in patients with a broad smile or who decline a dual-stage reanimation. It enables reliable single-stage facial reanimation in conjunction with a free muscle flap without interposition nerve grafting. Preoperative electromyography can identify patients who are likely to develop a spontaneous smile. The masseteric nerve is located 3 cm anterior to the tragus and 1 cm inferior to the zygomatic arch. It is transferred in a more superficial plane for direct coaptation to the motor branch of the free flap and leaves a minimal donor site morbidity. Visible muscle contractions are observed after 3–4 months.

14.1 Anatomy

The masseteric nerve is a terminal branch of the mandibular nerve (V3) and is therefore not compromised in its function in isolated facial palsy. It can contain over 2500 motor axons for coaptation and thus provides nearly 75% of axons compared to the facial nerve at the stylomastoid foramen. It traverses over the lateral pterygoid muscle, behind the tendon of the temporal muscle and through the mandibular notch before entering the masseteric muscle on its deep surface. After entering the muscle belly, the nerve travels diagonally towards the oral commissure at a 50° angle to the zygomatic arch. It releases a consistent branch behind the zygomatic bone before the main trunk splits into several terminating branches during its further course through the muscle. This proximal branch is usually preserved during facial reanimation surgery and partial denervation of the masseter muscle does not seem to lead to a clinically relevant donor deficit [1].

Anatomy of Masseteric Nerve

Key Points:

- Course of masseteric nerve through mandibular notch.
- Entry into masseter muscle on deep surface
- Release of proximal branch behind zygomatic arch and course of nerve within masseter muscle

D. Braig · S. U. Eisenhardt (✉)
Department of Plastic Surgery and Hand Surgery, University Medical Center Freiburg, Medical Faculty of the University of Freiburg, Freiburg, Germany
e-mail: david.braig@uniklinik-freiburg.de; steffen.eisenhardt@uniklinik-freiburg.de

© Springer Nature Switzerland AG 2021
C.-H. J. Tzou, A. Rodríguez-Lorenzo (eds.), *Facial Palsy*, https://doi.org/10.1007/978-3-030-50784-8_14

(Example; Reference: Klebuc PRS 2011: Facial Reanimation Using the Masseter-to-Facial Nerve Transfer)

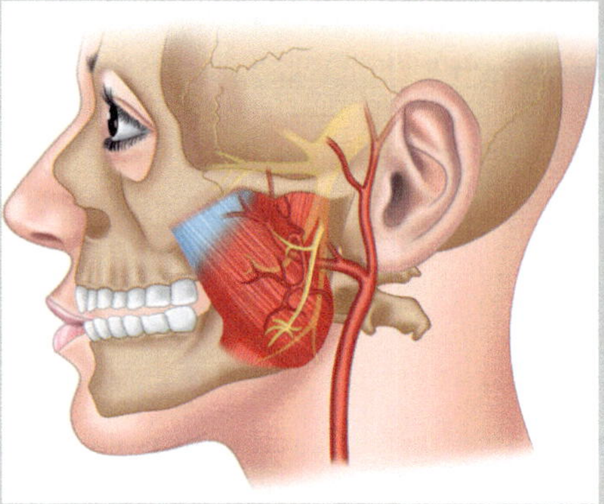

14.2 Diagnostics

Function of the masseter muscle is clinically evaluated by palpating the contracted muscle while the patient clenches his teeth. We additionally recommend an electromyography to quantitatively measure the muscle's activity and assess activation of the masseter muscle during normal smile production. This occurs in nearly 50% of individuals and may help to predict spontaneous smile development in subjects who are candidates for free muscle reanimation procedures with the masseteric nerve [2].

A needle electrode is placed bilaterally in the relaxed masseter muscle to evaluate the insertional activity and resting activity in the muscle, followed by teeth clenching to record the maximal voluntary contraction. The patient is then asked to smile to assess co-activation of the masseter muscle during smile production. Although needle electrodes are commonly used for electromyography, up-to-date surface electrodes perform sufficiently well to evaluate masseter function non-invasively (Fig. 14.1).

14.3 Indications

In long-standing facial paralysis with atrophy of the mimic musculature sole re-innervation does not lead to recovery of muscle function. It is thus necessary to transfer a free muscle flap in conjunction with a functional nerve. The masseteric nerve can be used in a one-step procedure to reanimate a face without an interposition nerve graft by direct coaptation to the motor nerve of the muscle transplant. This technique has been established in children with Moebius Syndrome, where it is not possible to use a CFNG due to bilateral facial palsy [3]. In patients with unilateral facial paralysis, the masseteric nerve can either be used alone, or in combination with a CFNG [4]. The differences and advantages of each donor nerve are summarized in Table 14.1. The main advantages of the masseteric nerve over a CFNG are a shorter re-innervation time of only 3–4 months, an increased number of motor axons, the lack of an additional donor site from harvesting a nerve transplant and the entire preservation of the contralateral facial nerve [5]. The masseteric nerve leads to increased symmetry while smiling due to the higher axon count [6]. This leads to the formation of a greater number of neuromuscular junctions in the muscle transplant, which in turn increases the contraction amplitude of the muscle. In contrast to a CFNG, it is even possible to obtain a symmetrical broad smile that requires extensive excursion of the oral commissures. In addition, the contraction amplitude of the muscle flap can be adjusted to the contralateral side by secondary thinning. In CFNG innervated muscle flaps, the possibility to adjust the contraction amplitude of a muscle flap by thinning is largely limited because of the reduced axon count [7].

Many authors favour the masseteric nerve over a CFNG in elderly patients, as results with a CFNG alone are frequently inferior to the results seen in the paediatric population. A major drawback is however the lack of spontaneity in approximately one-third of patients. Nowadays

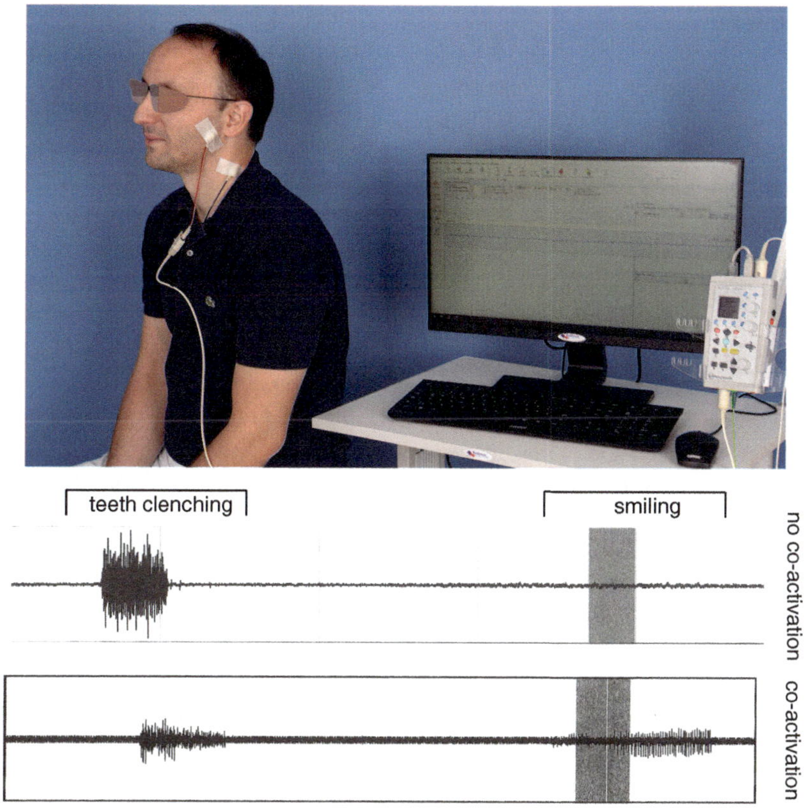

Fig. 14.1 Electromyography is performed to quantitatively measure the muscle's activity and assess activation of the masseter muscle during normal smile production. Surface electrodes are placed over the masseter muscle to record the resting activity of the muscle, followed by teeth clenching to record the maximal voluntary contraction. The patient is then asked to smile to assess co-activation of the masseter muscle during smile production. The depicted photo shows the set-up used for surface electromyography. Selected electromyograms show muscle activity in a patient with and without co-activation of the masseter muscle upon voluntary smile production

Table 14.1 Comparison of CFNG and masseteric nerve as donor nerves for facial reanimation surgery

	Masseteric nerve	CFNG
Stages	Single-stage	Dual-stage
Muscle contractions	3–4 months	9–12 months
Symmetry of smile	Frequent	Rarely
Donor site morbidity	Minor	Obvious
Spontaneity	Approximately 2/3	Always

these patients can be identified preoperative by selective electromyography and counselled accordingly. Whether dual innervation with an additional CFNG can add spontaneity to the powerful masseteric nerve is still open to debate [8].

Another advantage of the masseteric nerve is the single-stage nature of the operation. Whereas CFNG innervation of a muscle flap requires two separate operations with an interval of several months, coaptation of the masseteric nerve to a muscle flap is performed in a single operation. This is often the reason why elderly patients tend to favour the masseteric nerve over a CFNG [9].

Activation of the masseter muscle upon smiling in preoperative selective electromyography is a dependable predictor of spontaneous smile development. In these patients, the masseteric nerve should be preferred to innervate a free muscle flap due to its numerous advantages over a CFNG.

14.4 Technique

We perform a preauricular access extending from the helical root caudally to the mandibular angle. The incision is placed into existing pretragal wrinkles and commonly results in an inconspicuous scar. The soft tissue is mobilized until the anterior margin of the parotid gland is encountered. The preparation plane is performed under the SMAS in complete facial palsy to minimize adherences between the muscle flap and the skin. These might lead to unsightly retractions of the overlying skin upon smiling. In incomplete paralysis, the muscle is placed more superficially to avoid injury to functional facial nerve branches.

The masseteric nerve shows a very consistent course within the masseter muscle and can be reliably encountered 3 cm anterior of the tragus and 1 cm inferior of the zygomatic arch (Fig. 14.2) [1]. Intraoperative selective nerve stimulation can help to identify and preserve intact facial nerve branches in incomplete facial palsy. The fascia of the masseter muscle is incised and the muscle fibres divided along their course to identify the masseteric nerve deep within the muscle belly. Identification and dissection of the nerve is performed under repetitive nerve stimulation, which leads to strong muscular contractions upon direct stimulation of the nerve branches. The nerve is carefully dissected proximally and distally from the surrounding muscle tissue. Accompanying blood vessels require meticulous haemostasis with bipolar diathermy to avoid injury to the masseteric nerve. Generally about 2–3 cm of nerve length distally to the zygomatic arch can be obtained before the nerve splits into its terminal branches (Fig. 14.2). To avoid complete denervation of the muscle, the proximal branches beneath the zygomatic arch are preserved. Contrary to older approaches, this technique preserves most of the masseter function, as the muscle is not released from its origin and the proximal nerve branches are preserved [5, 10].

The nerve is divided shortly before it divides into its terminal branches and transposed in a more superficial plane to facilitate coaptation to the motor nerve of the muscle flap. The muscle flap is then inserted with its pedicle on the deep side and anchored slightly distally to the nasolabial fold. The proximal end of the flap is turned over to gain access to the neurovascular pedicle. Now the masseteric nerve is coaptated epineurally with 9-0 nylon to the motor nerve of the muscle flap. The nerve anastomosis is additionally stabilized with fibrin glue and covered by closure of the overlying SMAS with 4-0 Monocryl. In cases where a dual innervation with

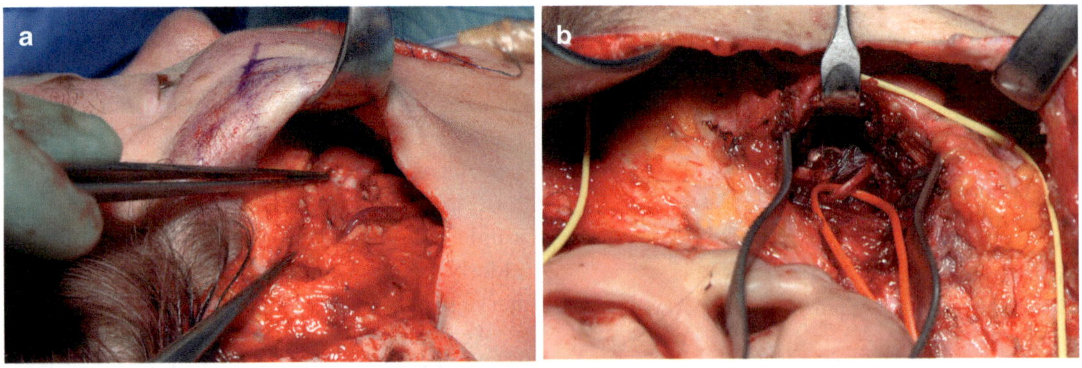

Fig. 14.2 (**a**) The masseteric nerve can be reliably identified 3 cm anterior to the tragus and 1 cm inferior to the zygomatic arch. Forceps show the inferior boarder of the zygomatic arch. The SMAS is incised at right angles and the masseter muscle divided along its muscle fibres to expose the masseteric nerve deep within the muscle belly (white dashed line). (**b**) The masseteric nerve is carefully dissected within the muscle under repetitive nerve stimulation, which generally yields about 2–3 cm of nerve length available for transposition before it divides into its terminal branches. The photograph shows the nerve within the muscle before it is divided at its distal end (red loop)

a CFNG is performed, the CFNG is additionally sutured to the motor nerve of the muscle flap. Subsequently anastomosis of the artery and vein are performed and the muscle is sutured onto the fascia of the temporal muscle under slight tension. First muscle contractions are usually encountered after 3–4 months and full reinnervation after 6 months. After this period evaluation of the muscle contraction amplitude and planning of additional thinning procedures can be planned (Fig. 14.3).

14.5 Summary

The masseteric nerve is an increasingly popular alternative to CFNG for facial reanimation surgery with free flaps. In comparison to a CFNG, it requires only a single-stage procedure and leads to enhanced muscle contractions and symmetry of smile due to its high axon count. On the downside only two-thirds of patients acquire a spontaneous smile. Its function can be evaluated clinically, and additional electromyography may

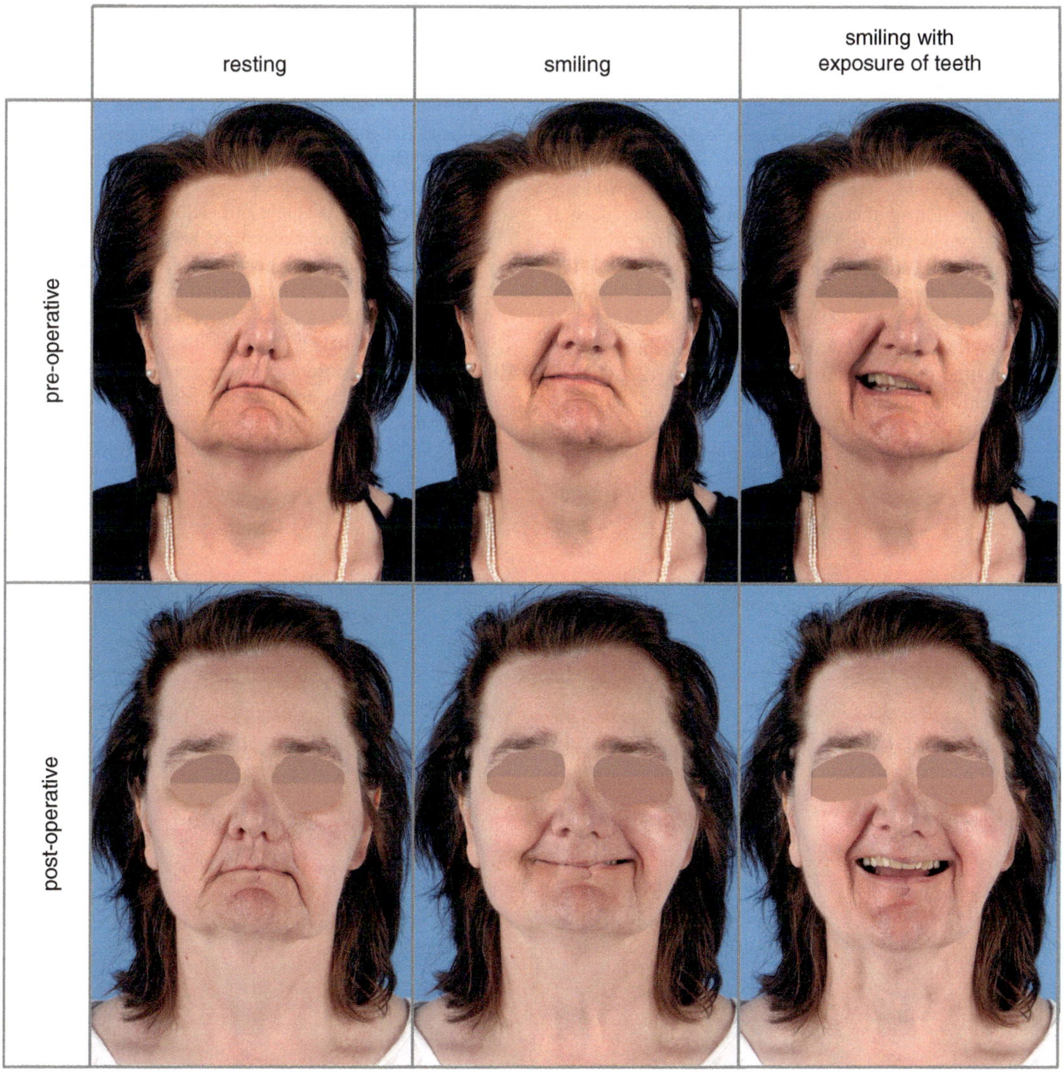

Fig. 14.3 The photos show a 53-year-old woman with complete facial paralysis of the left face. A free gracilis muscle flap was coaptated to the masseteric nerve of the affected side. Photographs were taken preoperative and 10 months post-operative

aid in selecting patients who are likely to produce a spontaneous smile.

Intraoperatively the nerve can reliably be visualized 3 cm anterior to the tragus and 1 cm inferior to the zygomatic arch by selective, repetitive nerve stimulation. Transposing the nerve in a more superficial plane facilitates coaptation to the motor nerve of the free flap. Muscle contractions become evident already 3–4 months after surgery.

References

1. Borschel GH, Kawamura DH, Kasukurthi R, Hunter DA, Zuker RM, Woo AS. The motor nerve to the masseter muscle: an anatomic and histomorphometric study to facilitate its use in facial reanimation. J Plast Reconstr Aesthet Surg. 2012;65(3):363–6. PubMed PMID: 21992936.
2. Schaverien M, Moran G, Stewart K, Addison P. Activation of the masseter muscle during normal smile production and the implications for dynamic reanimation surgery for facial paralysis. J Plast Reconstr Aesthet Surg. 2011;64(12):1585–8. PubMed PMID: 21798833.
3. Zuker RM, Manktelow RT. A smile for the Mobius' syndrome patient. Ann Plast Surg. 1989;22(3):188–94. PubMed PMID: 2735718.
4. Cardenas-Mejia A, Covarrubias-Ramirez JV, Bello-Margolis A, Rozen S. Double innervated free functional muscle transfer for facial reanimation. J Plast Surg Hand Surg. 2015;49(3):183–8. PubMed PMID: 25469588.
5. Klebuc MJ. Facial reanimation using the masseter-to-facial nerve transfer. Plast Reconstr Surg. 2011;127(5):1909–15. PubMed PMID: 21532419.
6. Bae YC, Zuker RM, Manktelow RT, Wade S. A comparison of commissure excursion following gracilis muscle transplantation for facial paralysis using a cross-face nerve graft versus the motor nerve to the masseter nerve. Plast Reconstr Surg. 2006;117(7):2407–13. PubMed PMID: 16772949.
7. Braig D, Bannasch H, Stark GB, Eisenhardt SU. Analysis of the ideal muscle weight of gracilis muscle transplants for facial reanimation surgery with regard to the donor nerve and outcome. J Plast Reconstr Aesthet Surg. 2017;70(4):459–68. PubMed PMID: 28159544.
8. Biglioli F, Colombo V, Tarabbia F, Pedrazzoli M, Battista V, Giovanditto F, et al. Double innervation in free-flap surgery for long-standing facial paralysis. J Plast Reconstr Aesthet Surg. 2012;65(10):1343–9. PubMed PMID: 22728067.
9. Eisenhardt SU, Thiele JR, Stark GB, Bannasch H. Comparison of cross face nerve graft with masseteric nerve as donor nerves for free functional muscle transfers in facial reanimation surgery. Handchir Mikrochir Plast Chir. 2013;45(4):223–8. PubMed PMID: 23970401.
10. Spira M. Anastomosis of masseteric nerve to lower division of facial nerve for correction of lower facial paralysis. Preliminary report. Plast Reconstr Surg. 1978;61(3):330–4. PubMed PMID: 625495.

Spinal Accessory Nerve-Innervated Gracilis (XI-Gracilis) for Facial Reanimation: Chang Gung Experience

15

David Chwei-Chin Chuang

15.1 Inroduction

The spinal accessory nerve(XI) has been a common choice of motor neurotizer in brachial plexus reconstruction. It was utilized either for nerve-to-nerve transfer(such as XI-to-suprascapular nerve for shoulder function) [1, 2], or for nerve-to-motor nerve of a free muscle (functioning free muscle transplantation, FFMT) for elbow [3] or finger function [4]. In the FFMT, the XI can be usually dissected more than 10 cm in length from neck to trunk back, transected and transferred to the infra-clavicular region for nerve coaptation. However, XI-innervated gracilis (XI-gracilis) for facial paralysis reconstruction has never been considered a popular choice. Terzis et al. [5] applied the XI nerve elongation with a nerve grafts to innervate a FFMT to treat Möbius syndrome. Chuang et al. [6] first applied the both sides of XI to directly innervate two gracilis muscles for bilateral Möbius syndrome patient in 2000. After a series of six bilateral Möbius syndrome patients reconstruction with very promising results [7], the authors started to use XI-gracilis to treat unilateral facial paralysis in 2007 (Fig. 15.1).

There are two major dysfunctions of the facial nerve injury: truly facial paralysis (incomplete or complete) [8] and postparalysis facial synkinesis [9]. Both can cause severe functional and aesthetic deficits, a serious affliction and devastating deformity to the victim. Truly facial palsy more than 1 year is called chronic facial paralysis. For chronic facial paralysis, although debate between local and free muscle transfer for facial reanimation persists [10], FFMT is still the main stream of surgical procedure for these deficits treatment [11–16]. For postparalysis facial synkinesis, treatment is also debated [9, 17]. Postparalysis facial synkinesis can occur after any cause of facial paralysis with many presentations. The synkinesis can occur not only always during facial expression, but also at rest because long-term unsolved synkinesis will result in permanent contracture, such as small eye, deep nasolabial fold, lower lip retraction, and platysma neck bands. Those symptoms and signs make patients distress with severe emotional sequelae. Past treatments with botulinum toxin, rehabilitation, or simple selective myectomy or neurectomy are inadequate. Currently surgical treatment proposed by the author [9] for the postparalysis facial synkinesis has been continuously performed. For mild type (Type I, good smile quality and mild synkinesis), conser-

Electronic Supplementary Material The online version of this chapter (https://doi.org/10.1007/978-3-030-50784-8_15) contains supplementary material, which is available to authorized users.

D. C.-C. Chuang (✉)
The Department of Plastic Surgery, Chang Gung Memorial Hospital, Chang Gung University, Taipei-Linkou, Taiwan

© Springer Nature Switzerland AG 2021
C.-H. J. Tzou, A. Rodríguez-Lorenzo (eds.), *Facial Palsy*,
https://doi.org/10.1007/978-3-030-50784-8_15

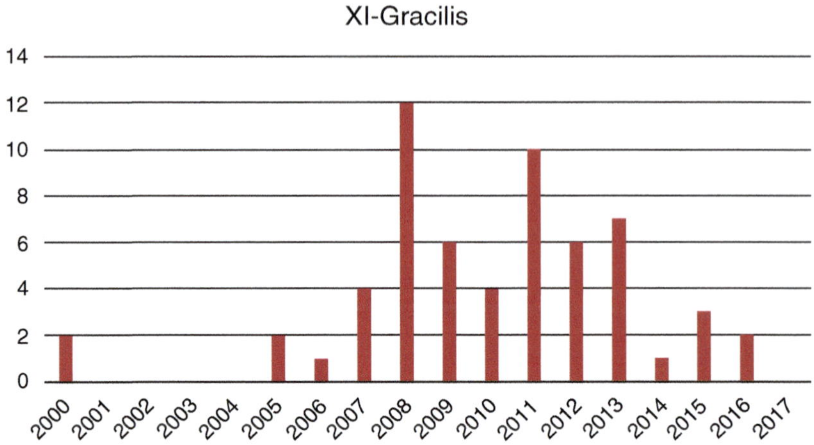

Fig. 15.1 The year patients received XI-gracilis for facial reanimation at one medical unit (Chang Gung Memorial Hospital)

vative treatment with rehabilitation, botulinum toxin injection, or selective myectomy are the treatment of choice. For the Type II, acceptable smile but severe synkinesis, and Type III, unacceptable smile but severe synkinesis, extensive myectomy and neurectomy of the synkinetic muscles and nerves, followed by FFMT in one- or two-stage procedures are our strategic treatment. The long-term results following such aggressive surgery are promising and permanent without requirement of any further botox injection or rehabilitation.

There are at least ten muscles utilized as FFMT for facial reanimation in the literature [18, 19]. However, gracilis muscle remains the preferred muscle by most reconstructive surgeons. Limited nerves were utilized for motor neurotizer in the literature, including contralateral facial nerve as a one [16] or two-stage procedure [11–15], or hypoglossal nerve [20], spinal accessory nerve [5, 6], masseteric nerve [21, 22], and others (such as phrenic [23], brachial plexus C7 [24]). Three methods of CFNG-, XI- and V3-gracilis have been the most popular in our medical center. This paper will focus on XI-gracilis.

15.2 Materials and Methods

Between 1985 and 2017, 392 patients received 403 gracilis FFMT for chronic facial paralysis and postparalysis facial synkinesis reconstruction at Chang Gung Memorial Hospital performed by the senior surgeon (DCC Chuang). Three hundred and twenty-one patients (82%) were chronic facial paralysis, and 71 (18%) were postparalysis facial synkinesis. Eight patients with bilateral Möbius syndrome received both gracilis muscles FFMT, 6 by XI- and 2 by V3-gracilis. Four patients with failed primary CFNG-gracilis and three received second gracilis for redo reconstruction 1 year after initial debridement: two by XI- and one by V3-gracilis. They were all included. Patients with FFMT innervated by ipsilateral facial nerve branches (8 patients), innervated by contralateral facial nerve branches as a one-stage procedure (4 patients), and history with incomplete or loss of follow-up (10 patients) were excluded. The etiology of the palsies was most commonly due to postoperative complications (47.4%), one third (29%) virus infection, and one fifth from trauma and congenital (Table 15.1).

299 FFMTs in 299 patients (299/403, 74%) were innervated by CFNG, 68 FFMTs in 60 patients by XI (18%), and 33 FFMT in 30 patients by V3 (33/403, 8%). Ninety-eight percent of FFMTs were gracilis. Mean of duration of palsy prior to FFMT was 16.8 years (range, 0.5–52) in CFNG-, 10.0 years (range, 0.5–52) in XI-, and 9.9 years (range, 1–27) in V3-gracilis group patients (Table 15.1). For thesis of XI-gracilis: 60 patients with 68 FFMT were enrolled.

In Chang Gung Memorial Hospital, We first started using the two-stage CFNG-gracilis for facial reanimation in 1985, adopted the one-stage

Table 15.1 Patient demographics

Period: 1985–2017		XI-gra	V3-gra	CFNG-gra
Gender		M: 28 F: 30	M: 15 F: 15	M: 115 F: 175
Total patients and muscles	*Total*			
	377 pts 389 FFMT	60 pts 69 FFMT (18%)	30 pts 33 FFMT (8%)	287 pts 287 FFMT (74%)
Age at day of FFMT (years)	Mean Range	37.5 4–68	0.4 4–72	30.9 3–68
Etiology	*Total (pts)*			
Virus infection (Bell's, herpes zoster)	108 (28.6%)	16	2	90
Suppurative otitis media	25 (6.6%)	4	1	20
(cholesteatoma)	154 (40.8%)	12	12	130
After tumor resection	51 (13.5%)	9	2	40
Trauma	39 (10.3%)	17	12	10
Congenital				
Duration of facial paralysis (year)	Mean Range	10.0 0.5–52	9.9 1–27	16.8 0.5–52
Onset of muscle contraction after transplantation (month)	Mean Range	5 3–12	3 2–6	9 6–18

V3-gracilis in 1995, and then the one-stage XI-gracilis in 2000. The reasons of such change from CFNG- and V3- to the XI-gracilis between 2000 and 2010 (Fig. 15.1) were XI- had benefits of CFNG-gracilis with characteristics of potentially to achieve spontaneous and synchronous smile, and also benefits of V3-gracilis with characteristics of one-stage surgery and quick result.

15.3 Anatomy Review

15.3.1 Spinal Accessory Nerve (XI)

The Accessory nerve (n. accessorius, 11th cranial nerve) is the only one cranial nerve which has its origins from the spine. It is a motor nerve, supplying somatic efferent fibers to the neck muscles and visceral efferent fibers which joins the vagus nerve for swallowing and phonation. Because it runs with the big vagus nerve in the cranium, it looks like an accessory to the vagus nerve. The accessory nerve has two origins: cranial and spinal. The cranial part, originating from medulla oblongata, has four or five delicate rootlets, running with the vagus nerve to the jugular foramen, becoming the internal branch of the accessory nerve. The spinal part, origining from cervical C1–C5 motor cells. Passes through the foramen magnum of the occipital bone into the cranial cavity. It penetrates the dura mater and passes through the jugular foramen, becoming the external branch of the accessory nerve. In the jugular foramen, Both join together and separate. The spinal part becomes spinal accessory nerve (XI). The XI nerve exits from the jugular foramen, in front of the internal jugular vein, and passes posterior to the stylohyoidues and digastricus muscle to the upper part of the sternocleidomastoideus. It pierces the muscle and locates behind. The XI nerve appears from behind the sternocleidomastoid, about one finger-width above the greater auricular nerve, or above the transverse branch of the external jugular vein (Fig. 15.2). It courses obliquely downward across the posterior triangle of the neck to the anterior border of the trapezius. In front of trapezius muscle, the XI nerve communicates with the second, third, and fourth cervical nerves which are sensory branches, coming from the anterior to join the XI nerve with a plexiform arrangement, and continues descending on the deep surface of the trapezius almost to its lower border [25, 26]. The XI innervates the sternocleidomastoid and trapezius muscles. The XI injury is common following neck dissection in head

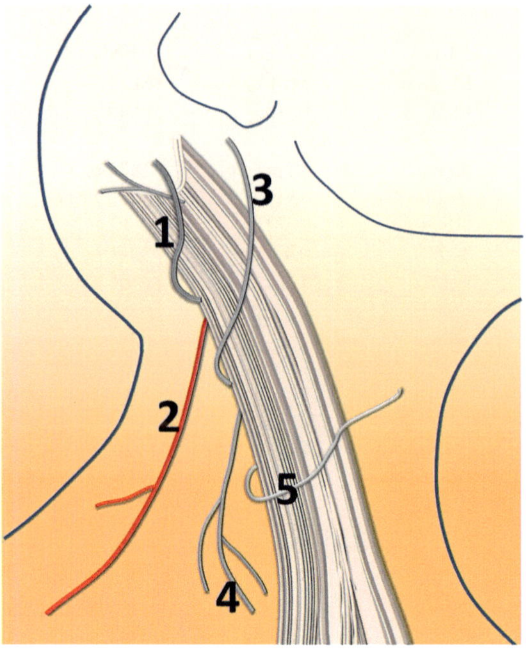

Fig. 15.2 The spinal accessory nerve (red line) appears out of the sternocleidomastoid muscle about one finger-width above the greater auricular nerve. (1) Lesser occipital nerve (posterior auricular nerves); (2) XI (spinal accessory nerve); (3) Greater auricular nerve; (4) Supraclavicular sensory nerve; (5) Transverse cervical nerve

and neck cancer survivors [27]. That is because it is covered only by the (superficial and deep) fascia and the skin between the sternocleidomastoid and trapezius.

15.4 Technique of XI-Gracilis for Facial Reanimation, One-Stage Procedure

15.4.1 Preoperative Evaluation

Patients' history and physical examination of the trapezius muscle are completed preoperatively. Every patient is required to have an accompanying person(s) to listen to the explanation. Benefits and pitfalls of different options and choice of neurotizer are explained and illustrated with photographs and/or videos of previous patients' results. Potential complications and donor site morbidity are described. Decisions are made in the next visit. Photos and videos are made preoperatively for later comparison.

15.4.2 Operative Method

General anesthesia with nasotracheal intubation is recommended to minimize the interference of the upper lip manipulation. Muscle relaxant drug is avoided during the XI nerve dissection. The operation is performed by two teams simultaneously: one team for recipient site of the paralytic face and neck, and the other team for donor site (the contralateral thigh) gracilis dissection.

(a) Key Points for Face Preparation and XI Exploration
   - A shoulder and head cushion to extend the operative neck to give more space in the face and neck dissection.
   - On the paralyzed face, three incisions are routinely performed on the face preparation (Fig. 15.3a). The first short incision along the white line of upper lip between philtrum and commissure is made to create a space above the oral mucosa. Four anchoring sutures with 4-0 Dexon are placed behind the orbicularis oris muscle. The second short incision on lower lip white line is made for preparation for lower lip suspension [28]. The third long preauricular incision is followed to allow for subcutaneous face-lift. Under the face-lift flap, a transverse incision down to the periosteum along the inferior zygomatic arch is made. Four anchoring 3-0 Dexon sutures are placed. For complete truly facial paralysis, soft tissue between the infrazygomatic margin down to the upper lip, including the zygomatic major muscle, buccal fat pad and facial nerve branches, is removed to create a recipient pocket. The Stenson's duct is identified and protected. For incomplete facial paralysis, the soft tissue removal is only soft tissue above the muscles and nerves without injury of the facial nerve branches. For postparalysis facial synkinesis, the

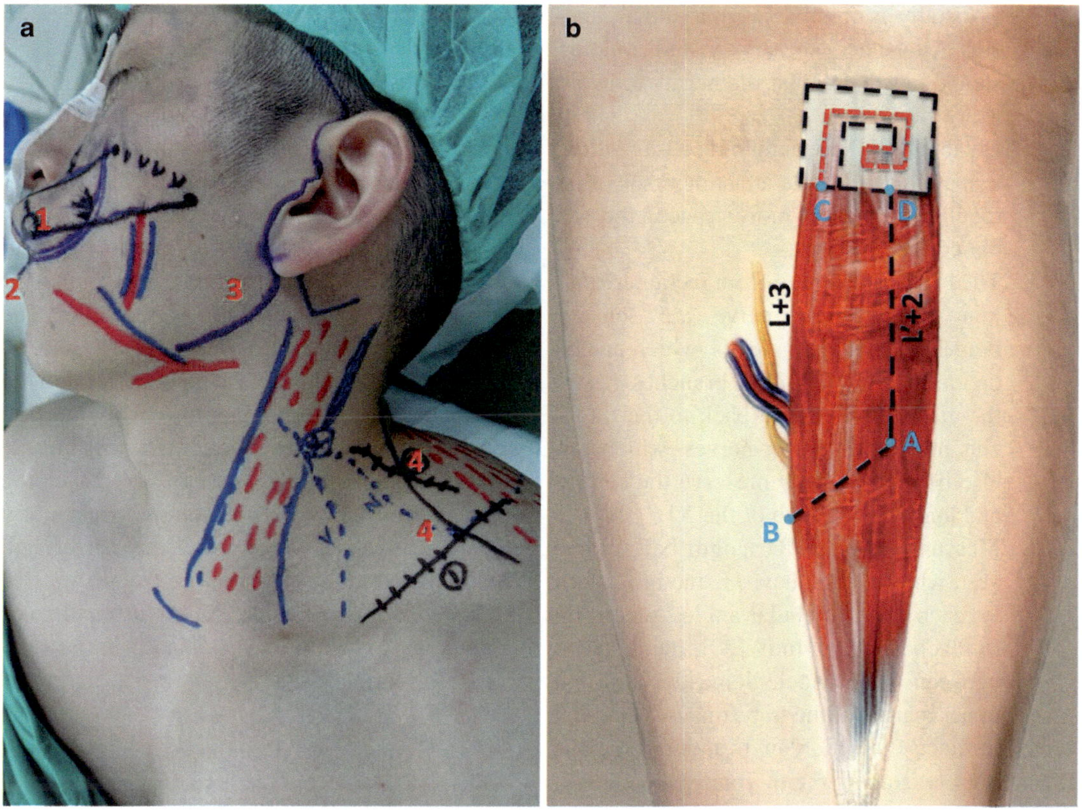

Fig. 15.3 (**a**) Three incisions for face recipient and one incision for neck XI dissection. (**b**) A potential trapezoid shape of gracilis based on the recipient face measurement under face-lift flap is drawn. Additional lengths are added: vessel side +3 cm, non-vessel side +2 cm to avoid postoperative contraction fold. The proximal aponeurosis, with 1 cm width in continuity with the muscle, is trimmed into a long tail

procedure here is similar to the complete facial paralysis, but the involved synkinetic and trigger muscles and nerves are removed as much as possible, including all zygomatic and buccal muscles and nerves, platysma and nasal muscles. After the soft tissue removal, four proposed lengths of the trapezoid shape of gracilis muscle harvest are measured. Through the experience revolution, two centimeters on the vessel-opposite and three centimeter on the vessel side are added (Fig. 15.3b) to avoid consequent lip contracture deformity.

- The fourth incision on the neck, either vertical along the course of the XI, or supraclavicular transverse incision (for cosmetic reason) is made (Fig. 15.3a). Either incision should be across the upper margin of the trapezius muscle.
- Expose the upper trapezius muscle. A sensory nerve over the lateral margin of the trapezius muscle can be seen and preserved to avoid postoperative numbness and pain.
- The XI, size similar to the leg sural nerve, can be found above and in front of the medial third of upper margin of the trapezius muscle in the posterior neck triangle. It is proved with help of nerve stimulator. Proximally, dissection upward to close to the sternocleidomastoid muscle to gain more length, but any branch goes back to the trapezius muscle should be protect to preserve upper trapezius muscle function. Distally, dissection along the course of XI

as distally as possible in front of the trapezius. All the nerve dissection and isolation should use the bipolar diathermy to avoid nerve damage.

- Detaching the trapezius muscle from the scapular and clavicle attachments is often required to give more space for XI dissection.
- The branches coming from the anterior to join in the main nerve are sensory branches of cervical plexus, which can be divided for traction. The branches out of the main branch going back to the trapezius muscle are motor nerves, which can also be divided, only preserve the central and long main branch of the XI.
- Measure the main XI length before harvest, which should have an enough length to reach the mandibular angle. According to Placheta et al. study [27], the distance between the sternocleidomastoid and the upper margin of the trapezius is 5 cm, and distance dissection in front of trapezius muscle is about 6 cm. Totally the enough length which can be transferred to the mandibular angle should be over 10 cm.
- The XI is transect, passing through a tunnel beneath the platysma muscle, and transferred to the mandibular angle to wait for inset of the trimmed gracilis muscle.

(b) Key Points for Upper Gracilis Dissection, Trimming, Harvest, and Transfer

The gracilis muscle anatomy, nerve innervation, and blood supply have been extensively described before [28]. The contralateral medial thigh upper gracilis muscle and its aponeurosis dissection, potential trapezoid shape of gracilis based on the recipient face measurement is drawn (Fig. 15.3b) and trimmed. The distal edge is drawn on two finger-breadths distal to the neurovascular pedicle. The transected edges are sutured with overlapping interrupted 3-0 nylons. The proximal aponeurosis, with 1 cm width in continuity with the muscle, is trimmed into a long tail. Maximal length of the vessel and nerve pedicles is obtained prior to division. The procedure has been also descried before [6, 9, 15].

Once the recipient face and donor thigh are finished in dissection, the trimmed gracilis is then harvested and transferred, which is placed under the cheek flap in reverse fashion: the proximal tendinous aponeurosis is anchored to the upper lip anchoring four stitches. The distal muscle cut edge is fixed to the anchoring four stitches at zygomatic periosteum which are set earlier. The tail of the fascia aponeurosis which is in continuity with the gracilis muscle is passing through the subcutaneous tunnel to the lower lip incision wound, and sutured to the orbicularis oris muscle in the lower lip wound under tension. Once the muscle is well set, vessel anastomoses (one artery and one vein) to the facial vessels are performed. Finally the obturator nerve of the gracilis muscle is coapted to the transferred XI in the mandibular angle area. A suction drain is placed in the neck wound for drainage.

15.5 Postoperative Cares and Rehabilitation

Patient will be extubated after the operation. Neck is immobilized with a pre-made neck splint for 3 weeks. Patient is transferred to the Microsurgery Intensive Care Unit for close monitoring for 3–5 days. A simple system to check swelling is used. Palpation of the nasojugal region to check face swelling is performed every hour in the ICU observation. There are four degrees of swelling which can be compared to the varying firmness of the thenar eminence with different finger-to-thumb opposition, from index to little finger. If the surface firmness is like as thumb-index opposition, it is soft and classified as 1° swelling. If the firmness is slightly firmer like as thumb-long finger opposition, it is 2° swelling. As thumb-ring finger opposition, it is 3°; and thumb-little finger, 4° swelling. 1–2° swelling is acceptable, 3° swelling is warrant for closer observation. 4° swelling is critical and requires bedside wound opening to assess the hematoma. Patient is usually hospitalized for a week.

Rehabilitation including massage and muscle stimulation, will begin 3 weeks after FFMT. Usually the muscle may start moving (M1 strength) in 4–6 months postoperatively. Induction exercise [2, 3] will start. Patient is instructed to perform shoulder elevation against resistance, a trigger movement that "jumpstarts" the movement of the transferred muscle. However, once the upper lip movement is noted and the lateral incisor is visible (M2 muscle strength), 6–12 months postoperatively, the induction exercise should be reduced and stopped. Smiling training in front of mirror (mirror therapy) to adjust and control the muscle movement, making symmetric smile to the healthy side, is begun with the goal to achieve natural smile. Surgical treatment of the residual deformity was usually performed a year and half postoperatively.

15.6 Outcome Assessment

The optimal results achieved at different timepoints for each methods: in general, CFNG-gracilis at the second to third year, XI-gracilis the first to second year, and V3-gracilis 6 months to 1 year. Therefore all patients who received XI-gracilis should be followed at least 1 year. Patients were photographed and videotaped during pre-and postoperative visits in a standardized fashion, including facial repose, mild, moderate, and maximal smile, as well as "tickle and joke test " to check its spontaneity. Five independent reviewers reviewed the collected photos and videos, and graded the functional and aesthetic outcomes.

Smile excursion score [6] is a score system to check the muscle strength from 0 to 4, based on how many teeth visible when performing maximal smile. Score 4 is when tour or more teeth are seen. A postoperative smile excursion score ≥2 is considered acceptable, ≥3 good, and ≥4 excellent result.

Cortical adaptation staging system [6] includes five stages of movement:

no-, dependent-, independent-, spontaneous-with synkinesis, and spontaneous movement with less or absent synkinesis. "Tickle and joke test" is routinely performed to test if the patient has spontaneous smile. Tickle test is tickling on the patient's axilla purposely, joke test is talking joke(s) to induce smile. Stage III is classified as independent and acceptable; stage IV and V showed its spontaneity and is classified good and excellent result.

A patient questionnaire was devised since 2012 in our center [6] for patient's satisfaction score. The questionnaire is performed via phone interview or by mailed written response. There are five scores: regrets, unacceptable but does not regret surgery, acceptable but needs major improvement, satisfied but needs minor improvement, and completely satisfied without revision.

We used Hadlock's "SMILE" (Smile Measurement of Improvement in Lip Excursion) scale system to quantitatively measure paralyzed lip excursion during smiling in postoperative photography [29] (Fig. 15.4a, b). "*X*" is horizontal excursion, "*Y*" vertical excursion, and "*Z*" overall excursion. The "*Z*" value is derived by $Z = \sqrt{x^2 + y^2}$, the larger the better.

Lastly, we used Terzis's Aesthetic and Functional Grading System [11] for general observation: Grade 1 (poor) to Grade 5 (excellent). Grade 4 (good) and 5 (excellent) were acceptable results. Grade 1 and 2 (fair) were unacceptable. Grade 3 (moderate) showed muscle contraction but not symmetric.

15.7 Statistical Analysis

Statistical analysis was performed using SPSS 21.0 software (SPSS, Inc., Chicago, Ill). Paired *t* test was used to determine whether the postoperative smile was significantly different from the preoperative one. Comparison was made based on smile excursion score and cortical adaptation stage. The Mann–Whitney test was used for two independent samples and the Kruskal–Wallis test was used for more than two independent groups. Data were presented as percentages or means with ranges or standard deviations (SD). *P* values <0.05 were considered statistically significant.

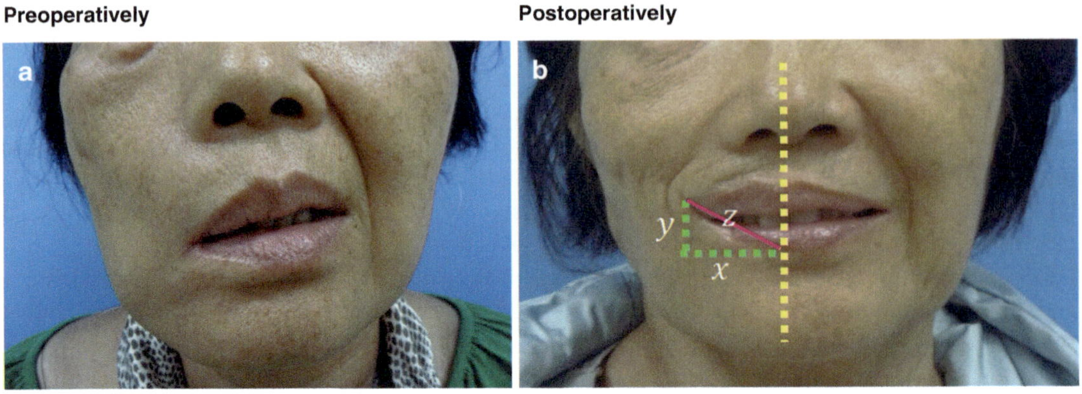

Fig. 15.4 Hadlock's SMILE Lip Excursion Scale: (**a**) Patient photo preoperatively. (**b**) Total lip excursion length (Z-length) after FFMT, derived by $Z = \sqrt{(x^2 + y^2)}$. The larger the better

15.8 Results

15.8.1 Denervation Time

Denervation time was defined between day of FFMT and onset of muscle contraction. Average denervation time was 5 months (range, 3–12) in the XI-group, but 9 months (range, 6–12) in CFNG-group, and 3 months (range, 2–6 months) in the V3-gracilis group. Denervation times for XI- and V3-groups were significantly shorter than for the CFNG-group (Table 15.1).

15.8.2 Ischemic Time for Gracilis Transfer

Ischemic time for three groups was usually within 1 h with no difference among three groups, because the gracilis harvest is always after the donor and recipient sites are well-prepared.

15.8.3 Complications

We had one patient did not show improvement in smile excursion for unknown reason. Mini-temporalis was turned over to the upper lip to enhance the result. One patient with bilateral facial palsy due to bilateral Möbius syndrome had the first left face gracilis failure in the first operation. He had undergone an additional operation 1 year later after the failed muscle removal, using the segmental rectus femoris innervated by the previous XI nerve and succeeded. In our series, the XI nerve transect did not cause significant motor or sensory symptoms and signs. If it has, shoulder soreness and pain was complained, but it is usually spontaneously resolved within 1 month.

15.8.4 Smile Excursion Score

In the first 2 years postoperatively, the XI- or V3-groups both showed significantly greater scores than the CFNG-group. However, in the third year, there was no difference among the three groups. All three group patients achieved a mean score of 3 with at least three teeth visible (Table 15.2, Fig. 15.5a, b). Preoperatively, CFNG-group had better dental show due to more synkinesis patients with incomplete paralysis.

15.8.5 Cortical Adaptation Stage

In the CFNG-group, nearly all achieved stage IV or V spontaneous smile. In the XI-group all achieved at least stage III (independent) smile, and nearly half patients showed potentially upgrade to spontaneous smile over time. In the V3-group, most achieved stage III or II smile, but

Table 15.2 Specific observation: smile excursion score (tooth visible, score 0–4)

	Pre-op			In the first Year Post-op			In the second Year Post-op			In the third Year Post-op			More than 3 years (>36 M)		
	XI	V3	CFNG	XI	V3	CFNG	XI	V3	CFNG	XI	V3	CFNG	XI	V3	CFNG
Mean ± SEM	0.325 ± 0.038	0.132 ± 0.047	0.55 ± 0.076	2.91 ± 0.161	3.11 ± 0.204	2.183 ± 0.048	3.687 ± 0.150	4.014 ± 0.224	2.567 ± 0.112	3.333 ± 0.135	3.500 ± 0.190	3.083 ± 0.108	3.835 ± 0.05972	3.600 ± 0.2449	3.160 ± 0.09274
t test, *P* value															
XI:V3	0.0094			0.4593			0.2767			0.4826			0.1315		
XI:CFNG			0.0245			0.0015			0.0002			0.1789			0.0001
CFNG:V3		0.0009			0.0013			0.0002			0.0772			0.3356	

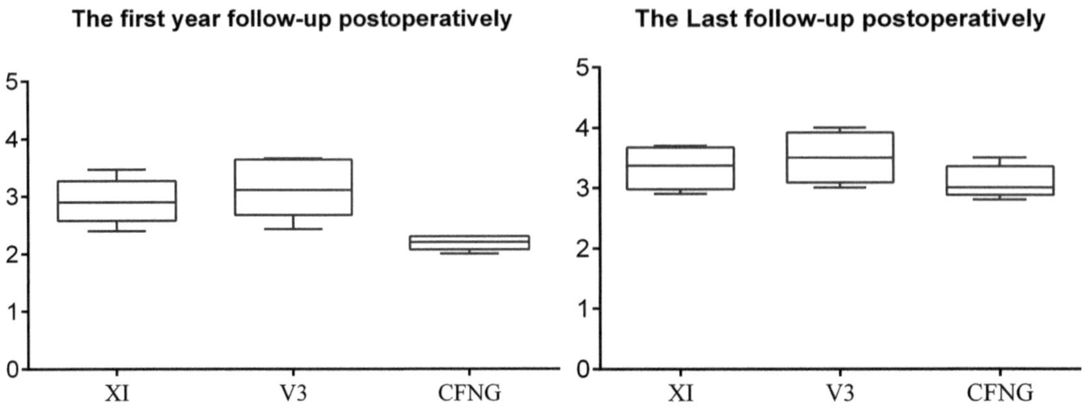

Fig. 15.5 : Smile excursion (teeth visible) score

Table 15.3 Specific observation: cortical adaptation stage

	XI-gra	V3-gra	CFNG-gra
Cortical adaptation stage (I–V)	• Most: ≥ stage 3 • 33%, stage IV • 12%, stage V • Tickle and joke test • Most pass	• Most: Stage I • Tickle and joke test • Failed to pass	• Stage IV–V • Tickle and joke test : All pass

Table 15.4 Patient Questionnaire (0–5)

	XI-gracilis	V3-gracilis	CFNG- gracilis
Final results (N = number of pts who were randomized chosen and answered)	• $N = 30$ • Mean score: 3.40 • Score 5: 3 • Score 4: 9 • Score 3: 15 • Score 2: 3 Score ≥ 3: 90%	• $N = 15$ • Mean score: 3.2 • Score ≥ 3: 67%	• $N = 50$ • Mean score: 3.46 • Score 5: 5 • Score 4: 22 • Score 3: 16 • Score 2: 6 Score ≥ 3: 86%

none had its spontaneity in unilateral facial palsy patients (Table 15.3).

15.8.6 Patient Questionnaire

To achieve the similar sample sizes of patients, we randomly chose 50 CFNG-patients, 30 XI-patients, and 15 V3-patients for this study. They all were reconstructed in the recent 10 years. A score ≥ 3 (acceptable and satisfied)was reported in 86% of the CFNG-, and 90% in the XI-group. Both were significantly higher than the V3-group at 67% (Table 15.4).

15.8.7 Hadlock's SMILE Lip Excursion Scale

Similarly we purposely chose the similar sample sizes from three groups for comparison: 30 from CFNG-, 30 from XI- and 14 from V3-group patients. Regardless no matter in the first year or the last follow-up, CFNG-group demonstrated significantly better lip excursion than the XI- and V3-groups (Table 15.5, Fig. 15.6a, b).

15.8.8 Terzis's Functional and Aesthetic Grading System

The CFNG-group demonstrated progressive improvement from an average score of 1.367 pre-operatively, to 3.117 after 1 year, 3.683 at 2 years, and finally 4.180 at last follow-up. The XI-group also had similar progressive improvement. In contrast, the V3-gracilis group demonstrated significant improvement at 1 year (from 1.037 to 3.738), but then decreased to 3.611 at second years, and then achieved a very slow improvement to 4.100 upon last follow-up (Table 15.6, Fig. 15.7a, b).

Table 15.5 Hadlock's SMILE Lip Excursion Scale

	Number	One-year follow-up	Last follow-up	Median follow-up time of last follow-up
XI	30	7.25 (4.15–13.26)	7.4 (3.75–13.68)	15
CFNG	30	12.73 (10.52–15.80)	14.12 (12.66–16.26)	32
V3	14	9.25 (2.49–16.40)	9.25 (1.81–18.05)	12
p value		0.04[a]	0.007[a]	

[a]The results are expressed as median + interquartile range (IQR)

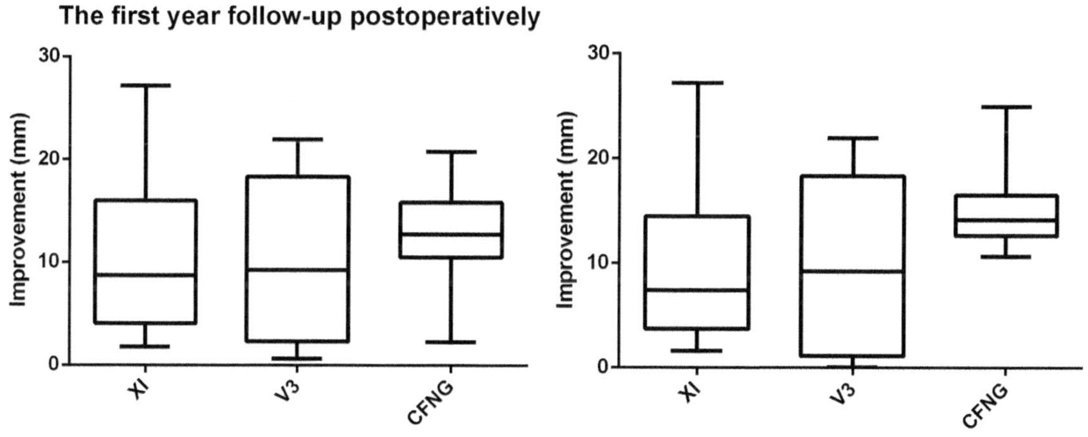

Fig. 15.6 : Hadlock's smile lip excursion

15.9 Discussion

15.9.1 Why Is the XI-Gracilis Not Popular?

An ideal motor nerve to innervate a FFMT for facial reanimation should (1) be a nearby nerve to avoid the requirement of a nerve graft, (2) be a strong nerve to provide adequate innervation, (3) provide a quicker recovery with a short rehabilitation time, (4) have minimal donor site morbidities, (5) provide universal application in different situation, and (6) have the potential to create a spontaneous smile which is the most important for the result. The reasons why V3-gracilis becomes popular since 2006 after Manktelow's report [21], because V3-gracilis provides many benefits as an ideal motor nerve. However, we found V3-gracilis is not good enough to gain spontaneous smile for unilateral facial paralysis. Patients after V3-gracilis are quite difficulty to have big smiling with mouth opening, easily forgetting to smile when smile is spontaneous initiated, and involuntary movement of the cheek is persistent during eating and biting.

The XI-gracilis shows a lots of benefits than pitfalls. The benefits include one-stage procedure, powerful innervation with quick recovery, and potential to create a spontaneous smile by time. However, why is the XI-gracilis not popular? There are some pitfalls: (1) one more neck wound for XI exploration, (2) rather difficulty of XI dissection in the neck deep wound to obtain a more than 10 cm length nerve, (3) postoperative neck splint immobilization for 3 weeks, and (4) postoperative donor site shoulder complications which are too much emphasized and concerned by otolarygology head and neck surgeons [30–32].

15.9.2 Sequelae by XI Transect

There are significantly different opinions regarding the sequelae of XI injury and palsy, especially found in ENT-, sport-, and head and neck surgery-

Table 15.6 Terzis's functional AND aesthetic grading

	Pre-op			In the first year Post-op			In the second year Post-op			In the third year Post-op			More than 3 years (>36 M)		
	XI	V3	CFNG	XI	V3	CFNG	XI	V3	CFNG	XI	V3	CFNG	XI	V3	CFNG
Mean ± SEM	1.347 ± 0.053	1.037 ± 0.023	1.367 ± 0.049	3.723 ± 0.163	3.738 ± 0.221	3.117 ± 0.128	4.040 ± 0.198	3.611 ± 0.200	3.683 ± 0.130	4.140 ± 0.185	4.067 ± 0.245	4.150 ± 0.115	4.439 ± 0.202	4.100 ± 0.245	4.180 ± 0.146
t test, *P* value															
XI:V3	0.0003			0.9569			0.1585			0.8127			0.3086		
XI:CFNG			0.7923			0.0151			0.1628			0.9649			0.3439
CFNG:V3		0.0001			0.0352			0.7686			0.7512			0.7863	

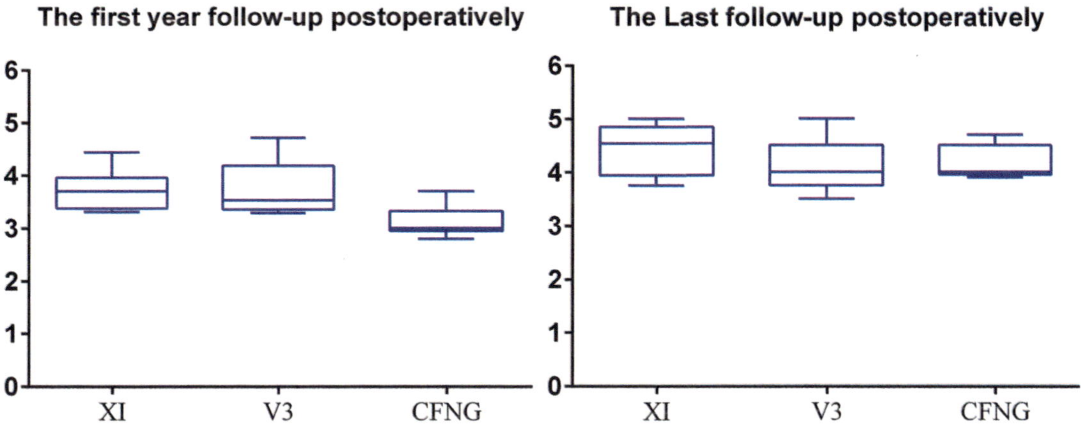

Fig. 15.7 Terzis's functional and aesthetic score

related journals. The XI injury, as described, will cause denervation of the trapezius and sternocleidomastoid muscles, compromise shoulder movement and lead to secondary sequelae, such as trapezius atrophy, shoulder girdle depression, scapular dyskinesis, causing loss of shoulder active abduction and shoulder/neck and myofascial pain [30, 31]. However, the XI nerve has been extensively applied in brachial plexus reconstruction. More than 1000 cases of XI transfer had been performed in our center. We haven't seen significant sequel occurrence. Wilgenet al [32] questioned " are all shoulder complaints after neck dissection due to the XI nerve injury alone in head and neck surgery ?", and reported the incidence of XI injury associated signs and symptoms is varied from 18 to 100% following a radial or modified radial neck dissection and lymph node dissection. Our XI harvest, the sternocleidomastoid and upper third trapezius are still preserved. The sequelae by XI nerve transfer were very minimal in our series. The common sign was atrophy of middle and lower parts of trapezius, and temporary shoulder soreness which usually disappeared spontaneously within 1 month. From the anatomy point of view, the trapezius muscle is only attached on the scapula, clavicle and acromion, but not across G-H joint to the humerus. It might mildly impact the shoulder stability and will not affect the shoulder elevation.

15.9.3 Why Patients of Postparalysis Facial Synkinesis Are Included?

All patients with postparalysis facial synkinesis in this series received extensive myectomy and neurectomy of the involved nerves and muscles (including cheek, nose, corrugator and platysma muscles, and all zygomatic and buccal facial nerve branches). It becomes a status of facial paralysis before FFMT. Their reconstructive procedure, postoperative care and rehabilitation were all the same as the truly facial paralysis without additional botox injection and extra rehabilitation. The only pitfalls is the patients after facial reanimation seemed to have higher revision rate, especially on the upper lip contracture, than truly facial paralysis.

15.9.4 Cortical Adaptation

Manktelow in 2006 [21] reported a series of 27 patients (9 with total bilateral, 9 with partial bilateral, and 9 with primarily a unilateral facial paralysis) received V3-gracilis for facial reanimation. He concluded 85% of patients learned to smile without biting, and the spontaneity occurred routinely in 59% and occasionally in 29% of patients. Brain plasticity of cortical connections between the cortical centers of the seventh and fifth cranial nerves was hypothesized. Since then, V3-gracilis becomes more popular because it provides more consistently powerful muscle contraction. In our series, this brain plasticity only occurred on bilateral Möbius syndrome patients.

For the unilateral facial paralysis, V3-gracilis does not show such benefits with spontaneity and synchrony.

15.9.5 Result Evaluation

Although some standardized evaluation systems for facial nerve paralysis and recovery have been established, such as House-Brackmann, Sunnybrook, or Sydney system [33], we found neither one could subjectively and objectively analyze our patients' results after FFMT reconstruction. On the contrary, our evaluation had multiplicity approach: teeth exposure score can test the transferred muscle strength;, cortical adaptation system with "tickle and joke test" can evaluate the emotional muscle movement, simple and not confusing;, Hadlock's "SMILE" lip excursion scale can quantitatively check the lip excursion;, and Terzis's functional and aesthetic evaluation system can quantitatively and qualitatively check the gross result. We additionally used patient questionnaire for more patients' subjective result. Those multiplicity approaches made the outcomes assessment more convincing.

15.9.6 Indication and Contraindication

XI-should be avoided in athletes, especially in those whom require much movement of the shoulder abduction and elevation, which will insult in embarrassingly involuntary motion of the cheek muscle during exercise. Low education or poor communication patients may also be contraindicated for XI- and V3-patients because they are difficult in smile training.

15.10 Summary

Although XI-gracilis for facial paralysis reconstruction has not yet considered a popular choice in the world, we continuously use this technique for facial reanimation due to its effectiveness, a one-stage procedure (like V3-gracilis), but a tendency to have a spontaneous smile (like CFNG-gracilis) by time. Involuntary movement of the muscle transplant on face also tends to reduce or disappear by time while shoulder elevation (Video 15.1). The classic two-stage CFNG-gracilis is still our first choice for facial reanimation. However, compared the benefits and pitfalls, the XI-gracilis has proven it a good alternative (Videos 15.2 and 15.3).

References

1. Allieu Y, Privat JM, Bonnel F. Paralysis in root avulsion of the brachial plexus neurotization by the spinal accessory nerve. Clin Plast Surg. 1984;11:133–6.
2. Chuang DCC. Neurotization procedures for brachial plexus injuries. Hand Clin. 1995;11:633–45.
3. Chuang DCC. Nerve transfer with functioning free muscle transplantation. Hand Clin. 2008;24:377–88.
4. Doi K, Sakai K, Kuwata N, Ihara K, Kawai S. Reconstruction of finger and elbow function after complete avulsion of the brachail plexus. J Hand Surg (AM). 1991;15(5):796–803.
5. Terzis JK, Noah EM. Dynamic restoration in Möbius and Möbius-like patients. Plast Reconstr Surg. 2003;111:40–55.
6. Chuang DCC, Lu JCY, Anesti K. One-stage procedure using spinal accessory nerve (XI)-innervated free muscle for facial paralysis reconstruction. Plast Reconstr Surg. 2013;132:117e–29e.
7. Lu JCY, Chuang DC. One-stage reconstruction for bilateral Mobius syndrome-simultaneous using bilateral spinal accessory nerve to innervate two free muscles for facial reanimation. Ann Plast Surg. 2013;70:180–96.
8. Melvin TAN, Limb CJ. Overview of facial paralysis: current concepts. Facial Plast Surg. 2008;24:155–63.
9. Chuang DCC, Chang TNJ, Lu JCY. Postparalysis facial synkinesis: clinical classification and surgical strategies. Plast Reconstr Surg Glob Open. 2015;3:e320–35.
10. Labbe D, Huault M. Lengthening temporalis myoplasty and lip reanimation. Plast Reconstr Surg. 2000;105:1289–97.

11. Terzis JK. Analysis of 100 cases of free muscle transplantation for facial paralysis. Plast Reconstr Surg. 1997;99:1905–21.
12. Manktelow RT. Free muscle transplantation for facial paralysis. Clin Plast Surg. 1984;11:215–20.
13. Harii K, Ohmori K, Torii S. Free gracilis muscle transplantation with microneurovascular anastomoses for the treatment of facial paralysis. Plast Reconstr Surg. 1976;57:133–43.
14. Zuker RM, Goldberg CS, Maktelow RT. Facial animation in children with Möbius syndrome after segmental gracilis muscle transplant. Plast Reconstr Surg. 2000;106:1–8.
15. Chuang DCC. Technique evolution for facial paralysis reconstruction using functioning free muscle transplantation – experience of Chang Gung Memorial Hospital. Clin Plast Surg. 2002;29:449–59.
16. Guelinckx P, Sinsel NK. Muscle transplantation for reconstruction of a smile after facial paralysis past, present and future. Microsurgery. 1996;17:391–401.
17. Terzis JK, Karypidis D. Therapeutic strategies in post-facial paralysis synkinesis in adult patients. Plast Reconstr Surg. 2012;129:925e–39e.
18. Freilinger G, Gruber H, Happak W, Pechmann U. Surgical anatomy of the minic muscle system and the facial nerve: importance for reconstructive and aenthetic surgery. Plast Reconstr Surg. 1987;80:686–90.
19. Hamilton SGL, Terzis JK, Carraway JH. Surgical anatomy of the facial musculature and muscle transplantation. In: Terzis JK, editor. Microreconstruction of nerve injuries. Philadelphia: Saunders; 1987. p. 571–86.
20. Ueda K, Harii K, Yamada A. Free neurovascular muscle transplantation for the treatment of facial paralysis using the hypoglossal nerve as a recipient motor source. Plast Reconstr Surg. 1994;94:808–17.
21. Manktelow RT, Tomat LR, Zuker RM, Chang M. Smile reconstruction in adults with free muscle transfer innervated by the masseter motor nerve: effectiveness and cerebral adaptation. Plast Reconstr Surg. 2006;118:885–99.
22. Klebuc MJ. Facial reanimation using the masseter-to-facial nerve transfer. Plast Reconstr Surg. 2011;127:1909–15.
23. Xu Y, Liu J, Li P, Donelan MB, Parrett BM, Winograd JM. The phrenic nerve as a motor nerve donor for facial reanimation with the free latissimus dorsi muscle. J Reconstr Microsurg. 2009;25:457–63.
24. Terzis JK, Konofaos P. Novel use of C7 spinal nerve for Möbius. Plast Reconstr Surg. 2010;126:106–17.
25. Gray H, Goss CM. 26th Edition of Gray's anatomy. Philadelphia: Lea & Febiger; 1955. p. 1020–1.
26. Kiemer AC, Zelenka I, Heller S, et al. Surgical anatomy of the spinal accessory nerve and the trapezius branches of the cervical plexus. Arch Surg. 2000;135:1428–31.
27. Placheta E, Tinhofer I, Schmid M, Reissig LF, Pona I, Weninger W, Rath T, Chuang DCC, Tzou CHJ. The spinal accessory nerve for functional muscle innervation in facial reanimation surgery- an anatomical and histomorphometric study. Ann Plast Surg. 2016;77:640–4.
28. Chuang DCC. Gracilis flap. In: Wei FC, Mardini S, editors. Flaps and reconstructive surgery, Chap. 29. Amsterdam: Saunders (Elsevier); 2009. p. 395–408.
29. Bray D, Henstrom DK, Cheney ML, Hadlock TA. Assessing outcomes in facial reanimation: evaluation and validation of the smile system for measuring lip excursion during smiling. Arch Facial Plast Surg. 2010;12:352–4.
30. Carenfelt C, Eliasson K. Occurrence, duration and prognosis of unexpected accessory nerve paresis in radical neck dissection. Acta Otolaryngol. 1980;90:470–3.
31. Kelley MJ, Kane TE, Leggin BG. Spinal accessory nerve palsy: associated signs and symptoms. J Orthop Sports Phys Ther. 2008;38:78–86.
32. Wilgen CP, Dijkstra PU, van der Laan BF, Plukker JT, Roodenburg JL. Shoulder complaints after neck dissection: is the spinal accessory nerve involved? Br J Oral Maxillofac Surg. 2003;41:7–11.
33. Coulson S, Croxson GR, Adams RD, O'dwyer NJ. Reliability of the "Sydney," "Sunnybrook," and "House-Brackmann" facial grading systems to assess voluntary movement and synkinesis after facial nerve paralysis. Otolaryngol Head Neck Surg. 2005;132:543–9.

One-Stage Latissimus Dorsi Muscle Transfer for Facial Reanimation: Comparison Between Single and Dual Innervation

16

Goo-Hyun Mun and Kyeong-Tae Lee

Key Points

- One-stage latissimus dorsi neuromuscular transfer is a viable option for dynamic smile reconstruction, with strengths including achievement of reliable and acceptable long-term outcomes and reduction of the operation frequency.
- Dual-innervation technique can reduce denervation time of the functional latissimus dorsi muscle by providing additional neural input from the ipsilateral masseteric nerve.
- More favorable outcomes showing stronger contraction of the transferred muscle as well as spontaneous movement can be achieved in the dual-innervation technique.
- Elaborate planning and technically demanding procedures are required for successful implementation of the dual-innervation technique.
- Compared to the conventional method, the dual-innervation technique is not associated with increasing donor morbidity including functional impairments.

G.-H. Mun (✉) · K.-T. Lee
Department of Plastic Surgery, Samsung Medical Center, Sungkyunkwan University School of Medicine, Seoul, South Korea

16.1 History of One-Stage Latissimus Dorsi Muscle Transfer

A two-stage dynamic reanimation technique consisting of cross-facial nerve grafting and subsequent free muscle transplantation has long been the dominant reconstruction option for enabling spontaneous smiles in patients with facial paralysis. This technique has generated superior outcomes both in repose and dynamic smiling compared to those of conventional methods. However, the technique's limitations are that it requires a two-stage operation with procedures approximately 8–12 months apart, and it takes up to 2 years to acquire transferred muscle contraction after the completion of the first-stage cross-facial nerve grafting. Another disadvantage of this method is the need for harvesting a long sural nerve for the cross-facial nerve graft, as this may lead to uncomfortable sequelae, including hypothesia or paraesthesia in the submalleolar and lateral foot regions.

To overcome the drawbacks of the two-stage method, Wei et al. and Harii et al. proposed a new one-stage latissimus dorsi neuromuscular transfer surgical technique [1, 2] in which the muscle motor nerve is directly crossed through the face and attached to the contralateral facial nerve branches. The latissimus dorsi muscle has distinct strengths over other conventionally used muscles. It provides a parallel-fibered muscle

© Springer Nature Switzerland AG 2021
C.-H. J. Tzou, A. Rodríguez-Lorenzo (eds.), *Facial Palsy*,
https://doi.org/10.1007/978-3-030-50784-8_16

that can generate sufficient contraction power to lift the nasolabial fold during smiling. A stalk of the thoracodorsal nerve long enough to easily reach the contralateral facial nerve branches can be obtained by a proximal dissection up to its origin through the posterior cord of the brachial plexus and the distal dissection of the muscle parenchyma. In addition, this one-stage method reduces the number of nerve coaptations and results in a shorter time to acquire the first contraction of the transferred muscle compared to the conventional two-stage method. According to the Takushima et al. study that contained the largest case series of latissimus dorsi neuromuscular transfers and reported comprehensive outcomes over a 15 year period [3], postoperative contraction of the transferred muscle was acquired at an average of 6.5 months, which was approximately one-third of the time of the two-stage method. Above all, over three-fourths of the patients treated with this method obtained good outcomes showing a grade 4 or 5 in their grading system, which demonstrates method reliability. With these strengths, the one-stage latissimus dorsi neuromuscular transfer has been established as a viable option in dynamic smile reconstruction.

16.2 Dual-Innervation Technique

16.2.1 Emergence of the Dual-Innervation Technique

Generally acceptable outcomes showing spontaneous and symmetric muscle movement at smile and balanced appearance at rest have been achieved in a majority of facial palsy patients treated with the one-stage latissimus dorsi neuromuscular transfer. However, suboptimal results with insufficient contraction of the transferred muscle are occasionally encountered in the long run, which may overshadow the strengths of this method and caution surgeons on its use. Suboptimal results are usually the result of the shrinking and atrophy of the transferred muscle during the denervated period, which is usually more than 6 months, and the resulting reduction in contraction power after re-innervation, which would not be sufficient for generating a symmetric smile.

To resolve this issue, Watanabe et al. introduced a new dual-innervation technique using the latissimus dorsi muscle. They innervated the transferred latissimus dorsi muscle by both neurorrhaphy to a buccal branch of the contralateral facial nerve with the thoracodorsal nerve, as done conventionally, and by neurotization via direct contact with the ipsilateral masseter muscle [4]. By virtue of an adjacent neural source from the ipsilateral masseteric nerve, the re-innervation of the transferred muscle can be relatively fast, occurring about 3 months after surgery in their study. This can reduce denervation atrophy of the transferred muscle during the period of axonal regeneration from the contralateral facial nerve branch, showing a modified 'baby-sitting' effect, and ultimately maintain the contraction power of the transferred muscle in smile. A reinforced neural input from the contralateral facial nerve branches combined with that from the ipsilateral masseteric nerve enables spontaneous and symmetric smile. In summary, the dual-innervation technique theoretically has the potential for a relatively faster and more powerful re-innervation of the transferred muscle via the ipsilateral masseteric nerve and spontaneous smiling via the contralateral facial nerve branch.

Building on the pioneering work of Watanabe et al., surgeons have performed the dual-innervation technique with a common goal of compensating the potential drawbacks of the conventional one-stage latissimus dorsi neuromuscular transfer. Several technical modifications have been attempted that are mainly focused on the methods for secondary innervation from the ipsilateral masseteric nerve. In our technique, instead of exposing the bare masseter muscle for direct neurotization as done by Watanabe et al., a distal runoff of the descending branch of the thoracodorsal nerve or a transverse branch is additionally harvested and is coapted directly with the ipsilateral masseteric nerve, which is similar to Takushima's [5] (Fig. 16.1).

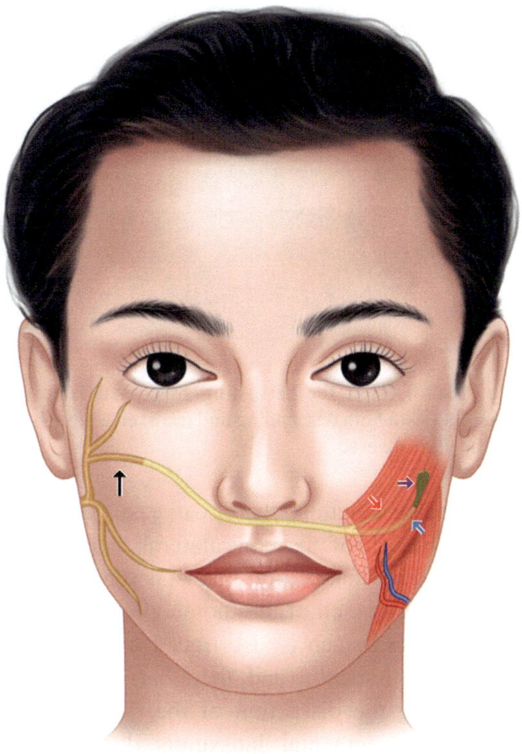

Fig. 16.1 Dual-innervation technique. Similar to the conventional single-innervation technique, a thoracodorsal nerve stalk is coapted with a buccal branch of the contralateral facial nerve. In addition, a transverse branch of the thoracodorsal nerve is pulled to the ipsilateral masseteric nerve and direct neurorrhaphy is performed between them

16.2.2 Surgical Technique

16.2.2.1 Preoperative Planning

Meticulous and elaborate preoperative planning is essential for achieving the best results in dynamic smile reconstruction. A patient's past medical history needs to be thoroughly vetted including cause and duration of symptoms, remnant function of facial nerves in the affected side, presence of synkinesis, and so forth. A physical examination to evaluate the length and vector of oral commissure movements in both the affected and unaffected sides in a sitting position is performed. Heaviness of the cheek soft tissue and overall contour in adjacent facial regions are carefully examined to avoid unintended cheek bulkiness after the muscle transfer and/or to correct concomitant contour deformities, if possible.

The required length of thoracodorsal nerve needed to reach a potential donor nerve of the contralateral facial nerve branches through a subcutaneous tunnel through the philtrum region is also estimated. The shape, position, and contractility of masseter muscle ipsilateral to the facial paralysis side are examined by palpation. The approximate thickness and contractility of the ipsilateral latissimus dorsi muscle below axilla also needs to be estimated.

16.2.2.2 Preparation of the Cheek Pocket

The procedures are carried out by two teams operating simultaneously including one for facial preparation and another for the latissimus dorsi muscle flap harvest. After marking the planned area of undermining on the cheek skin, a preauricular incision with extending cephalad along the sideburn hairline is made on the paralyzed face. The cheek flap is widely elevated above the superficial musculoaponeurotic fascia and parotid fascia to prepare a pocket for the subsequent muscle transfer. Undermining is advanced approximately 1–2 cm medially beyond the nasolabial fold. After creating the cheek pocket, five or six 3-0 polyethylene stitches are positioned across the residual fibers or traces of the orbicularis oris muscle with the checking position of a newly created nasolabial fold when pulling them.

The masseteric nerve, which is expected to be topographically located at a point approximately 3 cm medial from the tragus and 1 cm below the zygomatic arch, is identified beneath the masseter muscle with splitting the muscle fiber. The muscle is explored at a location 1 cm below the zygomatic arch and 1 cm medial to the posterior border of the muscle, and the motor nerve that usually lies 1.5–2 cm beneath the muscle surface is identified and prepared. This nerve stump serves as the secondary donor for a co-harvested nerve branch for the dual innervation.

Another small incision with a 1.5–2 cm length is made just below the submandibular angle of the paralyzed side and the facial artery and veins that are used as recipient vessels in a majority of cases are explored. On the healthy side, a small incision of approximately 12–14 mm long is made posterior to the lateral border of the zygomaticus major muscle and anterior to the margin of the parotid gland on the cheek to explore facial nerve branches that can be used for potential donor nerves. Typically, several zygomatic and/or buccal branches of the unaffected facial nerve are identified. Of these, the branches that show an adequate size and induce a sufficiently powerful contraction of the zygomaticus major muscle and/or levator labii superioris muscles on checking with a nerve stimulator are selected and prepared for the subsequent coaptation with the thoracodorsal nerve stump. For passage of the thoracodorsal nerve stalk, a small subcutaneous tunnel connecting the prepared cheek pocket on the affected side and the harvested contralateral donor nerve is made with a long scissor crossing the upper lip region.

16.2.2.3 Harvesting the Latissimus Dorsi Muscle Segment

A functional latissimus dorsi muscle flap is usually harvested on the same side as the paralyzed face with the patient in the supine position and a small pillow placed under their back. A lazy-S incision is made along the anterior margin of the latissimus dorsi muscle, which is usually identified at the posterior axillary line (Fig. 16.2), and the planned area of the latissimus dorsi muscle is dissected from the surrounding tissues. The neurovascular pedicle of the muscle is identified under the muscle, and the thoracodorsal nerve is carefully separated from the thoracodorsal vessels. An adequate length of the vascular pedicle is obtained, and the thoracodorsal nerve is further atraumatically traced toward its origin into the posterior cord of the brachial plexus as far as possible. Subsequently, a varying length of intramuscular dissection of the descending branch of the thoracodorsal nerve is performed to obtain additional nerve length so that it can easily reach the buccal branch of the contralateral facial nerve. For the dual innervation, a distal runoff of the descending branch of the thoracodorsal nerve or a transverse branch is also traced with an intramuscular dissection and then harvested. After completing the dissection of the neurovascular pedicle, a segmental latissimus dorsi muscle block is harvested in a trapezoid shape referring to the planned lengths in the face. If the muscle segment is very thick, its outer portion can be carefully thinned before pedicle division, and meticulous hemostasis is performed. The neurovascular pedicle is then divided, and the muscle flap segment is transferred to the recipient site (Fig. 16.3). The donor site is closed in the usual fashion with the placement of a suction drain.

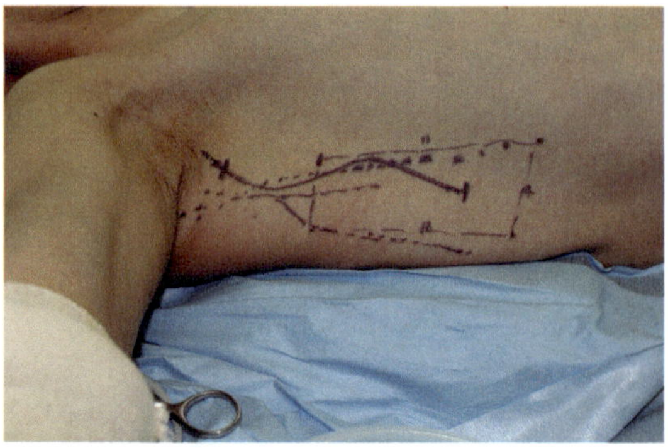

Fig. 16.2 Design for harvesting functional latissimus dorsi flap with both descending and transverse branch of a thoracodorsal nerve

16.2.2.4 Transfer of the Harvested Muscle

The harvested muscle flap is set into the prepared cheek pocket. Its proximal end is securely fixed to the nasolabial region using stay sutures anchored to the orbicularis oris muscle, which are prepared during the pocket preparation. The harvested thoracodorsal nerve stalk is transposed through the subcutaneous tunnel of the upper lip to reach the exposed contralateral facial nerve branches (Fig. 16.4). A co-harvested nerve branch, either a distal runoff of the descending branch or a transverse branch, is pulled to the prepared ipsilateral

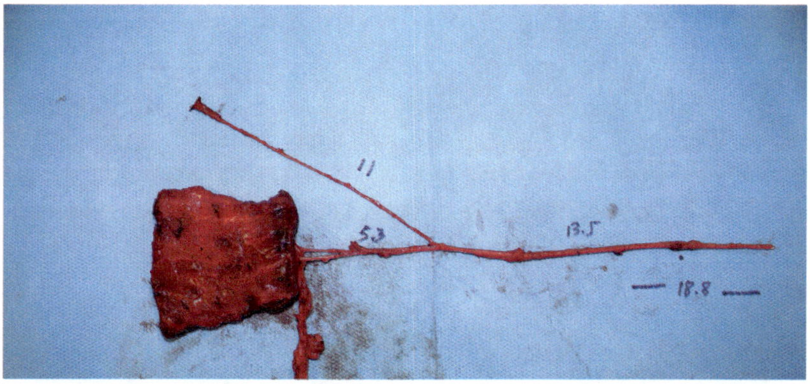

Fig. 16.3 Appearance of the harvested functional latissimus dorsi muscle with a descending and a transverse branch of the thoracodorsal nerve for dual innervation

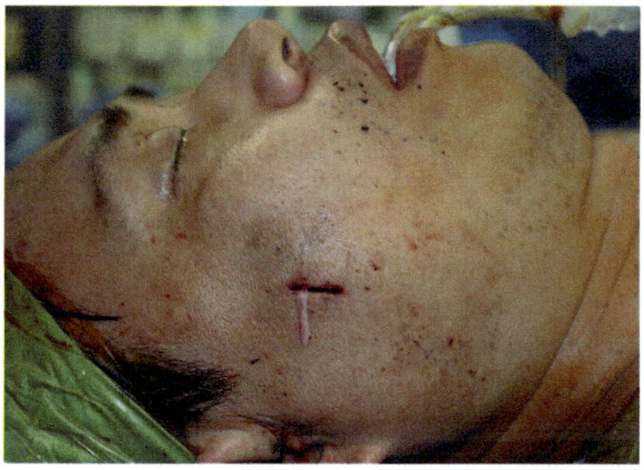

Fig. 16.4 After identifying a buccal branch of the contralateral facial nerve through small cheek incision, a long thoracodorsal nerve stalk is passed under the subcutaneous tunnel and retrieved through the incision, which has been prepared for neurorrhaphy

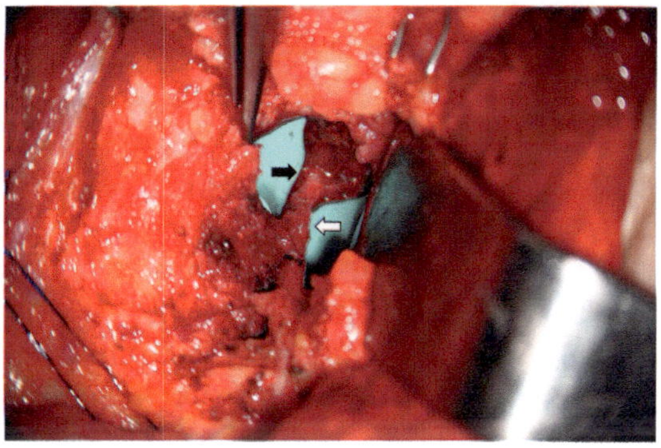

Fig. 16.5 Neurorrhaphy is conducted between a harvested transverse branch of the thoracodorsal nerve (white arrow) and ipsilateral masseteric nerve (black arrow)

masseteric nerve. In addition, the vascular pedicle is passed subcutaneously onto the prepared ipsilateral facial vessels in the submandibular region. After placing the muscle flap in a proper position, microvascular anastomoses are conducted between the facial vessels and the thoracodorsal vessels. Epineural sutures using 10-0 Nylon are then carried out in two sites; between the thoracodorsal nerve stump and the contralateral facial nerve branch, and between the transverse nerve branch and the ipsilateral masseteric nerve (Fig. 16.5). Lastly, the distal end of the latissimus dorsi muscle flap is fixed to the zygomatic region under appropriate tension with non-absorbable sutures considering the planned vector (Fig. 16.6). In patients with a strong contraction of the contralateral mimetic muscle and heavy soft tissue loading, a static sling using fascia lata or a dermal substitute product can be combined and placed under or beside the muscle segment. A shallow layer of malar fat pad is placed under the cheek flap and a small amount of buccal fat can be removed during or after the muscle placement if significant bulkiness is observed. The facial wounds are finely repaired with the placement of a small suction drain in the cheek pocket.

16.2.2.5 Postoperative Course

The drain is removed after a few days and the patient is discharged after removal of the stitches, usually 6 or 7 days after the operation. The patient is then followed at a 2- to 3-month interval. Any secondary procedures to improve the outcome are scheduled at least 18 months after the surgery.

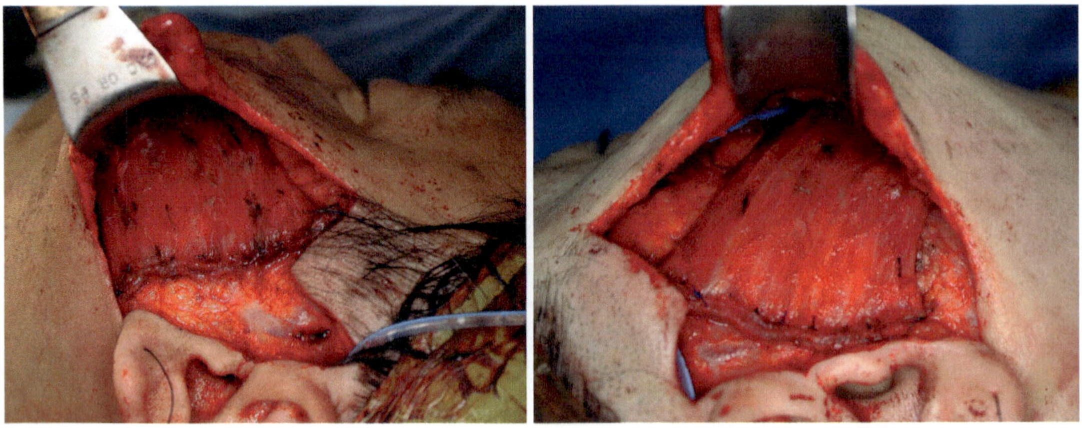

Fig. 16.6 Intraoperative images of the flap inset to the prepared cheek pocket after vessel anastomosis and neurorrhaphy

16.3 Comparison Between the Single and Dual-Innervation Technique

16.3.1 Clinical Efficacy of the Dual-Innervation Technique

The dual-innervation technique theoretically aims to obtain faster and more powerful contraction of the transferred muscle using an ipsilateral masseteric nerve source and to achieve a spontaneous smile using a contralateral facial nerve source. The most distinct characteristic of the dual-innervation technique compared to the conventional single-innervation technique is the supplementary neural input from the ipsilateral masseteric nerve. The ipsilateral masseteric nerve on the paralyzed side has long served as a valuable alternative option for the donor nerve, especially in cases of bilateral facial palsy. This nerve has abundant axonal loading and provides a strong neural input to the transferred muscle, which leads to a sufficiently powerful excursion during smile. In addition, spatial proximity to the transferred muscle allows for a relatively short re-innervation period and a reduction of possible denervation atrophy of the muscle, which contributes to the achievement of good muscle contraction. Given that one of the main weaknesses of the conventional single-stage latissimus dorsi neuromuscular transfer technique is the occasional and unexpected development of insufficient excursion of the muscle, potentially due to the long denervation period, the dual-innervation technique can compensate for this by the supplementation of neural inputs from the ipsilateral masseteric nerve. An additional neural input from the contralateral facial nerve allows for spontaneous contraction of the transferred muscle, which preserves the strength of the original technique.

According to the Watanabe et al. study [4], the first contraction of the transferred muscle was postoperatively observed at 3 months on average, which is relatively shorter compared to that of the conventional single-innervation technique (longer than 6 months). In addition, all three patients included in their study developed a spontaneous and symmetric smile and facial expression with minimum synkinesis. They conducted an electromyographic study on the transferred latissimus dorsi muscle and found that action potential was detected both on biting with the masseter muscle on the paralyzed side and on smiling with the zygomaticus major muscle on the non-paralyzed side. This implies that the muscle is dual-innervated by the ipsilateral masseteric nerve and contralateral facial nerve, which lends support to this technique. Biglioli et al. reported outcomes of the single-stage dual-innervation technique using the gracilis muscle for dynamic smile reconstruction [6]. In that study, the obturator nerve that was co-harvested with the gracilis muscle was coapted with the ipsilateral masseteric nerve and a cross-facial nerve graft was conducted between the contralateral facial nerve branches and the obturator nerve, which were anastomosed in an end-to-side manner. In spite of using a different technique of neurorrhaphy and muscle types, similarly favorable outcomes were observed in that the voluntary muscle contraction was first postoperatively observed at a mean 3.8 months and spontaneous contraction was achieved at a mean 7.2 months after operation.

16.3.2 Single-Innervation Versus Dual-Innervation Technique

Despite the suggested benefits and actual favorable outcomes of the dual-innervation technique as shown in the previous preliminary studies, there have been no published studies demonstrating the superiority of this technique to conventional ones using the single-innervation method. This is probably because it has not been long since the dual-innervation technique was first introduced, and the evaluation of dynamic reconstruction in facial paralysis generally requires a long follow-up period.

A total of 65 patients with a mean age of 37 years (range, 7–67) underwent a single-stage latissimus dorsi neuromuscular transfer for the treatment of long-standing facial paralysis in the authors' institution. Among them, the conventional single-innervation technique was used in 46 cases and the dual-innervation technique was used in 19 cases. Generally favorable outcomes, including relatively faster muscle contraction on biting, the first postoperative movement of the muscle at approximately 3 months, and subsequent spontaneous smiling were observed in the majority of cases using the dual-innervation technique (Fig. 16.7), which was consistent with the results of previous studies. In our crude analyses for overall reanimation outcomes using the Terzis Functional and Aesthetic grading system on the

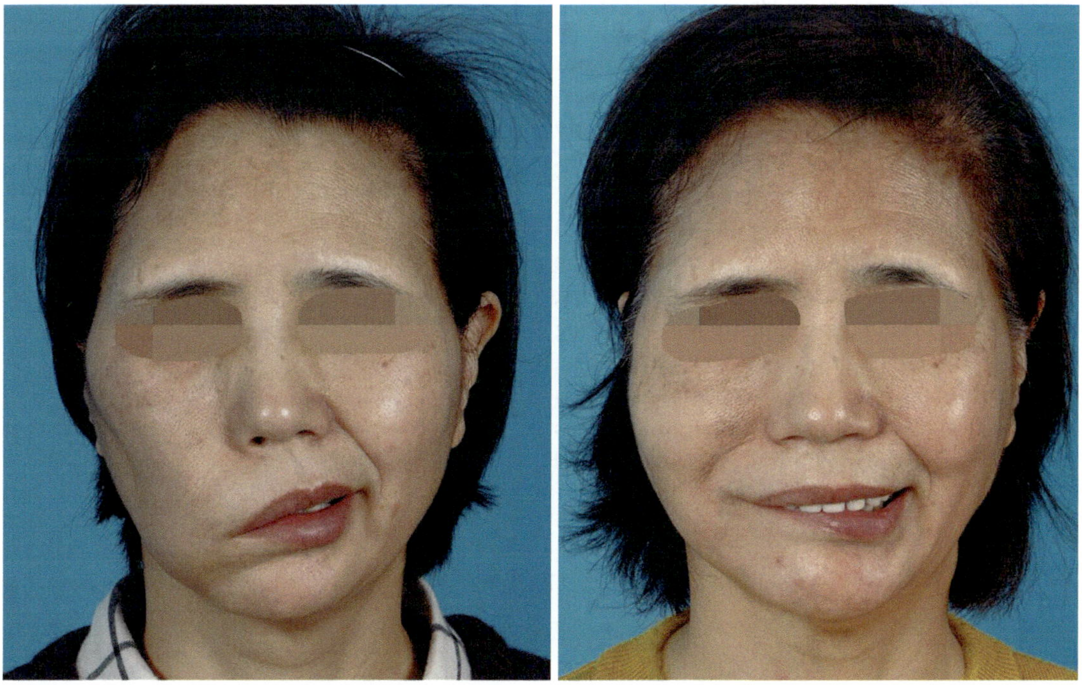

Fig. 16.7 A 55-year-old woman with established facial paralysis on her right hemiface, which developed following Bell's palsy. (Left) Preoperative appearance on smiling. (Right) She was treated with a functional latissimus dorsi muscle transfer using the dual-innervation technique. At 17 months without secondary procedure, she postoperatively developed a spontaneous and symmetric smile

mean follow-up period of 15 months, a good (IV) or excellent (V) grade was observed in 48.8% of cases using the conventional single-innervation technique and 71.4% in those using the dual-innervation technique. The observed dominance among the two neural inputs during smile varied depending on the patient. Although more favorable outcomes were achieved in the dual-innervation group, it would be too small a number of cases and too short a length of follow-up period to conduct an objective comparison and to generalize the results. Further studies are required to demonstrate the clinical efficacy of the dual-innervation technique and to consider it a more popular option for dynamic reconstruction.

16.3.3 Donor Morbidity

When using the dual-innervation technique, harvesting a transverse branch of the thoracodorsal nerve and a descending branch is required. A concern is that a further dissection of the latissimus dorsi muscle to harvest the transverse nerve branch may induce additional donor morbidity. However, according to our study (unpublished), cases using the dual-innervation technique did not show significantly higher donor morbidities, in terms of both complication rates and functional impairments, compared with those using the conventional single-innervation technique. Particularly in the survey of Quick-Disabilities of the Arm, Shoulder, and Hand questionnaire for evaluating postoperative function of the upper extremities, cases with dual innervation had similar scores compared to those with single innervation. This implies that harvesting both the descending and transverse branches of the thoracodorsal nerve might not have increased donor morbidities including functional deficits. To harvest a transverse nerve branch, splitting only the muscle cleavage through the course of the thoracodorsal nerve was sufficient without considerable transection of the latissimus dorsi muscle.

Financial Disclosure None.

References

1. Wang W, Chang T, Yang C, et al. Cross-face neurovascular latissimus dorsi for facial reanimating in one stage. Chin J Microsurg. 1989;12:155.
2. Harii K, Asato H, Yoshimura K, Sugawara Y, Nakatsuka T, Ueda K. One-stage transfer of the latissimus dorsi muscle for reanimation of a paralyzed face: a new alternative. Plast Reconstr Surg. 1998;102(4):941–51. Epub 1998/09/12.
3. Takushima A, Harii K, Asato H, Kurita M, Shiraishi T. Fifteen-year survey of one-stage latissimus dorsi muscle transfer for treatment of longstanding facial paralysis. J Plast Reconstr Aesthet Surg. 2013;66(1):29–36. Epub 2012/09/11.
4. Watanabe Y, Akizuki T, Ozawa T, Yoshimura K, Agawa K, Ota T. Dual innervation method using one-stage reconstruction with free latissimus dorsi muscle transfer for re-animation of established facial paralysis: simultaneous reinnervation of the ipsilateral masseter motor nerve and the contralateral facial nerve to improve the quality of smile and emotional facial expressions. J Plast Reconstr Aesthet Surg. 2009;62(12):1589–97. Epub 2008/11/18.
5. Takushima A. Double innervated latissimus dorsi muscle transfer for longstanding paralyzed face. In: 12th international facial nerve symposium. Boston: Harvard Medical School; 2013.
6. Biglioli F, Colombo V, Tarabbia F, Pedrazzoli M, Battista V, Giovanditto F, et al. Double innervation in free-flap surgery for long-standing facial paralysis. J Plast Reconstr Aesthet Surg. 2012;65(10):1343–9. Epub 2012/06/26.

17 Two-Stage Facial Reanimation Using CFNG

Terence Kwan-Wong, Gregory H. Borschel, and Ronald Zuker

17.1 Introduction

The first reported cases of free functional muscle transfer for facial reanimation were published by Harii et al. in 1976 [1], where a segment of gracilis was transferred and anastomosed to the superficial temporal vessels, with innervation provided by the temporal nerve. While cross face nerve grafting had been explored as early as 1971, its use was limited to providing a neural conduit from intact facial nerve branches to paralysed nerve branches.

In 1977, O'Brien et al. published a series of cases where two-stage facial reanimation was performed using a cross face nerve graft to innervate an extensor digitorum brevis muscle transplant [2]. Outcomes were suboptimal given limited excursion and inconsistent revascularization of muscle segments. Three years later, O'Brien published another series on their experience with two-stage facial reanimation, this time including a group of patients who received segmental gracilis muscle transfers, and found that excursion was superior to the EDB transfer [3]. Since that time, two-stage facial reanimation using a gracilis muscle transfer has had significant uptake as a reliable method for providing good, lasting results with minimal donor site morbidity.

The first stage procedure entails identifying a redundant zygomatic or buccal facial nerve branch from the contralateral, unparalysed side of the face to be used to provide neural input for the proposed muscle transplant. One end of a sural nerve graft is coapted to the donor nerve, while the opposite end is banked in the upper buccal sulcus adjacent to the canine on the paralyzed side. Six to 12 months elapse, during which axonal sprouting from the donor nerve proceeds toward the free end of the nerve graft. Finally, in the second stage procedure, the gracilis muscle transplant is performed, innervated by the cross face nerve graft. By staging the procedures, the time needed to reinnervate the motor end plates to the muscle transplant is minimized. Prolonged denervation of the transplanted muscle results in irreversible muscle atrophy and fibrosis, which adversely affects the reconstructive outcome.

Compared to muscle transplants powered by the motor nerve to masseter, the two-stage procedure using a cross face nerve graft provides less oral commissure excursion than one powered by the motor nerve to masseter—approximately 50–75% the excursion of the normal side, as

T. Kwan-Wong
Division of Plastic and Reconstructive Surgery, The Hospital for Sick Children, Toronto, ON, Canada
e-mail: tnwong@ualberta.ca

G. H. Borschel · R. Zuker (✉)
Division of Plastic and Reconstructive Surgery, Hospital for Sick Children (SickKids), University of Toronto, Toronto, ON, Canada
e-mail: gregory.borschel@sickkids.ca; ronald.zuker@sickkids.ca

© Springer Nature Switzerland AG 2021
C.-H. J. Tzou, A. Rodríguez-Lorenzo (eds.), *Facial Palsy*,
https://doi.org/10.1007/978-3-030-50784-8_17

opposed to 90% or more when powered by the masseteric nerve. This difference can be attributed to the difference in axonal density provided by the donor nerve [4–6]. Snyder-Warwick et al. demonstrated that the distal end of the cross face nerve graft had a 74% decrease in axonal density compared to the native facial nerve branch; by contrast, the motor nerve to masseter had a relative axonal density of 78% [7].

However, reconstructing the movement of the oral commissure only addresses part of the stigma associated with facial paralysis. The ability to generate a smile at appropriate times during social interaction is at least as important as the physical ability to form a smile. A spontaneous smile involves emotional and sensory integration by the frontal lobe which is effected by the motor nucleus of the facial nerve. By utilizing a branch of the intact contralateral facial nerve, two-stage facial reanimation using cross face nerve grafting reconstructs not only the physical ability to smile, but uniquely, also the ability to spontaneously generate a smile congruent with the patient's emotions.

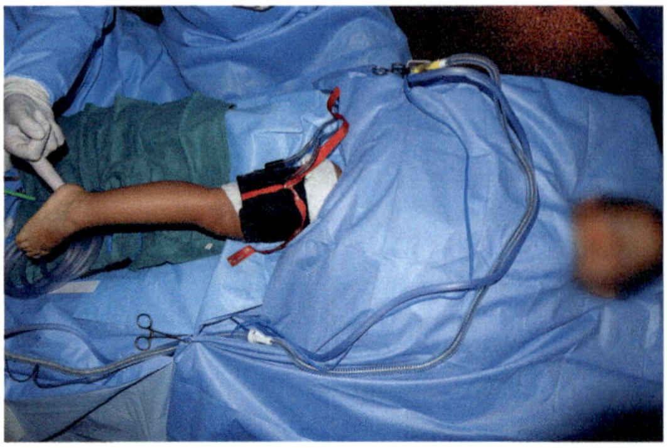

Fig. 17.1 The patient is positioned supine, permitting a two team approach to surgery

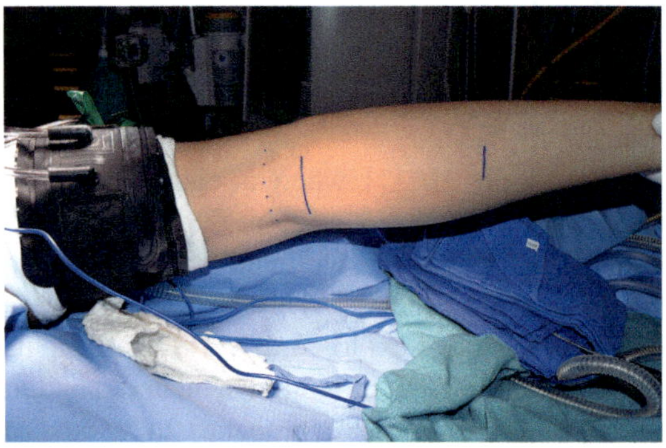

Fig. 17.2 Markings for the sural nerve procurement. A sterile tourniquet is used to optimize intraoperative visualization

17.2 Technique

17.2.1 Stage One: Cross Face Nerve Grafting

17.2.1.1 Sural Nerve Harvest

We prefer to perform our sural nerve harvest with the patient supine, which obviates the need to change positioning intraoperatively. Furthermore, this permits a two team approach with one team harvesting the sural nerve while the second team exposes and maps the donor facial nerve (Fig. 17.1). Access to the posterior leg for nerve harvest can be facilitated by flexing and internally rotating the hip and knee. If needed, a gel roll can be placed underneath the ipsilateral hip to improve visualization of the posterior leg. The donor leg is circumferentially prepared and draped to allow it to be repositioned as needed. A sterile pneumatic tourniquet is used to minimize bleeding and improve visualization during dissection.

The proximal incision is marked as a 4 cm line centered over the midline of the leg located 4 cm distal to the flexion crease of the knee (Fig. 17.2). The skin is incised with a 15 blade scalpel, and then dissection proceeds in the subcutaneous plane using tenotomy scissors and bipolar cautery down to the level of the fascia overlying the gastrocnemius muscle. Hemostasis should be meticulously maintained during the dissection to optimize visualization of tissue planes and anatomical structures.

The fascia is incised, and the medial and lateral heads of the gastrocnemius muscle are visualized. The sural nerve is located in the interval between the medial and lateral heads of the gastrocnemius, running adjacent to the lesser saphenous vein. The sural nerve is dissected proximally towards its takeoff from the tibial nerve. Occasionally, the sural nerve has significant

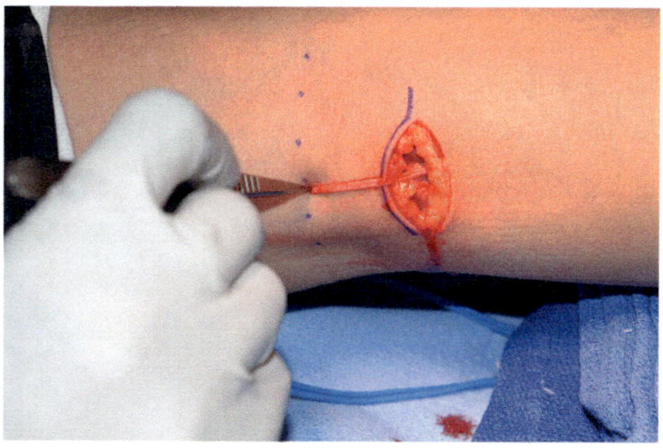

Fig. 17.3 The sural nerve is identified, isolated and divided proximally just distal to its takeoff from the tibial nerve

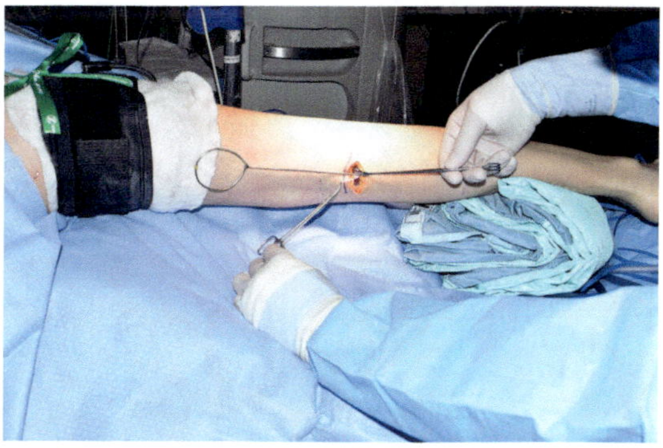

Fig. 17.4 The proximal end of the sural nerve graft passed through the nerve stripper. A hemostat is used to provide gentle proximal traction as the sural nerve is stripped to the level of the mid-calf

contribution from the lateral communicating branch—in these cases, the lateral communicating branch is also dissected proximally to its origin from the common peroneal nerve, and can be used for additional nerve graft if needed. The sural nerve is then dissected as distally as possible under direct vision.

The sural nerve is transected as proximally as safely possible from its takeoff from the tibial nerve (Fig. 17.3), and the free end of the sural nerve is passed through the loop of the nerve stripper. Traction is maintained on the nerve during the stripping process by applying a fine mosquito on the tip of the graft. The tip of the nerve stripper is passed deep to the fascia overlying the gastrocnemius, and gentle pressure is used to guide the stripper as distally as possible. If there is significant resistance to passage of the nerve stripper, the surgeon should confirm that the nerve stripper is in the correct plane and being guided in an axis parallel to the long axis of the leg.

Approximately 12 cm of sural nerve is needed for cross face nerve grafting in children 5 years and older. Once sufficient length has been stripped, the tip of the stripper can be palpated, and a counter incision made in this location to identify the distal end of the nerve graft. At this point, the sural nerve graft can be delivered from the distal incision using gentle traction, and removed from the end of the nerve stripper. If needed, the sural nerve can be dissected distally for additional length before being transected using sharp scissors. The proximal end of the sural nerve graft is marked with a surgical marker, and brought to a side table to be prepared. The graft is trimmed of adventitia, and the proximal end crushed by the mosquito during the stripping process is freshened using sharp scissors (Fig. 17.4). The graft is kept moist at all times with saline dampened surgical gauze.

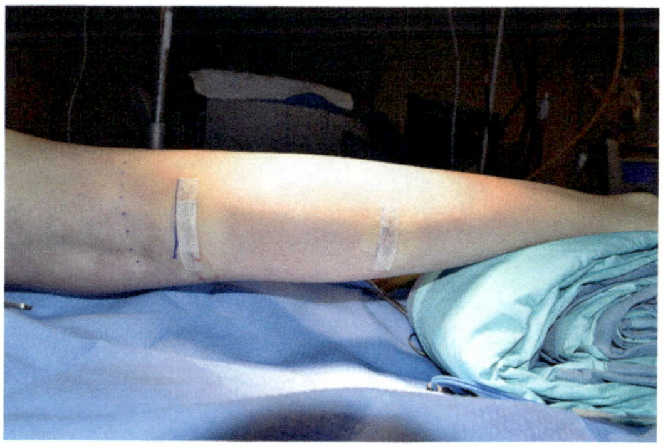

Fig. 17.5 After the skin incisions are closed, skin adhesive as well as wound closure tapes are applied over top to provide a robust, waterproof dressing over the surgical site

The tourniquet is let down before final closure in order to ensure hemostasis. Layered closure is performed using absorbable sutures. Finally, a layer of skin adhesive over top of the closed incisions to act as a waterproof barrier (Fig. 17.5).

17.2.1.2 Cross Face Nerve Grafting

A rhytidectomy incision with a short submandibular extension is marked on the non-paralyzed

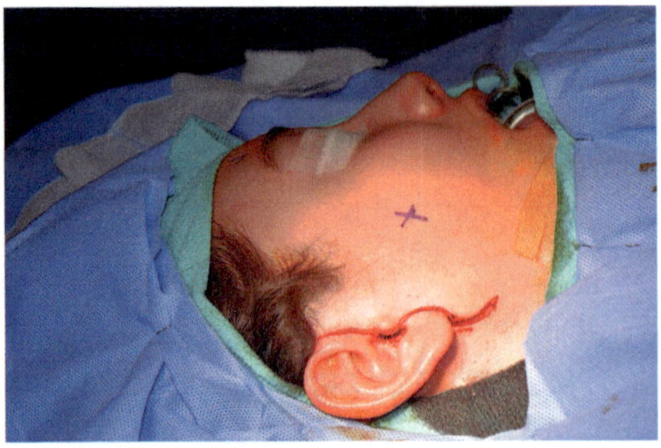

Fig. 17.6 Facial incision for cross face nerve grafting. The anticipated location of the donor facial nerve branch is marked midway between the lateral oral commissure and the root of the helix

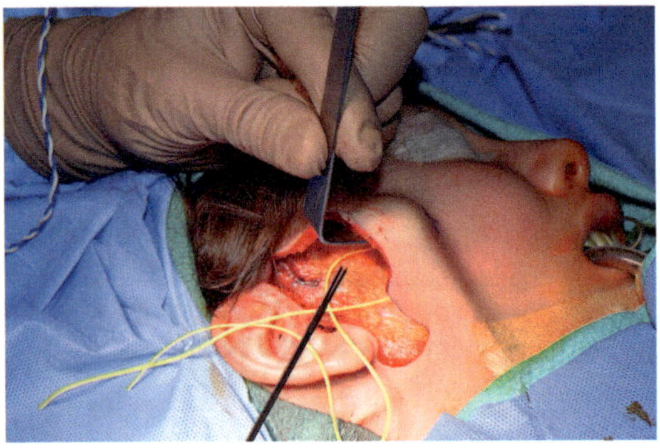

Fig. 17.7 The facial nerve branches have been identified and isolated. A nerve stimulator is used to create a map to determine appropriate donor nerves

side. It is useful to mark the approximate location of the donor facial nerve branch, which can be approximated by a point halfway between the helical root and oral commissure [8] (Fig. 17.6). The face is elevated in a subcutaneous plane, superficial to the parotid facia, until the anterior border of the parotid gland is reached. As dissection continues anteriorly, branches of the facial nerve are identified and dissected.

Facial nerve mapping is performed by stimulating facial nerve branches and noting the facial movements elicited (Fig. 17.7). The ideal donor facial nerve branch should be of similar caliber to the sural nerve graft, and effect strong activation of the zygomaticus major, zygomaticus minor, and levator angularis oris while minimizing distortion from the orbicularis oris (Fig. 17.8).

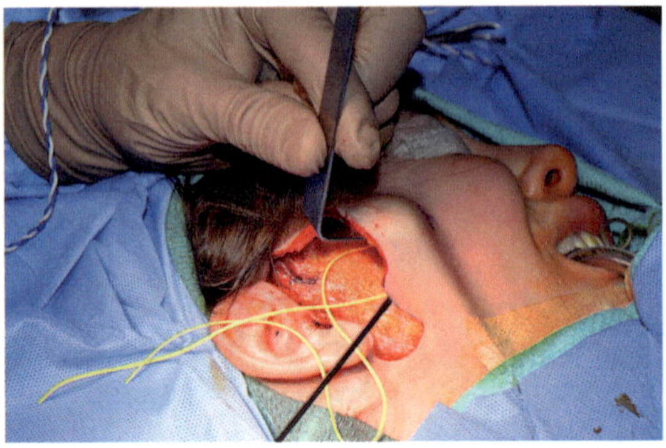

Fig. 17.8 The selected facial nerve branch is activated with the nerve stimulator, leading to appropriate facial muscle contraction—'a smile'

Nerve stimulation can also be used to confirm redundant innervation to the zygomaticus and lip levator musculature to ensure that the smile on the non-paralyzed side will not be adversely affected by dividing the donor nerve. The selected facial nerve branch is dissected retrograde into the substance of the parotid gland itself. This proximal dissection aids in optimizing the final reconstructive result by providing a better size match between the donor facial nerve and the sural nerve graft, increasing axonal counts in the donor nerve and improving visualization for the neurorraphy [9].

Low frequency electrical stimulation has been shown to improve peripheral nerve regeneration and axonal survival [10, 11]. Physiologically, this translates into more robust innervation of the muscle transplant, which clinically manifests as improved excursion of the reconstructed smile. At our center, we routinely perform electrical stimulation of the donor nerve for 1 h at 20 Hz prior to its division and coaptation to the sural nerve graft (Fig. 17.9). The nerve stimulator amperage is set to the lowest setting that elicits clinically evident contraction of the facial musculature. Once the electrical stimulation is complete, the donor facial nerve branch is transected.

A buccal mucosal incision is made at the level of the canine on the paralysed side, and blunt dissection is carried down to the level of the maxillary periosteum. During the dissection, terminal branches of the infraorbital nerve can be

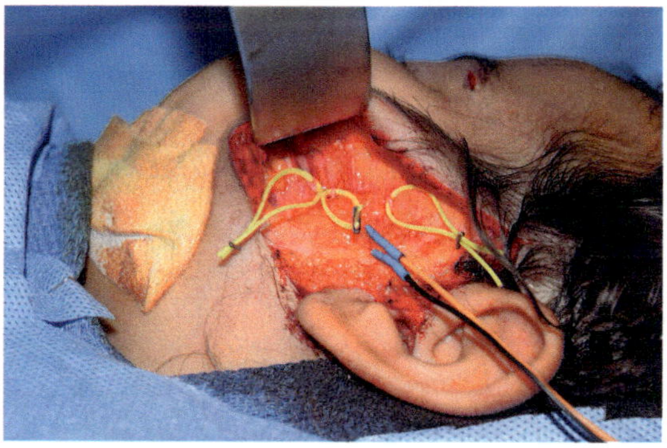

Fig. 17.9 Low frequency electrical stimulation is provided for 1 h to the donor facial nerve branch in order to enhance nerve regeneration

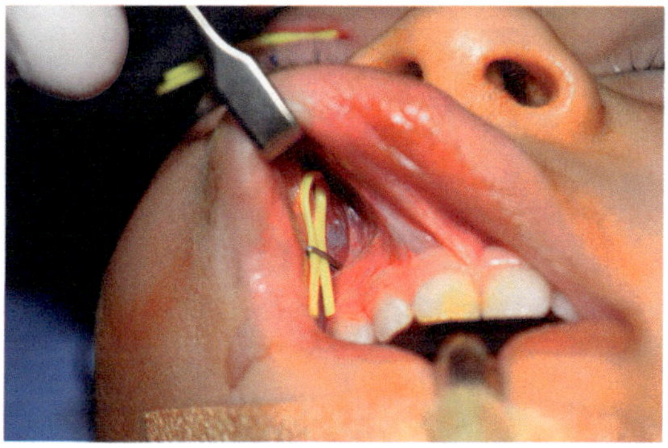

Fig. 17.10 A terminal branch of the infraorbital nerve is identified within the upper buccal sulcus, identified here using a yellow vessel loop. This will be coapted to the distal end of the cross face nerve graft

seen as they course anteriorly to provide innervation to the lip. We routinely dissect these nerve branches, identifying one or two branches that will provide a good size match for anastomosis to the banked end of the sural nerve graft (Fig. 17.10). In an animal model of cross face nerve grafting, end to side anastomosis of a sensory nerve to a nerve graft demonstrated enhanced motor nerve regeneration, and ultimately, improved functional outcomes [12].

The selected infraorbital nerve branches are divided in order to improve exposure within the upper buccal sulcus incision. Fine Jake forceps are used to create a supraperiosteal tunnel connecting the upper buccal sulcus incision with the rhytidectomy exposure. The sural nerve graft is reversed, and passed through the previously made

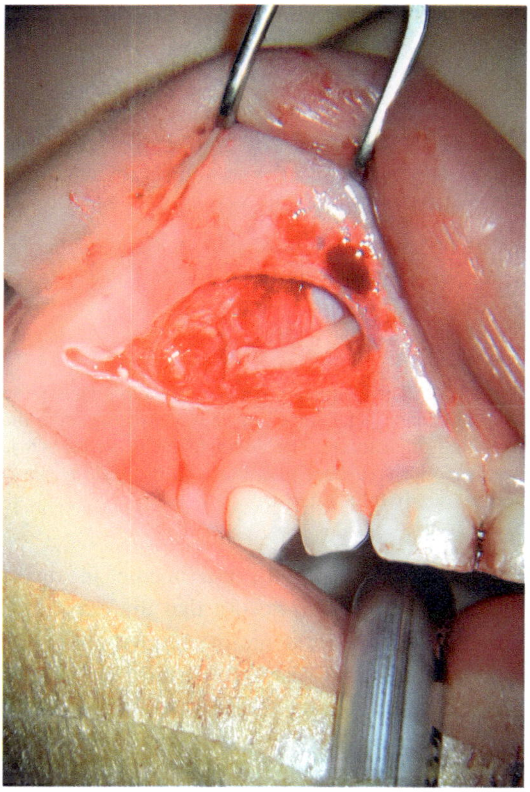

Fig. 17.11 The cross face nerve graft is secured in the upper buccal sulcus on the paralyzed side

tunnel. The nerve graft is positioned to ensure that the coaptations can be done under no tension. The location of the distal end of the nerve graft in the upper buccal sulcus incision can be marked using a vascular clip, non-resorbing suture, or both to aid with identification of the distal cross face nerve graft in the second stage procedure (Fig. 17.11).

The operating microscope is brought in at this point, and the ends of the sural nerve graft are inspected and trimmed back to a healthy fascicular pattern. Coaptation of the nerve graft to the donor facial nerve proximally, and to branches of the infraorbital nerve distally, are performed using a combination of 10-0 nylon sutures and fast set fibrin glue (Fig. 17.12).

The facial incision is closed using deep dermal sutures followed by a running subcuticular suture using an absorbable monofilament suture. We do not routinely use silastic drains for our facial closures. The oral incision is closed using

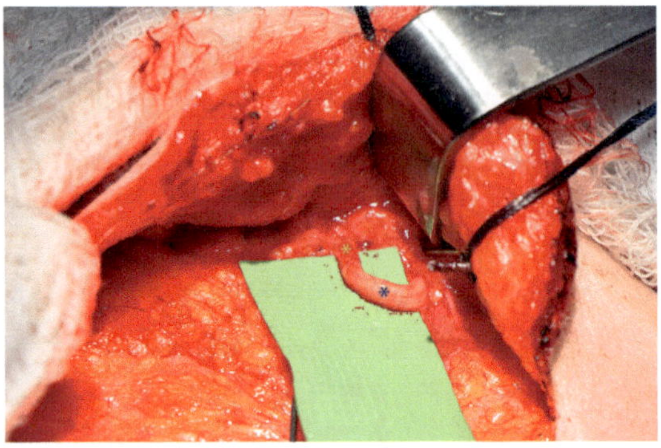

Fig. 17.12 The coaptation between the cross face nerve graft and donor facial nerve branch is completed under the operating microscope. The donor facial nerve branch is seen superiorly (yellow asterisk), and the sural nerve is seen inferiorly (blue asterisk)

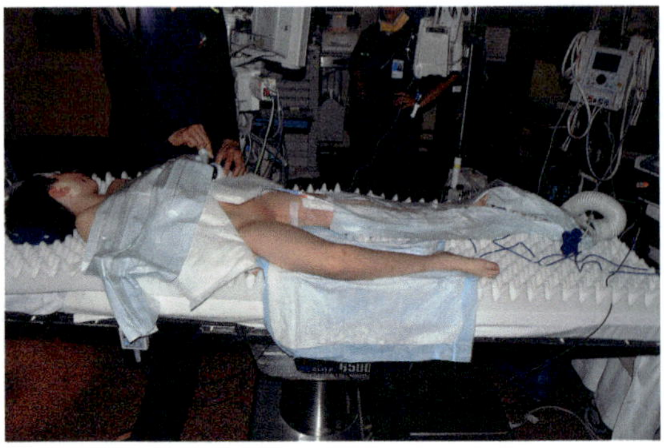

Fig. 17.13 A two team approach is also used for the second stage procedure. One team prepares the face to receive the muscle transplant while the second team procures the gracilis from the thigh

absorbable sutures with the needle in direct vision at all times to ensure that the cross face nerve graft is not accidentally captured within the mucosal closure. Wound closure strips are applied over top of the facial incisions.

A reminder is written on a strip of medical tape and applied over the donor side cheek to remind the patient, caregivers and health care team to avoid applying pressure over the surgical site. Postoperatively, patients are placed on a soft diet for 3 weeks, a week of oral antibiotics, and a course of 0.12% chlorhexidine mouthwash four times a day to maintain oral hygiene and minimize the likelihood of wound healing complications. We routinely admit patients for 24–48 h postoperatively to monitor analgesic needs and ensure that they are fully ambulatory prior to discharge.

17.2.2 Stage 2: Free Functional Muscle Transfer

Generally, we wait around 6–12 months following the cross face nerve graft to perform the muscle transplant, depending on the length of nerve graft utilized. The regeneration front of the cross face nerve graft can be tracked by the progression of a Tinel's sign across the upper lip.

Similar to the first stage procedure, we utilize a two team approach to improve efficiency. One team is responsible for exposure and preparation of the recipient side of the face, while the second team dissects and procures the segmental gracilis muscle with its neurovascular supply (Fig. 17.13).

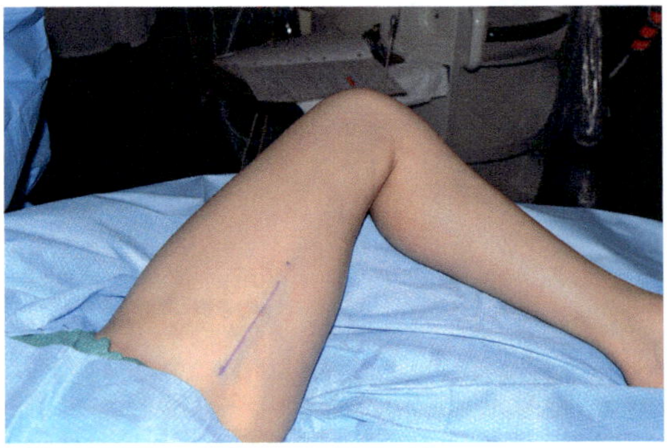

Fig. 17.14 Markings for the incision on the medial thigh for gracilis procurement

17.2.2.1 Gracilis Harvest

The gracilis is harvested with the patient supine, and with the knee flexed, and the hip flexed and externally rotated. In this position, the course of the adductor longus can be visualized or palpated. In older children, the gracilis itself is sometimes palpable. The incision is marked as a 10 cm line that lies 1–2 cm posterior to the axis of the adductor longus, and centered over the estimated location of the major pedicle entering the gracilis, which is located approximately 10 cm inferior to the muscle origin at the pubic symphysis (Fig. 17.14).

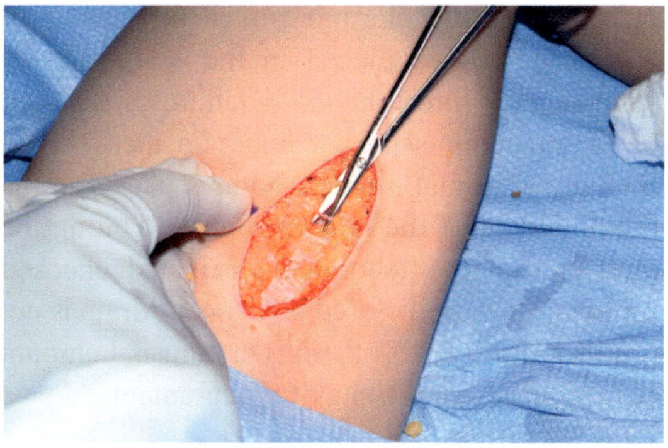

Fig. 17.15 Occasionally, a perforator can be seen traversing the thigh incision. When present, this serves as an excellent guide to the location of the pedicle supplying the gracilis

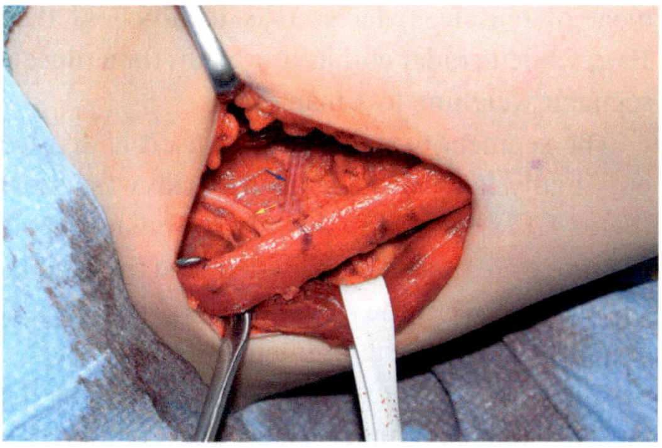

Fig. 17.16 The gracilis can be segmentally dissected in order to minimize muscle bulk. The anterior one-third of the muscle will be utilized, and the neurovascular pedicle can be seen entering this segment (yellow arrow—obturator nerve; blue arrow—vascular bundle). The posterior two-third of the muscle will be left behind in the thigh

The skin incision is made using a 15 blade scalpel, and subcutaneous dissection is performed using tenotomy scissors. Meticulous hemostasis should be maintained throughout the dissection to optimize visualization of structures. Dissection proceeds to the level of the gracilis fascia. Sometimes, a perforator can be seen running obliquely across the incision; in these cases, the perforator is a useful landmark for approximating the location of the vascular pedicle to the gracilis (Fig. 17.15). The fascia overlying the gracilis is incised, and reflected anteriorly to expose the interval between the gracilis and adductor longus. Retracting the gracilis and adductor longus from each other, dissection proceeds deep into this interval to identify the vascular pedicle to the gracilis, and its takeoff from the medial circumflex femoral system. The obturator nerve enters the muscle proximal to the vascular pedicle, and travels in an oblique trajectory, as opposed to the more transverse lie of the vessels. Dissection of the vascular pedicle proceeds as proximal as possible towards its takeoff from the deep femoral artery in order to maximize length. Often, ligation and division of vascular branches entering the adductor longus and adductor magnus is necessary in order to provide sufficient pedicle length. The nerve supplying the gracilis is dissected proximally to its takeoff from the obturator nerve.

The segment of gracilis to be procured is determined by the location of the vascular pedicle, and also by the donor nerve used to innervate the muscle transplant. In two-stage facial reanimation, where the gracilis will be innervated by a cross face nerve graft, the gracilis is harvested such that the pedicle is eccentrically biased towards the proximal portion of the muscle segment. This permits the nerve to the gracilis to be positioned closer to the cross face nerve graft located in the upper buccal sulcus, facilitating subsequent coaptation and decreasing the distance for nerve regeneration. The length of gracilis is determined by the team operating on the patient's face by measuring the distance between the helical root and the oral commissure, and adding 2 cm to this number to account for placement of anchoring sutures. The required length is marked on the gracilis, accounting for positioning of the pedicle slightly closer to the proximal end of the muscle.

The relationship between the entry of the pedicle relative to the gracilis determines what segments of the muscle can be procured to minimize bulk. Often, the posterior 2/3 of the gracilis can be excluded from the segment to be harvested (Fig. 17.16). If this selected segment is still too large, a further removal of an anterior strip can be performed, although dissection must be done carefully to ensure the neurovascular supply to the segment to be used is not damaged or inadvertently excluded. In young children, the segment of muscle to be used is ideally less than 10 g, while in older children, we aim for a muscle segment weighing less than 20 g.

The segment of gracilis to be used is divided proximally and distally using heavy scissors (Fig. 17.17). Following this, the vascular pedicle and nerve are ligated and divided, and the gracilis is delivered from the donor site. If desired, the obturator nerve to the segmental gracilis muscle can be stimulated ex vivo to confirm that the muscle remains innervated and contractile. Horizontal mattress sutures are placed 1 cm away from the proximal end of the muscle in order to minimize the risk of pull through of the sutures that will be subsequently placed to anchor the gracilis to the oral commissure and upper lip (Fig. 17.18). The number of horizontal sutures placed is usually one more than the number of anchoring sutures placed in the oral commissure—e.g., if three anchoring sutures are placed in the oral commissure and upper lip, there should be four horizontal mattress sutures placed in the proximal end of the gracilis muscle. During the gracilis inset, the donor site is irrigated, checked for hemostasis and closed in layers. A drain is not routinely used unless there is an unusual amount of bleeding from the site of procurement.

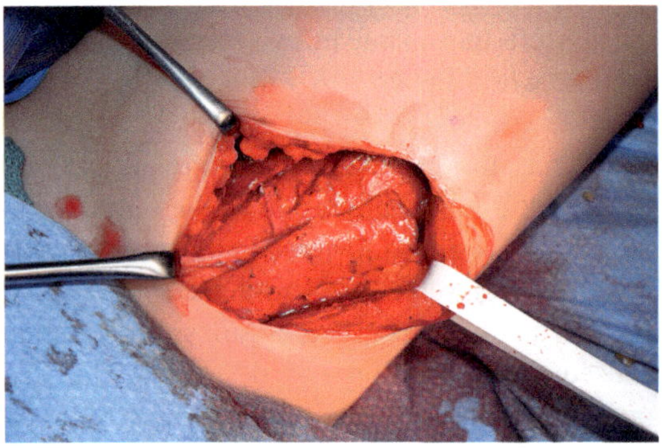

Fig. 17.17 The segment of the gracilis to be used is divided, and the neurovascular pedicle is appropriately ligated and divided

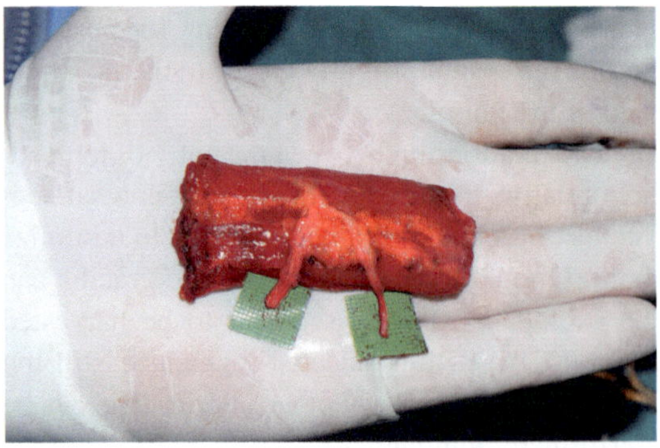

Fig. 17.18 The gracilis muscle is shown here, ready for transplantation into the facial pocket. Horizontal mattress sutures will be placed into the distal end of the muscle to provide anchor points for the oral commissure sutures

17.2.2.2 Muscle Transplantation to Face

Facial exposure to the paralysed side is provided via an extended rhytidectomy incision with a submandibular extension. The superior extent of the incision extends a short distance into the sideburn area to permit exposure to the temporal fascia, while the submandibular component parallels the inferior border of the mandible far enough anteriorly to provide access to the facial vessels. Similar to the facial exposure for the cross face nerve graft, the flap is raised in the subcutaneous plane, superficial to the parotid fascia. The dissection proceeds anteriorly until the oral commissure is reached.

Once the skin flap has been elevated, the recipient vessel can be identified and dissected in preparation for the muscle transplant. Our preferred recipient vessels are the facial artery and vein for its good size match to the vessels supplying the gracilis, and for its favorable location for anastomosis relative to the cross face nerve graft. Occasionally, especially in children with Moebius syndrome, the facial vein may be absent. In these situations, a transverse facial vein is present, and can be dissected and reflected inferiorly for use. The facial artery is almost always present, and can be localized preoperatively by digital palpation and then marking the location of the pulse with a surgical marking pen. Dissection of the facial vessels is facilitated by removal of the buccal fat pad, which has ancillary benefit by reducing excess bulk in the cheek following muscle transplantation (Fig. 17.19). As the facial vein courses over the inferior border of the mandible, it takes a relatively vertical course, travelling parallel and anterior to the masseter. The facial artery is located anterior to the vein, but takes a more oblique course towards the oral commissure.

Reconstruction of the nasolabial fold on the paralysed side is a critical step in providing a good outcome. Meticulous placement of sutures is paramount, and the surgical team should not hesitate to remove sutures that do not provide the desired vector or depth of pull. In cases of unilateral facial paralysis, the nasolabial crease on the normal side should be marked in the preoperative area, and used intraoperatively as a template for reconstructing the nasolabial fold on the paralysed side. We typically place three anchor sutures—one in the oral commissure, and two into the region of the upper lip / lower cheek—using heavy, absorbable suture such as a #1 Vicryl (Fig. 17.20). In instances where there is significant lower lip droop, an extra anchor suture can be placed into the lower lip to help normalize the resting position of the lower lip (Figs. 17.21 and 17.22).

Proper depth of suture placement is equally vital to creating a natural and aesthetically pleasing nasolabial fold. In cases of acquired facial paralysis, the native perioral musculature provides a useful guide for placement of the anchor sutures, whereas these anatomic landmarks are often absent in congenital cases. If sutures are placed too close to the dermis, this will pucker the overlying skin, and produce upper lip eversion. Conversely, sutures placed too deep will produce inversion of the upper lip on animation. Once the surgical team is happy with the vector, position and appearance of the reconstructed smile and nasolabial fold, the distance between

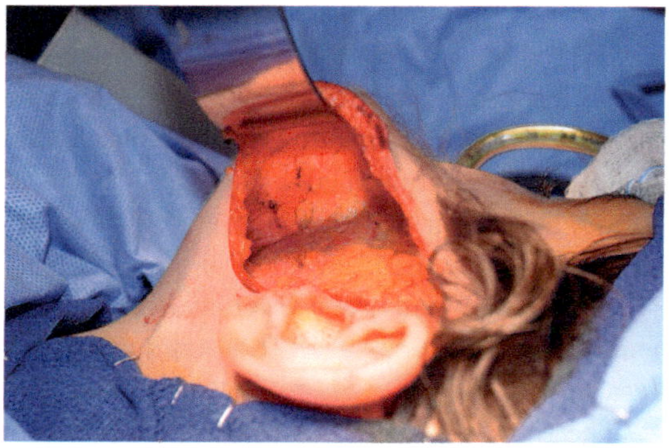

Fig. 17.19 The facial pocket created for the muscle is seen here. The recipient vessels have been identified and prepared, and the pocket is ready for placement of the anchor sutures to reconstruct the nasolabial fold

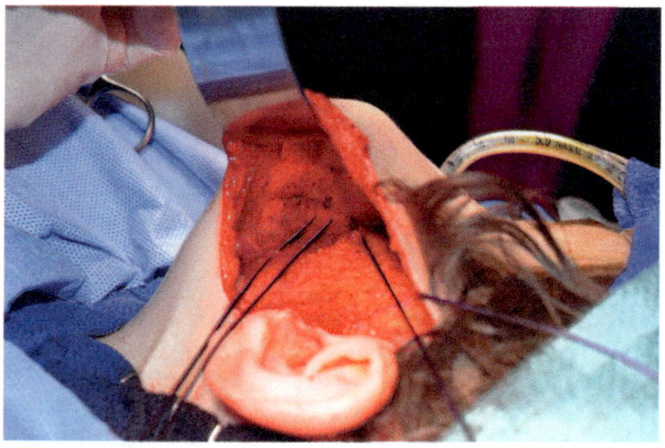

Fig. 17.20 Meticulous placement of anchoring sutures in the nasolabial fold is critical for a favourable outcome

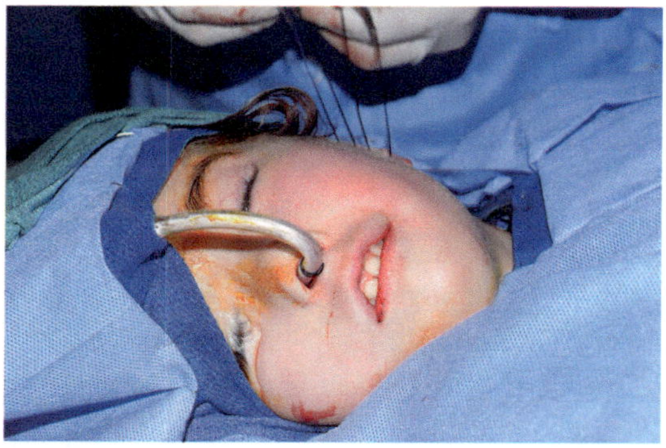

Fig. 17.21 Anchoring sutures placement—no traction applied

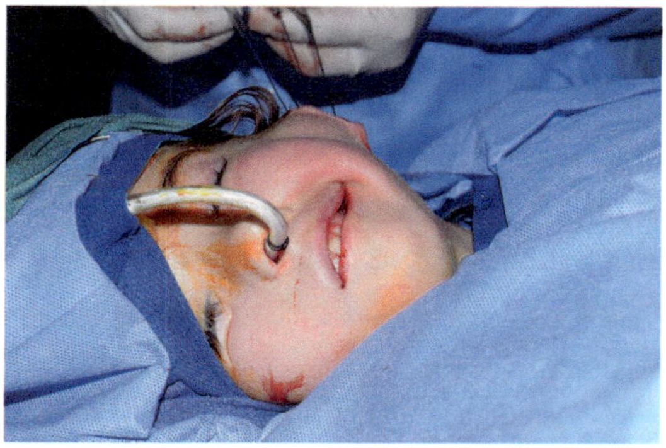

Fig. 17.22 Anchoring suture placement—traction applied. Attention is directed to creating a natural, symmetrical nasolabial crease without creating unwanted inversion or eversion of the lip

the anchor sutures and ipsilateral helical root is measured and communicated to the team responsible for procuring the gracilis muscle (Fig. 17.23).

The deep subcutaneous fat in the cheek flap is trimmed in order to further minimize soft tissue bulk overlying the muscle. Care should be taken to avoid overaggressive thinning of this flap, as exposure of the dermis to the transplanted muscle will result in undesired cutaneous distortion during animation. The gracilis is oriented such that the neurovascular hilum is biased toward the oral commissure to facilitate anastomosis of the nerve and vessels. The anchor sutures are passed behind the horizontal mattress sutures previously placed in the gracilis (Fig. 17.24), back through the perioral tissues and then back through the gracilis in a figure of eight manner. This method provides precise fixation of the muscle while minimizing the likelihood of delayed malposition of the muscle (Fig. 17.25).

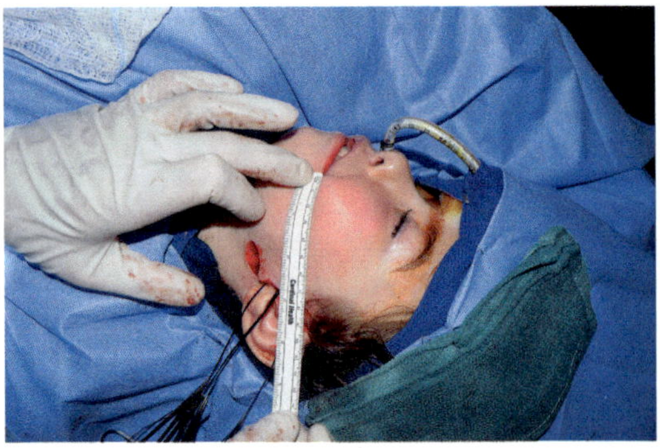

Fig. 17.23 The length of gracilis to be procured is determined by measuring the distance from the commissure to the root of the helix, and then adding one centimeter onto each end to permit suture placement

The upper buccal sulcus adjacent to the canine root on the paralysed side is incised, and dissection proceeds to identify the banked cross face nerve graft. If the distal cross face nerve was anastomosed to infraorbital nerve branches in the first stage procedure, this is divided. Fine Jake forceps are used to create a subcutaneous tunnel connecting the facial exposure to the upper buccal sulcus, and the obturator nerve supplying the gracilis muscle is passed through this tunnel into the upper buccal sulcus pocket in preparation for neurorraphy.

The operating microscope is brought in, and the ends of the donor and recipient nerve and vessels are carefully inspected, sharply trimming back to healthy anatomy as needed. At this point, excess vessel and nerve is resected, balancing the need for tension free anastomosis with elimination of redundant length. We usually anastomose the facial vein before turning our attention to the facial artery. Vascular inflow to the transplanted muscle can be confirmed using Doppler ultrasound, and empirically corroborated by visually inspecting the muscle for color and contractility (Fig. 17.26). Finally, neurorraphy is performed using a combination of 10-0 nylon sutures and fast set fibrin glue.

The free end of the gracilis is secured to the temporal fascia just superior to the zygomatic arch using heavy absorbable sutures placed in a horizontal mattress fashion (Fig. 17.27). The reconstructed commissure should lie symmetrically to the unparalysed side at rest. If there

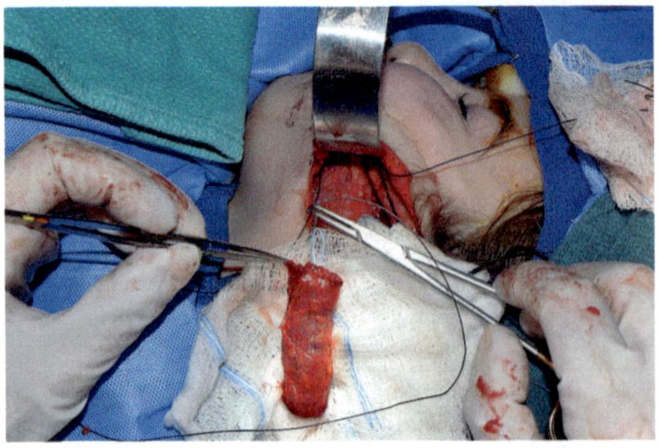

Fig. 17.24 The muscle is secured using anchoring sutures passed behind the previously placed horizontal mattress sutures

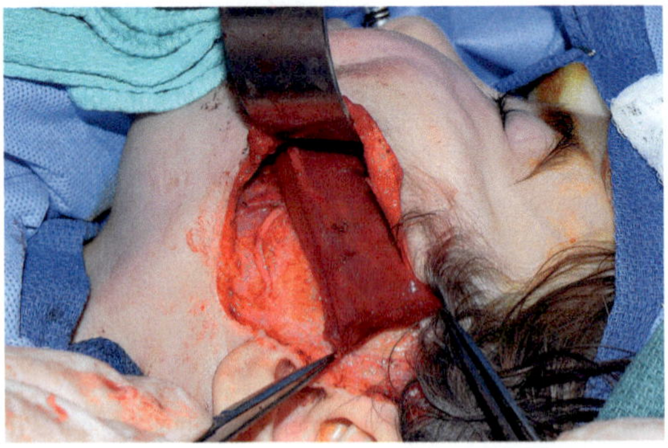

Fig. 17.25 The muscle is carefully positioned in the facial pocket, and the anchoring sutures secured

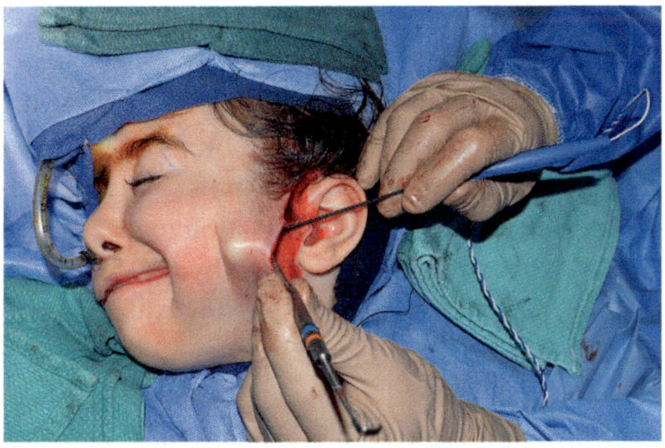

Fig. 17.26 After revascularization and neurorraphy, the viability, contractility and position of the transplanted muscle can be assessed by stimulating the neural supply to the gracilis with a nerve stimulator

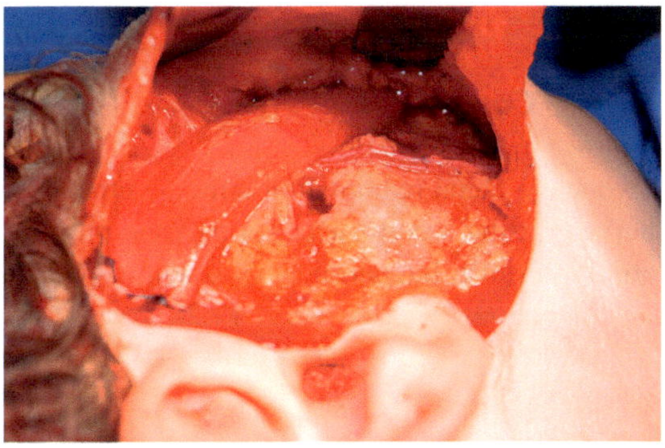

Fig. 17.27 The transplanted muscle is seen here, anchored to the oral commissure distally and to the temporalis fascia proximally

is any small discrepancy in the position of the commissure, this can be fine-tuned by slightly adjusting the origin of the transplanted muscle in a craniocaudal plane. Proper tensioning of the gracilis helps restore the physiologic actin-myosin relationship of the transplanted muscle, which maximizes muscle excursion postoperatively. Overtensioning of the muscle is undesirable, and does not resolve over time.

Once the position of the muscle and vector of pull is confirmed to be satisfactory, the surgical sites are irrigated and checked for hemostasis. The rhytidectomy incision is closed in layers with absorbable sutures, over top of a Penrose drain which is brought out through a separate postauricular stab incision. The intraoral exposure is closed under direct vision using absorbable monofilament suture, ensuring that the nerve is not inadvertently incorporated into the wound closure.

All our patients undergoing gracilis muscle transplantation have custom thermoplastic oral hooks made by occupational therapy. After all incisions are closed, the fit of the hook is confirmed, and adjusted as needed. The splint should be tensioned to provide a small degree of posterolateral traction to the oral commissure to offload tension on the reconstruction, and is anchored to the hair bearing scalp using a combination of elastics and silk suture.

As in the first stage cross face nerve graft, a labeled strip of tape is applied as a reminder to avoid applying pressure to the surgical site. Postoperatively, patients are placed on a caffeine free soft diet, prophylactic antibiotics and chlorhexidine mouthwash. A Foley catheter is kept in place overnight to monitor urine output, and children are usually kept on bed rest for 24 h before beginning graduated ambulation. Most patients are discharged on postoperative day 3–5.

17.3 Complications

The incidence of postoperative complications is relatively uncommon. Early complications include hematoma, seroma, and infection. There should be a low threshold for treating these issues in an open matter in the operating theatre. If left untreated, these issues have the potential to severely compromise muscle function and the overall cosmetic result in the long term.

Late complications are difficult to address secondarily, and as such, every effort should be made in the primary surgery to minimize the likelihood of these issues arising in the first place. The most common late complication is facial bulk in the region of the transplanted muscle. This can be avoided primarily by excluding the anterior and posterior segments of the gracilis, judicious lipectomy of the deep subcutaneous fat in the cheek flap, and excision of the buccal fat pad. In the late period, this bulk must be addressed by carefully re-elevating the cheek flap, and then carefully tangentially excising the subcutaneous flap and muscle.

Disruption of the muscle insertion at the oral commissure and inappropriate tensioning of the muscle are especially challenging, and the benefits of repositioning the muscle should be balanced with the expectation of reduced commissural excursion. Secondary correction of these issues requires careful elevation of not only the cheek flap, but the muscle as well. Dissection of the deep surface of the muscle must be done carefully to avoid compromising the neurovascular supply to the transplanted muscle. Where the muscle insertion has been disrupted, it may be possible to release the muscle from its scarred attachments, and reanchor it to the commissure. In some cases, reinserting the muscle will cause overtensioning of the oral commissure. In these situations, a short tendon or fascial graft may be needed in order to span the distance from the gracilis to the oral commissure.

Inadequate muscle excursion is probably the most difficult complication to correct secondarily. Mild deficiencies in muscle excursion can potentially be corrected by therapy alone. However, moderate to severe restrictions in excursion are most effectively addressed by excising the previously transplanted muscle and performing a new muscle transplant. If inadequate neural input is the suspected cause for the issues, then it may be useful to biopsy of the distal end of the cross face nerve graft to assess axonal density. If there is any question regarding the quality of neural input provided by the cross face nerve graft, there should be a low threshold to excise the existing nerve graft, and perform a repeat sural nerve harvest and cross face nerve grafting. In these cases, great care must be taken to avoid creating iatrogenic facial weakness on the normal side. Innervation using the ipsilateral motor nerve to masseter should remain a consideration for these cases, accepting the fact that complete spontaneity may not be possible.

17.4 Conclusion

Two-stage facial reanimation utilizing cross face nerve grafting reconstructs not only the physical ability to smile, but permits the patient to do so in a spontaneous manner (Figs. 17.28 and 17.29). By employing techniques described in this chap-

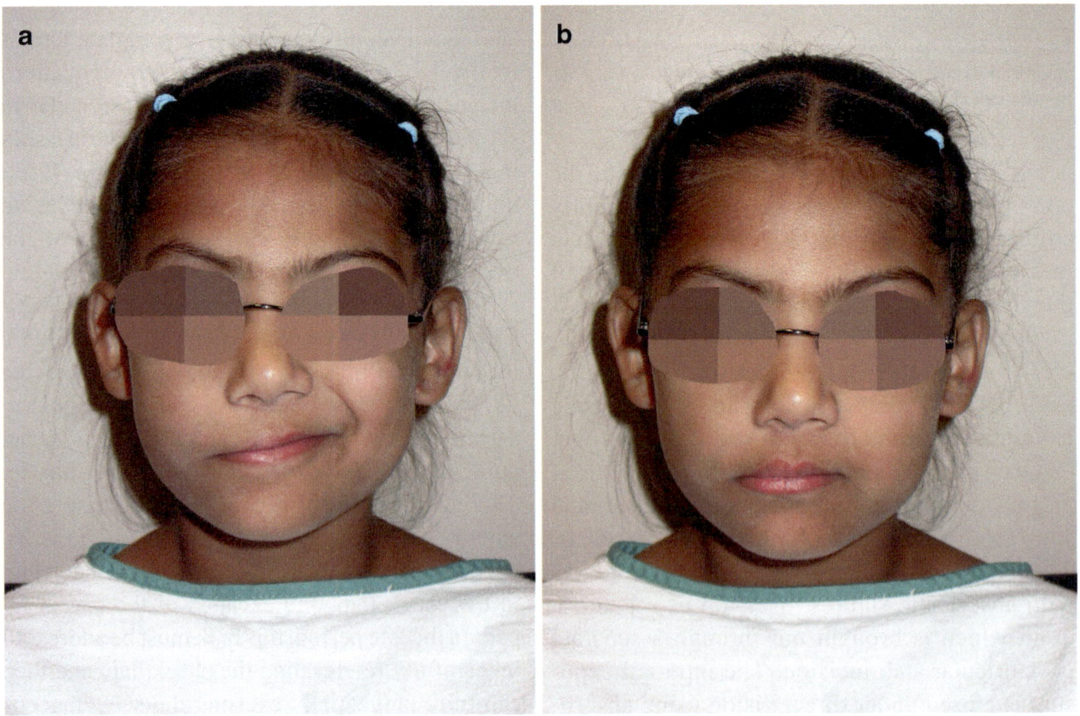

Fig. 17.28 (**a**) Preoperative view—at rest. (**b**) Preoperative view—patient attempting to smile

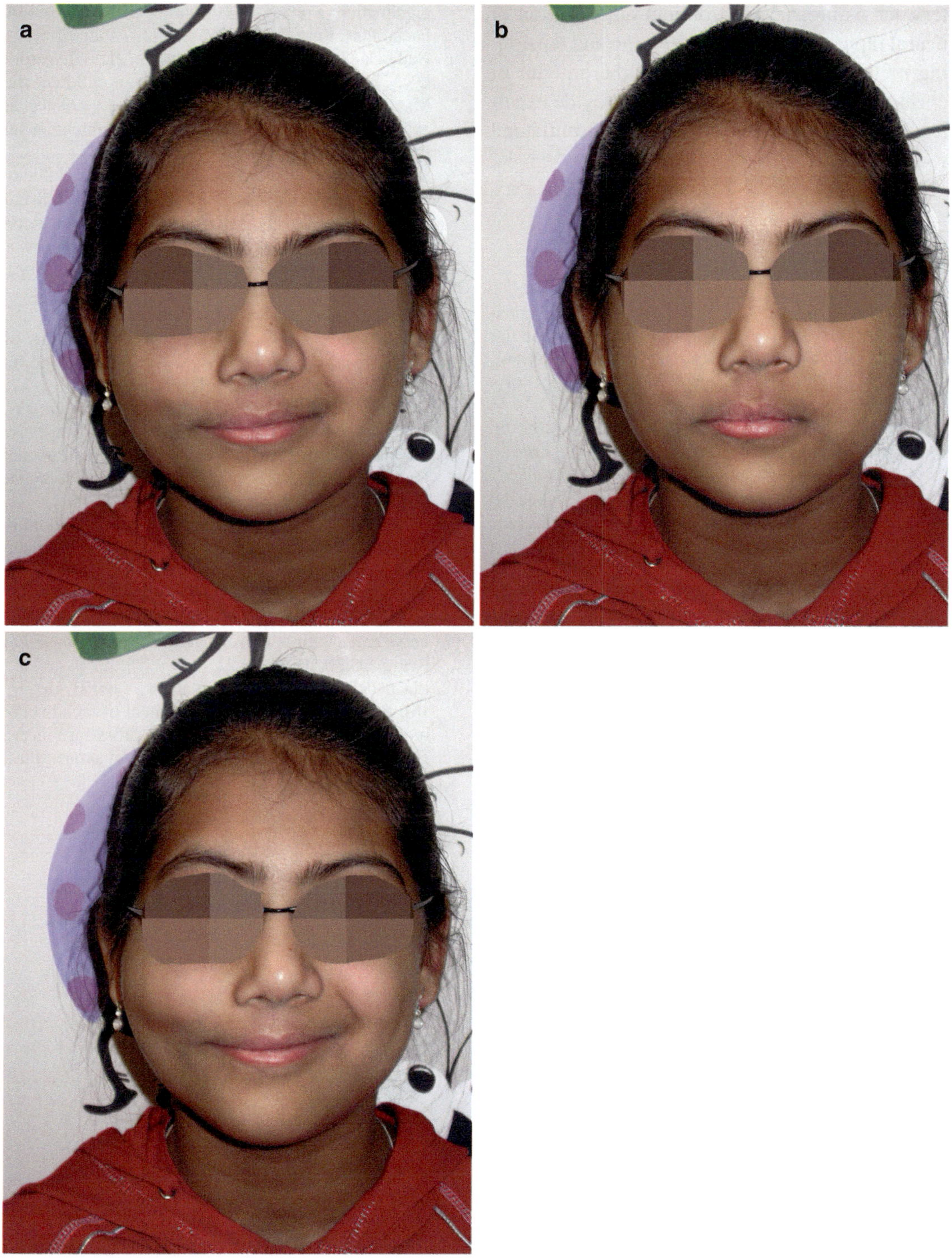

Fig. 17.29 (**a**) Postoperative view—at rest. (**b**) Postoperative view—patient asked to generate a small smile. (**c**) Postoperative view—patient asked to generate a full smile

ter such as proper selection and optimization of neural input, appropriate positioning and tensioning of the muscle, and reducing the amount of cheek bulk, clinicians can reliably provide excellent results for patients suffering from unilateral facial paralysis.

References

1. Harii K, Ohmori K, Torii S. Free gracilis muscle transplantation, with microneurovascular anastomoses for the treatment of facial paralysis. A preliminary report. Plast Reconstr Surg. 1976;57(2):133–43.
2. O'Brien BM. Microvascular free muscle transfer. In: O'Brien, editor. Microvascular reconstructive surgery, Chap. 15. London: Churchill Livingstone; 1977.
3. O'Brien BM, Franklin JD, Morrison WA. Cross-facial nerve grafts and microneurovascular free muscle transfer for long established facial palsy. Br J Plast Surg. 1980;33(2):202–15.
4. Bae YC, Zuker RM, Manktelow RT, Wade S. A comparison of commissure excursion following gracilis muscle transplantation for facial paralysis using a cross-face nerve graft versus the motor nerve to the masseter nerve. Plast Reconstr Surg. 2006;117(7):2407–13.
5. Bhama PK, Weinberg JS, Lindsay RW, Hohman MH, Cheney ML, Hadlock TA. Objective outcomes analysis following microvascular gracilis transfer for facial reanimation: a review of 10 years' experience. JAMA Facial Plast Surg. 2014;16(2):85–92.
6. Hadlock TA, Malo JS, Cheney ML, Henstrom DK. Free gracilis transfer for smile in children: the Massachusetts eye and ear infirmary experience in excursion and quality-of-life changes. Arch Facial Plast Surg. 2011;13(3):190–4.
7. Snyder-Warwick AK, Fattah AY, Zive L, Halliday W, Borschel GH, Zuker RM. The degree of facial movement following microvascular muscle transfer in pediatric facial reanimation depends on donor motor nerve axonal density. Plast Reconstr Surg. 2015;135(2):370e–81e.
8. Dorafshar AH, Borsuk DE, Bojovic B, Brown EN, Manktelow RT, Zuker RM, et al. Surface anatomy of the middle division of the facial nerve: Zuker's point. Plast Reconstr Surg. 2013;131(2):253–7.
9. Hembd A, Nagarkar PA, Saba S, Wan D, Kutz JW, Isaacson B, et al. Facial nerve axonal analysis and anatomical localization in donor nerve: optimizing axonal load for cross-facial nerve grafting in facial reanimation. Plast Reconstr Surg. 2017;139(1):177–83.
10. Al-Majed AA, Neumann CM, Brushart TM, Gordon T. Brief electrical stimulation promotes the speed and accuracy of motor axonal regeneration. J Neurosci. 2000;20(7):2602–8.
11. Gordon T, Brushart TM, Chan KM. Augmenting nerve regeneration with electrical stimulation. Neurol Res. 2008;30(10):1012–22.
12. Placheta E, Wood MD, Lafontaine C, Liu EH, Hendry JM, Angelov DN, et al. Enhancement of facial nerve motoneuron regeneration through cross-face nerve grafts by adding end-to-side sensory axons. Plast Reconstr Surg. 2015;135(2):460–71.

18 Bilateral Facial Reanimation in Möbius Syndrome

Alexander Cardenas-Mejia, Jose E. Telich-Tarriba, and Alexandro Aguilera-Salgado

Key Points

- Single-stage dynamic facial reanimation surgery with gracilis muscle transfer is a safe and effective procedure in patients with classic Möbius syndrome.
- The masseteric nerve is the optimal motor donor in Möbius syndrome due to its proximity to the surgical site, low donor morbidity and ease of dissection.
- The accessory spinal nerve is the second preferred motor donor owing to its high axonal load and constant anatomical location.
- An experienced team is necessary prior to performing simultaneous harvest and insetting of two free functional muscle transfers.
- Each patient's treatment plan should be individualized, based on their specific clinical and electrophysiological characteristics.

18.1 Introduction

In 1880, Von Graefe reported the association between congenital paralysis of the facial and abducens nerves; however, it was not until 1892 that German neurologist Paul Julius Möbius published his landmark paper describing of 43 patients with congenital facial paralysis associated with other malformations, effectively describing the syndrome that would later bear his name [1].

Möbius syndrome is a rare disorder, approximately 300 cases have been described in international literature; it is estimated to have an incidence of 1 case per 50,000 newborns. Our group has recently published the largest series worldwide, including 115 patients managed over 5 years [1].

The syndrome is classically defined as combined bilateral abducens and facial nerve paralysis; it can be accompanied by involvement of other nerves, such as the hypoglossus, trigeminal or the accessory spinal; other malformations commonly encountered in this group of patients are limb malformations, cleft palate and congenital heart disorders [1].

Due to the heterogeneity in the clinical manifestations of the syndrome, Terzis et al. proposed a simple classification in order to identify key diagnostic elements and establish reconstructive strategies [2]:

- Classic Möbius: Bilateral paralysis of the sixth and seventh cranial nerves.
- Incomplete Möbius: Bilateral paralysis of the sixth cranial nerve, and unilateral residual function of the facial nerve.

A. Cardenas-Mejia (✉) · J. E. Telich-Tarriba
A. Aguilera-Salgado
Plastic and Reconstructive Surgery Division Hospital General "Dr. Manuel Gea González", Mexico City, Mexico

Postgraduate Division of the Medical School, Universidad Nacional Autonoma de Mexico, Mexico City, Mexico

© Springer Nature Switzerland AG 2021
C.-H. J. Tzou, A. Rodríguez-Lorenzo (eds.), *Facial Palsy*,
https://doi.org/10.1007/978-3-030-50784-8_18

- Möbius-like: Unilateral facial paralysis accompanied by paralysis of another cranial nerve, excluding the sixth.

Several surgical procedures may be needed in order to treat the whole spectrum of clinical manifestations that afflict patients with Möbius syndrome, the most common procedures include surgical correction of strabismus, congenital hand malformations and facial reanimation procedures [1].

Facial reanimation surgery has remained a challenge for years, yet, it holds a special place among this group of patients, due to its capacity to bring movement to an otherwise inexpressive face. Several procedures have been described in order to achieve dynamic facial reanimation, nevertheless, owing to advances and standardization of microsurgical techniques, the gracilis free functional muscle transfer (FFMT) has become the procedure of choice [3].

Patients with classic Möbius syndrome require the use of extra-facial donor nerves to innervate the gracilis muscle; the masseter nerve has become the donor of choice by authors such as Zuker and Cardenas, however other authors such as Terzis and Noah advocate the use of the rarely affected accessory nerve, other options include the hypoglossus nerve, and in very select cases the C4 or C7 motor nerves [2].

Facial reanimation surgery in patients with Möbius syndrome has usually been performed in stages, starting with the reanimation of one side of the face with the FFMT in the first stage, and performing a second contralateral flap a few months later [4].

Current controversies include the time that must awaited between surgeries, and the selection of donor nerves; for example, Terzis reports performing a four-stage reconstruction [5], while Zuker has published his experience doing a two-stage procedure [6]. Currently, only three groups have published reports on single-stage bilateral facial reanimation in Möbius syndrome: Chuang's, Woolard's and our own [4, 7, 8].

In this chapter, we present the senior author's experience performing single-stage bilateral facial reanimation surgery in patients with classic Möbius syndrome.

18.2 Preoperative Evaluation

Every patient is evaluated at the peripheral nerve clinic, the diagnosis of classic Möbius syndrome is confirmed by a multidisciplinary team after a thorough clinical and neurophysiological evaluation, and the patients are grouped according to Terzis' classification [2]. A detailed neurological evaluation is performed, including any of the possible motor donor nerves in order to develop a customized surgical plan. Photography and video recordings are mandatory, they should document the face at rest and during maximum contraction both pre and postoperatively.

18.3 Surgical Technique

Two surgical teams work simultaneously during the procedure. The first team begins the operation on the right side of the face using a preauricular incision with temporal and mandibular extensions; the cheek flap is dissected in a subcutaneous plane above the parotid fascia. Dissection is carried anteriorly until finding the anterior border of the masseter muscle, the zygoma corresponds to the superior limit of dissection, while the mandibular border is the lower limit. At the anterior border of the masseter the facial vein is identified and dissected toward the oral commissure. The buccal fat pad is extracted carefully using blunt dissection, and afterwards the facial artery is dissected. Should the facial vessels be absent or small, then the superficial temporalis artery and vein are identified and dissected; once the artery and vein have been identified and dissected surgical clips are applied distally.

The surgeon then identifies the orbicularis muscle, the modiolus and zygomatic muscles, a 0 vicryl suture is applied to each of these landmarks, applying a figure-of-eight anchoring suture. Once the sutures have been positioned, one should verify that a nasolabial fold is recreated when traction is applied.

The next step is to identify and dissect the chosen donor nerve. When the masseteric nerve is selected, the border of the zygomatic arch is followed until the mandibular notch is reached, at that point a 2 cm incision parallel to the zygomatic arch is performed, and blunt dissection is performed rejecting the parotid gland until reaching the masseter muscle fibers; once the nerve is has been isolated it is transected at its most distal portion and directed outwards (Fig. 18.1). If the accessory spinal nerve is selected we perform a longitudinal incision over the posterior border of the ipsilateral sternocleidomastoid muscle, the great auricular nerve is identified as it travels cranially over the sternocleidomastoid muscle, parallel and posterior to the external jugular vein, with careful blunt dissection just deep to the investing fascia, the accessory nerve will be found at approximately 1 cm cranially. The nerve is dissected until branching begins, at this point it is transected and directed toward the mandibular angle through a subcutaneous tunnel (Fig. 18.2).

Meanwhile, the second surgical team begins harvesting the gracilis muscle. A short 7 cm skin incision over the posterior border of the adductor longus muscle is made, approximately 3 cm below the inguinal crease. Blunt dissection is performed until the gracilis muscle belly is identified. Circumferential dissection of the muscle begins by surrounding its proximal and distal edges using a penrose drain to use for traction. The obturator nerve is identified and stimulated to verify adequate contraction of the muscle, and it is followed until its emergence at the foramen obturatum; afterwards, the adductor longus muscle is rejected and the vascular pedicle is identified, it is carefully dissected until its origin at the femoral vessels.

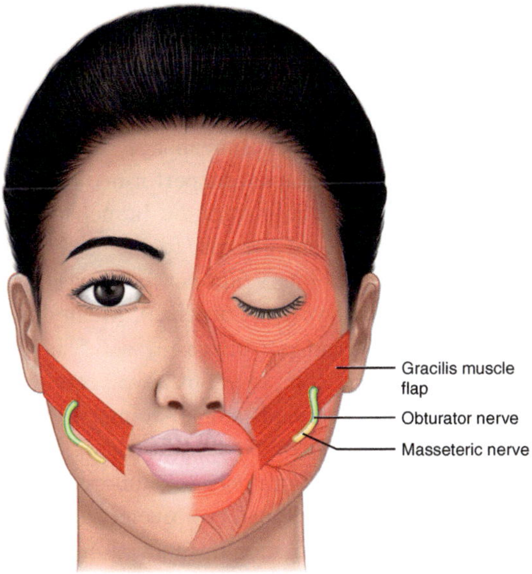

Fig. 18.1 Diagram of a bilateral gracilis FFMT with neurotization of the obturator nerve to the masseteric branch of the trigeminal nerve

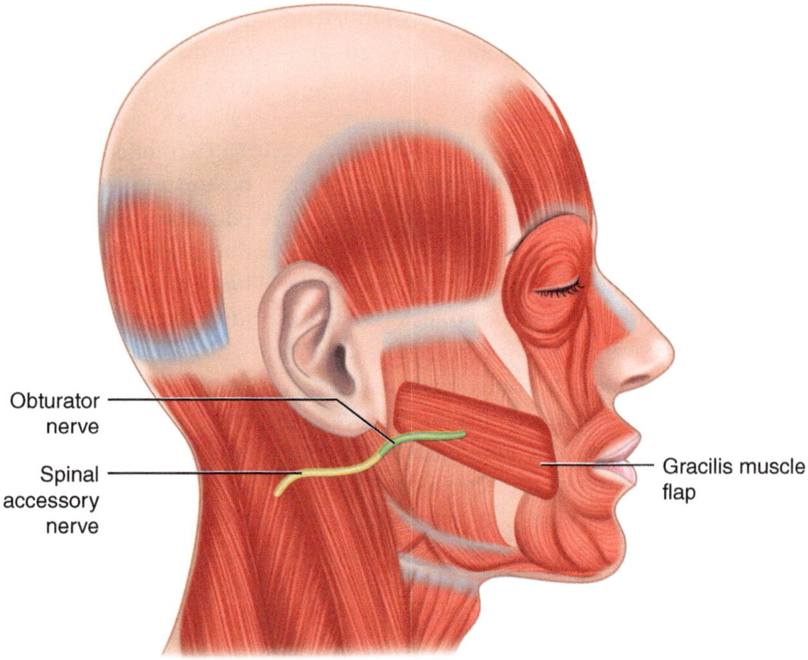

Fig. 18.2 Diagram of a bilateral gracilis FFMT with neurotization of the obturator nerve to the accessory spinal nerve

Once the neurovascular pedicle has been adequately identified and isolated, the gracilis muscle is trimmed into a trapezoid shape based on the measurements made by the face team, adding one extra centimeter to allow suturing at the edges. Transection of the muscle is made using two passes of a GIA 60 mm intestinal stapler (MEDTRONIC, Minneapolis, US), one in longitudinal and the other one in transverse direction. Once dissection on the face has been completed the vascular pedicle is divided using surgical clips and the nerve is transected.

The muscle is transferred to the first team and an incision is made at the proximal tendon, creating a V-shaped end. Using the stitches previously anchored to the nasolabial fold the extremes and center of the V are sutured and lowered to position the muscle. Following this, the neurorrhaphy is performed to the donor nerve using an end-to-end technique with two 10-0 nylon sutures and applying fibrin gel once it is completed. Finally, the artery and veins are anastomosed in an end-to-end fashion with 10-0 nylon sutures. After the neurovascular repairs, the distal end of the muscle is anchored to the preauricular fascia with mattress sutures, if there is any redundant muscle tissue it should be removed to achieve adequate tension, which is seen as a slight pull of the commissure.

At this time the leg team proceeds to harvest the second gracilis muscle from the contralateral leg, and the rest of the procedure proceeds in a similar fashion to the contralateral side.

18.4 Postoperative Period and Follow-Up

After the procedure the patients remain in the recovery room for 1–2 h and are transferred to the plastic surgery ward. They *are* hospitalized for 5 days and are evaluated hourly with a Doppler probe to verify the permeability of the vascular anastomosis. Prophylactic antibiotics, analgesia, and *thromboprophylaxis* are administered.

Follow-up is done at the peripheral nerve clinic from our hospital. A rehabilitation regime tailored to the donor nerve begins 3 weeks after the procedure, first by repetition of the movements associated to the motor donor, and once commissure excursion is detected the patient should practice in front of a mirror (Figs. 18.3 and 18.4).

18.5 Results

The protocol has been applied to four patients (2 males, 2 females) with a mean age of 9 years (range 4–22). Eight flaps were performed in total, four connected to the masseteric branch of the trigeminal nerve, and the rest to the accessory spinal. All surgical interventions were performed by the senior author (Dr. Cardenas). Mean duration of the surgical procedures was 6.5 h. No short or mid-term complications have been identified, all flaps survived and no reinterventions were necessary.

The rehabilitation protocol was tailored to the donor nerve used: masticatory movements for the masseteric nerve and shoulder elevation for the accessory spinal. Mean time to obtain muscle contraction has been 12 weeks for the right side (range 10–24 weeks) and 15 weeks for the left side (range 12–30 weeks). Once contraction is seen we initiate a smile rehabilitation protocol in front of a mirror, in order for the patient to identify the movements that trigger commissure contraction. Mean follow-up has been 43 months (39–48).

Two independent surgeons analyzed pre and postoperative photographs and recordings of the patients and use Terzis'scale to evaluate aesthetic and functional outcomes. Every patient had an initial score of I, and got to a level III after the procedure and rehabilitation. Chuang's scale was used as well, every patient improved from a basal score of 0.25 to a grade 2. Better results were obtained in patients whose muscle was connected to the accessory spinal nerve. A satisfaction questionnaire was applied to all patients using Likert scale, mean satisfaction value was 3.

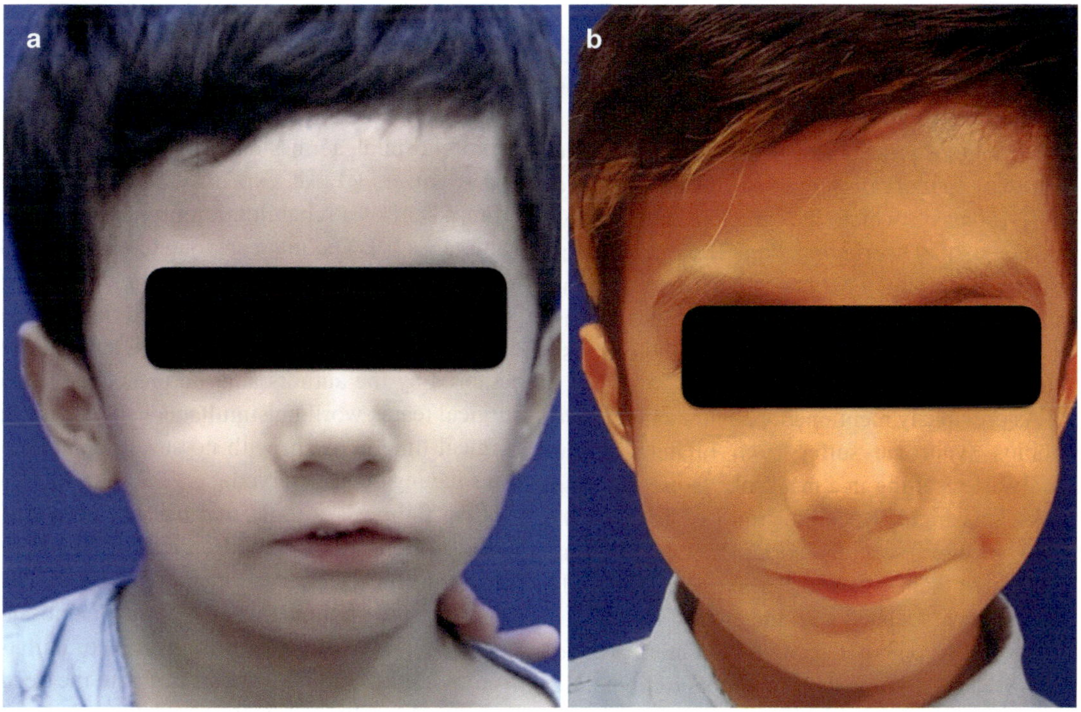

Fig. 18.3 (**a**) Preoperative clinical photography of a patient with classical Möbius syndrome. (**b**) 48-month follow-up photography after single-stage bilateral gracilis transfer neurotized to the masseteric nerve

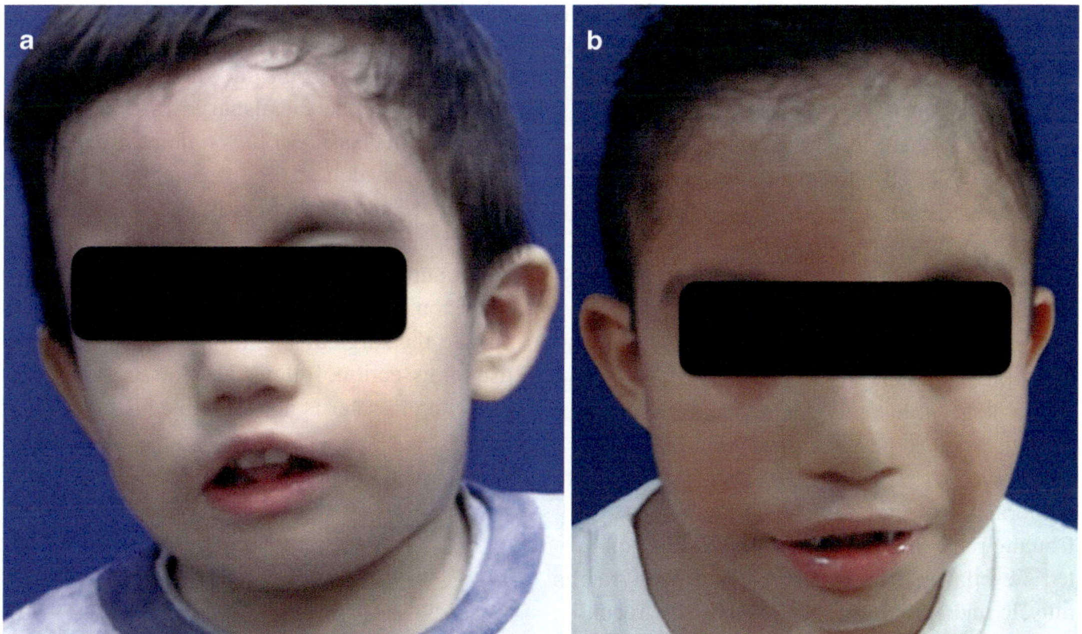

Fig. 18.4 (**a**) Preoperative clinical photography of a patient with classical Möbius syndrome. (**b**) 39-month follow-up photography after single-stage bilateral gracilis transfer neurotized to the spinal accessory nerve

18.6 Discussion

Dynamic facial reanimation in Möbius syndrome has been extensively described and includes a wide range of procedures: from regional muscle transfers (temporalis, masseter, platysma) to FFMT, out of which the gracilis muscle has become a "the" workhorse flap. The main objectives in this group of patients are to obtain a symmetrical, aesthetically pleasing and spontaneous smile through adequate excursion of the transferred muscle [1].

As previously mentioned, patients with classic Möbius syndrome suffer from bilateral facial paralysis, resulting in a mask-like expressionless look. This highly specific group of individuals will require several surgical interventions throughout their lives in order to correct the malformations associated with the entity [1].

Several reconstructive surgery centers around the world have shared their protocols for dynamic facial reconstruction in Möbius syndrome, each with differing opinions as to the number of surgeries required and the amount of time to wait between procedures. Terzis reported six cases of patients with Möbius syndrome, each reconstructed in four stages, two for elongation of the donor nerves and two for flap harvesting, with a period between 7 months and 2 years between procedures. Zuker reported using a two-stage protocol with and interim of 3 months between procedures. Lischez uses a similar protocol, but awaits 1 year between procedures [6, 9].

Regardless of any author's preferences, staging of dynamic facial reanimation has been a common practice around the world. As of today only three centers have proposed performing single-stage bilateral facial reanimation in Möbius syndrome: Woollard operated on 8 patients using the masseter nerve to reanimate bilateral segmental *lattissimus dorsi* flaps [8]; Chuang published a series of six patients submitted to bilateral reanimation using the gracilis muscle and spinal accessory nerve [7]; recently, in 2018 Aguilera-Salgado and Cardenas published their initial experience in four patients performing bilateral gracilis flaps connected to the masseter or spinal nerves [4]. All authors reported satisfactory results.

Single-stage bilateral facial reanimation has several potential advantages: it reduces the number of hospital admissions and anesthetic episodes, lowers global expenses and allows the prompt start of a rehabilitation protocol for both hemi faces [9]. The main critique to our protocol has been the theoretical increase in the rate of complications owing to the extended duration of the procedure, however thanks to the experience acquired by the authors and the presence of two surgical teams working simultaneously our mean surgical time is 6½ h, with no severe complications having been observed.

Flap failure is a topic that has not been discussed. In our clinic orthodromic transfer of the temporalis muscle, as described by Dr. Viterbo, is the procedure of choice when the gracilis muscle is not available [10]. However, in cases of unilateral failure the surgeon should evaluate the need to dismantle both gracilis flaps and do the Viterbo procedure bilaterally, as to avoid major asymmetry of the traction vector and volume of the cheeks.

Selection of a donor nerve continues to be a highly debated topic. Unlike patients with incomplete Möbius syndrome in whom the contralateral branch of the facial nerve as donor nerve, patients with classic Möbius require use of extra-facial donors such as the masseter branch of the trigeminal nerve, hypoglossal, spinal nerve, phrenic, and even cervical motor branches. In the senior author's experience, the masseter nerve has become the donor of choice due to its proximity to the surgical site, minimal morbidity and ease of dissection, followed by the accessory spinal if the masseter is not available [10].

18.7 Summary

Single-stage dynamic facial reanimation surgery with gracilis muscle transfer has proven to a safe and effective procedure in patients with classic Möbius syndrome. Each patient's treatment plan should be individualized, based on their specific clinical and electrophysiological characteristics. An experienced team is necessary prior to performing simultaneous harvest and insetting of two free functional muscle transfers.

References

1. Arrieta-Joffe P, Perez-Dosal M, Ortiz-de-Zarate G, Cardenas-Mejia A. Estudio clínico, citogenético, molecular y de imagen de los pacientes con Síndrome de Moebius del Hospital General "Dr. Manuel Gea González", Ciudad de México. Cir Plast Iberolatinoam. 2017;43(4):395–400.
2. Terzis JK, Noah EM. Möbius and Möbius-like patients: etiology, diagnosis and treatment options. Clin Plast Surg. 2002;29:497–514.
3. Palafox D, Arrieta-Joffe P, Cardenas MA. Tratamiento quirúrgico reconstructivo actual del sindrome de Moebius. Cir Plast. 2014;24(3):136–44.
4. Aguilera-Salgado A, Cardenas-Mejia A. Reanimación facial en síndrome de Möbius completo mediante transferencia en un solo tiempo de gracilis libre bilateral. Cir Plast Ibarolatinoam. 2018;44(1):75–84.
5. Leung MKS, Dieu T, Cleland H. Surgical approach to the accessory nerve in the posterior triangle of the neck. Plast Reconstr Surg. 2004;113(7):2067–70.
6. Terzis JL, Olivares FS. Long-term outcomes of free muscle transfer for smile restoration in children. Plast Reconstr Surg. 2009;123(2):543–55.
7. Lu C, Chuang CC. One-stage reconstruction for bilateral Möbius syndrome. Simultaneous bilateral spinal accessory nerve to innervate 2 free muscles for facial reanimation. Ann Plast Surg. 2013;70(2):1011–21.
8. Woollard AC, Harrison DH, Grobbelaar AO. An approach to bilateral facial paralysis. J Plast Reconstr Aesthet Surg. 2010;63:1557–60.
9. Lischez SD, Matloub HS, Gosain AK. Cortical adaptation to restoration of smiling following free muscle transfer innervated by the nerve to the masseter. Plast Reconstr Surg. 2005;115:1472–9.
10. Cardenas-Mejia A, Palafox D. Facial reanimation surgery in Möbius syndrome: experience from 76 cases from a tertiary referral hospital in Latin America. Ann Chir Plast Esthet. 2017. (Epub ahead of print).

Dual Innervation of Free Muscle Transfer with Masseter and CFNG

19

Alexander Cardenas-Mejia
and Jose E. Telich-Tarriba

Key Points

- Dual innervation of the gracilis muscle flap with a CFNG and the masseter nerve is a safe and effective procedure in patients with long-standing unilateral facial paralysis.
- The dual innervation technique takes advantage of the symmetry and spontaneity derived from the use of the CFNG and the strong contraction and quick reinnervation from the masseter nerve.
- Dual innervation procedures can be performed in one or two stages; no technique has proven to be superior.
- Timing between surgical stages and configuration of the nerve anastomoses should prioritize axon sprouting from the CFNG, therefore we recommend a two-stage procedure anastomosing the CFNG close to the hilum
- An intense postoperative rehabilitation protocol is mandatory.

A. Cardenas-Mejia (✉) · J. E. Telich-Tarriba
Plastic and Reconstructive Surgery Division, Hospital General "Dr. Manuel Gea González"; Postgraduate Division of the Medical School, Universidad Nacional Autonoma de Mexico, Mexico City, Mexico

19.1 Background

Facial paralysis is a deeply disabling condition; adequate function of the mimetic musculature is essential for both verbal and non-verbal communication. Furthermore, the facial nerve is also responsible for providing ocular protection, adequate nasal airflow, articulation of speech, and oral continence. Etiology of long-standing unilateral facial paralysis can be heterogeneous, ranging from developmental defects like craniofacial microsomia, to traumatic, infectious, or iatrogenic causes [1].

Smile restoration surgery has been thoroughly proven to improve quality of life, however, decision-making in the surgical management of long-standing facial paralysis remains challenging owing to the variety of facial reanimation procedures available nowadays. Despite this, the goals of all procedures remain constant: restoration of facial symmetry at rest, and achievement of a spontaneous and symmetric smile [1].

The earliest surgical procedures for facial paralysis correction were aimed toward static repositioning of facial tissues. Dynamic facial reanimation was born in 1879 when Drobnik executed a facial to spinal-accessory nerve anastomosis, later, Werner Körte performed the first hypoglossal to facial nerve transfer in 1901. These procedures were further developed by Sir Charles Ballance, who published his findings in 1931. Modern facial nerve microsurgery was

© Springer Nature Switzerland AG 2021
C.-H. J. Tzou, A. Rodríguez-Lorenzo (eds.), *Facial Palsy*,
https://doi.org/10.1007/978-3-030-50784-8_19

started by Sir Terrence Cawthorne who did the first repair of a facial nerve using an operative microscope in 1938. The cross-face nerve graft (CFNG) was developed independently by Scaramella and Smith, and later popularized by Anderl in the seventies. In 1976, Harii first published his experience on gracilis muscle transfer for facial reanimation; later on O'brien proposed a modified technique coapting the obturator nerve to a CFNG *in lieu* of the deep temporal nerve.

Free Functional Muscle Transfer (FFMT) is currently the gold standard in treatment for long-standing unilateral facial paralysis. The gracilis muscle has become the most used flap, owing to its constant neurovascular anatomy, acceptable donor-site morbidity, and adequate excursion. Most surgeons prefer applying the traditional two-stage technique described by O'brien, in which a CFNG connected to a contralateral facial nerve branch is performed in the first procedure, and a gracilis muscle transfer is done in a second procedure once the regenerated axons in the graft have reached the paralyzed side [2].

Use of the contralateral facial nerve connected to a CFNG has the advantage of allowing synchronic and spontaneous movement, however, the main drawback of the technique is the low number of axons that reach the target muscle, resulting in weak contraction. Extra-facial donors have usually been reserved to cases in which the contralateral facial nerve is not available, such as patients with Möbius syndrome; these motor donors have the advantage of possessing a high axonal count, resulting quick reinnervation and strong contractions, however they require the patient to perform concurrent voluntary movements in order to activate the flap [3].

Among extra-facial donors, Zuker popularized the use of the trigeminal's nerve to the masseteric muscle. This nerve has several advantages that make it well suited for facial reanimation surgery, such as its proximity to the surgical site, consistent location, limited donor-site morbidity, high-density axonal load, and ease for rehabilitation, therefore it has become the standard source of innervation for FFMT in several hospitals around the world, including ours. Some authors have hypothesized that the similarity between the biting and smiling movements, as well as the proximity of the cortical representation of the facial and masseter muscles might be able to generate a spontaneous smile due to cerebral plasticity, however this has not been fully demonstrated in the clinical setting [4].

Thus, selection of an ideal donor nerve in unilateral facial paralysis reconstruction remains an issue, it would seem like the surgeon is forced to choose between a technique that ensures the reliable recovery of function, or one that achieves symmetry and spontaneity [2].

Dual innervation or axonal supercharge is a technique that aims to obtain innervation from multiple neural sources in order to gain a more reliable recovery of the target musculature; Yamamoto et al. first published its use for facial reanimation by combining input from the hyoglossus nerve and the facial nerve to treat recent onset paralysis. The idea of combining the use of the facial and masseter nerve stimulus seeks to take advantage of the strengths of both neural sources: symmetry and spontaneity from the former and quick reinnervation and contraction force from the latter [5].

In this chapter we present the senior author's experience using a dually innervated gracilis muscle fabricated in two stages.

19.2 Surgical Technique

19.2.1 First Stage

The goal of the first stage of the procedure is to perform a CFNG using the contralateral buccal branch of the facial nerve.

A preauricular incision is made on the healthy side of the face, a cheek flap is dissected anteriorly until the buccal branch of the facial nerve is identified with help of an electrostimulator and transected. Simultaneously, a 20–25 cm sural nerve graft is harvested by a second team and transferred to the face, placing it in an orthodromic fashion. An end-to-end anastomosis to the previously identified buccal branch is performed, then the distal end of the graft is tied to a blunt tendon passer and is passed to the contralateral side through the upper lip, where it is banked beneath the nasolabial fold.

19.2.2 Second Stage

The second stage of the operation is carried out once reinnervation of the CFNG has been confirmed by Tinnel sign and neuroconduction studies, three to four months later.

Two surgical teams work simultaneously. The head team begins the operation by making a preauricular incision on the paralyzed side; the cheek flap is dissected in a subcutaneous plane above the parotid fascia. Dissection is carried anteriorly until the anterior border of the masseter muscle is found; the zygoma corresponds to the superior limit of dissection, while the mandibular border is the lower limit. At the anterior border of the masseter the facial vein is identified, and directly anterior to it is the facial artery. Both vessels are dissected toward the oral commissure, divided and pulled toward the incision (If the facial vessels are absent or small, the superficial temporalis artery and vein are dissected). The buccal fat pad is extracted carefully using blunt dissection in an attempt to decrease tissue bulk.

The surgeon then identifies the orbicularis oris, the modiolus and zygomatic muscles, and applies 0 vicryl sutures to each landmark, using figure-of-eight stitches as anchoring technique. Once the sutures have been positioned the nasolabial fold should be recreated when traction is applied.

The next step is to identify and dissect the banked CFNG and the masseteric nerve. The CFNG should be harvested from the spot where it was planted; the masseteric nerve is identified by performing blunt dissection at the mandibular notch, rejecting the parotid gland and the masseter muscle fibers; once the nerve has been isolated it is transected at its most distal portion and directed outwards.

While the first team works on the head, the second surgical team harvests the gracilis muscle. A short 7 cm skin incision over the posterior border of the adductor longus muscle is made, approximately 3 cm below the inguinal crease. Blunt dissection is performed until the gracilis muscle belly is identified. Circumferential dissection of the muscle begins by surrounding its proximal and distal edges using a penrose drain to use for traction. The obturator nerve is identified and stimulated to verify adequate contraction of the muscle, and it is followed until its emergence at the foramen obturatum; afterwards, the adductor longus muscle is rejected and the vascular pedicle is identified, it is carefully dissected until its origin at the femoral vessels.

Once the neurovascular pedicle has been adequately identified and isolated, the muscle is trimmed into a trapezoid shape based on the measurements made by the face team, adding one extra centimeter to allow suturing at the edges. The muscle is transected with a GIA 60 mm intestinal stapler (MEDTRONIC, Minneapolis, US). Once dissection on the face has been completed the vascular pedicle is divided using surgical clips and the nerve is transected.

The muscle is transferred to the face and an incision is made at the proximal tendon, creating a V-shaped end. Using the stitches previously anchored to the nasolabial fold the extremes and center of the V are sutured and lowered to position the muscle. An end-to-end anastomosis is performed between the distal end of the CFNG and the obturator nerve, and then an end-to-side coaptation from the masseteric nerve to the obturator nerve about 1 cm proximal to the gracilis muscle hilum. Finally, the vascular anastomoses are made in an end-to-end fashion (Fig. 19.1).

After the neurovascular repairs, the distal end of the muscle is anchored to the preauricular fascia with mattress sutures, any redundant muscle tissue is removed to until adequate tension is achieved, which is seen as a slight pull of the commissure.

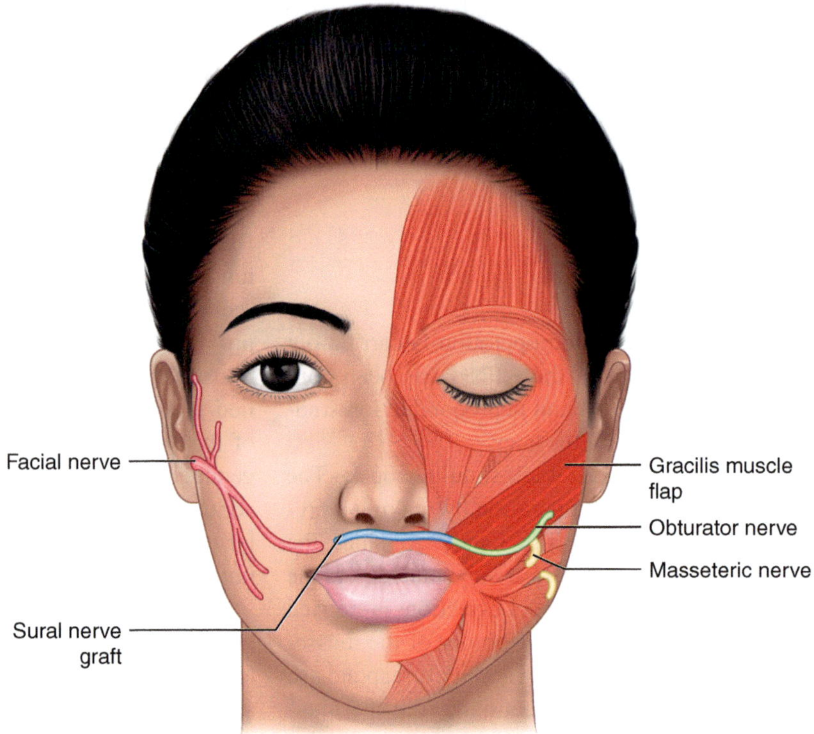

Fig. 19.1 Diagram of a dually innervated gracilis FFMT with neurotization of the obturator nerve to the masseteric branch of the trigeminal nerve and the contralateral facial nerve

19.3 Postoperative Period and Follow-Up

After the procedure the patients remain in the recovery room for a couple of hours and are transferred to the plastic surgery unit afterwards. They remain hospitalized for 5 days and are evaluated hourly with a Doppler probe to verify the permeability of the vascular anastomosis. Prophylactic antibiotics, analgesia, and thromboprophylaxis are administered.

Follow-up is done at the peripheral nerve clinic from our hospital. Rehabilitation is started 3 weeks after the procedure by making masticatory exercises, once the gracilis shows signs of contraction the smile rehabilitation protocol is started in front of a mirror, so the patient identifies the triggers for symmetric and independent commissure contraction (Figs. 19.2 and 19.3).

19.4 Discussion

Dual innervation for muscle flaps in facial reanimation is an idea that has been scarcely researched. The first report of such a technique was published by Labbé in 2002, who supercharged a temporalis myoplasty with a CFNG connected to the deep temporalis nerve [6]. However, Wantanabe was the first to attempt dual innervation of a free flap, by anastomosing a latissimus dorsi to the contralateral facial nerve, and positioning its ilium in close contact with a denuded area of the masseter muscle [7], the technique was later modified by Okazaki [8] by doing a true anastomosis to the masseter nerve. Use of the gracilis muscle flap transfer with a dual neural source has been previously reported and studied by few peripheral nerve clinics around the globe [2, 9, 10] (Table 19.1).

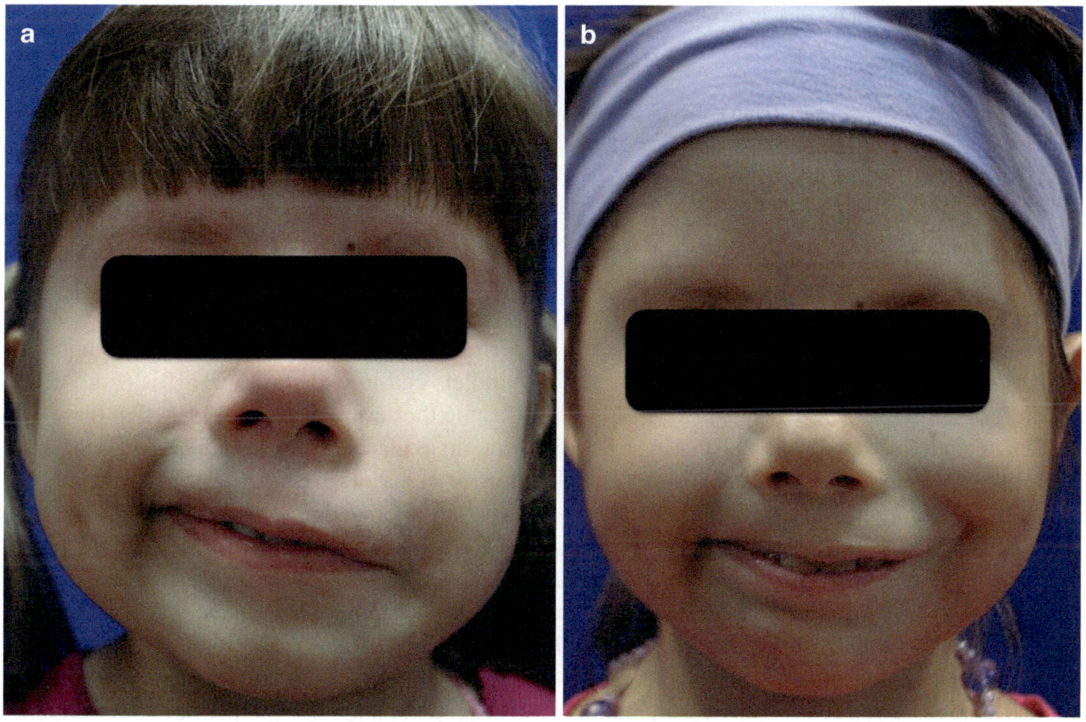

Fig. 19.2 (**a**) Preoperative clinical photography of a child with incomplete Möbius syndrome. (**b**) 3-year follow-up photography after dually innervated gracilis FFMT

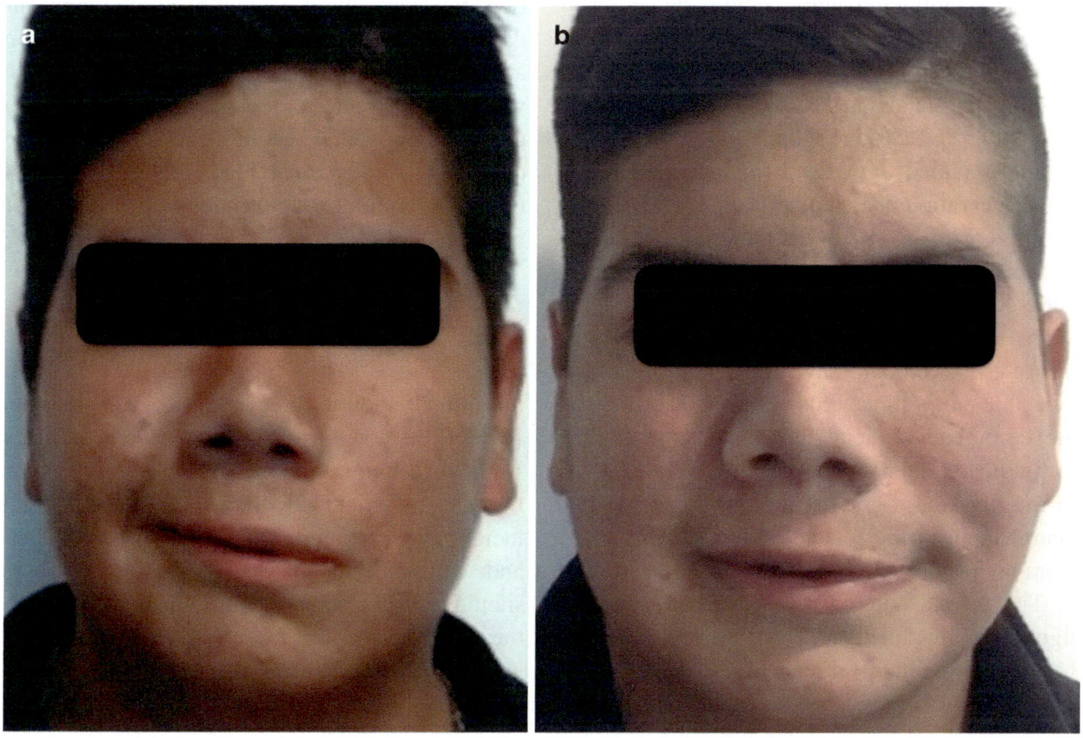

Fig. 19.3 (**a**) Preoperative clinical photography of a male patient with unilateral facial paralysis. (**b**) 12-month follow-up photography after single-stage bilateral gracilis transfer neurotized to the spinal-accessory nerve

Table 19.1 Summary of the dual innervated facial reanimation techniques reported in the literature

Author	Patients (n)	Flap	Stages
Labbe (2003)	5	Temporalis	Two
Wantanabe (2009)	3	Lattissimus dorsi	One
Biglioli (2012)	4	Gracilis	One
Cardenas (2014)	9	Gracilis	Two
Mutsumi (2015)	4	Lattissimus dorsi	One
Sforza (2015)	13	Gracilis	One
Dusseldorp (2018)	26	Gracilis	Two

Our technique was developed in an effort to treat patients who failed to show contraction of the transplanted muscle after a conventional two-stage procedure with a CFNG, these patients were taken to the operating room to perform a masseteric nerve transfer to the obturator nerve in order to avoid complete denervation. A second source of inspiration were patients with incomplete Möbius syndrome, who have residual motor function on one side of the face, but not enough to power a free flap. We have currently extended the use of the technique to most patients treated for long-standing unilateral facial paralysis [9].

Two controversies arise from the several dual innervation techniques published. The first is the amount of stages necessary to complete the reconstruction; despite good and reproducible results obtained with the two-stage procedure, dual innervation one-stage procedures have been reported in an attempt to get the same results in a shorter time frame [2, 7], however in this scenario it is possible that by the time the CNFG axons reach the gracilis, nerve sprouts from the masseter nerve could have already occupied the available motor units, thus negating the effects of the contralateral facial nerve. In contrast, our technique requires two stages, involving a CFNG in the first and a gracilis muscle flap with dual neural input in the second, thus allowing axons from both sources to recruit major motor units.

The second controversy pertains to the configuration in which the nerve anastomoses are built. Most techniques tend to combine end-to-end and end-to-side neurorrhaphies, following the recommendations made in from Dr. Viterbo's research [9]. In our series a CFNG to obturator nerve end-to-end coaptation is done first, while a masseteric to obturator nerve anastomosis is performed in an end-to-side configuration; Dr. Biglioli reported a reverse setup, with the masseteric nerve connected in an end-to-end fashion and the CFNG anastomosis done end-to-side [2]; in a preliminary report Dr. Hadlock described performing coaptation of both motor donors in a parallel end-to-end fashion [10] (Fig. 19.4). Despite the several setups described in the literature, no evidence exists proving a one configuration is superior to the rest. In our opinion a two-stage procedure and anastomosing the CFNG close to the muscle hilum could maximize the number of neuromuscular junctions innervated by the contralateral facial nerve, leaving the remainder to be repopulated by the masseter nerve.

Future challenges in the field are centered upon comparing the dual innervated technique against single-innervated gracilis flap, as well as evaluating the differences between single versus two-stage procedures, ideally by employing standardized tools. New sources of dual innervation are currently being evaluated for patients in whom the masseteric nerve is unavailable, with the accessory spinal becoming a strong candidate due to its high axonal load and capability of obtaining excursion independently from shoulder movement.

19.5 Summary

Dual innervation for gracilis muscle transfer with a CFNG and the masseter nerve is a reproducible surgical technique that yields consistent results for the treatment of long-standing unilateral facial paralysis. Timing between surgical stages and configuration of the nerve anastomoses should prioritize axon sprouting from the CFNG, therefore we recommend a two-stage procedure anastomosing the CFNG close to the hilum.

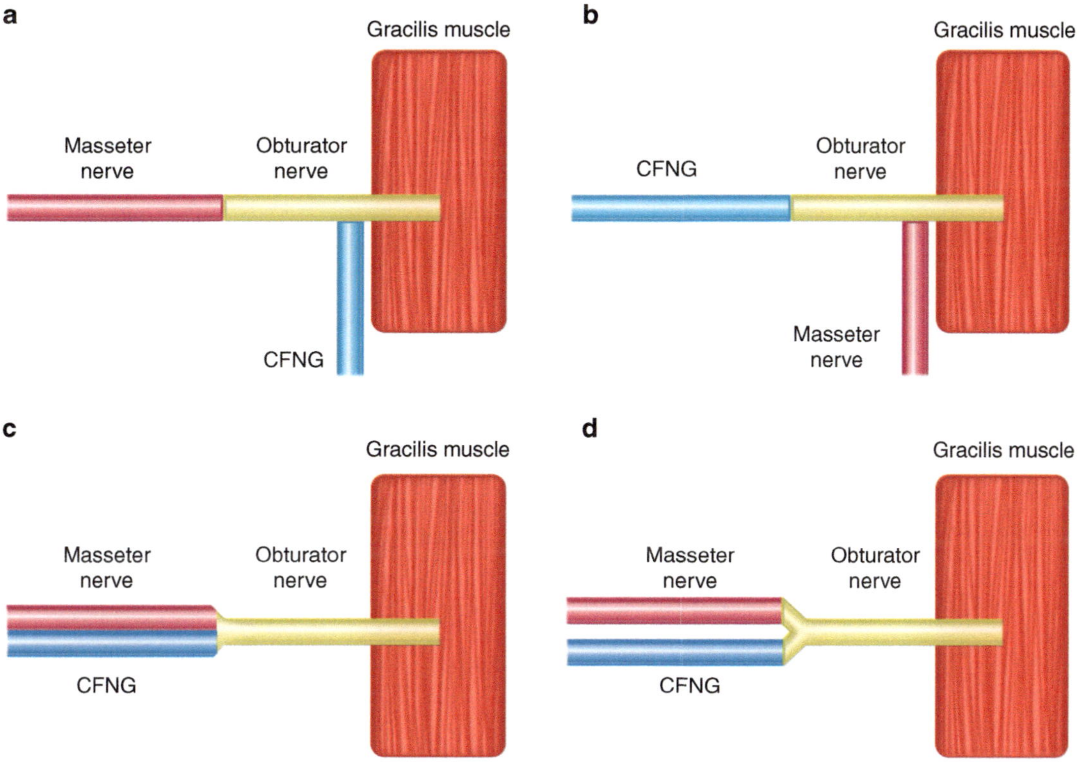

Fig. 19.4 Diagrams of the described neurorrhaphy configurations. (**a**) Biglioli's configuration. (**b**) Cardenas' configuration. (**c**) V-shaped anastomosis. (**d**). Y-shaped anastomosis

References

1. Tate JR, Tollefson TT. Advances in facial reanimation. Curr Opin Otolaryngol Head Neck Surg. 2006;14(4):242–8.
2. Biglioli F, Colombo V, Tarabbia F, Pedrazzoli M, Battista V, Giovanditto F, Dalla Toffola E, Lozza A, Frigerio A. Double innervation in free-flap surgery for long-standing facial paralysis. J Plast Reconstr Aesthet Surg. 2012;65(10):1343–9.
3. Terzis JK, Noah EM. Möbius and Möbius-like patients: etiology, diagnosis and treatment options. Clin Plast Surg. 2002;29:497–514.
4. Cardenas-Mejia A, Palafox D. Facial reanimation surgery in Möbius syndrome: experience from 76 cases from a tertiary referral hospital in Latin America. Ann Chir Plast Esthet. 2017. (Epub ahead of print).
5. Yamamoto Y, Sekido M, Furukawa H, et al. Surgical rehabilitation of reversible facial palsy: facial–hypoglossal network system based on neural signal augmentation/neural supercharge concept. J Plast Reconstr Aesthet Surg. 2007;60:223–31.
6. Labbé D, Hamel M, Bénateau H. Lengthening temporalis myoplasty and transfacial nerve graft (VII-V). Technical note. Ann Chir Plast Esthet. 2003;48(1):31–5.
7. Watanabe Y, Akizuki T, Ozawa T, Yoshimura K, Agawa K, Ota T. Dual innervation method using one-stage reconstruction with free latissimus dorsi muscle transfer for re-animation of established facial paralysis: simultaneous reinnervation of the ipsilateral masseter motor nerve and the contralateral facial nerve to improve the quality of smile and emotional facial expressions. J Plast Reconstr Aesthet Surg. 2009;62(12):1589–97.
8. Okazaki M, Kentaro T, Noriko U, Satoshi U, Tsutomu H, Alisa O, Mayuko H, Hiroki M. One-stage dual latissimus dorsi muscle flap transfer with a pair of vascular anastomoses and double nerve suturing for long-standing facial paralysis. J Plast Reconstr Aesthet Surg. 2015;68(6):e113–9.
9. Cardenas-Mejia A, Covarrubias-Ramirez JV, Bello-Margolis A, Rozen S. Double innervated free functional muscle transfer for facial reanimation. J Plast Surg Hand Surg. 2015;49(3):183–8.
10. Dusseldorp JR, Jowett N, Hadlock TA. Dually innervated free gracilis transfer in smile reanimation. In: ASPN annual meeting, Phoenix; 2018.

Simultaneous Use of Static Support and Free Muscle Transfer

20

Anouk J. M. Cornelissen and Shai M. Rozen

Key Points

- With the end in mind, aesthetic reconstruction should always be ultimate treatment goal in facial palsy patients.
- Optimizing aesthetic results requires combining both dynamic and static techniques addressing both symmetry at rest and in motion.
- Restoring symmetry at rest is no less important than restoring motion since most human interactions and time spent are in repose rather than smiling.
- Non-facial donor nerves for either nerve transfer or for neurotization of a free functional muscle in the flaccid facial palsy patient don't usually provide tone, therefore the use of static support is generally necessary to restore symmetry at rest.
- While the flaccid facial palsy patient benefits from static support, the synkinetic facial palsy patients does not require static support but rather targeted weakening of antagonistic muscles.

A. J. M. Cornelissen · S. M. Rozen (✉)
Department of Plastic Surgery, The University of Texas Southwestern Medical Center, Dallas, USA
e-mail: Anouk.cornelissen@mumc.nl; shai.rozen@utsouthwestern.edu

20.1 Introduction

Regardless of technique, the way patients feel about themselves and how they are perceived by society, are the most important goals for the patient and subsequently the reconstructive surgeon. To obtain this goal, the surgeon must recognize the importance of optimizing both function and aesthetics. Psychological distress as a result of social facial discrimination, has been suggested as the main reason facial palsy patients undergo surgery [1]. Facial discrimination stems from facial asymmetry both during expression due to loss of motion and at rest due to loss of tone.

The literature is abundant in descriptions of dynamic reanimation techniques, but less detailed on addressing asymmetry at rest. Restoring smile symmetry is without a doubt important in normalizing expression; however, restoring symmetry is paramount in patients with facial palsy since the majority of the time spent by humans is in repose. Moreover, slight smile asymmetries are considered within normal range in humans while asymmetry at rest is more often considered abnormal and often mimics the appearance of a stroke patient. Also, smile asymmetry can be hidden by simply minimizing either frequency or degree of smile in contrast to rest asymmetry which is immediately noticeable and difficult to camouflage [2].

© Springer Nature Switzerland AG 2021
C.-H. J. Tzou, A. Rodríguez-Lorenzo (eds.), *Facial Palsy*, https://doi.org/10.1007/978-3-030-50784-8_20

Facial palsy treatment should therefore not solely focus on restoring facial motion but also tone to obtain an optimal result. In the attempt to achieve this, surgeons must not limit themselves to a single approach but rather consider all available surgical tools despite the traditional tendency to classify dynamic vs. static or aesthetic vs. functional procedures. The exact chosen surgical approach depends on several variables as patient presentation (flaccid vs. partial vs. synkinesis), palsy duration (acute vs. subacute, vs. longstanding) and etiology (cancer vs. benign vs. infectious), nerve continuity (residual vs. reconstructed nerve continuity vs. no nerve continuity), and more. Also, depending on the donor nerve, the balance between motion and tone may differ. In addition to the facial nerve providing more spontaneity than a non-facial nerve, it also provides more tone than non-facial donor nerves. Yet, if the axonal input is supplied via a cross facial nerve graft, muscle power and excursion may decrease and likely provide less strength than an ipsilateral non-facial nerve. Conversely, non-facial nerve donor nerves tend to provide less tone and therefore concomitant static procedures are usually necessary. This chapter will focus on the simultaneous use of dynamic and static procedures and their suitability based on patient presentation.

20.2 Patient Presentation

Nearly all patients present at first as complete, flaccid facial palsy. However, the flaccid presentation may change within weeks to months depending on etiology and patient characteristics. Some patients remain with complete flaccid facial palsy, while others develop incomplete facial palsy or might even reach full recovery. Incomplete facial palsy patients may further divide into two groups—incomplete weak facial palsy patients who regain some facial tone and varying degrees of weaker motion, or incomplete synkinetic facial palsy patients presenting with a "tight face" i.e., hypertonicity and synkinetic motion also known as paradoxical facial movement.

The synkinetic patient is characterized by facial hypertonicity, often with an exaggerated pull toward the palsied side, and associated with involuntary motion in one area of the face while attempting to move the other. The flaccid and partial weak patients should be viewed differently from the synkinetic patients since presentation and treatment are different and often opposing.

20.2.1 Complete Flaccid Facial Palsy

Since the facial nerve carries within it parasympathetic, sensory, special sensory, and motor fibers, palsy of the facial nerve may affect all aspects of innervations, including decreased lacrimation, loss of taste in the anterior two-thirds of the tongue, loss of sensation in a small portion of the external auditory canal, and of course facial motion. It is beyond the scope of this chapter to review the entire macro and microanatomy of the facial nerve but it is highly suggested that readers familiarize themselves with the anatomy of the facial nerve from its cortical representation to the brain stem (upper motor neuron) and from the facial nerve nuclei in the brain stem, via the internal auditory canal through the intratemporal bony portion until it leaves the skull through the styloid foramen and divides into its peripheral branches and reaches the mimetic muscles (lower motor neuron). Complete loss of tone and motion is seen in these patients (Fig. 20.1) and they are characterized by a hemi flaccid face often drawn to the contralateral side due to the unopposed pulling forces of the normal side. In most patients with lower motor neuron injury the entire hemi face is affected (unless singular peripheral branches are injured) while in the less commonly seen upper neuron palsy patients the contralateral forehead is often spared.

20.2.1.1 Mid and Lower Face

Midface paralysis is characterized by the inability to move the lips and cheek. The failure to smile and express happiness often concerns patients the most, directly impairing social communication. Additionally, patients will also often

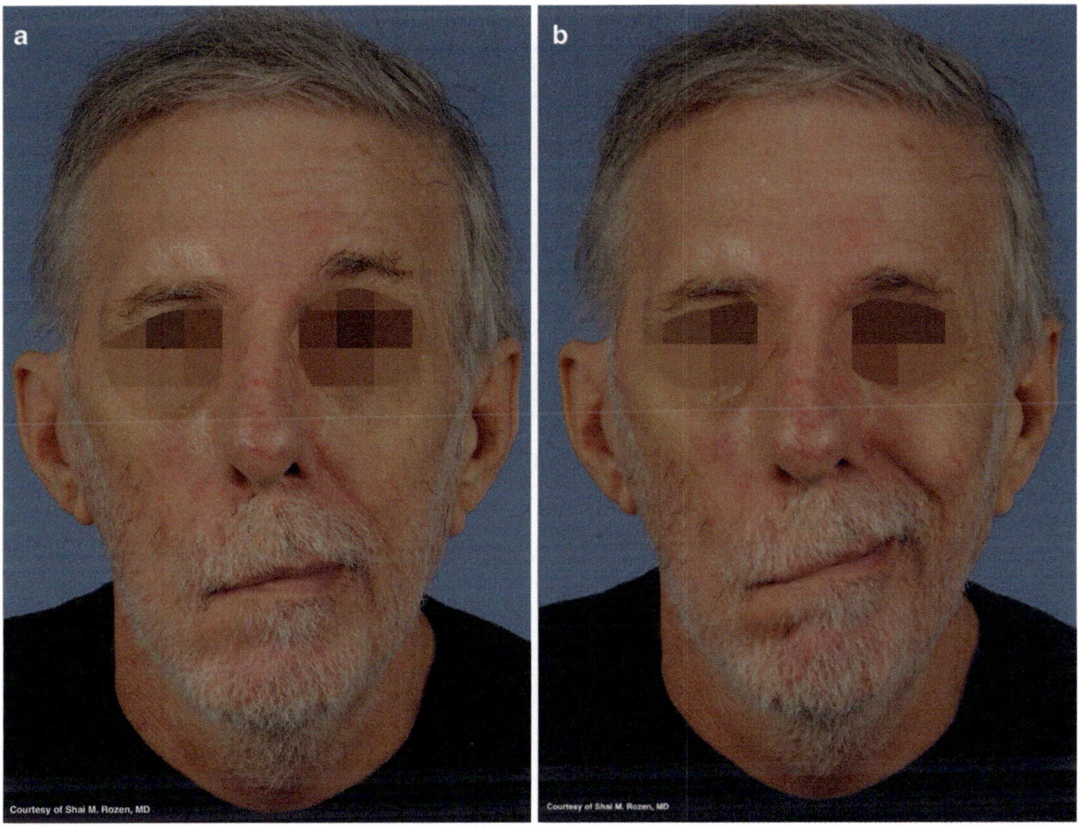

Fig. 20.1 A 67-year-old man 7 months after resection of hemangiopericytoma prior to reanimation with a masseter to facial nerve transfer. (**a**) Repose, (**b**) Animating

complain of slurred speech, drooling, and food boluses collecting in the buccal sulcus. In repose, asymmetries increase as patients' further age, likely due to a combination of volume loss, weakening of the true and false facial ligaments, and loss of skin tone (Fig. 20.1). Philtral deviation is typically seen toward the healthy side, while increased philtrum to oral commissure distance due to orbicularis oris muscle loss of tone, a flattened nasolabial fold and collapsed nasal vestibule causing obstruction of the nasal airway are all present on the paralyzed side. In motion during speech or smile the asymmetry tends to worsen due to increased pull from the contralateral healthy side and lower lip asymmetries are considerably more noticeable when the depressors of the lip pull the lip downward on the healthy side while the lip remains elevated on the palsied side.

20.2.1.2 Periorbital

The periorbital region is significantly affected by paralysis and takes high priority in the treatment scheme. The cornea of palsy patients is at great risk for keratitis, which may further develop into ulcerations, scarring, and in severe cases blindness. Complete facial palsy patients are unable to close their upper eyelid due to paralytic lagophthalmos and loose tone of the lower eyelid resulting in lower lid malposition or ectropion. Additionally, patients usually complaint of dry eyes due to decreased tear production from the lacrimal gland combined with excessive tearing due to an inferior clearing of tears due to lower lid malposition and malfunctioning lacrimal sac "pump" normally created by the orbicularis occuli muscle [3]. Perhaps one of the most apparent signs identifying flaccid palsy patients is the widened palpebral aperture and increased sclera

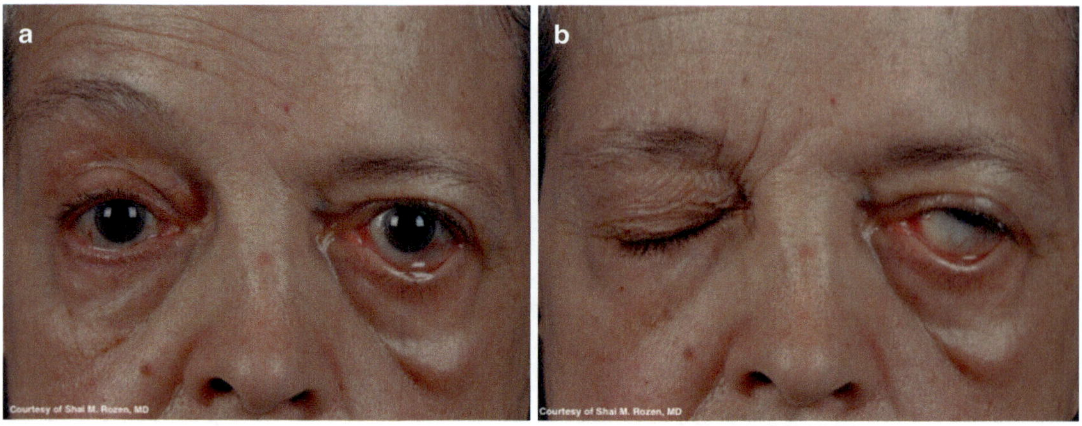

Fig. 20.2 A 73-year-old woman approximately 6 months after acoustic neuroma resection performed at outside hospital. (**a**) Ectropion, (**b**) paralytic lagophthalmos

show which is all too often neglected in treatment (Fig. 20.2a, b).

20.2.1.3 Forehead

Although forehead asymmetry is the less common complaint of palsy patients it can be a significant contributor to asymmetry. At rest severe brow ptosis may not only obstruct vision, but also suggest the impression of an unhappy or serious face which may in turn hinder communication. This asymmetry can be accentuated by increased activity of the frontalis muscle of the unparalyzed side during conversation or emotional interactions (Fig. 20.2a).

20.2.2 Incomplete Facial Palsy

Partial facial paralysis patients can be seen in two types of presentations: Less commonly, in patients with partially normal and partially injured facial nerve branches as seen after trauma or surgery or more commonly, in patients with pan facial weakness who reach this stage after a period of recovery from a complete palsy yet fail to reach complete recovery. The latter group of patients usually present in two typical appearances: incomplete weak facial palsy or incomplete synkinetic facial palsy. Common to all of these patients, is that their facial nerve is by definition anatomically intact.

20.2.2.1 Incomplete Weak Facial Palsy

Incomplete weak facial palsy patients are similar to complete facial palsy patients aside from some remaining tone and movement. The degree of tone and movement may vary and therefore treatment strategy may vary. Treatments may include small balancing procedures of the contralateral healthy side in cases of very mild weakness or incorporate the full array of options used in patients with complete paralysis. For these reasons, the treatment of these patients will not be discussed separately and is quite similar to that of complete facial palsy patients.

20.2.2.2 Incomplete Synkinetic Facial Palsy

Synkinesis is defined as involuntary and uncoordinated mimetic muscle motion creating paradoxical facial movements. Around 15% of incomplete facial palsy patients will develop synkinesis [4]. Synkinesis may be a result of abnormal nerve sprouting during recovery, although the exact mechanism remains unclear. The time until onset of synkinesis after facial nerve injury can vary between 3.5 and 12 months [5].

The spectrum of synkinetic motion varies by facial subunit and by severity. The most common synkinetic motion observed is oral-ocular synkinesis (involuntary eye closure during voluntary mouth movement) (Fig. 20.3b) and ocular-oral

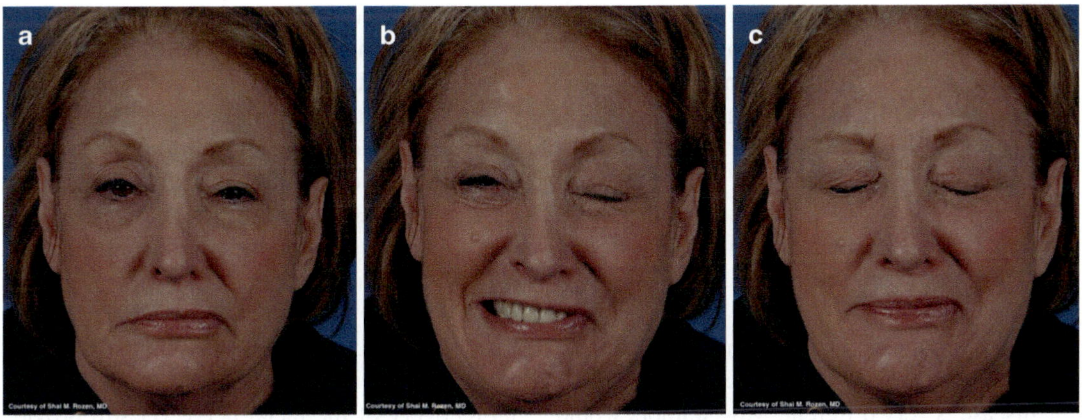

Fig. 20.3 A 67-year-old patient years after partial recovery from Bell's palsy with synkinesis. (**a**) Repose—note hypertonicity on palsied left side, (**b**) oral—ocular synkinesis, (**c**) ocular—oral synkinesis

synkinesis (involuntary mouth movement during voluntary eye closure) (Fig. 20.3c). Another paradoxical facial motion also seen is strong antagonistic muscle activity of the depressor anguli oris (DAO) and platysma during attempted smile, often preventing a full unopposed lifting of the lip (Fig. 20.3b).

The spectrum of synkinesis severity is also broad; some patients might only show mild to moderate involuntary movements, while others will experience continuous painful spasm of the face.

20.2.2.3 Mid and Lower Face

As opposed to flaccid palsy, the nasolabial fold is often more pronounced on the paralyzed side. Additionally, patients with synkinesis will often have a tight "frozen" paralyzed midface sometimes appearing as a constant grin often with pulling of the upper lip and modiolus toward the paralyzed side (Fig. 20.3a). The lower lip depressors in most of these patients are similar to complete flaccid palsy patients yet the depressor anguli oris and platysma muscles may be hyperactive which may hinder a smile because they counteract the upward and lateral movement of the oral commissure (Fig. 20.3b).

20.2.2.4 Periorbital

Differing from flaccid facial palsy, patients are mostly able to close their eyes. In fact, because the orbicularis oculi muscle is tight most patients have a smaller palpebral aperture with decreased scleral show (Fig. 20.3a). As previously mentioned, the most common form of synkinesis is oral-occular synkinesis.

20.2.2.5 Forehead

The forehead in patients with synkinetic spasm often looks symmetric. However, sometimes the position of the eyebrow might be a bit lower like in flaccid patients, especially during repose (Fig. 20.3a) although the mechanism causing this is completely different; in flaccid patients it is caused by ptosis due to weakness, whereas in synkinetic patients it may be caused by spasm of the orbicularis oculi muscle which is stronger than the frontalis muscle. Conversely, some patients present with a high brow to abnormal increased tightness of the ipsilateral frontalis muscle or as seen in the same patient, during attempted eye closure as part of a synkinetic motion (Fig. 20.3c).

20.3 Patient Selection

Preoperative patient assessment is key since facial palsy treatment is tailored to each individual patient. This should include a thorough history including duration of paralysis, continuity of facial nerve, presenting symptoms, course of onset, possible etiology including history of malignancies, and the patient's main complaints typically including smile asymmetry, speech impediment, eating, and drinking difficulties. A comprehensive physical examination including all cranial nerves including both motor and sensory components is paramount.

20.3.1 Duration: Subacute vs. Longstanding

The duration of facial palsy symptoms is important as the approach of subacute and longstanding disease is very different. Most authors would consider mimetic muscles to be salvageable up to 18 months after onset of palsy and would likely use nerve transfers as part of the treatment strategy. This period of salvageability might be longer in incomplete weak facial palsy patients due to continued innervation of the muscles. In longer durations of palsy, irreversible damage to motor end plates and atrophy of facial musculature occurs and a transplant of a new neurovascular muscle unit is necessary.

20.3.2 Etiology

Etiology is important to assess. Often patients are sent with a diagnosis of Bell's Palsy yet provide a history of a slowly progressive facial nerve weakening. This type of progression is typical to cancer unless proven otherwise. Recurrent bouts of palsy should direct investigations to either recurrent infections as seen in patients with Ramsay-Hunt syndrome (herpes zoster oticus) or slow growing neoplasms. Only when the diagnosis is unclear and other etiologies are ruled out, is diagnosis of Bell's palsy warranted. Also, if the patient's prognosis is not favorable, certain approaches as one-stage procedures may be preferable over techniques requiring multiple stages.

20.3.3 Facial Nerve Continuity

Facial nerve continuity may refer to either an originally intact facial nerve or a reconstructed facial nerve but implies that some degree of regeneration might occur in patients with subacute facial palsy durations of up to 18 months. This is important not because full motion is always expected, especially if little to no motion is seen at 6 months after onset, but rather that there is still a small chance the nerve regeneration which may result in some facial tone and improved symmetry at rest. In these cases, if nerve transfers are chosen as part of the treatment, they should be performed more distally on select facial nerve branches, as to enable potential recovery of the facial nerve yet still provide power. Conversely, if no facial nerve continuity exists, nerve transfers may be performed more proximally and the use of static procedures will more likely be needed. More details are provided in the Chap. 8.

20.3.4 Patient's Demographics: Age and Facial Features

Other important factors in determining a treatment plan are patient's demographics such as age and anatomical structure of the face. Over time, skin tone decreases and the true and false facial ligaments weaken. In addition, subcutaneous volume will diminish accentuating asymmetry in repose. In patients with heavier anatomical facial features, asymmetry might also appear more obvious. Therefore, older patients and patients with "heavy faces" with complete flaccid facial palsy will benefit from additional static support [2]. Patients should not be excluded from treatment based on only their age since dynamic techniques have been demonstrated to be effective in older patient groups. Proper evaluation of the patient is necessary to make a decision based on risk-benefit analysis [6].

20.3.4.1 Patient's Wishes

Lastly, as with any treatment plan, patient's wishes and expectations should be taken into consideration. If their expectations are not realistic they need to be adjusted. In addition, patient's motivation should be evaluated before initiating complex reconstructive surgery that has to be performed in several phases and requires long-term commitment of the patient.

20.4 Treatment Options

The treatment for flaccid and synkinetic facial palsy patients has both similarities and dissimilarities. In complete facial palsy, in addition to dynamic reanimation, improving symmetry at rest is one of the main treatment goals. Similarly, in the synkinetic patient obtaining symmetry in motion as well as symmetry at rest are critical but approached very differently and usually asymmetry at rest in synkinetic patients is less severe than in flaccid palsy patients. In practice, most patients with synkinesis present with a mix of symptoms of weakness, hyperactivity, and hypertonicity and will need treatment for both.

20.4.1 The Flaccid Complete Facial Palsy Patient

As we have learned over the years, dynamic reanimation alone rarely resolves all symptoms with a satisfactory result. Therefore, an increasing number of authors have developed different techniques to allow simultaneous static support in addition to dynamic solutions, whether they be nerve transfers in the subacute population or free functional muscle transplant (FFMT) in the long-standing palsy patient, in order to provide not only motion, but also improve symmetry at rest. Treatment options discussed below are also relevant to most patients with weak non-synkinetic partial facial palsy patients with some differences depending on the degree of tone or motion individual patients might have. Treatment options will be discussed by anatomical region of the face.

20.4.1.1 Mid and Lower Face

Treatment Goals

The main treatment objectives in the mid and lower face is to provide improved facial expression, enhanced nasolabial fold definition, improved nasal breathing, better oral competence, and improved aesthetics. This can only be achieved by combining both static and dynamic techniques.

Static Support

Oral Commissure, Nasolabial Fold, and Alar Support

Many techniques providing static support to the midface have been described. Detailed preoperative markings are crucial to assess the correct fold placement and desired vector. The preferred method of the senior author (SR) in patients with long-standing facial palsy is the use of four or five fascia lata strips, each with individual insertions and slightly different vectors. The plain of dissection is sub-SMAS. The most important strip is attached to the modiolus, which even in long-standing facial palsy patients with muscle atrophy, is readily identified in the confluence of the zygomatic major muscle and the orbicularis oris muscle fibers. Two additional strips are inserted into the mid lip and slightly medial to it. The alar base is then palpated, slightly more medially and superiorly, where an additional strip is inserted with the purpose of lateralizing the paralyzed alae. Once the vector is determined and a pleasing natural nasolabial fold is created, the slings are secured to the deep temporal fascia under very slight tension either superficial or deep to the zygomatic arch. The strips can be inserted through a pre-auricular incision or an additional nasolabial incision. The senior author does not commonly use a separate nasolabial fold for the medial insertion unless the patient is old and has significant nasolabial folds which hide the nasolabial incisions extremely well as demonstrated in Fig. 20.4. It is important to realize that the new nasolabial fold is not created by inserting the strips into the previous nasolabial fold but rather more medially on the orbicularis muscle fibers to improve the symmetry of the lips. The lateralization of the modiolus and upper lip creates an inflection at the nasolabial crease providing a natural fold.

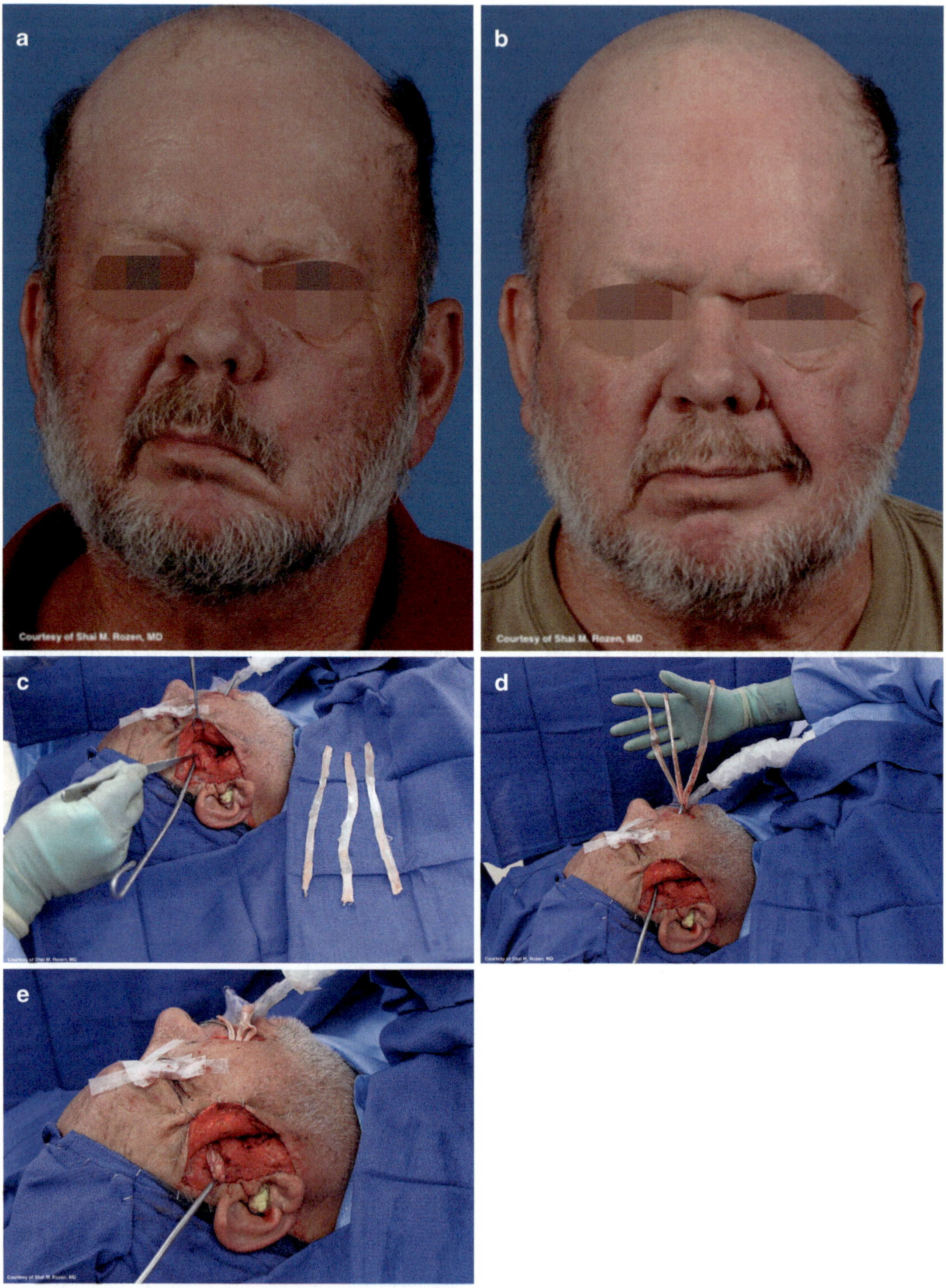

Fig. 20.4 A 61-year-old man after gunshot wound to the left temporal bone. (**a**) Repose, (**b**) repose 11 months after insertion of four tensor fascia lata strips and gracilis muscle innervated by the masseter nerve, (**c–e**) Intraoperative photos of insertion of fascia lata strips deep to the zygomatic arch (taken from another patient for demonstration purposes)

Lower Lip

The lower lip deformity is more obvious during animation. In long-standing facial paralysis patients reinnervation of the lower lip isn't possible, though dynamic reanimation techniques have been described, but not commonly used due to inconsistent results. In patients with a full tooth smile especially of the lower teeth, or in patients who are animated during speech, the lower lip on the healthy side tends to strongly pull downwards due to the depressor labii inferioris muscle. Because of contralateral lower lip paralysis, the paralyzed lower lip tends to remain elevated, creating an abnormal lower lip shape. This bothers patients both during smile and often more during speaking. Therefore, several techniques have been described, which attempt to balance the lower paralyzed lip by pulling it downward. This can be done by a T-shape double fascia graft; one fascia sling is placed horizontally at the lower lip to correct the static position, and the other is grafted obliquely at the lateral side by folding and crossing the horizontal fascia. This has showed promising result regarding improved symmetry especially when opening the mouth [7] but as with any static technique, may also create excessive pull, hence caution is recommended.

Dynamic Solutions

Oral Commissure, Nasolabial Fold, and Alar Support

The above-mentioned static support procedures improve symmetry at rest however do not provide movement. Dynamic reconstruction options depend on the duration of paralysis and the potential salvageability of the facial musculature. In subacute facial palsy, nerve transfers might be useful to dynamically reanimate mimetic muscles, whereas for longstanding facial palsy free functional muscle transplants or regional muscle transfers are needed.

Subacute Facial Paralysis

These options are discussed in more detail including figures in the chapter on nerve transfers and therefore only a brief overview will be provided in this chapter. In subacute facial palsy, the native facial musculature can be reinnervated. The exact duration of facial palsy after which the native facial musculature is still salvageable is up for debate. However, nerve transfers can likely be performed successfully up to 18 months with some reports even at 24 months, but it seems that earlier transfers confer improved excursion. In patients with weak incomplete facial palsy the window of opportunity may be longer. The senior author does not advise performing nerve transfers in synkinetic patients. The addition of cross facial nerve grafts to possibly improve tone and synchroneity is also often used and described in more detail in the nerve transfer chapter.

Longstanding Facial Paralysis

In longstanding facial palsy, the mimetic musculature is no longer salvageable and a new neurovascular muscle unit must be introduced, either in the form of a free functional muscle transplant (FFMT) or regional muscle transfer.

Free Functional Muscle Transplant

Gracilis muscle with the obturator nerve is the most used free functional muscle transfer in facial palsy because of the low donor site morbidity and easy dissection. The gracilis muscle can be innervated by a contralateral redundant branch of the facial nerve or by an ipsilateral non-facial nerve. Traditionally, if a cross-face nerve graft is used, the procedure is performed in two stages: a cross-facial nerve graft followed by a FFMT. The same advantages and disadvantages of using facial vs. non-facial innervation as discussed in nerve transfer choices apply for FFMT. Innervation with the facial nerve presents the advantage of obtaining an emotional and spontaneous smile, yet with the reported drawback of decreased excursion and sometimes no motion at all.

A one-stage approach using a FFMT coapted to an ipsilateral non-facial nerve is also a common technique, in which the most frequently used donor nerve is the masseter nerve. The most apparent disadvantage with using a non-facial nerve is unreliable spontaneity and involuntary motion [8]; the advantages include a shorter time to achieve motion, higher reliability, and increased excursion likely because of increased axonal load, shorter regenerative distance, and perhaps the need for only one coaptation [9] (Figs. 20.5 and 20.6a, b).

Regional Muscle Transfer

Midface

Many types of regional muscle transfers have been described. However, the temporalis lengthening myoplasty, also known as the Labbé proce-

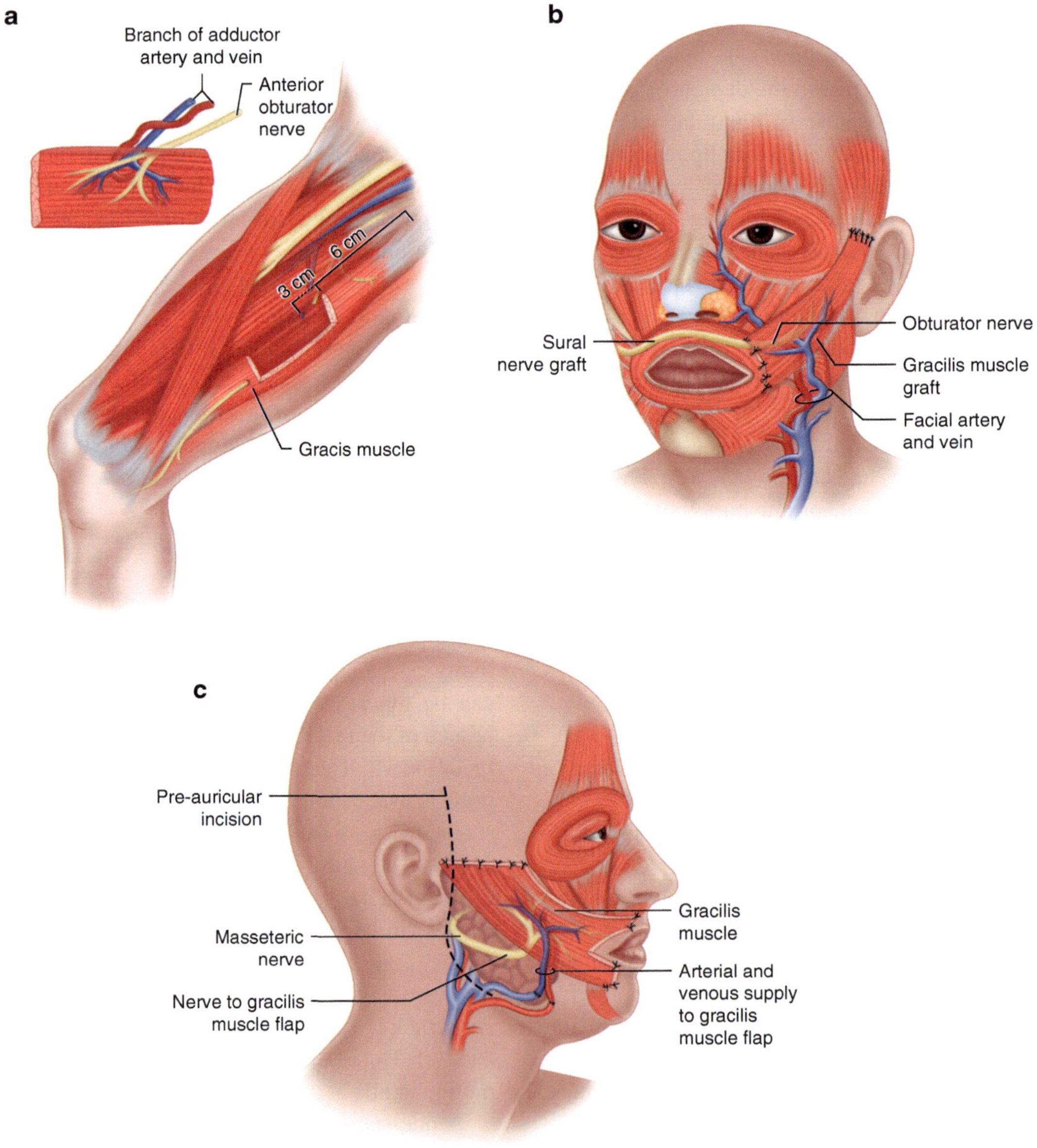

Fig. 20.5 Drawing of a free gracilis muscle flap. (**a**) Harvest from medial thigh, (**b**) the gracilis muscle innervated by the contralateral facial nerve via a cross facial sural nerve graft, (**c**) The gracilis muscle innervated by an ipsilateral masseter nerve

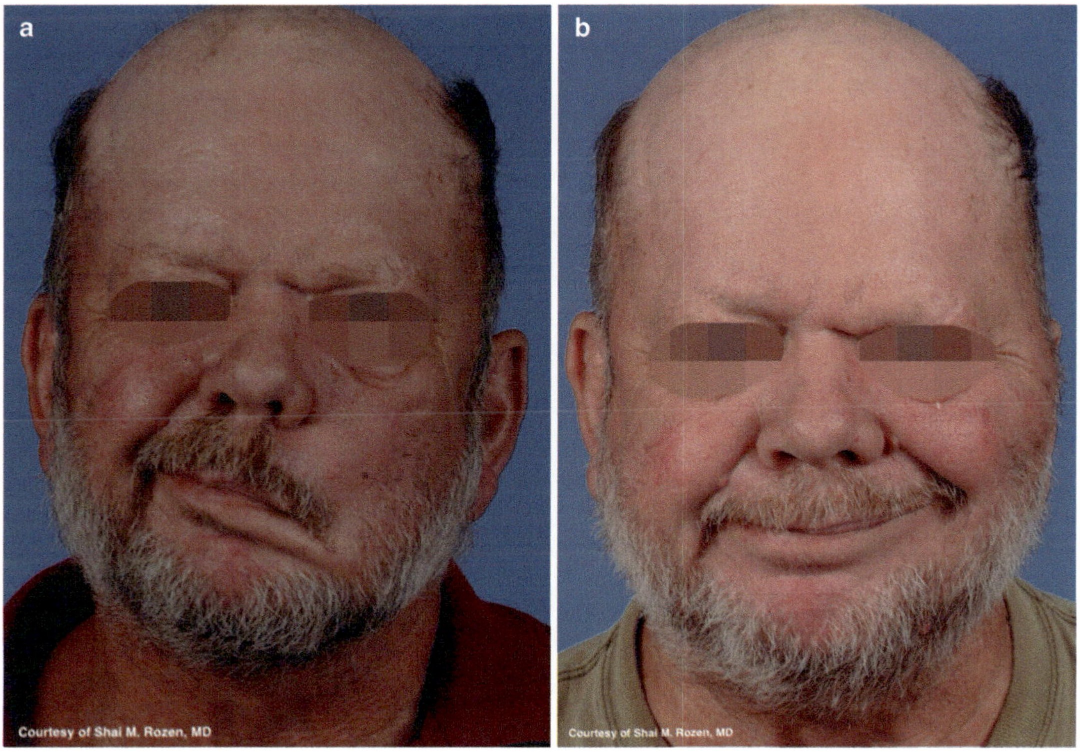

Fig. 20.6 The man from Fig. 20.4 during animation. (**a**) Before, (**b**) after combined static TFL slings and free gracilis muscle transplant innervated by the masseter nerve

dure, has recently gained popularity. The advantage of the transfer of the temporalis muscle is that it offers a quick recovery of motion since no reinnervation is needed, no microsurgical techniques are needed, and it provides satisfactory smile excursion as well as decent static support. Unlike with FFMT the use of an additional static sling is less frequently needed, likely because of the increased tendinous portion in the muscle. However, with the temporalis lengthening myoplasty procedure excursions are lower than with free functional muscle transplants and vector control seems more limited [6, 10]. The reader is advised to read the chapter dedicated to this procedure for full details.

20.4.1.2 Lower Lip

Many techniques have been described for dynamic lower lip reanimation but none have become mainstream, likely due to very low reproducibility and unreliability. These historically included digastric muscle transposition, free functional platysma transplant, and others. In reality, the best opportunity to reinnervate the lower lip is during the acute and subacute period either via nerve grafting or nerve transfer. A separate chapter is dedicated to this approach.

20.4.1.3 Periorbital

Treatment Goals

As previously mentioned one of the highest priorities in the care of facial palsy patients is ocular protection. Regardless of the technique used for corneal protection it is almost always necessary to provide additional protection in the form of lubrication with drops during the day time and ointment at night. In some patients in whom recovery is expected, this may suffice if the patient is compliant. In the other cases static interventions are most commonly used but in the subacute palsy patients attempts at reinnervation of the orbicularis oculi muscle should be attempted.

Static Procedures for the Eye

Upper Eyelid Lagophthalmos

Upper eyelid lagophthalmos occurs because of the paralysis of the orbicularis oculi muscle leaving the action of the levator palpebrae muscle unopposed (See Fig. 20.2b). The most common technique used for correction of paralytic lagophthalmos is insertion of a weight in the upper eyelid, which allows improved corneal protection at night when the levator palpebrae muscle is relaxed. One should remember that during the day when the levator muscle is active, a weight is not intended to perform quick voluntary closure. For this reason, most patients will need to continue lubricating the cornea, and try to avoid exposure to moving air experienced in a car AC, ceiling fan, or winds that might increase dryness.

Traditionally, a weight is placed in the pretarsal position however, the senior author (SR) suggests to place a heavier weight in the post-septal position laying on the levator palpebrae aponeurosis just cranial and sutured to the superior border of the tarsus [11]. This technique allows the weight to be better hidden, decreases the chances of extrusion, and prevents entropion as is commonly seen with a pretarsal positioning (Figs. 20.7 and 20.8).

Lower Eyelid Ectropion

Lower lid ectropion can be surgically addressed by procedures on the lower eyelid. In young patients with no horizontal laxity a lateral canthoplasty can be performed. In older patients with existing horizontal laxity a lateral tarsal strip will be more suitable. The senior author also likes to add a small orbicularis muscle sling for additional support. If support is needed both laterally and medially the use of a palmaris tendon or fascia lata sling to support the lower eyelid by securing it to both the lateral and medial canthal ligament regions is also effective.

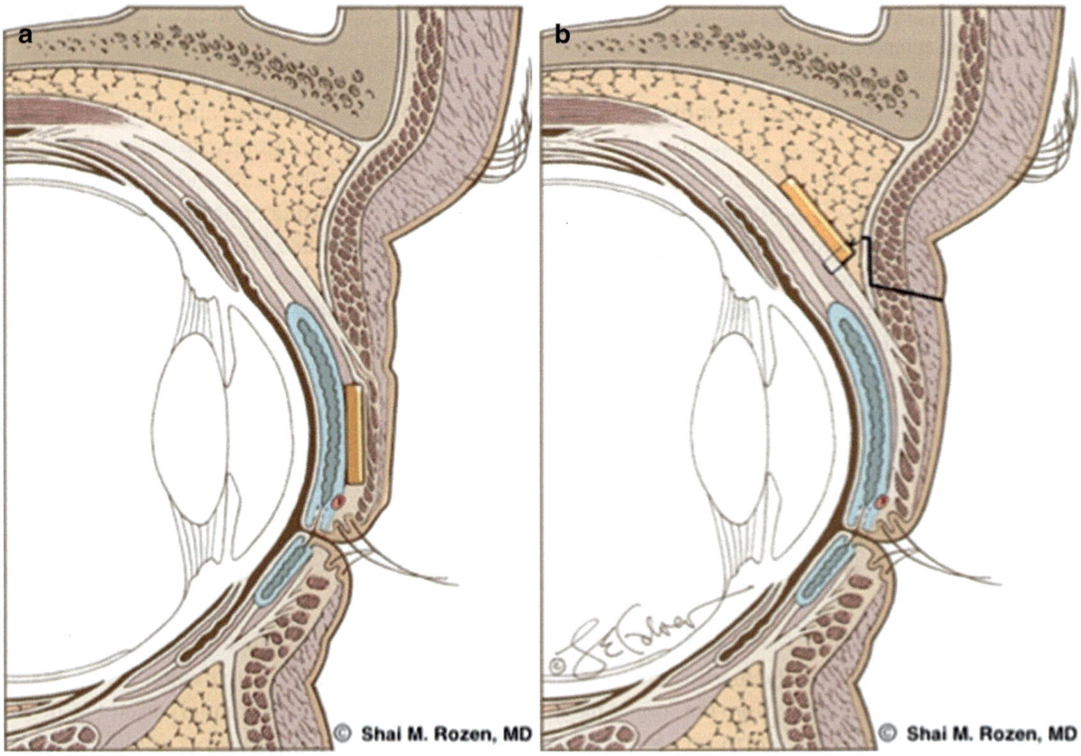

Fig. 20.7 Drawing of the upper eyelid gold weight placement in a sagittal view of the eyelid. (**a**) The commonly used pretarsal weight technique, (**b**) the right post-septal weight technique

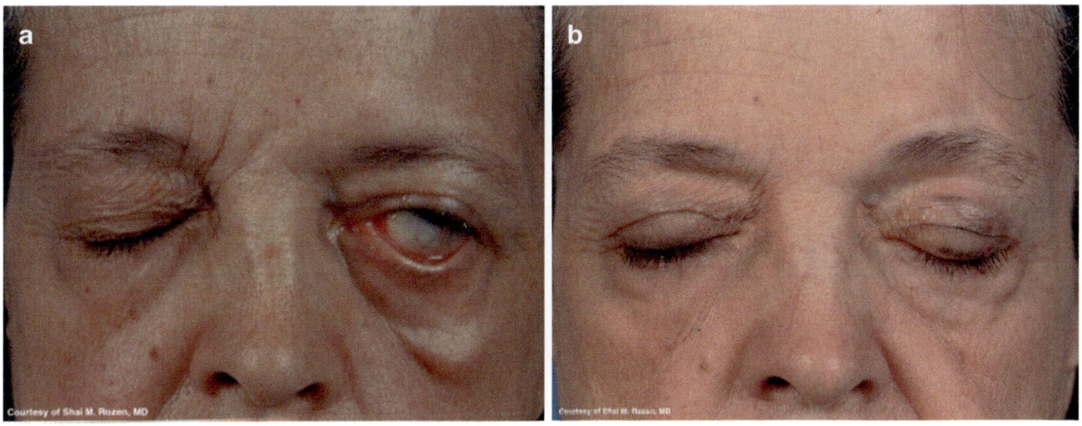

Fig. 20.8 The woman from Fig. 20.2. (**a**) Lagophthalmos prior to insertion of gold weight, (**b**) improved palpebral closure after upper lid loading in the post-septal technique and lower lid tarsal strip

Malar Soft Tissue

Laxity of the malar soft tissue, especially in older patients may further worsen lower lid malposition. Although treatment of ectropion should not be relegated to a midface lift, the latter could make the techniques previously mentioned more durable over time. The senior author prefers to elevate the midface lift via a high smas approach as described by other authors [12, 13]. This technique enables lifting the midface in a near superior vector via distributing the support over a wider surface rather than in techniques used to lift the midface via a lower eyelid approach.

Dynamic

Dynamic reanimation of the periorbital reanimation relies on the same principles as mentioned previously in the midface. The duration of palsy should not exceed the point in which irreversible orbicularis oculi muscle atrophy occurs. The exact period in which this occurs in complete facial palsy is not known but most authors consider this around 18 months. Orbicularis oculi innervation may be performed via nerve transfers, ipsilateral nerve grafts, or contralateral nerve grafts known as cross facial nerve grafts. The exact technique of reinnervation depends on the specific patient scenario but in the senior authors opinion and work and based on some previous work by other authors [14], the most important component if reinnervation is via nerve transfers which provides voluntary palpebral closure. Any added innervation by the facial nerve either via intratemporal nerve graft or cross facial nerve graft may provide additional resting tone and even a more synchronous and spontaneous blink. In addition, the senior author demonstrated that reinnervation of the orbicularis oculi muscle confers additional corneal protection to static procedures alone.

20.4.1.4 Forehead

Brow Lift

Treatment for brow ptosis is aimed at static support. Lifting the brow can be done using several different techniques. Likely the most effective is direct excision of skin directly above the brow (Figs. 20.2a and 20.9). The advantage of this technique is that the elevating force and securing of the new position is closest to the brow that needs elevation. The main disadvantage, although minimal in the senior authors' opinion, is the scar, that is very well hidden in Caucasians. This may be less conspicuous in darker skin patients who may experience more scar hypertrophy, and therefore a thorough history and exam regarding previous scarring experience should be performed. In order to hide the brow scar several techniques may be performed. The senior author prefers a very small limb, zig-zag incision performed with an 11 blade that may help brake and better hide the scar, and uses it in cases of severe brow ptosis in older patients. Other authors have

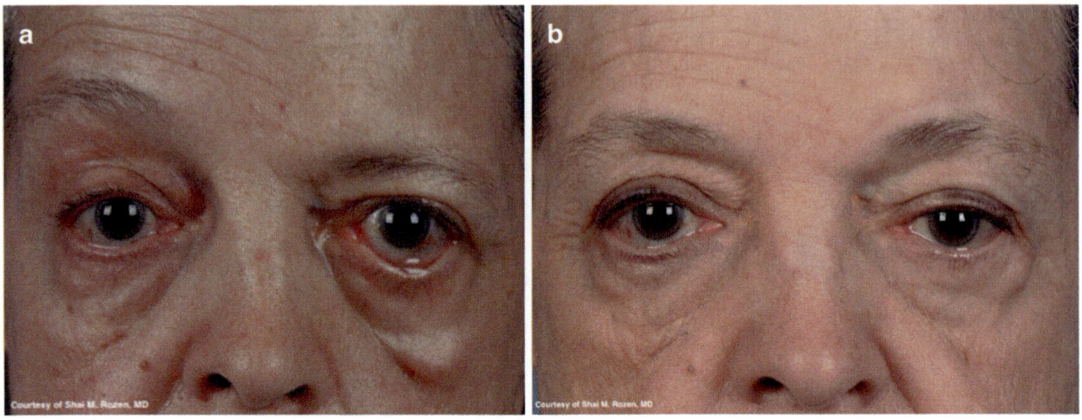

Fig. 20.9 The woman from Fig. 20.2. (**a**) Ectropion prior to lower lid correction, (**b**) improved lower lid position after tarsal strip

suggested placing incisions at the patients' natural rhytides, although this will usually slightly increase the pull distance from the brow. Another technique, preferred by the senior author in most cases in younger patients or those without heavy facial features, is elevation of the brow via four incision placed above the brow, in similar zig-zag incisions but without skin resection. In this technique, the deep dermis of the brow is pulled in different superior vectors based on the different brow portions, and secured to the periosteum. Special care should be given to avoid injury to the supraorbital and supratrochlear nerves as to avoid painful neuromas.

Additional described techniques include brow lifting via a coronal incision or via endoscopic techniques, but surgeons should consider that these are palsy patients and that the caudal forces of gravity are unopposed by frontalis elevation, hence these techniques may be less durable over time, since the distances between the target brow to the points of fixation are considerably increased. To further help with symmetry, the contralateral frontalis muscle might be weakened using Botox.

20.4.2 Incomplete Synkinetic Facial Palsy

The treatment of patients with synkinesia considerably varies depending on the severity of the synkinesia, which facial subunit is affected most, and whether the chief complaint is that of paradoxical facial motion, inability to produce an effective motion due to hypertonicity, or most commonly the combination of both. The treatment principles aim at reducing synkinesia, reducing hypertonicity, and improving motion. The means in which this is achieved also vary considerably and include both medicinal interventions, surgical interventions, and physical therapy. Within an individual patient, treatments may be opposing—weakening certain portions of the face while strengthening others. What should be realized is that as opposed to the flaccid facial palsy patient in which the treatment is directed at afflicted facial zone, in the synkinetic patient, treatment may not only be needed in the afflicted area but also in a distant area that effects the area of concern. Synkinesis is an area in facial palsy that has recently seen new developments and will likely see more advances in the near future.

20.4.2.1 Perioorbita, Midface, and Lower Face

Two of the main features in patients with synkinesia are abnormal synkinetic motions mostly seen in the periorbital region and hypertonicity that limits normal motion more often seen in the midface and neck region. In synkinetic patients, the problem is not a lack of innervation but rather abnormal innervation, whether strong or weak.

Periorbital Synkinesis

The most common type of synkinesis is oral-ocular or ocular-oral synkinesia. This presents as closure of the palpebral aperture when the patient attempts to smile and conversely when a patient attempts to close the eyes they will smile. It is most bothersome, when patients are eating (see Fig. 20.3b, c).

Botulinum toxin injection is an important treatment modality used in the periorbital region. Injections are given into the orbicularis oculi muscle and sometimes very conservatively in the orbicularis oris. The exact locations may vary by patient but more-so by surgeons' preference and experience. Most physicians would inject 6–12 units to the lower half of the orbicularis oculi muscle in the pretarsal and preseptal portions. Some would add 2.5 units in the superior orbicularis oculi muscle. Excess injection may cause ectropion or ptosis if it diffuses to the levator palpebrae muscle, although both are rare. Orbicularis oris muscle injection should be performed with caution as this may cause temporary excess midface paralysis and remind patients of where they started, creating stress. A comprehensive discussion is important prior to the first injection session and the senior author recommends beginning conservatively and explaining to the patient that it may take several sessions until the optimal dosages and placements are reached. The repeated nature of the treatment is also important to emphasize. Other common areas of paradoxical facial motions are in the chin area which may benefit from 5 of 7.5 units of botox (see Fig. 20.10).

Physical therapy with a specialized facial nerve therapist is also advisable and may be helpful in most patients. The main emphasis is trying to concentrate on activating certain groups of muscles while suppressing others. Also, certain stretching exercises, especially in the buccinator and cheek zone are recommended. Patience compliance is important to the success of physical therapy.

Surgery in the periorbital region for synkinesis is not common and is usually confined to very severe cases. Surgery for blepharospasm has been described decades ago. The main problems

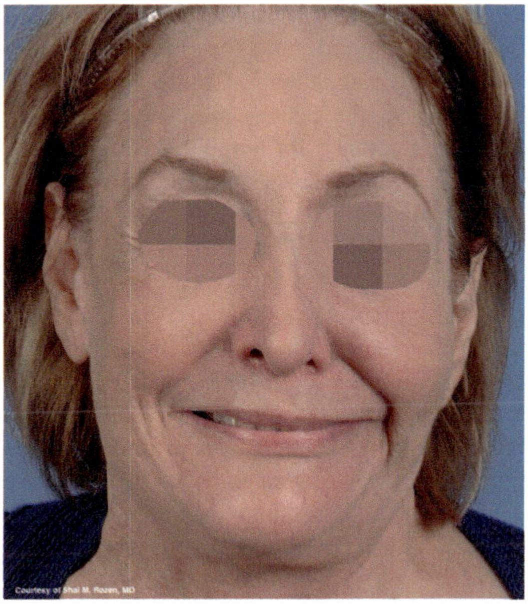

Fig. 20.10 The woman from Fig. 20.3 with synkinesis after combining a free functional gracilis muscle flap and botox injection into the left periorbital region

encountered were recurrence over time, likely because of the multidirectional innervation of the orbicularis oculi muscle. Yet surgery is perhaps correctly advocated in the periorbital area in most severe cases of spasm when patients literally have a frozen face with complete inability to move. The principle in these surgeries is the combination of aggressive neurectomies and myectomies, to a point of almost converting the patient to a flaccid facial paralysis and then proceeding with reconstruction as they were a flaccid palsy patient. These types of surgery should be reserved to the most sever patients and performed by experienced facial palsy surgeons [15].

Midface and Lower Face Synkinesis and Hypertonicity

One of the more unrecognized areas in patients with synkinesia is the hypertonicity and hyperactivity of antagonistic muscles. The main culprit muscle groups currently recognized are the depressor anguli oris, the platysma, and to some extent the buccinator muscle and to a lesser extent the elevators of the lip. It is increasingly acknowledged that due the excessive tone of these muscles at rest and antagonistic action while attempting to smile, they inhibit symmetry at rest and during attempted smile. As described previously in the patient presentation portion, these patients may not initially seem paralyzed when observing them at rest and may actually appear weak on the healthy side (see Fig. 20.3a).

Botulinum toxin injections in the platysma can be helpful in decreasing the feeling of tension in the midface especially at the end of the day, and some patients even report some improvement in the smile, albeit mild to moderate. Injection of the platysma may range from 25 to 50 units and the senior author recommends injecting a small portion also above the mandibular border into the extensions of the fibers into the midface.

Botox injection in the depressor anguli oris (DAO) muscle is helpful as well, although in the senior authors experience DAO resection is more beneficial and is discussed below.

Physical therapy is also recommended. The emphasis is mainly stretching exercises especially in the cheek area including the buccinator muscle.

Surgery is discussed more commonly today but long-term results still need to be reported. There is increasing interest is DAO resection on the affected side. At rest the patients usually present with a downward pull of the corner of the mouth giving an appearance of a sigmoid smile pattern that further increases when attempting to smile (sigmoid smile) [16]. The surgeon should ask the patient to smile strongly and then palpate the DAO, which feels like a string. A 3 cc injection of 1% lidocaine with 1:100,000 0f epinephrine is given and a return visit within 30 min to clinic will provide both patient and surgeon the ability to assess the possible negative affect the DAO has on the smile. If a patient has significant improvement in smile and greater tooth exposure, they may be a good candidate for DAO myectomy [17].

There is also increasing interest in platysma myectomy, with similar principles as with DAO resection, except here both myectomy and neurectomy are performed. This is a more controversial surgery since recurrences are more likely due to the nature of the multidirectional platysma innervation, and orbicularis oris muscle weakening has been observed in some patients. Still this option should be further explored [15].

Synkinetic patients who are less responsive to tension relief for smile restoration or wish an even stronger smile, might also benefit from dynamic treatment with a FFMT similar to that described for complete flaccid facial palsy (see Fig. 20.10).

In incomplete weak facial palsy a redundant ipsilateral branch of the facial nerve might be used to transfer to the FFMT instead of a cross-face nerve graft as described in a recent article with promising results [18] but further investigations are needed to further define which patients would benefit most from the procedure.

20.5 Summary

With an aesthetic end result in mind, treatment of facial palsy should not only focus on function but should always bear in mind form in its most aesthetic sense. This means not only optimizing motion but also optimizing the patient's appearance at rest. To achieve an optimal outcome, all available reconstructive and aesthetic surgical tools and the combination thereof must be considered despite of their perceived "classification" as static, dynamic or aesthetic and all facial subunits should be assessed and addressed.

References

1. Bradbury ET, Simons W, Sanders R. Psychological and social factors in reconstructive surgery for hemi-facial palsy. J Plast Reconstr Aesthet Surg. 2006;59(3):272–8.
2. Rozen SM. Discussion: symmetry restoration at rest after masseter-to-facial nerve transfer: is it as efficient as smile reanimation? Plast Reconstr Surg. 2017;140(4):802–4.
3. Dartt DA. Neural regulation of lacrimal gland secretory processes: relevance in dry eye diseases. Prog Retin Eye Res. 2009;28(3):155–77.
4. Husseman J, Mehta RP. Management of synkinesis. Facial Plast Surg. 2008;24(2):242–9.
5. Placheta E, Tzou CH, Hold A, Pona I, Frey M. Facial synkinesia before and after surgical reanimation

of the paralyzed face. Plast Reconstr Surg. 2014;133(6):842e–51e.
6. Hembd A, Harrison B, Rocha CSM, Rocha FS, Chamseddin K, Labbe D, Cardenas-Mejia A, Rozen SM. Facial reanimation in the seventh and eighth decades of life. Plast Reconstr Surg. 2018;141(5):1239–51.
7. Hayashi A, Yoshizawa H, Natori Y, Suda S, Mochizuki M, Nishimuta Y, Tanaka R, Mizuno H. Assessment of T-shape double fascia graft for lower lip deformity from facial paralysis: a questionnaire survey. J Plast Reconstr Aesthet Surg. 2016;69(3):427–35.
8. Rozen S, Harrison B. Involuntary movement during mastication in patients with long-term facial paralysis reanimated with a partial gracilis free neuromuscular flap innervated by the masseteric nerve. Plast Reconstr Surg. 2013;132(1):110e–6e.
9. Garcia RM, Hadlock TA, Klebuc MJ, Simpson RL, Zenn MR, Marcus JR. Contemporary solutions for the treatment of facial nerve paralysis. Plast Reconstr Surg. 2015;135(6):1025e–46e.
10. Labbe D, Bussu F, Iodice A. A comprehensive approach to long-standing facial paralysis based on lengthening temporalis myoplasty. Acta Otorhinolaryngol Ital. 2012;32(3):145–53.
11. Rozen S, Lehrman C. Upper eyelid postseptal weight placement for treatment of paralytic lagophthalmos. Plast Reconstr Surg. 2013;131(6):1253–65.
12. Marten TJ. High SMAS facelift: combined single flap lifting of the jawline, cheek, and midface. Clin Plast Surg. 2008;35(4):569–603, vi–vii.
13. Trussler AP, Hatef D, Broussard GB, Brown S, Barton FE. The viscoelastic properties of the SMAS and its clinical translation: firm support for the high-SMAS rhytidectomy. Plast Reconstr Surg. 2011;128(3):757–64.
14. Terzis JK, Bruno W. Outcomes with eye reanimation microsurgery. Facial Plast Surg. 2002;18(2):101–12.
15. Chuang DC, Chang TN, Lu JC. Postparalysis facial synkinesis: clinical classification and surgical strategies. Plast Reconstr Surg Glob Open. 2015;3(3):e320.
16. Paletz JL, Manktelow RT, Chaban R. The shape of a normal smile: implications for facial paralysis reconstruction. Plast Reconstr Surg. 1994;93(4):784–9; discussion 790–781.
17. Labbe D, Benichou L, Iodice A, Giot JP. [Depressor anguli oris sign (DAO) in facial paresis. How to search it and release the smile (technical note)]. Ann Chir Plast Esthet. 2012;57(3):281–5.
18. Gur E, Zuker RM, Zaretski A, Leshem D, Barnea Y, Arad E, Yanko R, Meilik B, Kedar DJ, Fliss E. Incomplete facial paralysis - the use of the ipsilateral residual facial nerve as a donor nerve for facial reanimation. Plast Reconstr Surg. 2018;142:202.

21 Temporal Muscle Transposition for Smile Reanimation of the Paralyzed Face (Modified McLaughlin-Procedure)

Ahmet Bozkurt, Lara Küenzlen, and Ulrich Rieger

21.1 Introduction and Indication

An individual and tailored concept is the key for an optimal and effective treatment strategy for patients with a facial nerve paralysis. This includes restoration of mimetic functions, aesthetic facial symmetry at rest and protection of the eye by complete eyelid closure. The surgical goals require both an exact analysis of (1) the aetiology or underlying pathology, (2) duration of illness, (3) degree of clinical symptoms, (4) coexisting diseases and life expectation, and, in particular, (5) the expectations of the patient [6].

Current gold standards [7] are mainly based on nerve reconstruction strategies and/or cross facial nerve grafts (CFNG) combined with free muscle transplantation. If these procedures are not feasible or requested for a number or reasons, regional muscle transplantation or transposition of masticatory muscles (Fig. 21.1) like the temporalis muscle (TM) and/or masseter muscle (supplied by the trigeminal nerve) is an effective alternative for dynamic restoration. Therefore, despite modern and sophisticated microsurgical techniques, muscle transposition procedures have their relevance and are still powerful techniques, either as single procedure or in combination with the CFNG to bridge the time until nerve regeneration enables free functional muscle transplantation. To perform movements like smiling or eye closure, patients have to clench their teeth for muscle activation. After the first description by Gillies in 1935 [8], a number of modifications and techniques have been published [1–6, 9, 10] (Figs. 21.2 and 21.3). On the basis of the vector, the TM can provide a certain degree of both static suspension at rest (e.g., oblique lift of the mouth) and dynamic voluntary movement (e.g., smiling), but not involuntary and without control of the direction of movement. In principle, the TM can be transposed in an anterograde or retrograde way. For retrograde transposition [10], the TM is released from the temporal fossa, turned over the zygomatic arch and extended mouth (and to the eye) (Fig. 21.2b). To gain length and to reach the mouth, the TM can be elongated with its fascia or with additional fascial or tendon grafts. Beside the mouth region, the eye can also be addressed by the TM transposition. Shortly, for the treatment of the upper lid (lagopthalmus) and lower lid (ectropium), a strip of TM with its overlying fascia is elevated from its origin, turned over and tunneled to the lateral canthus. The fascia is partially ele-

A. Bozkurt (✉)
Department of Plastic and Aesthetic Surgery, Hand and Burn Surgery, Helios University Hospital, University Witten/Herdecke, Wuppertal, Germany
e-mail: ahmet.bozkurt@helios-gesundheit.de

L. Küenzlen · U. Rieger
Department of Plastic and Aesthetic, Reconstructive and Hand Surgery, Agaplesion Markus Hospital, Frankfurt, Germany
e-mail: lara.kuenzlen@fdk.info; ulrich.rieger@fdk.info

© Springer Nature Switzerland AG 2021
C.-H. J. Tzou, A. Rodríguez-Lorenzo (eds.), *Facial Palsy*,
https://doi.org/10.1007/978-3-030-50784-8_21

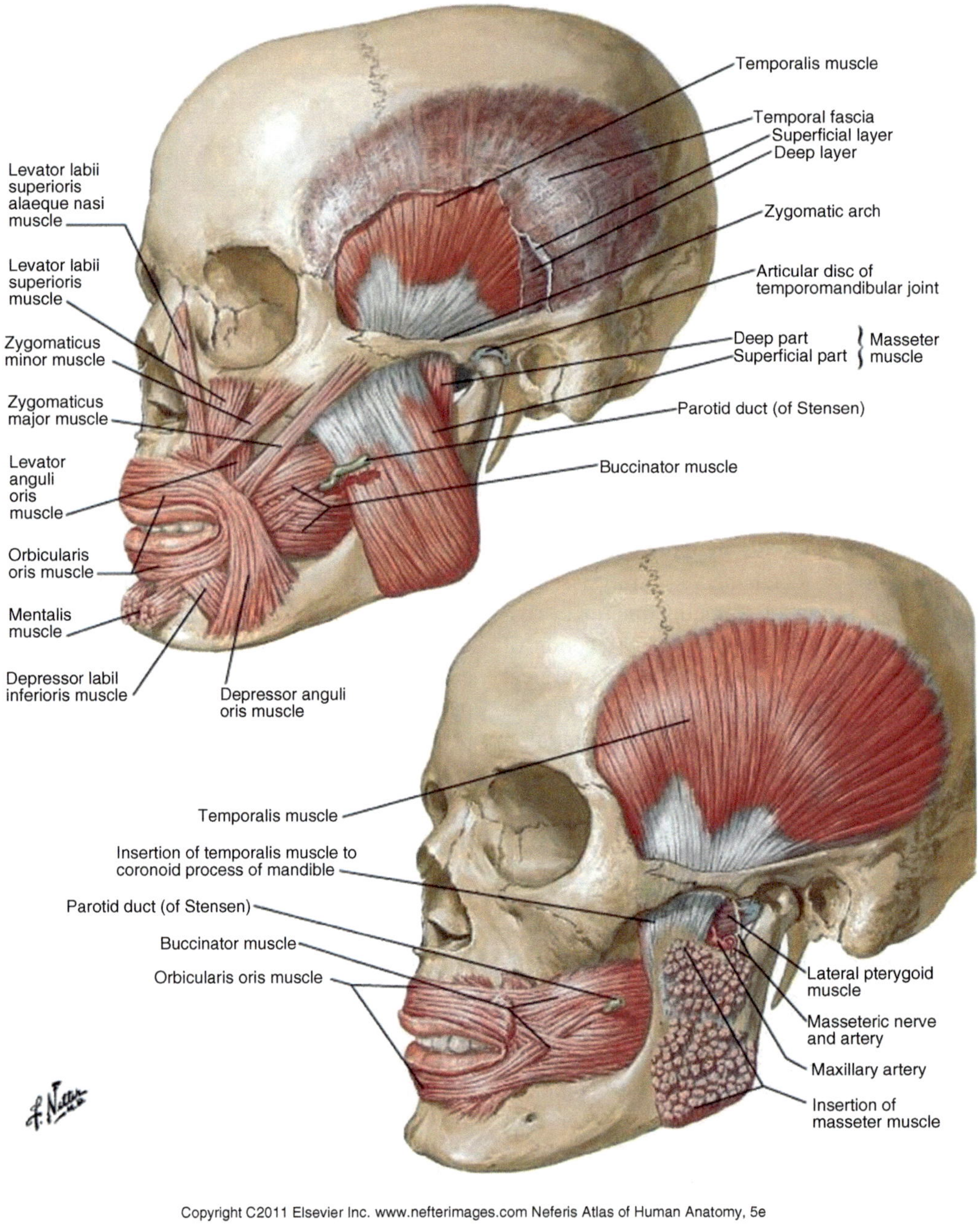

Copyright C2011 Elsevier Inc. www.nefterimages.com Neferis Atlas of Human Anatomy, 5e

Fig. 21.1 Anatomy of the temporalis muscle

vated from the muscle flap and passed along the upper and lower lid to the medial canthal ligament. With contraction of the TM, the fascial strips are pulled tight closing the eye. A disadvantage of this procedure is that movements of the eyelids are observable while chewing (Fig. 21.2b). We, therefore, prefer lid implants (platinum/iridium lid chain implants: Fig. 21.4b) for the upper lid and lateral tarsorrhaphy /canthopexy. A further disadvantage of the retrograde procedure is a contour deformity with a volume deficit (visible hollow) in the temporal fossa and a volume excess (muscle bulge) over the zygomatic arch [6]. We, therefore, prefer the much more widespread anterograde TM transfer [1, 2], where the TM is detached from its insertion, either at the bony

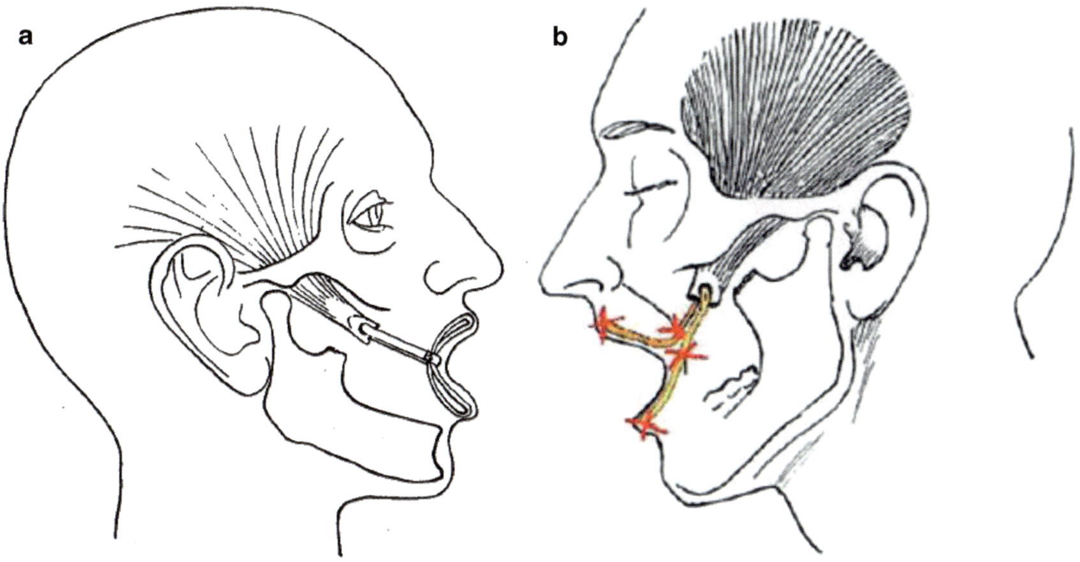

Fig. 21.2 Scheme of original temporal muscles transfer according to McLaughlin [1] in (**a**) and the presented modified procedure in (**b**) according to Exner and Kuhn [2]

insertion or with osteotomy of the coronoid process of the mandibule (Figs. 21.2 and 21.3).

As a further masticatory muscle, the masseter can be rotated and transferred either completely or partially to the mouth [9], but this can only lead to a limited degree of dynamic movement of the mouth region or a limited "smile" due to lack of force and muscle excursion. Therefore, a combined approach using both the TM (→upper lip and nasolabial fold) and the masseter muscle (→commissure and lower lip) has also been described. Further modifications of functional TM transfer with both dynamic and static components have been suggested by Olivari [4].

After the first descriptions by Gillies [8], about 20 years later McLaughlin [1] popularized the transposition of the temporal muscle in combination with fascia lata for reanimation of the paralyzed oral sling. More than six decades later, this procedure is still a highly effective and successful treatment strategy and should be considered as a component or an alternative in the toolbox of any surgeon treating facial nerve paralysis [2].

Since the first publication by McLaughlin, a number of modification have been introduced including extraoral, preauricular (Fig. 21.3), and enoral approaches [2–6].

The goal of the current chapter is to provide a didactic instruction in a step-by-step manner with practical tricks and guidance supported by anatomical and schemes as well as intraoperative pictures.

21.2 Anatomic Consideration

The temporalis muscle (TM) is one of the muscles of mastication (masseter, medial, and lateral pterygoid muscles) (Fig. 21.1). The origin of this broad and fan-shaped muscle is the temporal fossa as well as the temporal fascia. The muscle fibers descend deep to the zygomatic arch forming a tendon-like structure. The insertion of the TM is the coronoid process of the mandible, where the TM is the most powerful muscle of the temporomandibular joint. The TM is mainly supplied by the deep temporal arteries (anterior and posterior) arising from the maxillary artery. As one of the masticatory muscles the TM is responsible for elevation and retraction of the mandible. The TM is innervated by the deep temporal nerves arising from the mandibular nerve (trigeminal nerve; V3).

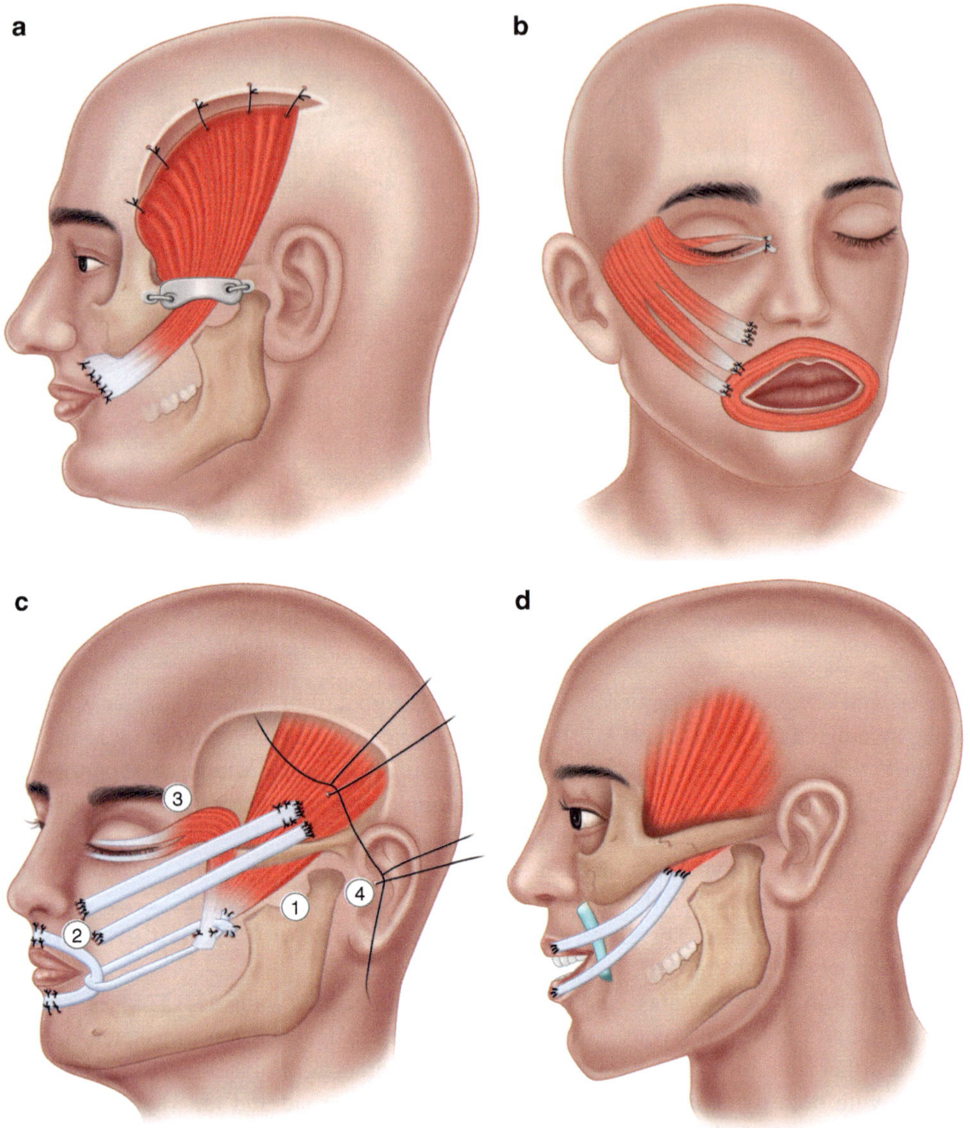

Fig. 21.3 Modifications of the muscle temporalis transfer. See the temporalis muscle lengthening procedure according to Labbé and Huault [3] in (**a**), the retrograde temporalis muscle transfer according to Rubin adapted from Olivari [4] (**b**), the combined technique or static and dynamic techniques according to Olivari [4] in (**c**) and the modified techniques of Greulich [5] using cartilage anchor in the nasolabial fold in (**d**)

21.3 Operative Technique of the Modified McLaughlin Temporalis Muscle Transfer: A Step-by-Step Instruction

For reanimation of the mouth region, McLaughlin initially suggested a two-step procedure with a perioral fascial sling and subsequent TM transposition [1] (Fig. 21.2a). This has been abandoned and, like others [2–6, 9, 10], we prefer a modified one-step approach (Fig. 21.2b). Before surgery, the functioning of the TM has to be controlled. Preoperatively, patients receive 500 mg metronidazole and 1.5 g cephazolin. Then we trace anatomical landmarks and structures like the (1) nasolabial crease, (2) the modiolus, (3) the midline as well as the (4) vermilion border between the lip and the adjacent normal skin as well as (5) the zygomatic arch and (6) localization of the coronoid process (Fig. 21.4a, b). After contralateral nasal intubation and intraoral block of the throat, we infiltrate the cheek and the periorbital region using local anesthetic solution with epinephrine (1:200,000) in case of patients with a partial facial nerve palsy; in patients with a complete facial nerve palsy we additionally use lidocaine.

If a preexisting scar (in contrast to the presented case; (Fig. 21.4a, c)) is not present, we use a typical preauricular facelift incision with preparation in the sub-SMAS plane. The skin flap should be elevated with a respective thickness not only due to skin perfusion, but also to avoid visible movements of the fascia lata. Furthermore, during flap elevation and tunneling it is of upmost importance to prevent injury of the parotid duct (Stenon-duct) as well of facial nerve branches in cases of partial facial nerve palsy. In the latter case, as mentioned above, we do not use infiltration solutions with local anesthetics. Furthermore, in these cases an extraoral approach to the coronoid process along the ascending branch of the mandibule is an alternative to the external approach.

After cheek skin flap elevation and sub-SMAS tissue preparation from the preauricular region below the zygomatic arch toward the coronoid process, we insert the nondominant hand of the surgeon into the mouth and open/close the mouth to palpate and verify the location of the coronoid process with the dominant hand. Then, the coronoid process is freed from surrounding tissue and Farabeuf or Langenbeck wound retractors are placed and the insertion of the temporal muscle as well as the incisura mandibulae are identified (Fig. 21.4c, d). Then, the point of the drill hole (3.2–3.5 mm) is defined in the center of the coronoid process: caudally to the tendon-like insertion of the TM and cranial to the plane of the incisura mandibulae. Before osteotomy two zero-vicryl sutures are inserted into the drill hole as safety threads to prevent cranial and deep retraction or sliding of the coronoid process due to the traction of the TM (Figs. 21.4c, d and 21.5b). After incision and deepithelialization of the nasolabial crease in a crescent-shaped fashion, both the upper and lower lips are tunneled toward the midline. Thus, a continuous tunnel between the zygomatic arch, the modiolus, and the lips is provided. Then, a chevron-like osteotomy is performed taking care not to splitter the coronoid process and not to damage the drilled hole (Figs. 21.5b and 21.6).

In the meantime, a second team harvests the fascia lata from the ipsilateral thigh. Depending on the respective facial dimensions or geometry of the patient, usually a length of approximately 25–30 cm with a width of 5–8 mm is recommended. Starting with an incision 3–4 cm cranial from the lateral edge of the patella, the fascia is harvested from distal to proximal with short multiple transverse incisions in a stepwise fashion using an atraumatic tendon stripper (Fig. 21.5a).

Basically, the idea behind the temporal muscle transposition is the mechanism of a pulley. The harvested fascia lata is pulled up to half the length through the drill hole of the coronoid process (Fig. 21.2b). Recently, we use the Mini-Tendon Shuttle (QuickPass Tendon Shuttle; Arthrex®; https://www.arthrex.com/products/AR-8090S) to help facilitate passage of the fascia lata through the drill hole (Fig. 21.6). This two-component device has (1) an elastic net to insert and fix the fascia lata working like a finger trap and (2) a flexible, but stable tip to pass the drill hole (Fig. 21.6a). Then, the most critical part is the positioning and fixation of the fascia lata. Both ends of the fascia lata are diverted to the incised nasolabial fold and corner of the mouth (Fig. 21.7a–c). The cranial check rein is fixated with deep non-resorbable monofile 3-0 and/or 4-0 sutures at the modiolus and the corium of the deepithelialized nasolabial crease. The corium in combination with the modiolus offers a stable anchorage. Others suggest harvest a cartilagineous strip from the ear and insert it subcutaneously in front of the nasolabial fold as cartilage anchor, both in free functional muscle transfer and in muscle transposition procedures [5] (Fig. 21.3d).

Then, with an appropriate traction at the caudal end of the opposite fascia lata, a cranio-lateral elevation of the corner of the mouth in overcorrection is established, i.e., approximately

6–8 mm above the resting position of the contralateral position of the corner of the mouth and nasolabial crease, respectively. In this position the caudal fascia lata sling is fixated in the same way as the cranial sling. Using the mini-tendon shuttle, both ends of the fascia lata are tunneled to the upper and lower lip, respectively. After skin incisions at the vermillion, these ends are fixated with the orbicularis oculi muscle sling with deep non-resorbable monofile 4-0 sutures (Figs. 21.7d and 21.8). Before extubation, 500 mg prednisolone administered intravenously. For safety reasons, i.e., risk of suture fistula and/or transmitted infections, we avoid extraoral incisions of the oral mucosa. Initially, these skin incisions and deep sutures may result in unaesthetic retractions, but will diminish if the sutures are placed deeply enough.

Since the nasolabial fold has been deepithelialized in a crescent-shaped pattern, wound closure will lead to an additional elevation of the angle of the mouth and nasolabial fold. The additional nasolabial incisions can be skipped in male patients due to occurrence of hair follicle cysts and ingrown stubbles.

The postoperative treatment includes antibiotics and antimicrobial mouth rinsing (e.g., hexetidine) as well soft food for 5–7 days. We start the exercises directly at the first postoperative evening. Using a hand mirror patients are instructed to clenching the teeth (molars) over a wooden spatula.

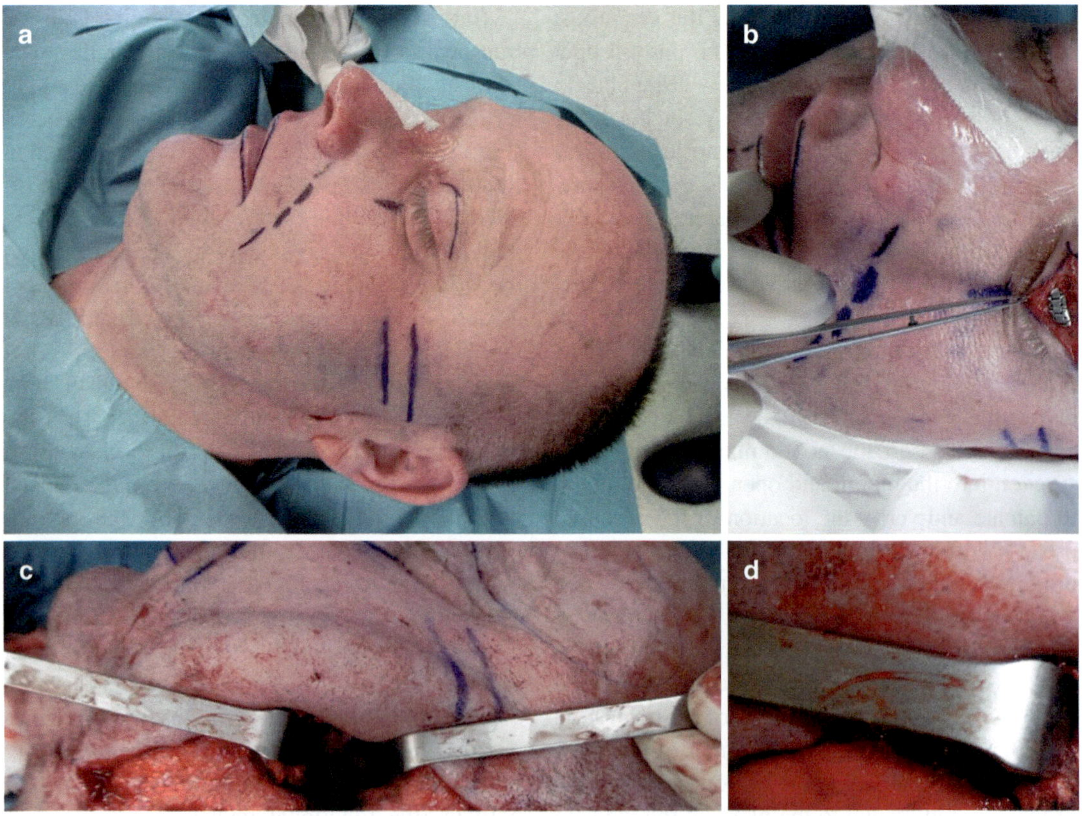

Fig. 21.4 Intraoperative images of the temporalis muscle transfer-*Part I*. Marking of anatomical landmarks (midline, nasolabial fold, modiolus, vermilion, zygomatic arch, and localization of the coronoid process) in (**a**). Platinum/iridium upper eye lid chain implant (weight: 1.2 g; size: 13.9 × 5.0 × 1.4 mm) in (**b**). Coronoid process freed from surrounding tissue in (**c**, **d**)

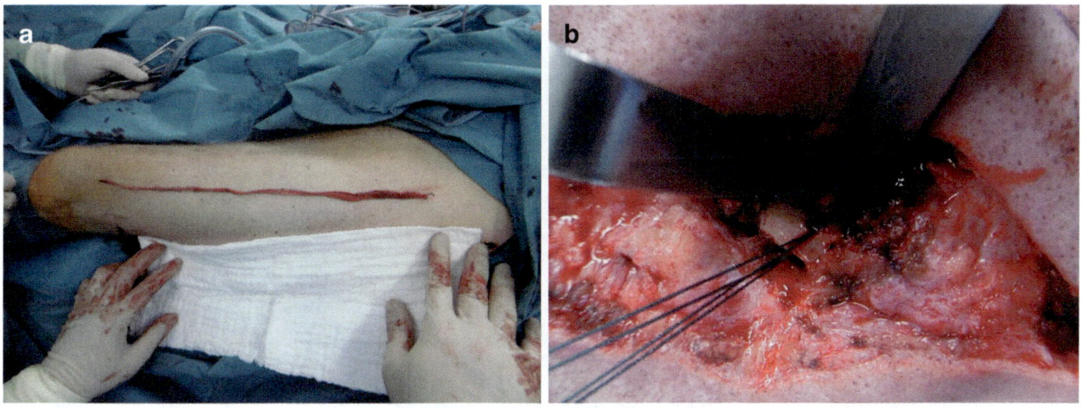

Fig. 21.5 Intraoperative images of the temporalis muscle transfer-*Part II*. Harvest of the fascia lata from the ipsilateral thigh in (**a**) and chevron-like osteotomy of the coronoid process with a drilled hole in (**b**)

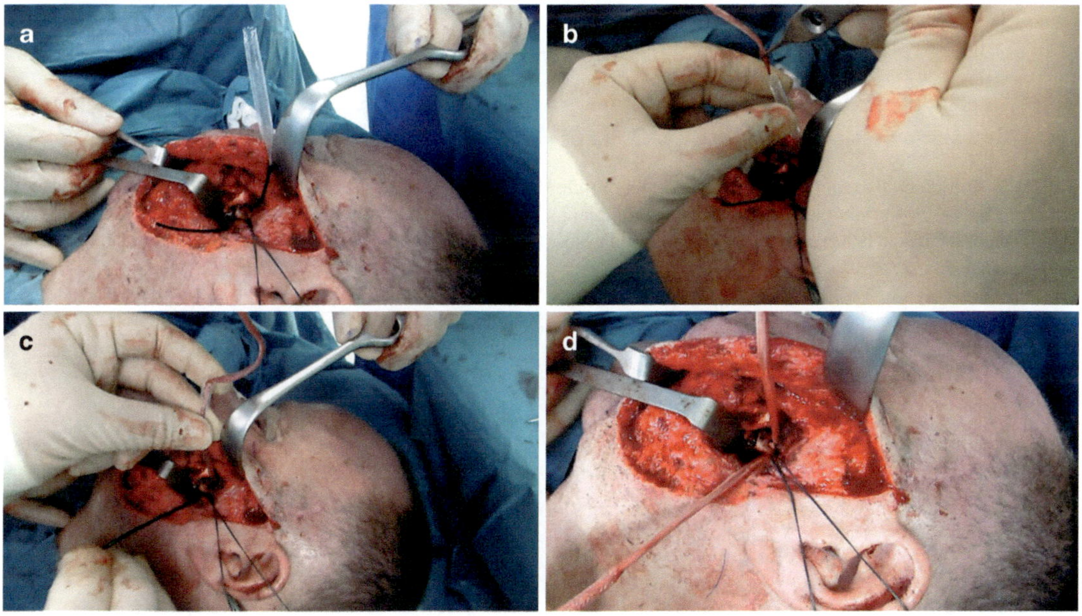

Fig. 21.6 Intraoperative images of surgical steps (**a–d**) of the temporalis muscle transfer-*Part III*. Use of a mini-tendon shuttle (QuickPass Tendon Shuttle; Arthrex®) to help facilitate passage of the fascia lata through the drill hole

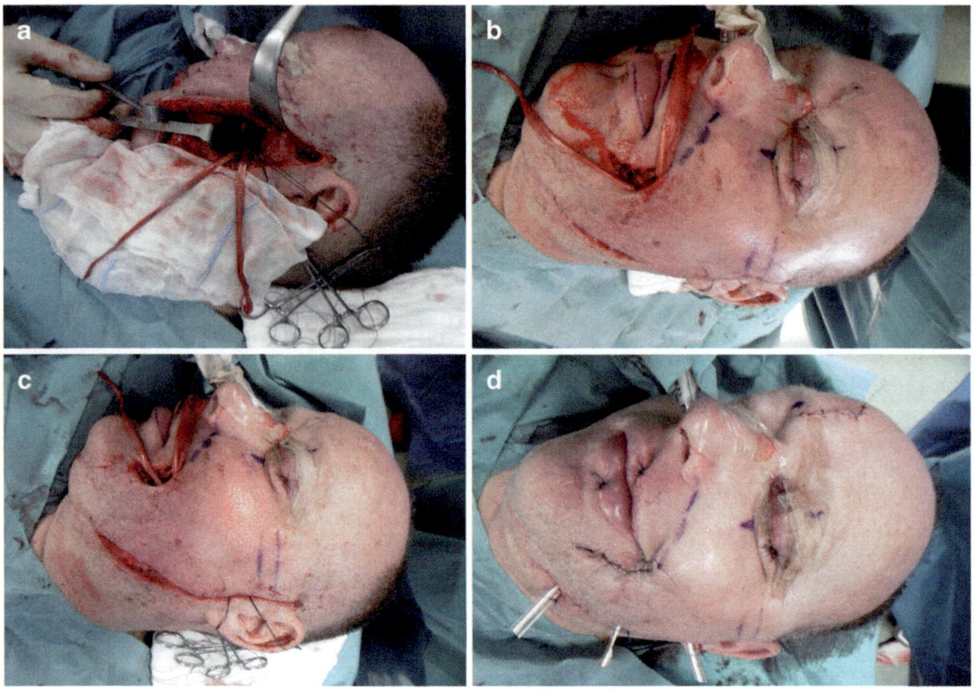

Fig. 21.7 Intraoperative images of the temporalis muscle transfer-*Part IV*. Positioning and fixation of the fascia lata. Both ends of the fascia lata are diverted to the incised nasolabial fold and corner of the mouth and are fixated with deep non-resorbable monofile sutures at the modiolus and the corium of the deepithelialized nasolabial crease (**a–d**)

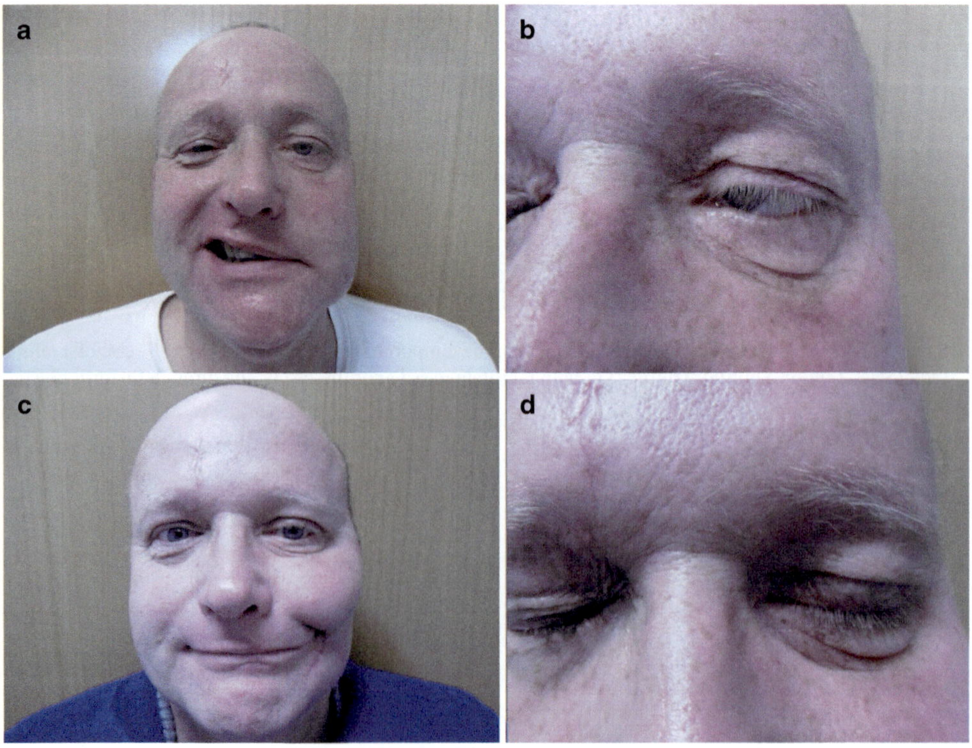

Fig. 21.8 Preoperative (**a**, **b**) and postoperative (**c**, **d**) pictures

21.4 Summary

After the first descriptions by Gillies, about 20 years later McLaughlin popularized the transposition of the temporal muscle in combination with fascia lata for reanimation the paralyzed oral sling. More than six decades later, this procedure is still a highly effective and successful treatment strategy and should be considered as a component or an alternative in the toolbox of any surgeon treating facial nerve paralysis. Since the first publication by McLaughlin, a number of modification have been introduced including extraoral, preauricular (Labbe, Greulich, Exner), and enoral approaches. The goal of the current chapter is to provide a didactic instruction in a step-by-step manner with practical tricks and guidance supported by anatomical and schemes as well as intraoperative pictures.

Advantages of temporalis muscle transfer for facial reanimation:

- One-stage procedure
- Short operation time
- Independent from patients age and duration of palsy
- Predictable surgical outcome
- Immediate effect
- Successful reconstruction of symmetry at rest and voluntary movements (smiling, oral contiguity, lid closure) without synkinesis
- Bridging the time during multi-staged free muscle transfer

Disadvantages of temporalis muscle transfer for facial reanimation:

- No involuntary, emotionally, emotionally-linked, and no spontaneous smiling
- Only one vector for reanimation

References

1. McLaughlin CR. Surgical support in permanent facial paralysis. Plast Reconstr Surg. 1953;11:302–14.
2. Exner K, Kuhn T. Gillies and McLaughlin's dynamic muscle support in irreversible facial palsy. Handchir Mikrochir Plast Chir. 2010;42(2):102–8.
3. Labbé D, Huault M. Lengthening temporalis myoplasty and lip reanimation. Plast Reconstr Surg. 2000;105(4):1289–97.
4. Olivari N. Practical plastic and reconstructive surgery: an atlas of operations and techniques. Heidelberg: Kaden Publishing; 2004.
5. Greulich M. The cartilage anchor--a helpful tool for precise control of the nasolabial fold. Handchir Mikrochir Plast Chir. 2010;42(2):90–4.
6. Pallua N, Bozkurt A. Nerve injuries in traumatic head injury: when to explore/suture/transplant? In: Pape H-C, Sanders R, Borrelli Jr J, editors. The polytraumatized patient with fractures. Berlin: Springer; 2011.
7. Frey M, Michaelidou M, Tzou CH, Hold A, Pona I, Placheta E. Proven and innovative operative techniques for reanimation of the paralyzed face. Handchir Mikrochir Plast Chir. 2010;42(2):81–9.
8. Gillies H. Experiences with fascia lata grafts in the operative treatment of facial paralysis. London: Proceedings of the Royal Society of Medicine; 1935.
9. Baker DC, Conley J. Regional muscle transposition for rehabilitation of the paralyzed face. Clin Plast Surg. 1979;6:317–31.
10. Rubin L. Temporalis and masseter muscle transposition. In: May M, editor. The facial nerve. New York: Thieme; 1986.

Lengthening Temporalis Myoplasty for Smile Reanimation: Labbé Technique

22

Daniel Labbé and Pierre Guerreschi

Key Points

- Dynamic reanimation.
- Pedicle muscle flap: Temporalis muscle is entirely mobilized.
- No aponeurotic material is required to lengthen the muscle transfer and to reach the labial commissure.
- Brain plasticity allows the muscle to change its function thanks to specific rehabilitation within 6 months in average.

22.1 Introduction

Facial paralysis sequelae can drive patients to isolation, unemployment, and/or depression [1]. The facial asymmetry observed at rest is aggravated by mimics. The management of facial paralysis sequelae remains a challenge for the surgeon. One of the mainstream technique use the temporalis muscle to reanimate the upper lip and the labial commissure.

Lengthening Temporalis Myoplasty (LTM), first described by Labbé in 1997 [2, 3], ensures the transfers of the entire temporalis muscle from the coronoid process to the upper lip without interposition of aponeurotic tissue. The pinnate nature of the temporal muscle allows the lengthening of its posterior fibers. The temporalis muscle, like all the other dynamic muscle transfers, changes its function because it is entirely mobilized towards another effector: the upper lip and the labial commissure. Thanks to brain plasticity [4], the muscle loses its chewing function and after 6 months of speech rehabilitation it acquires its new smiling function.

22.2 Preoperative Planning

The refined preoperative study of the patient's smile on the healthy side helps determine the respective insertions of the zygomatic muscles, superficial and deep elevator muscles of the upper lip and also helps refine the type of smile that needs to be achieved. We refer to the Rubin's classification of the three types of smiles [5]. A close examination of the smile on the healthy side can highlight the cutaneous insertions of the elevator muscles or the orbicularis oris that transmits the movements of elevator muscles. These cutaneous insertions are identified by a slight shadowed area on the white lip when smiling.

Electronic Supplementary Material The online version of this chapter (https://doi.org/10.1007/978-3-030-50784-8_22) contains supplementary material, which is available to authorized users.

D. Labbé
Plastic Surgery Department, Centre Hospitalier Privé Saint-Martin, Ramsay - Générale de Santé, Caen, France

P. Guerreschi (✉)
Plastic Surgery Department, University Hospital of Lille, Lille, France

© Springer Nature Switzerland AG 2021
C.-H. J. Tzou, A. Rodríguez-Lorenzo (eds.), *Facial Palsy*, https://doi.org/10.1007/978-3-030-50784-8_22

These key points will be reported onto the paralyzed side as a mirror image to locate precisely the anchor points of the temporalis muscle [6].

The nasolabial fold and its exact shape is designed by passively lifting up the upper lip and moving it backwards. This is performed when the patient is sitting down, then controlled again with the patient lying down.

22.3 Surgical Technique

1. The entire temporalis muscle is exposed by a zigzag Cairns approach (Fig. 22.1). The scalp flap is dissected in a subgaleal plane after hydrodissection with serum and adrenaline.
2. 2 cm above the orbital rim, the periosteal is incised and the dissection continues in a subperiosteal plan along the external orbital margin with a large periosteal elevator (Fig. 22.2). This elevator is then used to put the tissues in tension to help the splitting of the superficial aponeurosis of the temporalis muscle.
3. Passing through the two sheets of the superficial aponeurosis of the temporalis muscle is a key step to reach the zygomatic arch. The dissection goes through the two sheets of the superficial aponeurosis (Fig. 22.3) that contains the fat pad and the median temporal vascular pedicle. The fat must be left attached to the scalp flap. If this fat is left on the temporalis muscle side, it will impair the lowering of the muscle. Furthermore, this fat would be missing at the end of the surgery, creating an unsightly temporal notch as well as a curve above the zygomatic arch.
4. The retrozygomatic dissection frees the superficial side of the temporalis muscle from its insertions on the zygomatic arch. It is a subperiosteal dissection on the deep side of the zygomatic arch performed with a periosteal elevator (Fig. 22.4).

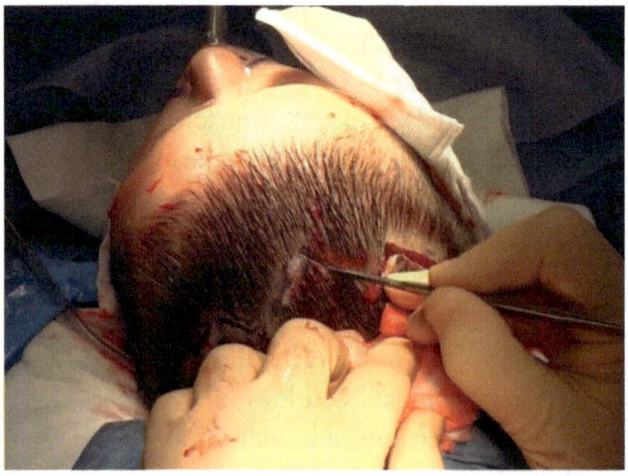

Fig. 22.1 Zigzag Cairns approach

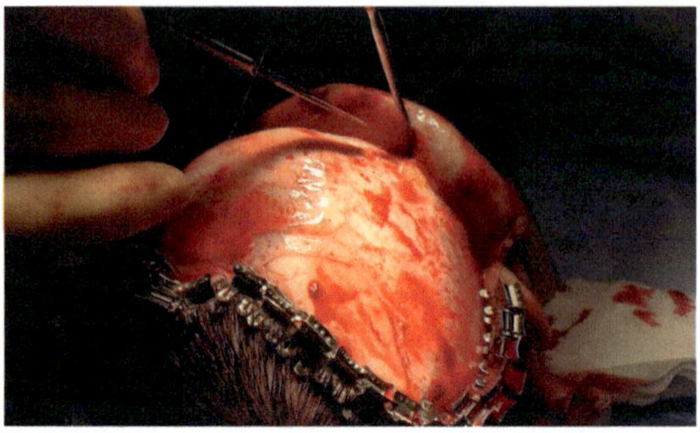

Fig. 22.2 Periosteal elevator on the orbital column

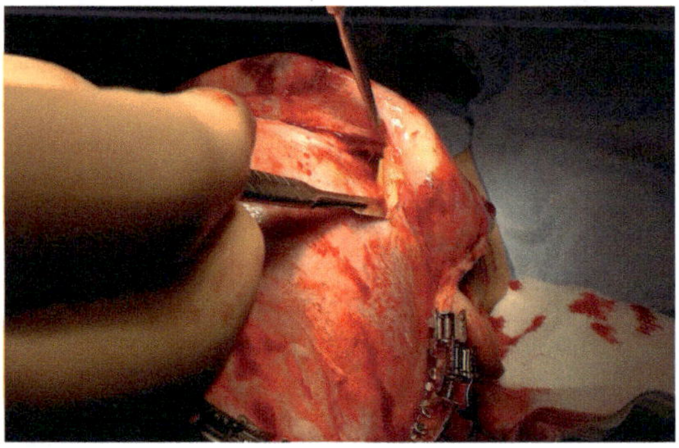

Fig. 22.3 Aponeurosis splitting

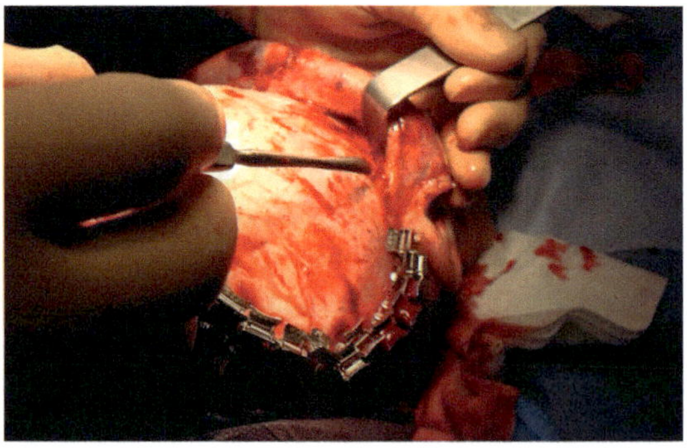

Fig. 22.4 Retrozygomatic dissection

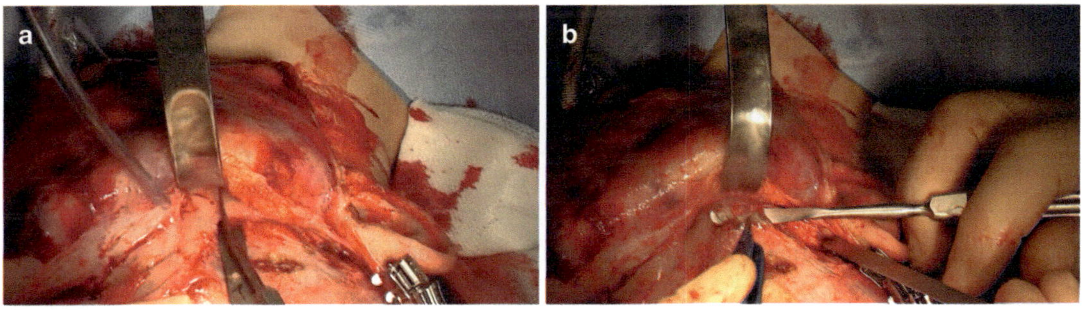

Fig. 22.5 (**a**) Zygomatic arch osteotomy. (**b**) Residual fibers of the masseter

5. The temporalis muscle is protected with a malleable retractor to perform the osteotomy of the zygomatic arch (Fig. 22.5a). The zygomatic arch is tilted backwards along with its masseter insertions. This gesture is completed by freeing the residual fibers of the masseter muscle (Fig. 22.5b)., inserted on the deep surface of the superficial aponeurosis of the temporal muscle.
6. After the subperiosteal dissection of the sigmoid notch, a malleable retractor is placed on the internal side of the upper branch of the mandible to perform the osteotomy of the coronoid process. An oblique osteotomy is performed backwards and forwards with a sagittal saw (Fig. 22.6). This mandibular bone fragment bears the insertions of the temporalis tendon.
7. The deep dissection progresses between the muscle and the skull using a periosteal elevator (Fig. 22.7). First the incision of the aponeurosis of the temporalis muscle has to leave a 5 mm strip of this aponeurosis inserted into the temporal crest to allow the reinsertion of the muscle at the end of the procedure. This step ends by a cautious dissection around the deep temporal pedicles.
8. Via the nasolabial approach, the anchor points on the upper lip are positioned according to the preoperative drawing. Commonly, three Prolene 4.0 sutures are tested during the procedure to ensure the correct shape of the smile (Fig. 22.8).
9. The dissection is then performed backwards above the superficial musculoaponeurotic system (SMAS) on 2 cm before plunging

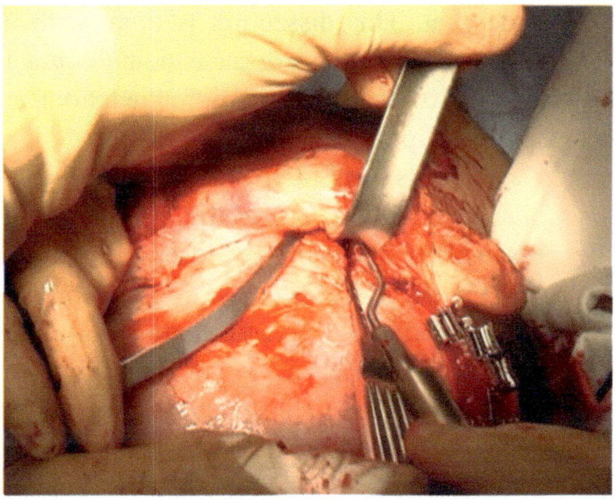

Fig. 22.6 Osteotomy of the coronid process

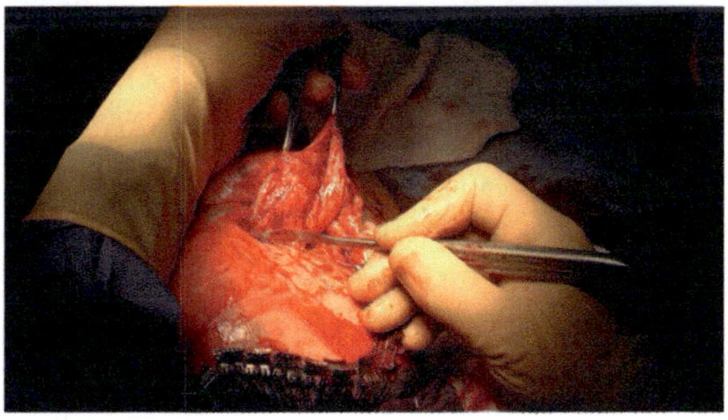

Fig. 22.7 Deep dissection of the temporal muscle

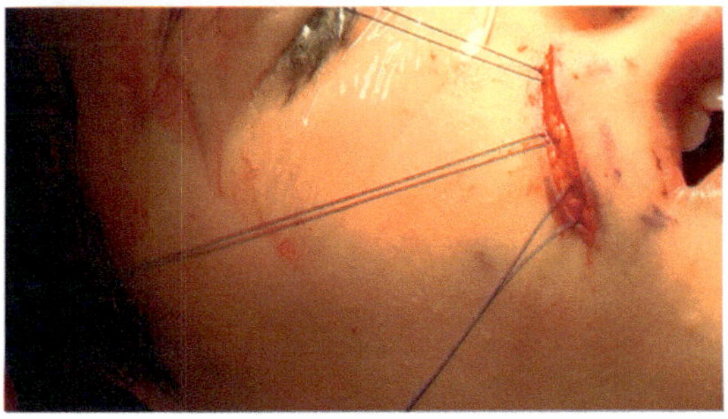

Fig. 22.8 Three anchor points on the upper lip

towards the buccal fat pad to reach the coronoid process (Fig. 22.9). The dissection is done with Mayo scissors without any section. The tunnel is enlarged in opening the Mayo scissors. Then the coronoid process is grasped, via this approach, with a Kocher forceps.

10. At this stage, it is normal for the temporalis muscle to resist. It is necessary to free the tendon of the temporalis muscle from its additional permanent insertions of the masseter and pterygoid muscles, which prevent its descent. This dissection is done with a large periosteal elevator at tendon's contact (Fig. 22.10). It allows to expose the tendon at the upper lip level.
11. The tendon is then seized with a Satinsky vascular clamp backwards of the coronoid process, which can then be freed from the tendon with a blade. The coronoid process is thrown away. The clamp is then partially released in order to stretch the tendon and then tightened again to hold the tendon before attaching it permanently to the key points with nonabsorbable threads (Fig. 22.11). The external fibers of the tendon correspond to the muscle fibers of the posterior part of the temporalis muscle. Reinserted preferably on the commissure, they help give a proper horizontal direction to the labial commissure traction vector. We pay attention not to wrinkle the skin and the tendon's insertion is secured with a running suture of 3.0 barbed thread.
12. Through the Cairns approach, the temporalis muscle is reinserted in the temporal area on the aponeurotic strip left in place in the anterior part of the temporal crest to obtain a symmetric result using separate Flexocrin 3.0 sutures (Fig. 22.12). The surgeon's assistant monitors the absence of elevation of the labial commissure during the fixation of the muscle on the temporal crest.
13. The smile-related outcomes of this new distal insertion are evaluated by stretching the upper-posterior part of the muscle or via electrical stimulation (Fig. 22.13) with a needle (20 Hz and 4 mA) as described by Har-

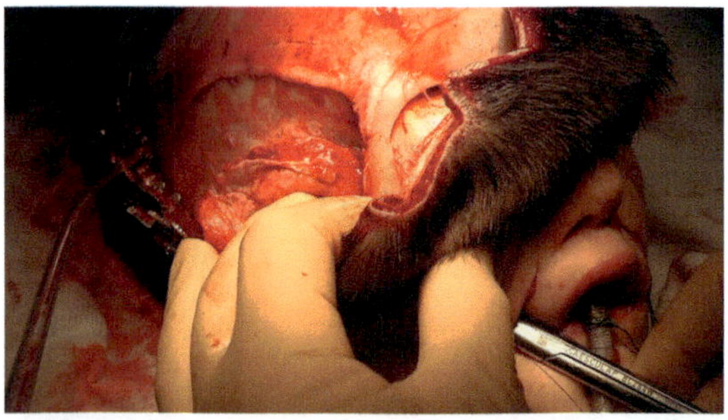

Fig. 22.9 Through the buccal fat pad

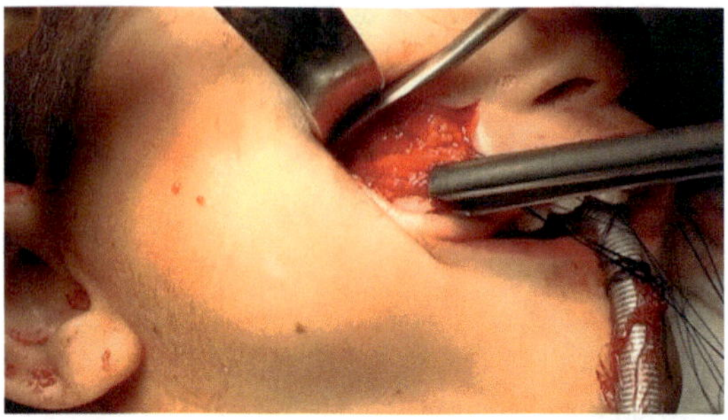

Fig. 22.10 Pulling the temporalis tendon

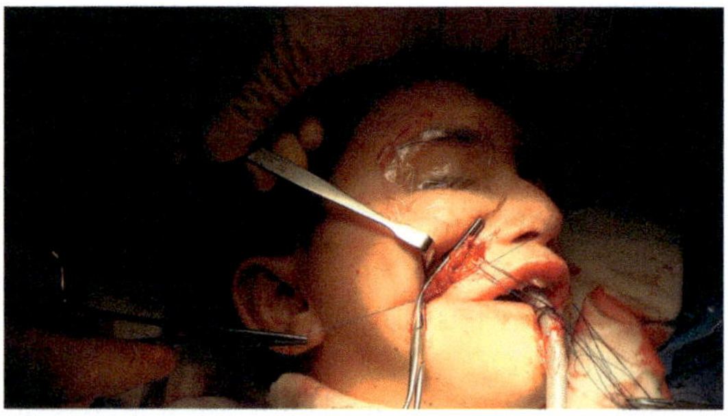

Fig. 22.11 Tendon reinsertion

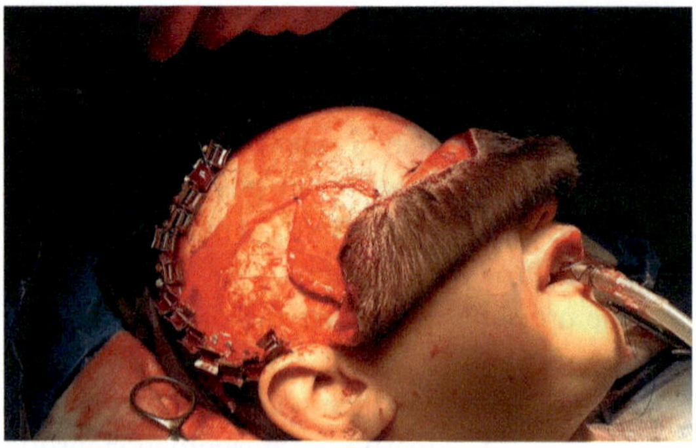

Fig. 22.12 Temporal reinsertion to the aponeurotic strip

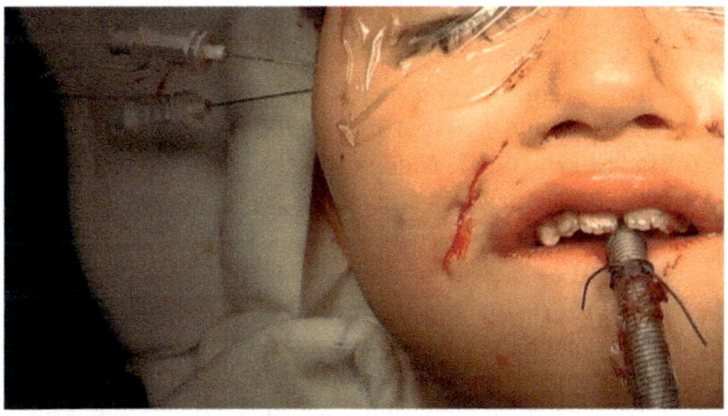

Fig. 22.13 Smile outcome tested

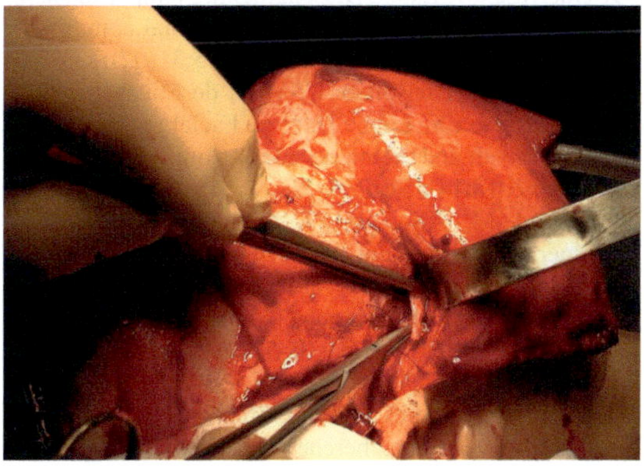

Fig. 22.14 Osteosynthesis of the zygomatic arch

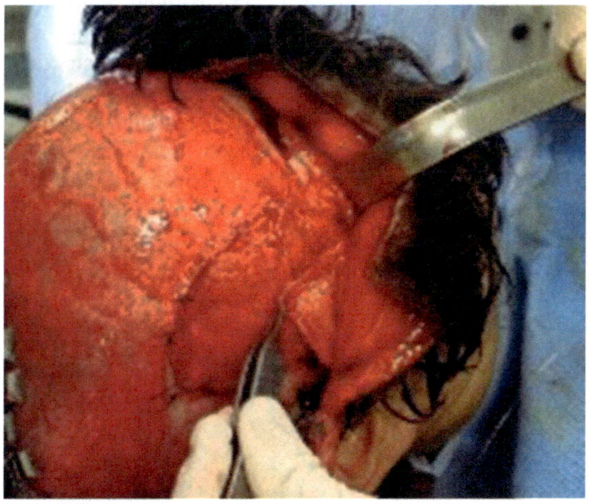

Fig. 22.15 Fat pad reinsertion

Shaï [7]. The posterior part of the muscle is refixed with loose sutures.

14. Osteosynthesis of the zygomatic arch with non-resorbable thread (Fig. 22.14).
15. It is essential to reinsert the fat pad from the split aponeurosis (Fig. 22.15) on the top of the temporal crest with a U-shaped suture to avoid the hollowing of the temporal area. Surgical closure while placing two silicon surgical drains, one in the transjugal opening and the other in the temporal area. Surgical closing of the scalp by staples, or resorbable sutures especially in children.

22.4 Rehabilitation

Lengthening temporalis myoplasty (LTM) requires a specific rehabilitation protocol in order to have perfect control of the muscle's new function via brain plasticity [8].

Rehabilitation can start before surgery to make the patient aware of the voluntary contraction of the temporalis muscle [9].

During the postoperative period, rehabilitation starts 3 weeks after the surgery; first with deep massages of the tendon insertion into the commissure to fight local adhesions. Afterwards, the patient follows a standardized protocol in three steps to move from a mandibular smile to a voluntary smile, and a spontaneous smile. The functional change of the temporalis muscle can be achieved step-by-step over a few months but only if the patient understands the stakes, is motivated and has a strong will to communicate [10].

The third step of the spontaneous temporal smile can be hard to achieve. The symmetric rehabilitation technique developed by Martin et al. aims at reinforcing cortical control of the smile [8]. To perform these rehabilitation exercises patients are placed in front of a computer mirror that reconstructs in real-time their face by symmetrically copying the healthy side and deleting the paralyzed one. Positive feedback reinforces brain plasticity capacities to "facialize" the temporalis muscle.

22.5 Conclusion

Labial commissure reanimation is one element of the complete therapeutic management of facial paralysis. As a matter of fact it is important to take into account the entire facial expression to propose a comprehensive project. Muscle overactivity, spasms, or synkinesis can affect the upper or lower level of the face on the paralyzed side and/or on the healthy side and must be treated [11–13].

Lengthening temporalis myoplasty is particularly relevant in the difficult treatment of peripheral facial paralysis, even in case of congenital bilateral facial palsy such as Moebius syndrome (Case 1: Data 1, Video 1). In one surgical procedure we can implement an active muscle transfer to reanimate the labial commissure and recreate a mobile nasolabial fold [14] (Case 2: Data 2, Video 2). This reliable and reproducible technique respects the donor site [15]. The passage of the temporal muscle under the zygomatic arch into the buccal fat pad ensures its sliding into the cheek avoiding any zygomaticomaxillary deformation.

References

1. Dey JK, Ishii M, Boahene KDO, Byrne PJ, Ishii LE. Changing perception: facial reanimation surgery improves attractiveness and decreases negative facial perception. Laryngoscope. 2013;124(1):84–90.
2. Labbé D. Myoplastie d'allongement du temporal et réanimation des lèvres. Note technique. Ann Chir Plast Esthet. 1997;42(1):44–7.
3. Labbé D, Huault M. Lengthening temporalis myoplasty and lip reanimation. Plast Reconstr Surg. 2000;105(4):1289–97. discussion 1298
4. Garmi R, Labbé D, Coskun O, Compère J-F, Bénateau H. Lengthening temporalis myoplasty and brain plasticity: a functional magnetic resonance imaging study. Ann Chir Plast Esthet. 2013;58(4):271–6.
5. Rubin LR. The anatomy of a smile: its importance in the treatment of facial paralysis. Plast Reconstr Surg. 1974;53(4):384–7.
6. Aljudaibi N, Bennis Y, Duquennoy-Martinot V, Labbe D, Guerreschi P. Lengthening temporalis myoplasty: virtual animation-assisted technical video. Plast Reconstr Surg. 2016;138(3):506e–9e.
7. Har-Shai Y, Gil T, Metanes I, Labbe D. Intraoperative muscle electrical stimulation for accurate positioning of the temporalis muscle tendon during dynamic, one-stage lengthening temporalis myoplasty for facial and lip reanimation. Plast Reconstr Surg. 2010;126(1):118–25.
8. Blanchin T, Martin F, Labbé D. Lengthening temporalis myoplasty: a new approach to facial rehabilitation with the "mirror-effect" method. Ann Chir Plast Esthet. 2013;58(6):632–7.
9. Guerreschi P, Labbe D. Lengthening temporalis myoplasty: a surgical tool for dynamic labial commissure reanimation. Facial Plast Surg. 2015;31(02):123–7.
10. Hembd A, Harrison B, CSM R, de Souza Rocha F, Chamseddin K, Labbe D, et al. Facial reanimation in the seventh and eighth decades of life. Plast Reconstr Surg. 2018;141(5):1239–51.
11. Risoud M, Aljudaibi N, Duquennoy-Martinot V, Guerreschi P. Long-term sequelae treatment of peripheral facial paralysis with botulinum toxin type A: repartition and kinetics of doses used. Ann Chir Plast Esthet. 2016;61(1):10–5.
12. Labbé D, Bénichou L, Iodice A, Giot J-P. Signe du Depressor Anguli Oris (DAO) dans les parésies faciales. Comment le rechercher et libérer le sourire (note technique). Ann Chir Plast Esthet. 2012;57(3):281–5.
13. Salles AG, da Costa EF, Ferreira MC, do Nascimento Remigio AF, Moraes LB, Gemperli R. Epidemiologic overview of synkinesis in 353 patients with longstanding facial paralysis under treatment with botulinum toxin for 11 years. Plast Reconstr Surg. 2015;136(6):1289–98.
14. Nduka C, Hallam M-J, Labbe D. Refinements in smile reanimation: 10-year experience with the lengthening temporalis myoplasty. J Plast Reconstr Aesthet Surg. 2012;65(7):851–6.
15. Panciera DT, Sampieri C, Deganello A, Danesi G. Lengthening temporalis myoplasty: objective outcomes and site-specific quality-of-life assessment. Otolaryngol Head Neck Surg. 2017;157(6):966–72.

Part IV

The Paretic Eye

23 Clinical Care from the Perspective of the Eye Doctor

Eva Stifter

Key Points

- First examination of patients with facial nerve palsy should be focused on establishing the underlying cause and ruling out severe neurological diseases.
- Lagophthalmos is defined as difficulties in or the impossibility to close the eyelids.
- Protection of cornea and ocular surface is crucial in all patients suffering from facial nerve paralysis.
- Therapy should take care for intensive eye lubrication, particularly during night.
- All ages may be affected.
- Management of the eye in patients suffering from facial nerve palsy needs to start early with medical and surgical techniques specifically tailored to the individual patient.

23.1 Background

Ocular protection is the main objective of optimized clinical care of patients with facial paralysis from the perspective of the eye doctor. Exposure keratopathy and corneal ulceration are potential complications of facial nerve palsy that should be prevented by optimized care of the eye as long as eyelid closure deficits are present [1, 2].

The facial nerve plays an important and dominant role in vivid communication and mimic expression of sensations in the human face. It is responsible for motor supply to the muscles of facial expression (*M. frontalis*, *M. orbicularis* oculi, *M. buccinator*, and *M. orbicularis* oculi) and stapedius, parasympathetic supply to the lacrimal and submandibular glands, and conveyance of sensory input from the anterior two-thirds of the tongue [2].

Facial paralysis may have numerous effects on facial expression and function, e.g. eyelid closure, oral continence, and speech. The orbicularis oculi muscle is the protractor of the eyelid. The eyelid retractors, the levator palpebrae superioris muscle of the upper eyelid, and the capsulopalpebral muscle of the lower eyelid oppose the actions of the orbicularis oculi muscle. Weakness of the orbicularis oculi muscle results in unopposed action of the eyelid retractors, lagophthalmos, and lower eyelid retraction with ectropion. This may lead to epiphora caused by eversion of the inferior lacrimal punctum, insufficient tear film protection, and increased corneal exposure. Blink rate and upper eyelid excursion are also typically compromised [1, 2].

A critical criterion for the intensity of ocular protection therapy is the absence or presence of Bell's phenomenon, which is the rolling up of the eye globe when efforts are made to close the

E. Stifter (✉)
Department of Ophthalmology, Medical University of Vienna, Vienna, Austria

© Springer Nature Switzerland AG 2021
C.-H. J. Tzou, A. Rodríguez-Lorenzo (eds.), *Facial Palsy*,
https://doi.org/10.1007/978-3-030-50784-8_23

lids. If Bell's phenomenon is missing, the risk of corneal injury is relevantly higher and more intensive corneal lubrication and protection is required [1].

Conclusively, patients with facial nerve palsy present typically with symptoms of an insufficient eyelid closure, dry eye, reduced corneal reflex, drooling, hyperacusis, altered taste, otalgia and speech articulation difficulties. In peripheral facial palsy, the missing innervation of facial muscles results in an inability to close the eyelids on the affected side appropriately. Impairment of the function of the facial nerve may thus severely reduce a patient's quality of life and irreversibly harm visual function of the affected eye by weakening eyelid closure and consequently increasing the risk of corneal infections due to less eye lubrication. Eye protection is therefore mandatory if lid closure is impaired [3, 4].

The sequelae range from poor cosmesis, simple eye irritation and epiphora to corneal ulceration and consequent blindness [1].

Lagophthalmos is defined as difficulties in or the impossibility to close the eyelids. Lid closure may be complete or incomplete and the degree of lagophthalmos can be measured in millimetres (mm) [5].

The major concern at the first presentation of a patient with facial nerve palsy should be focused on establishing the underlying cause and ruling out severe neurological diseases such as strokes or malignant tumours [4]. All ages may be affected. More female than male patients have presented with facial nerve paralysis in large evaluations of incidence [6].

Correct management within the first few days can effectively prevent long-term complications. After identifying the affected side, it is mandatory to evaluate if an upper motor neuron lesion is responsible for the facial weakness. A bilateral innervation of that part of the facial nuclei supplying the forehead, and consequently preserving forehead movement in the upper motor lesions is described in classic neurology. However, this sign has been considered unreliable. By contrast, a lower motor neuron disorder of the main nerve trunk results in weakness of the entire side of the face [4, 7].

The steps recommended to be taken at the initial check-up are a complete clinical neurological status investigation, brain magnetic resonance imaging (MRI), and an extensive evaluation of the general cardiovascular risk factors for stroke. This is of highest importance because an urgent referral to a specialized neurological care unit is needed to assess the need for thrombolysis for all patients suspected of having had a stroke attack. From the ophthalmological side, checks of the patients' visual acuity, pupillary reaction, ocular motility and visual field function to reveal neuro-ophthalmological deficits, which are important to rule out a possible different diagnosis, are recommended. These are baseline examinations, not requiring much time or specific equipment.

The risk factors for stroke include age over 60 years, arterial hypertension, diabetes, high cholesterol levels, smoking habits, any history of previous stroke or transient ischaemic attacks and atrial fibrillation. A full evaluation of the function of the other cranial nerves as well as the peripheral nervous system is also recommended, including testing tone, limbal weakness, hyperreflexia, upgoing plantars and sensory loss [4, 8].

When an upper motor neuron lesion is suspected, it is helpful to determine whether it is located in the brainstem or cerebral cortex. Brainstem disease may present with vertigo, ataxia or crossed neurology signs such as ipsilateral cranial nerve involvement, which may lead to paralytic strabism and diplopia, and sensomotoric contralateral hemiplegia. A cortical lesion often presents with weakness of the contralateral limbs. By contrast, involuntary movements of the face, such as spontaneous smiling, may be spared. All these symptoms have to be considered carefully for correct planning of the diagnosis and consequent therapeutic approaches [4, 8].

During this first-line check-up after the initial diagnosis of facial nerve palsy, an extensive eye evaluation of the globe and the periocular region is helpful to clarify the full extent of the symptoms and should include complete testing of visual function, including a standardized evaluation of visual acuity at a near and far distance and a basic neuro-ophthalmological check.

Slit-lamp examinations of the anterior and posterior eye segment are basic for further evaluation including measurement of the intraocular pressure. Eyelid malposition and eyelid closure deficits should be quantified precisely and compared with the fellow-eye for long-term follow-up.

Orthoptic motility testing to ascertain the oculo-motor function of the cranial nerves NIII oculomotorius, NIV trochlearis and NVI abducens is needed to rule out paretic strabismus, which may be combined with diplopia. In children, paretic strabismus can cause irreversible amblyopia and therefore requires special care and amblyopia treatment. In cases of combined cranial nerve deficiencies, intense evaluation of the pupillary reaction of both eyes, any presence of pupillary abnormalities and screening even for distinct anisocoria is also strongly recommended.

Where a stroke is suspected, a perimetric visual field test is important to rule out significant scotomas. As an alternative for patients with poor general health status, a basic confrontation perimetry can be quickly performed, without technical equipment, and is nevertheless of high relevance for further neuro-ophthalmological diagnosis if there is a typical quadrant or hemifield visual field loss or significant constriction of the visual field of the affected or contralateral eye.

Fundus examination with dilated pupils may reveal retinal disease as well as diabetic long-term co-morbidities. Evaluation of the optic disc can reveal signs of increased intracerebral pressure causing a swelling of the optic nerve that requires further examination. All tests have to be specifically orientated to the clinical symptoms of the individual patient to avoid missing important clinical information at the beginning relevant for correct disease management as well as any therapy if necessary.

As soon as a central cause for the facial palsy has been excluded, a focused examination of the ears, mastoid area, oral cavity, scalp and parotid glands should be initiated [2, 4].

The facial nerve is considered to be special among all cranial nerves because of its long tight bone canal that traverses the temporal bone with only little room for swelling. When inflamed, a compressive neuropathy may manifest with a reversible or irreversible nerve dysfunction [2].

Bell's palsy is the most common neurologic condition affecting the cranial nerves and is defined as an idiopathic lower motor neuron facial nerve paralysis that accounts for most of the newly diagnosed cases and shows no specific changes during extensive check-ups. However, Bell's palsy remains a diagnosis of exclusion. The complete medical evaluation should be undertaken mindfully that 30–41% of patients with lower motor neuron facial nerve weakness will have another underlying cause that requires specific management and is often associated with a poorer long-term prognosis [4, 7, 9].

Typically, Bell's palsy becomes fully acute within 24–48 h. Most cases are associated with mild postauricular pain. Its incidence does not significantly differ with sex or ethnicity. Diabetes is associated with as many as 10% of cases. In pregnancy, Bell's palsy is seen typically in the last trimester. It may also be associated with a herpes simplex virus infection causing a benign self-limiting inflammatory condition [2].

Incomplete facial nerve paralysis at presentation with some residual muscle movement activity and partial closure of the eyelid is considered a good prognostic sign for full recovery. Oral steroids should be started within 72 h of first presentation to significantly increase the chance of a complete recovery [2, 4, 10].

The recommendation for clinical diagnosis of Bell's palsy is a systemic evaluation of all five branches of the facial nerve representing five anatomic zones: (1) the temporal and frontal (forehead), (2) the zygomatic (upper midface, oral commissure), (3) the buccal (cheeks and nasolabial region), (4) the marginal mandibular (lower face and oral depression), and (5) the cervical (neck). True Bell's palsy encompasses all five nerve branches. However, they may be variably involved during the first 72 h, resulting in a typically flaccid face from the hairline to the clavicle [2]. Bilateral or recurrent facial paralysis

Table 23.1 List of possible causes of facial paralysis

Idiopathic Bell's palsy
Trauma
Herpes zoster
Congenital
Tumour
Benign lesions
Diabetes
Infection/Otitis media
Lyme disease
Acoustic neuroma resection/surgery
Iatrogenic accident/injuries

is rarely associated with Bell's palsy. Extensive evaluation is mandatory [2].

The possible causes of facial paralysis are summarized in Table 23.1 [2, 6, 7].

Independent of the underlying cause of the facial palsy, which may be idiopathic or result from trauma, surgery or malignant disease, the reduced or absent function of the orbicularis oculi muscle results in exposure of the cornea and may be exacerbated by an eyelid malposition [5]. By contrast, in central facial palsy, the *M. frontalis* and the *M. orbicularis* oculi are supplied supranuclearly by both hemispheres of the brain so that their function is normally not reduced and eyelid closure unaffected. Consequently, ocular protection is predominantly needed in lower motor neuron facial palsy cases.

Bacterial infections are responsible for 1–4% of new cases of lower motor neuron facial palsy. Acute otitis media accounts for most and is typically associated with systemic sepsis, a bulging tympanic membrane, conductive hearing loss and pinna lateralization. Malignant otitis externa may affect the external auditory canal and the tempory bone. Typically, the infection begins as an external otitis that may progress into an osteomyelitis of the temporal bone. These cases are characterized by a lack of sleep due to otalgia and are more likely to be seen in patients who are older, immunocompromised, or have poorly controlled diabetes. The condition may be associated with *Pseudomonas aeruginosa* infections and requires microbiological testing [2].

Lyme disease from a tick bite is a bacterial infection that can result in facial nerve palsy in one of 10 seropositive patients. Serological tests are recommended if Lyme disease is suspected. While positive Lyme titres may be helpful for diagnosis, negative or equivocal results in an endemic area showing typical Lyme symptoms may justify empiric antibiotic therapy with doxycycline even when there was no tick bite reported in medical history. Lyme-associated facial paralysis has a relevantly high rate of bilaterality in contrast to Bell's palsy. Normally it arises in the second phase of Lyme disease, several weeks or months after the initial tick bite. Additionally, cardiac abnormalities and neurologic symptoms including meningitis may occur [2].

Other conditions that may present with bilateral facial paralysis include rare autoimmune diseases such as Guillain-Barré syndrome (GBS), Melkersson–Rosenthal syndrome (MRS) and sarcoidosis. Although rare GBS is a serious autoimmune disorder in which the immune system attacks healthy nerve cells in the peripheral nervous system. This may lead to symptoms of weakness, numbness or tingling, and can eventually cause ascending paralysis that may involve some or all of the cranial nerves. In these cases, analysis of cerebrospinal fluid is recommended, which may show elevated protein levels without pleocytosis and specific ganglioside autoantibodies. The cause of this condition is still unknown, but it is typically triggered by an infectious illness such as severe gastroenteritis or a respiratory infection. With intensive neurological medical care, symptoms usually evolve over several weeks and recover over the next 4–6 months [2].

MRS is a neurological disorder characterized by recurrent, long-lasting swelling of the face, particularly of one or both lips (granulomatous cheilitis), recurrent and alternating facial palsy and a fissured tongue. Some affected individuals have all three of these features and others only one or two. Granulomatous cheilitis can be diagnosed by lid biopsy [2].

Neurosarcoidosis occurs in only 5–15% of all patients with sarcoidosis. It may manifest in an unusual manner and involves three cranial nerves resulting in anosmia (NI), facial palsy (NVII) and hearing loss (NVIII). When cranial nerve dysfunction occurs, it is critical to take neurosarcoidosis into consideration. Laboratory tests should include an evaluation of angiotensin-converting enzyme (ACE) and lysozyme. In addition, a chest X-ray is necessary to identify hilar lymphadenopathy. If conjunctival nodules are revealed, a tissue biopsy of the conjunctiva under local anaesthesia can be helpful to obtain histological proof of the suspected diagnosis [2, 11].

A test for the rheumatoid factor (RF) and antinuclear antibodies (ANA) is useful to rule out rheumatological diseases such as rheumatoid arthritis and lupus erythematosus. If the chronic autoimmune disease Sjögren syndrome is suspected, Sjögren-specific antibodies (SS-A/Ro and SS-B/La) should be included in the blood test [2].

A slow progressive onset of facial weakness is suggestive of cancer. However, the presence of pain or partial hemifacial paralysis may also suggest tumour disease, even when the onset of symptoms is fast, mimicking Bell's palsy. The patient's anamnesis needs to be rigorously checked for any history of regional cancer. In addition, a thorough examination of the head and neck region is necessary to look for cervical lymphadenopathy, in particular a parotid mass or a scalp lesion. The following imaging should be organized for further evaluation as soon as a clinical suspicion of tumour disease emerges: Computed tomography (CT) of the temporal bone and parotid area as well as magnetic resonance imaging (MRI) with and without gadolinium of the brain and the internal auditory canal, with special attention to the entire course of the facial nerve [2, 4].

Acoustic neuromas are known to account for about 80% of cerebellopontine angle lesions and most cases of tumour-related lower motor neuron facial palsy. These cases differentiate from other causes with ipsilateral sensorineural hearing loss and the absence of the corneal reflex sensitivity, which has also to be checked routinely during the ophthalmic check-up [4]. A combination of inadequate Bell's phenomenon, corneal anaesthesia and severe dry-eye syndrome should be aggressively managed with high-frequency lubricating eye care, consequent closure during the night and frequently performed eye checks to prevent corneal complications [1].

Iatrogenic or postsurgical infections may be sequelae of any tumour resection in the anatomic course of the facial nerve including parotid tumours and acoustic neuromas, but can also result from other surgery in the face in general, or after rhytidectomy (face-lift surgery). Traumatic causes such as temporal bone fractures or soft tissue injuries to the facial nerve should also be taken into consideration and are important for estimating the anticipated duration of the paralysis itself [2].

Facial weakness is less likely in children than in adults to be due to Bell's palsy. Therefore, urgent paediatric referral is required for children, who need extensive general paediatric and subsequent neuro-paediatric evaluation to establish the possible causes of the facial paralysis. Congenital abnormalities have to be carefully considered in new-born babies and differentiated from birth-related disorders. However, rarer causes including thalidomide toxicity, syphilis (Treponema pallidum), mononucleosis (Epstein–Barr virus), otitis media, CHARGE syndrome (including coloboma, heart defect, atresia choanae, retarded growth, genital hypoplasia, and ear anomalies with/without deafness), Moebius syndrome (i.e. rare complete congenital facial paralysis combined with paralytic strabismus due to cranial nerve paralysis), craniofacial microsomia and oculo-auriculo-vertebral dysplasia must also be ruled out [2, 12].

The major complications of untreated exposure keratopathy are corneal and conjunctival lesions related to dryness and infection. Pain and dry-eye symptoms such as foreign body sensations may be caused by an impaired blinking reflex. Prevention of exposure keratopathy is paramount to avoid corneal breakdown, irreversible scarring, and permanent visual loss or impairment because significant exposure keratopathy may be complicated by reduced corneal sensitivity leading to neurotrophic corneal ulceration. Intensive lubricating local therapy with eye drops and ointment of various viscosities is therefore mandatory to prevent serious eye complications. Cosmetic deformities from enduring epiphora, paralytic ectropion and eyelid retraction may impair a patient's quality of life and should always be addressed with special care.

23.2 Basic Assessment by the Eye Doctor

An extensive eye examination should be performed in all patients with facial palsy at initial diagnosis (see Table 23.2). Subsequent short-term controls should be planned for each patient individually at least every one to two weeks depending on the clinical course of the palsy. Daily controls may be needed if the corneal complications are severe and corneal perforation is likely.

Initially, an extensive medical history is required including information about the onset and duration of symptoms, visual performance of both eyes before facial palsy occurred, any history of previous eye diseases, eye surgery, trauma, use of contact lenses, long-term eye medication, and relevant allergies against eye therapy

Table 23.2 Overview of the recommended eye examinations in all patients with facial palsy

Anamnesis	Acute symptoms	Onset and duration of ocular symptoms and eyelid closure deficiency
		Dryness
		Epiphora
		Pain
		Redness
		Signs of inflammation
		Additional systemic or neurological disease
		Photophobia
		Functional deficits
	Medical history	Previous eye disease(s)
		Visual acuity on both eyes in youth respectively before the onset of facial palsy
		Previous ocular or eyelid surgery
		Previous trauma of eyelids or bulbus
		Previous demand for medication or eye drops
		Systemic diseases including cancer, diabetes
		History of severe or recurrent herpes simplex or herpes zoster of the face, eye or ear
		History of Lyme borreliosis or other infectious diseases
		Any allergy (particularly against eye medication and antibiotics)
		History of regional cancer
Inspection	Lid closure deficit	Extent of lagophthalmos at normal and forced lid closure attempts
	Upper and lower eyelid position	Ectropion (eversion of the eyelid away from the eye globe)
		Upper and lower eyelid retraction
		Attenuate blink with decreased excursion of the upper eyelid
	Bell's phenomenon	Up-rotation of the eye bulb at lid closure attempts for better lubrication of the cornea, absence is defined as a poor prognostic sign for the risk of epithelial corneal injury
	Ocular motility	Additional neurological symptoms
	Pupillary reaction	
	Lacrimal apparatus	Decreased tear production (Schirmer's tests)
		Lacrimal punctum malposition
Visual acuity examination	Best-corrected visual acuity	Evaluation of distance and near vision
Slit-lamp examination	Conjunctiva	Signs of dryness
	Cornea	Epithelial defects
		Corneal staining with fluorescein
		Corneal and limbo corneal scars

Table 23.2 (continued)

	Extensive tear film evaluation	Break-up time, staining, eversion of the lower lacrimal punctum
	Anterior chamber	Signs of uveitis or previous eye diseases
Photographic documentation	Slit-lamp images	Corneal pathologies for follow-up, combined with fluorescein staining in cases of corneal epithelial defects
Corneal sensitivity	Corneal anaesthesia	Deficiency indicative of acoustic neuroma
Microbiological swaps	Eyelids and conjunctiva	In cases of sever conjunctivitis and corneal ulcer
		Before onset of local antibiotic therapy
Intraocular pressure		Baseline and recurrent measurements during corticoid therapy mandatory to rule out secondary glaucoma and cortisone response
Fundus examination		Optic nerve evaluation
		Macula and peripheral retina
		Rule out diabetic retinopathy
		Retinal vessels

or antibiotic agents [5, 13]. The mode of onset of symptoms may be helpful to distinguish between viral palsy (with typically acute onset) and malignancy (which normally progresses slowly) [2]. Visual acuity in the near and far distance has to be assessed as it is a very sensitive marker for corneal changes [1]. To target therapy, the cause of the facial palsy has to be identified. The most common infectious causes include a history of herpes zoster or Lyme disease and require serological blood tests.

Infection with the varicella-zoster virus may cause geniculate ganglionitis with a prodrome of otalgia and vesicular eruption within the ear canal, which may spread to the oral cavity (*herpes zoster oticus*). Facial paralysis may follow the prodromal symptoms and is then called Ramsay Hunt syndrome (RHS), which is associated with sensorineural hearing loss and in 40% of cases vertigo owing to the involvement of the seventh cranial nerve (NVIII). It has to be considered that patients with RHS have a poorer long-term prognosis: only 21% of patients recover fully after 12 months of disease. In cases of RHS, oral steroid therapy should always be combined with antiviral acyclovir or valaciclovir therapy. Additional systemic analgesic medication may be needed because of the possible development of herpes zoster neuritis [2, 4].

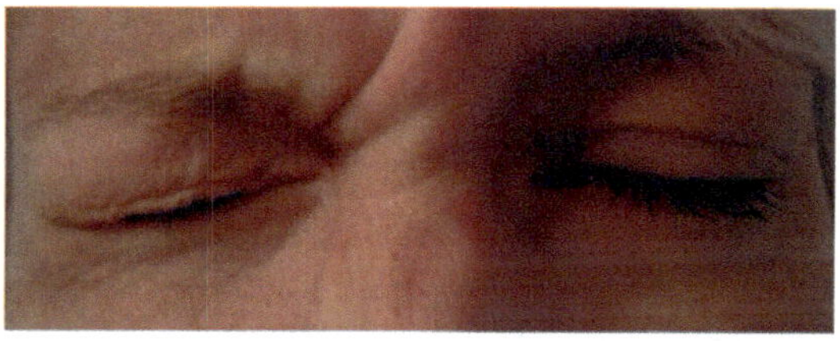

Fig. 23.1 Forced lid closure with peripheral facial palsy on the patient's left side. Note the relevantly less intense muscle action causing skin folds compared with the healthy right fellow-eyelids

The orbicularis oculi muscle strength should be fully examined in a blink attempt and with forced eye closure while the face is in repose. Forced lid closure activity is essential during inspection of the patient's active lid closure ability to evaluate the amount of lagophthalmos. With peripheral facial palsy and clinically relevant lagophthalmos, the lid rim may stay wide open. In cases of partial difficulty in closing the lids, the eyes lashes stay more visible compared with the healthy side (Fig. 23.1).

Cases of unilateral facial paralysis are ideal for comparison with the unaffected contralateral side/eye. As a systemic approach, starting with the wrinkling of the forehead is recommended, which should be evaluated semi-quantitatively. Then the brow should be examined for ptosis and the upper eyelid for the degree and strength of lid closure as well as for lagophthalmos, each of these evaluations has to be quantified and compared with the unaffected fellow-eye. Lagophthalmos should be checked in the upright and supine body position, especially after lid loading surgery [2].

In paretic lagophthalmos, upper eyelid retraction may be observed because of the levator muscle being unopposed by the paralysed orbicularis oculi muscle. The lower eyelid may show paralytic retraction and ectropion. Both findings can increase the risk of exposure keratopathy and should be thoroughly evaluated [2]. All reported symptoms of ocular surface irritation have to be noted precisely including burning sensations, redness, tearing, sticky secretions, or foreign body sensations. This is important for follow-up of the efficacy of lubrication therapy as pain sensations and ocular surface irritation are sensitive indicators for insufficient local therapy and care [5]. Corneal sensation and staining should be quantified to assess dry-eye syndrome and exposure keratopathy. The Schirmer test may be used to quantify the watery component of tear production. Slit-lamp examination is mandatory to diagnose corneal thinning or corneal ulceration early [2].

In all cases of lagophthalmos, an eye examination is also intended to exclude eye diseases other than peripheral facial palsy. Incomplete eyelid closure during sleep may be physiologic if the patient is showing normal and symmetrical forced eyelid closure when awake. A mechanic reason for lagophthalmos may be any extensive growing of the eye bulbus itself as in congenital glaucoma (called buphthalmos), high axial myopia or extensive staphyloma. Therefore, measurement of intraocular pressure and fundus examination preferably with dilated pupils is recommended for all eye assessment examinations in patients with facial palsy.

The presence of adequate Bell's phenomenon has to be meticulously examined and documented for follow-up evaluations [1].

Corneal exposure may be caused by substantial lid defects after trauma, surgery or radiation therapy leading to scar-induced ectropium of the eyelids. These defects are permanent. Surgical therapy has to be considered early.

Exophthalmos caused by Graves' disease is one of the most frequent different diagnoses and is characterized by significant lid retraction and a permanent eye closure deficit. Laboratory evaluation of thyroid antibodies and the thyroid-stimulating hormone (TSH) is useful to diagnose thyroid eye disease. This is a condition in which the eye muscles, eyelids, tear glands and fatty tissues behind the eye become inflamed. The eyes and eyelids may become red, swollen and uncomfortable. This diagnosis has to be ruled out during ophthalmic check-ups because a totally different therapy is needed [2]. Diabetic eye complications also have to be ruled out by ophthalmoscopy in all routine eye checks because of its high prevalence in patients with facial nerve palsy [12].

Establishing whether patients are following good ocular hygiene cleaning the eyelids regularly with clear water at least two times daily is strongly recommended. This is of high clinical relevance because bacterial blepharitis may significantly increase the risk of severe infectious complications of the cornea [1]. The function of the contralateral eye should also be assessed because patients with pre-existing monocular vision have to be treated more aggressively to preserve their stronger functioning single eye. Regular eye checks are recommended to prevent ocular complications as well as to follow recovery and continuously adapt ocular therapy to the patient's individual needs. Photographs may be valuable for documentation purposes.

The clinical grading system of cornea, asymmetry, dynamic function and synkinesis (CADS), which was developed to grade and evaluate measurements of ophthalmic sequelae in patients with facial nerve paralysis, is based on four different aspects of functional and morphological deficits: the corneal status, static facial asymmetry, dynamic function and synkinesis are semi-quantitatively assessed to facilitate objective evaluation and follow-up of patients suffering from facial nerve paralysis. Absent corneal sensation and absent Bell's phenomenon are included as negative prognostic indicators. Low tear production with Schirmer's test values of 5 mm or less may be considered. Monocular vision on the affected eye can be assessed as well [2, 14].

23.3 Prognosis

In general, recovery from facial paralysis varies greatly and is strongly influenced by the cause and completeness of paralysis at initial presentation. Idiopathic Bell's palsy is expected to recover spontaneously several weeks after onset but salvage may take more than 3–6 months. In these patients, no long-term surgical intervention is needed and they may fully recover their facial function [2]. Therefore, ocular protection is only needed until the blink rate is normal again and complete lid closure is achieved during the day and during sleep.

An evaluation of the clinical course of 2500 patients with facial nerve paralysis found that 94% of patients with initially partial facial paralysis achieved full functional recovery. By contrast, only 61% of patients with dense and more flaccid paralysis achieved full functional recovery. However, it should be kept in mind that 4% of the patients with partial recovery suffered from severe complications. Older patients and those with diabetes, hypertension, postauricular pain, impairment of corneal sensitivity and taste had a poorer long-term prognosis [2, 7].

Patients suffering from RHS secondary to the varicella-zoster virus also had a generally poorer prognosis with just 50% achieving a complete recovery. Only 21% of these patients were found to regain their full facial function, whereas 24% had severe sequelae and 4% recovered no function at all [2]. Recovery after tumour and trauma is often disappointing. In many tumour cases, surgical removal of the tumour necessitates sacrificing the facial nerve for surgical success causing a permanent and complete facial paralysis that requires nerve grafting for surgical facial nerve rehabilitation [2].

23.4 Ocular Therapy

After a comprehensive basic ophthalmic assessment, management of the eye in patients suffering from facial nerve palsy needs to start early with medical and surgical techniques specifically tailored to the individual. Initial therapy should focus on corneal lubrication by intensive application of artificial tear drops and lubricant ointment, preferably free from conservative agents. To prevent ulceration or dehydration of the cornea, artificial tears should be applied every 1–2 h during waking hours, depending on the severity of ocular surface disease. Preservative agents such as benzalkonium chloride used in artificial tear drops may cause a severe local allergy reaction as well as significant irritation of the ocular surface, particularly if long-term use is needed, and should therefore be avoided. Artificial tears with preservative agents may also have significant toxic effects on the corneal epithelium if used more than 3–4 times a day. Tear drops free from preservative agents have been shown to be safe for more frequent application [1, 2, 4, 5].

In cases of severe ocular surface disease, more viscous solutions and lubricant eye gels and creams may be an option. However, the disadvantage of blurry vision during the day has to be taken into account. If possible, lubricant ointment should only be applied during sleep at night to avoid a disturbance of normal vison during the day. Adding an artificial tear ointment during sleep may further protect the eye when it is most vulnerable [13].

As long as eyelid closure is deficient, intensive therapy including covering the eye during night with a central transparent shield fixed with a plaster, comparable to an adhesive moisture chamber, is mandatory. Its correct application is shown in Fig. 23.2. The intention is to provide

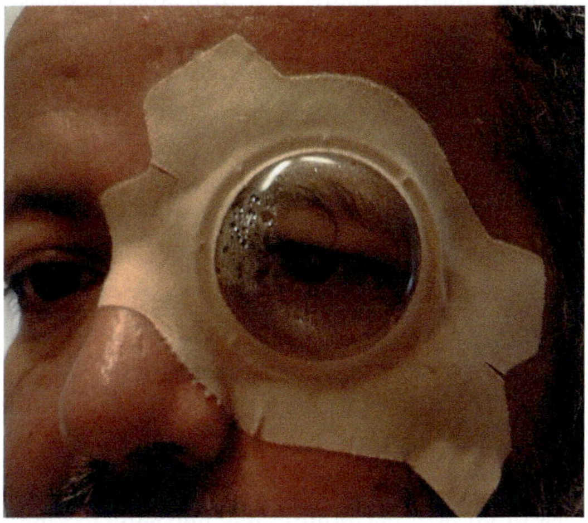

Fig. 23.2 Correct application of a protective plaster for creating a humid chamber

a humid chamber for effective protection of the eye surface against dryness. A thin strip of eye gel or ointment including vitamin A for increased epithelial healing should be applied to the lower eyelid fornix before covering the eye. Simply patching the affected eye is not sufficient because of the tendency for the eyelid to open under the patch due to the force of the unopposed levator muscle. Direct contact of the ocular surface to the patch may result in painful erosion [2].

Taping the eyelids for lid closure using skin-friendly plaster stripes should only be considered if a specially designed plaster with a central transparent shield is not available or not tolerated because of skin irritation. There is a high risk of inadequate closure when the ointment may interfere with the adhesion of the plaster stripe tape, exposing the cornea to irritation from the tape itself. Therefore, plasters building a moisture chamber should generally be preferred over direct taping of the lids [1, 2]. Scleral contact lenses providing a precorneal tear reservoir and protecting the cornea may be an alternative to tarsorrhaphy. These special contact lenses work as a liquid bandage to protect the cornea from eyelid interaction and exposure in addition to improving vision [15].

A special problem is an additional lack of corneal sensitivity in patients with facial nerve palsy. Corneal sensitivity is the primary factor for preserving the corneal epithelium intact and it initiates the blink reflex. A failure to maintain corneal integrity results in neuropathic keratopathy including degenerative changes in the cornea and conjunctiva. Patients with facial paralysis and an anaesthetic cornea are at an even greater risk for developing a corneal disorder because an inability to completely close the eyelids leads to chronic exposure, severe dry eye, keratitis and finally a permanent loss of clarity. One surgical option for unilateral cases is direct corneal neurotization using the contralateral supratrochlear or the supraorbital nerve as the donor sensory nerve, which may be performed in combination with facial reanimation procedures [16, 17]. In cases of corneal ulceration, there is always a high risk of corneal perforation and subsequent endophthalmitis with severe inflammation of the vitreous and complete loss of visual function.

Scheduling ophthalmic consultations at short intervals is mandatory for all patients with eye irritation, clinical symptoms or visual loss. It is particulary important for patients with concurrent corneal anaesthesia because the pain sensation may be missing as a leading symptom of severe ocular complications.

23.5 Surgical Management

In patients who will have permanent facial paralysis, for example after parotid tumour resection or due to vestibular schwannoma, surgical management may be considered early. More conservative treatment is typically warranted in patients with acute Bell's palsy or possible neuropraxia following surgery [1].

As soon as the ocular surface has been stabilized by the initial lubrication therapy, surgical treatment options may be considered depending on the severity and persistence of the eyelid malposition and ocular status. Surgical management for ocular protection can be divided into procedures that involve the entire eyelid complex, or the upper and lower eyelids separately [1].

The decision for surgical intervention should always be taken after exhaustive consideration of the cause of the palsy, the degree of neurological impairment, the patient's age and general medical condition, and the clinical setting available [2]. Temporary or permanent tarsorrhaphy are options as well as upper eyelid weight placement to treat eyelid retraction. Tarsorrhaphy is the traditional approach for surgical ocular protection. The palpebral fissure is shortened and the exposed ocular surface reduced. It is an effective procedure but can obscure peripheral vision and is cosmetically unappealing. Although tarsorrhaphy is intended to be reversible, notching, ectropion, trichiasis and epithelial cysts are possible complications. Therefore, tarsorrhaphy should not been attempted as a first-line approach but may be necessary where other methods of ocular protection have failed [1].

Gold or platinum implants for upper eyelid loading are valuable options for paralytic lagophthalmos treatment. The benefits of the implant technique are its reversibility and that eyelid loading can be performed under local anaesthesia. In patients with pre-existing paralytic lagophthalmos, weights may be taped to the upper eyelid to determine the appropriate weight resulting in a maximum eyelid closure while minimizing visually significant ptosis. The weight may be placed through a supratarsal lid crease incision, underneath the orbicularis oculi muscle, secured to the tarsal plate with partial thickness bites approximately 2–5 mm from the lid margin. Gold and platinum weights are both relatively biologically inert and generally well tolerated. However, although rare, complications can arise including local inflammation, capsule formation, infection, migration, extrusion, induced corneal astigmatism, ptosis and cosmetic bulge deformity when the implant is placed in a pretarsal position. As platinum density is higher than gold, platinum implants are relevantly thinner and are more cosmetically appealing in the pretarsal position [1, 18]. To minimize the risk of extrusion, the lid loading implant can be covered by the aponeurosis of the levator palpebrae muscle or a fascia lata graft [18, 19]. Nevertheless, the number of revision surgeries is relatively high.

Eyelid magnets are currently in the development stage. In future they could be taped to the upper and lower eyelid and implanted to improve eyelid closure, independent of gravity in the upright and supine body position. This should be an improvement compared with gold and platinum implants. Because of the impaired blink rate and residual lagophthalmos, particularly present in the supine position, gold weight implants can in fact worsen corneal exposure in the supine position [2].

Lengthening of the levator palpebrae superioris muscle using a fascia lata graft may also be used to achieve eye closure [1, 20].

For lower eyelid retraction, medial and/or lateral canthoplasty may be performed with and without a middle lamellar spacer for optimum repositioning of the eyelid. Midface suspension is a surgical alternative. The intention is always fast protection of the ocular surface and maintenance of corneal integrity by optimizing the eyelid position [1, 5].

Brow ptosis can lead to skin rubbing against the cornea and shedding of brow cilia directly on the ocular surface. Paralytic brow ptosis with a significant brow asymmetry requires powerful lifting because there is no frontalis function to assist. Browpexy or a direct brow lift may be considered as well as brow suture suspension [2].

Alternative rehabilitation methods include physical therapy with facial retraining exercises, transcutaneous electrical stimulation, biofeedback and acupuncture. Botulinum toxin A injections may be used to reduce facial muscle contractures, synkinesis and hemifacial spasm. Chemo-denervation of the levator palpebrae superioris muscle can be used to induce temporary ptosis to protect the cornea. Transconjunctival injection of low-dose botulinum toxin into the lacrimal gland has been described to be successful in reducing excessive tearing often associated with gustation [2, 21–23].

23.6 Summary

Damage to the eye is the most serious functional injury that may result from facial nerve impairment. Facial nerve palsy has a severe impact on a patient's quality of life. One of the most clinically relevant sequelae is the risk of corneal surface disease with the potential risk of blindness caused by deficient eyelid closure, insufficient eye lubrication and infectious complications. Therefore, all patients suffering from facial paralysis should be referred for ophthalmological diagnosis and early therapy for ocular protection. Moreover, extensive diagnostic evaluation and prompt diagnosis may be lifesaving in some patients with facial nerve paralysis.

References

1. Bhama P, Bhrany AD. Ocular protection in facial paralysis. Curr Opin Otolaryngol Head Neck Surg. 2013;21(4):353–7. https://doi.org/10.1097/MOO.0b013e32836239cf.
2. MacIntosh PW, Fay AM. Update on the ophthalmic management of facial paralysis. Surv Ophthalmol.

2019;64(1):79–89. https://doi.org/10.1016/j.survophthal.2018.06.001.
3. Coulson SE, O'Dwyer NJ, Adams RD, Croxson GR. Expression of emotion and quality of life after facial nerve paralysis. Otol Neurotol. 2004;25(6):1014–9.
4. Masterson L, Vallis M, Quinlivan R, Prinsley P. Assessment and management of facial nerve palsy. BMJ. 2015:351.
5. Sohrab M, Abugo U, Grant M, Merbs S. Management of the eye in facial paralysis. Facial Plastic Surg. 2015;31(2):140–4. https://doi.org/10.1055/s-0035-1549292.
6. Hohman MH, Hadlock TA. Etiology, diagnosis, and management of facial palsy: 2000 patients at a facial nerve center. Laryngoscope. 2014;124(7):E283–93. https://doi.org/10.1002/lary.24542.
7. Peitersen E. Bell's palsy: the spontaneous course of 2,500 peripheral facial nerve palsies of different etiologies. Acta Otolaryngol Suppl. 2002;549:4–30.
8. Donnan GA, Fisher M, Macleod M, Davis SM. Stroke. Lancet. 2008;371(9624):1612–23. https://doi.org/10.1016/s0140-6736(08)60694-7.
9. Baugh RF, Basura GJ, Ishii LE, Schwartz SR, Drumheller CM, Burkholder R, Deckard NA, Dawson C, Driscoll C, Gillespie MB, Gurgel RK, Halperin J, Khalid AN, Kumar KA, Micco A, Munsell D, Rosenbaum S, Vaughan W. Clinical practice guideline: Bell's palsy executive summary. Otolaryngol Head Neck Surg. 2013;149(5):656–63. https://doi.org/10.1177/0194599813506835.
10. Sullivan FM, Swan IR, Donnan PT, Morrison JM, Smith BH, McKinstry B, Davenport RJ, Vale LD, Clarkson JE, Hammersley V, Hayavi S, McAteer A, Stewart K, Daly F. Early treatment with prednisolone or acyclovir in Bell's palsy. N Engl J Med. 2007;357(16):1598–607. https://doi.org/10.1056/NEJMoa072006.
11. Loor RG, van Tongeren J, Derks W. Multiple cranial nerve dysfunction caused by neurosarcoidosis. Am J Otolaryngol. 2012;33(4):484–6. https://doi.org/10.1016/j.amjoto.2011.10.019.
12. Burk A, Burk R. Blauer Teil. Lider. In: Burk A, Burk R, editors. Checkliste Augenheilkunde. 5th ed. Leipzig: Georg Thieme Verlag; 2014. https://doi.org/10.1055/b-002-94105.
13. Burk A, Burk R. Grauer Teil. Ophthalmologische Basisuntersuchung. In: Burk A, Burk R, editors. Checkliste Augenheilkunde. 5th ed. Leipzig: Georg Thieme Verlag; 2014. https://doi.org/10.1055/b-002-94105.
14. Malhotra R, Ziahosseini K, Litwin A, Nduka C, El-Shammah N. CADS grading scale: towards better grading of ophthalmic involvement in facial nerve paralysis. Br J Ophthalmol. 2016;100(6):866–70. https://doi.org/10.1136/bjophthalmol-2015-307167.
15. Weyns M, Koppen C, Tassignon MJ. Scleral contact lenses as an alternative to tarsorrhaphy for the long-term management of combined exposure and neurotrophic keratopathy. Cornea. 2013;32(3):359–61. https://doi.org/10.1097/ICO.0b013e31825fed01.
16. Elbaz U, Bains R, Zuker RM, Borschel GH, Ali A. Restoration of corneal sensation with regional nerve transfers and nerve grafts: a new approach to a difficult problem. JAMA Ophthalmol. 2014;132(11):1289–95. https://doi.org/10.1001/jamaophthalmol.2014.2316.
17. Terzis JK, Dryer MM, Bodner BI. Corneal neurotization: a novel solution to neurotrophic keratopathy. Plast Reconstr Surg. 2009;123(1):112–20. https://doi.org/10.1097/PRS.0b013e3181904d3a.
18. Yu Y, Sun J, Chen L, Liu L. Lid loading for treatment of paralytic lagophthalmos. Aesthet Plast Surg. 2011;35(6):1165–71. https://doi.org/10.1007/s00266-011-9740-x.
19. Lessa S, Nanci M, Sebastia R, Flores E. Treatment of paralytic lagophthalmos with gold weight implants covered by levator aponeurosis. Ophthal Plast Reconstr Surg. 2009;25(3):189–93. https://doi.org/10.1097/IOP.0b013e3181a13d72.
20. Pirrello R, D'Arpa S, Moschella F. Static treatment of paralytic lagophthalmos with autogenous tissues. Aesthet Plast Surg. 2007;31(6):725–31. https://doi.org/10.1007/s00266-007-0074-7.
21. Chen N, Zhou M, He L, Zhou D, Li N. Acupuncture for Bell's palsy. Cochrane Database Syst Rev. 2010;(8):Cd002914. https://doi.org/10.1002/14651858.CD002914.pub5.
22. de Carvalho VF, Vieira APS, Paggiaro AO, Salles AG, Gemperli R. Evaluation of the body image of patients with facial palsy before and after the application of botulinum toxin. Int J Dermatol. 2019. https://doi.org/10.1111/ijd.14414.
23. van Landingham SW, Diels J, Lucarelli MJ. Physical therapy for facial nerve palsy: applications for the physician. Curr Opin Ophthalmol. 2018;29(5):469–75. https://doi.org/10.1097/icu.0000000000000503.

24 Oculoplastic Techniques and Gold Weight Implant

Bernardo Hontanilla

24.1 Correction of Lagophthalmos

Gold eyelid implants are designed for the gravity-assisted treatment of the functional defects of lagophthalmos resulting from facial paralysis. Placing a weight on the upper eyelid to increase the effects of gravity to close the upper eyelid is a very useful procedure for the patient with eye symptoms resulting from exposure and drying of the cornea. This surgical procedure has been established as a treatment for lagophthalmos [1–3]. However, various problems beset this technique, even though it frequently provides adequate symptom relief [4, 5]. For aesthetic purposes, the gold weight should not be visible when the eye is open. If the portion of the upper eyelid containing the tarsal plate is not exposed when the eye is open, the bulge of the weight will not be visible, giving pleasant aesthetic results. Nevertheless, the placement of the gold weight close to the border of the upper eyelid favors better closure of the eye despite worse aesthetic results and frequent extrusion of the implant. The optimum weight is selected by attaching a trial gold weight or a sizing weight to the upper eyelid of the patient with an adhesive tape and observing the eyelid closure.

The minimum weight that will bring the upper lid within 2–4 mm of the lower lid should be chosen [4]. However, in almost 30% of cases, the choice of the gold weight implant is inappropriate to cause the closure of the eye after its definite placement on the tarsal plate [9]. The reason could be the high position of the gold weight on the tarsal plate. This placement implies a different angle between the vertical line and the axis of the weight when it is placed on the outside of the skin of the upper eyelid (as performed in the trial) as opposed to being laced inside on the tarsal plate (final location after surgery). These two different outcomes might be caused by the different anatomical angles that influence the force acting on the weight in the upper eyelid when the head of the patient is in a vertical position (Fig. 24.1, left).

The force of an object falling obeys the following formula: mg (in which m is the mass and g is the gravity). If an object falls at an angle, the formula is as follows: $mg\cos\alpha$ (Fig. 24.1, left). If we match both forces when the upper eyelid falls with the gold weight on the skin surface in the trial and on the tarsal plate after the surgery, the formula is as follows: $m_1g\cos\alpha = m_2g\cos\beta$, in which m_1 is the weight of the gold implant located in the tarsal plate, α is the angle between the vertical axis and the implant on the tarsal plate, m_2 is the estimation of the implant weight placed on

B. Hontanilla (✉)
Department of Plastic, Aesthetic and Reconstructive Surgery, Clínica Universidad de Navarra, Pamplona, Spain
e-mail: bhontanill@unav.es

© Springer Nature Switzerland AG 2021
C.-H. J. Tzou, A. Rodríguez-Lorenzo (eds.), *Facial Palsy*,
https://doi.org/10.1007/978-3-030-50784-8_24

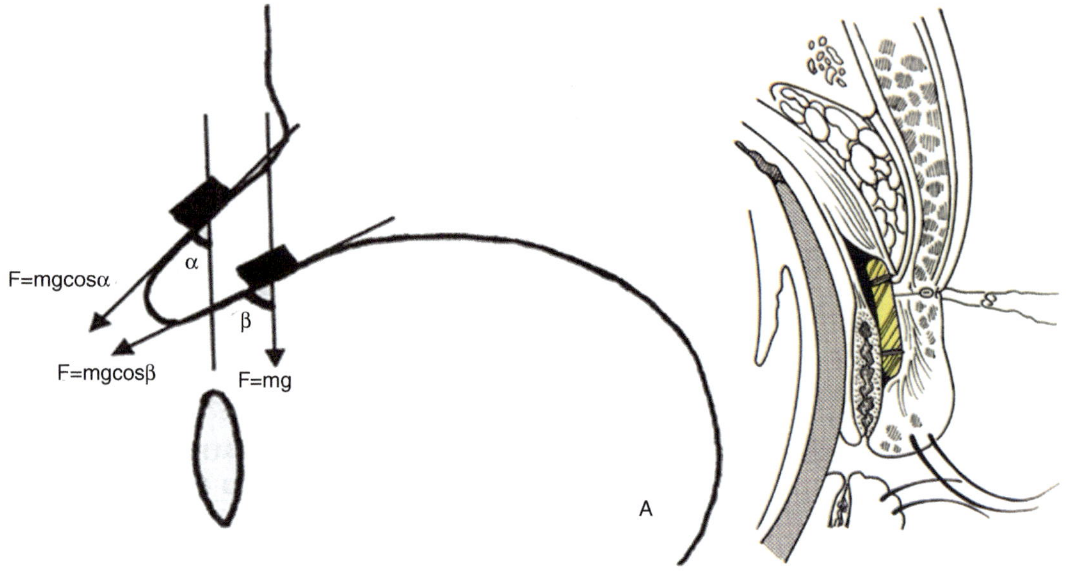

Fig. 24.1 (Left) A schematic drawing of the different forces that act over the upper eyelid after the gold weight is placed on the surface of the skin or on the tarsal plate. (Right) Figure shows a lateral view drawing of the lids and eyeball. Note the correct location of the implant

the surface of the upper eyelid from the trial, and β is the angle between the vertical line and the weight located on the surface of the upper eyelid. Then, $m_1 = m_2\cos\beta/\cos\alpha$.

Thus, the weight of the gold implant to be finally placed on the tarsal plate must be the weight of the implant placed on the upper lid multiplied by the ratio between the cosine of both angles.

The choice of the optimum weight placed on the patient's upper eyelid through the fixation of a trial gold weight or a sizing weight with an adhesive tape is evaluated by observing eyelid closure. The smallest weight which will provide good covering of the cornea should be used because large weights are more likely to migrate. As suggested by Manktelow, the minimum weight that will bring the upper lid within 2–4 mm of the lower lid should be chosen [4]. It has been emphasized, however, that an under-dosage gold weight implant is chosen to produce the same closure of the eye when it is finally placed on the tarsal plate in almost the 30% of cases [2]. Compared with the speed of the normal blink reflex, the eye closure that is produced by the gold weight is very slow. To make the weight work, it is required that the patient should close the eyes and keep them closed for 1 or 2 s to give time for the lid to descend. Moreover, the same gold weight selected often results in a delayed eye closure when it is placed on the tarsal plate as opposed to the surface of the skin of the upper eyelid. Given the high position of the gold weight on the tarsal plate, the reason could be the different angle formed between the vertical line and the axis of the weight when it is placed on the skin of the upper eyelid (as performed in the trial) and when it is placed inside on the tarsal plate (final location after surgery).

These distinct effects are presumably caused by the different angles that influence the force acting over the upper lid when the head of the patient is in a vertical position. According to the results observed in this study, the value of the angle between the vertical line and the gold implant on the superficial eyelid skin is 22° when the eye is open and 0° when it is closed. However, these results are 40 and 18°, respectively, for the angle between the vertical line and the weight on the tarsal plate. This variation leads to a different overall force acting on the eyelid when the gold implant is placed on the surface of the skin or on the tarsal plate.

Thus, as previously mentioned, a constant must be multiplied by the mass of the implant estimated in the trial to achieve the same closure of the eye after the final location of the gold implant. Although skin laxity during taping may alter the effect of the weight on lid closure, it is not affected when the gold weight chosen is placed on the tarsal plate in cases in which no skin recession is needed or no elevation of the eyebrow is performed. If it were the case, it should be necessary to add to the gold implant the weight of the skin resected. Moreover, care should be taken when the eyebrow is lifted because some quantity of skin is repositioned out of the upper eyelid, and it is necessary to test preoperatively the action of the gold weight carrying out the elevation of the eyebrow with the finger. However, recession of the levator muscle should be considered at surgery to avoid the possibility of postoperative ptosis of the upper eyelid [10]. Thus, mild ptosis is present in four patients of our series after placing a heavier gold weight. Anyway, according to data presented, a gold weight implant 0.2 g heavier than expected should be chosen to obtain better eye closure in terms of quantity and time of closure for lagophthalmos in facial paralysis. Therefore, if a 1.2-g implant results in eyelid closure in the trial, one should use a 1.4-g implant to obtain the best results.

24.2 Correction of Ectropion

Ectropion leads to inappropriate contact between the lower tear duct and the eyeball. This situation causes epiphora, which may be increased by the aberrant re-innervation of the lachrymal gland. Various surgical techniques are used to correct this condition, including tarsorrhaphy, external canthoplasty, and canthopexy [6]. In external canthoplasty, the external canthal ligament is taken out and then re-inserted higher in the periosteum of the frontal bone to ensure that the tendon is more stable. The use of a tendinous strap [7], or less frequently, alloplastic material, in the free edge of the lower lid is a common practice. The objective of this procedure is to support the lower eyelid against the eyeball to avoid epiphora. Alloplastic material is not recommended because of the high risk of infection and extrusion [6]. Long-term studies show that anchoring the tendon strap to the internal canthal ligament usually produces a loss of the graft tension so that the ectropion often reappears, and the epiphora worsens due to the loss of contact between the tear duct and the sclera. In this chapter, we describe a modification of the classical technique of suspension using tendons. Anchoring of the tendon to the internal canthus and external orbital bone is presented as an effective procedure to improve epiphora.

Different techniques have been described for the surgical treatment of ectropion and epiphora in patients with facial paralysis. Among these, tarsorrhaphy, canthoplasty, and canthopexy were the most commonly used, as mentioned above [7]. Tarsorrhaphy can interfere with the temporary field of vision, and external canthoplasty offers a poor aesthetic result, as it closes the lateral portion of the palpebral opening. Finally, in canthopexy, the recurrence of epiphora is frequent because the tear duct loses contact with the eyeball due to the lateral traction to which the eyelid is submitted.

Several techniques using suture anchors have been described [8–10]. On the one hand, it has been described a technique using just one anchor with 3/0 non-absorbable sutures. These authors do not use tendons to support the lower eyelid, but a muscle transfer or hypoglossal-facial nerve was performed in five and one of the seven patients used by theses authors, respectively. The anchor is inserted in a hole at the frontal process of the maxillary bone, and the sutures are anchored to the periosteum of the zygoma after passing though the lower eyelid. Others use a tendinous graft which is fixated medially and only anchored laterally using the Mitek system. In their study, the authors used other procedures such as free muscle transfers, direct neurotization, and cross-facial nerve to correct the ectropion, which could enhance the long-term results achieved using the Mitek system. Thus, the mini-tendon graft is presented as a supplementary technique in combination with dynamic techniques. The new technique described in our article uses two screw anchors, medially and laterally, which allows us to displace both anchorage points of the lower eyelid in the cranial direction. This displacement favors contact between the tear duct of the lower eyelid and the eyeball to facilitate lachrymal drainage. The increased elevation, especially in the medial portion of the lower eyelid, prevents the reappearance of the ectropion and epiphora. Moreover, in our study, no dynamic procedures were performed in any patients which could modify the results obtained when the anchoring system is used. Thus, we present a technique with good results using an isolated procedure.

The use of suture screw anchors requires three surgical incisions (Fig. 24.2 left). The first incision is made 0.5 cm above the medial canthal ligament, the second is located laterally to the external canthus, and finally the last incision is performed 1 cm lateral to the upper eyelid in the external orbital bone. The surgeon makes a tunnel in the lower eyelid using a keith 14F needle. The tendon graft is inserted along the tunnel (Fig. 24.2 center and right). Then, the tendon (the *palmar longus* tendon or the *fascia* lata) is attached to the inner canthal ligament. Once the tendon has been attached, the lateral portion of the tendon is attached also to the external orbital bone with an anchor. We move up the anchor point of the lower eyelid, especially in the medial portion, obtaining better contact between the tear duct and the sclera. This contact facilitates the drainage of the tear and prevents epiphora. Finally, the free border of the lower eyelid should be located 1.5 mm above the pupil with more tension than required in anticipation of lowering of the lower eyelid over the following few weeks.

24.3 Conclusion

The use of the gold weight is an established procedure in the treatment of lagophthalmos and usually produces successful results. The critical technical issues are the firm suture fixation to the tarsal plate and the high location of the weight on this plate. However, the estimated weight of the implant from the trials on the skin of the upper lid fails to obtain the expected eye closure outcomes after surgical implantation on the tarsal plate. One of the main reasons could be the different curvature on the skin and on the tarsal plate of the upper eyelid. In this chapter, the angles between the vertical line and the surface of the outer (skin) and inner (tarsal plate) part of the upper eyelid have been analyzed when the eye is opened and closed. The results show that an addition of 0.2 g to the gold weight estimated in the trial is required to achieve a similar closure of the eye by means of the gold implant on the tarsal plate.

On the other hand, the patients treated by the technique described presented adequate resolution of ectropion and epiphora in the postoperative evaluations. There was no recurrence of ectropion in the group of patients treated with screw anchors after 2 years of follow-up. A surgical revision was necessary in two patients to correct hypertension detected 1 month postop-

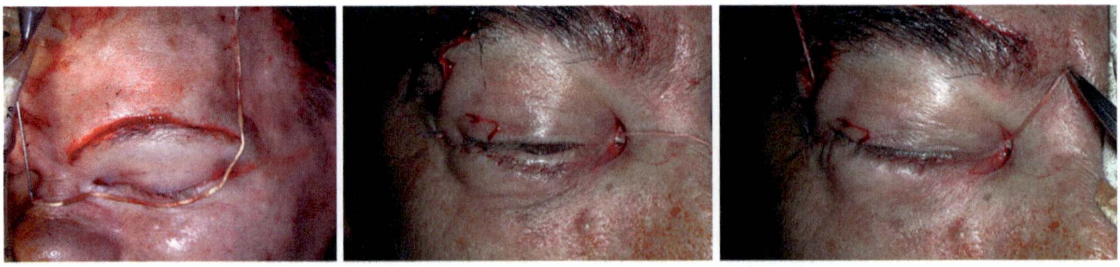

Fig. 24.2 (Left) Shows the plantaris tendon for the free border of the lower eyelid and the three incisions to pass the tendon. Note the elliptical excision of the frontal skin to rise the eyebrow. (Center) Once the tendon is passed through the free border of the lower eyelid and attached to the medial cantus, it is possible to rise the lid (right)

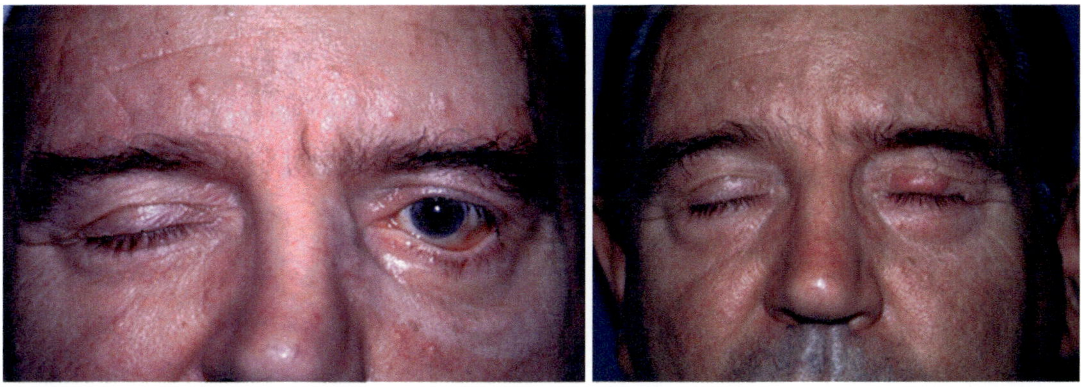

Fig. 24.3 A patient presenting a left-side facial paralysis. The patient is impeded to close the left eye and presents ectropion of the left lower eyelid and ptosis of the eyebrow. A 1.2-g gold weight was chosen in the trial and a 1.6-g implant was placed on the tarsal plate to correct the lagophthalmos. We performed the correction of the ectropion by using a static support with a sling of plantaris tendon and external canthoplasty. We also performed a cutaneous excision of the upper eyelid and elevation of the eyebrow with a cutaneous excision of the frontal skin. The same patient is shown 6 months after surgery with the eyes closed. The resolution of the ectropion is visible, elevation of the eyebrow is noticeable, and no ptosis of the upper eyelid is present

eratively. Lagophthalmos and epiphora were not found in any patient after surgical repair. The patients were asked about any interference of the lower eyelid in the visual field, and no patients were found to have problems of this kind (Fig. 24.3).

References

1. Jobe RP. A technique for lid loading in the management of the lagophthalmos of facial palsy. Plast Reconstr Surg. 1974;53:29.
2. Manktelow RT. Use of the gold weight for lagophthalmos. Oper Tech Plast Reconstr Surg. 1999;6:157.
3. Hontanilla B. Weight measurement of upper eyelid gold implants for lagophthalmos in facial paralysis. Plast Reconstr Surg. 2001;108:1539–43.
4. Muller-Jensen K, Jansen M. 6 years experience with reversible and surgical upper eyelid weighting in lagophthalmos. Ophthalmologe. 1997;94:295.
5. Gladstone GJ, Nesi FA. Management of paralytic lagophthalmos with a modified gold-weight implantation technique. Ophthal Plast Reconstr Surg. 1996; 12:38.
6. Hontanilla B, Aubá C. Surgical approach the correction of the paralysed eyelid in facial paralysis. Cir Plást Iberlatinamer. 2004;30:275–84.
7. Glat PM, Jelks GW, Jelks EB, et al. Evolution of the lateral canthoplasty: techniques and indications. Plast Reconstr Surg. 1997;100:1396–405.
8. Hontanilla B, Marre D. Eyelid reanimation with gold weight implant and tendon sling suspension: evaluation of excursion and velocity using the Facial Clima system. J Plast Reconstr Aesthet Surg. 2013;66:518–24.
9. Qian JG, Wang XJ, Wu Y. Severe cicatrical ectropion: repair with a large advancement flap and autologous fascia sling. J Plast Reconstr Aesthet Surg. 2006;59:878–81.
10. Hontanilla B, Gómez-Ruiz R. Surgical correction of lower eyelid paralysis with suture screw anchors. J Plast Reconstr Aesthet Surg. 2009;62:1598–601.

Dynamic Eye Closure

25

Holger Jan Klein, Andrés Rodríguez-Lorenzo, and Chieh-Han John Tzou

Key Points

- Dynamic concepts of ocular reanimation involve the creation of active eye closure via nerve and/or muscle transfer and usually apply to long-standing, irreversible facial palsy or congenital absence of the facial nerve or muscles.
- Regional muscle transposition aims at reliable and immediate return of eye closure, but does not account for spontaneous mimetic nature, whereas free tissue transfer allows for synchronous, mimetic movement, but requires a prolonged time to achieve the desired function.
- Temporalis muscle transposition is a straightforward, reliable approach in adults providing immediate function, but lacks responsiveness to emotion and spontaneous blinking reflex.
- Frontalis muscle transposition should be considered in young facial palsy patients with severe ocular involvement.
- Free muscle transfer provides a high amplitude of movement, blink restoration, and potential simultaneous multi-level restoration of the completely paralyzed hemi face.

25.1 Introduction

Functional problems around the eye due to facial palsy are usually addressed with priority to compensate for the reduced or missing eye sphincter closure. Besides permanent application of artificial tears, ointment, or occlusion with a wet chamber, impaired vision, corneal ulceration, conjunctivitis, tearing, and an increased sensibility of the eye to light, wind, or sun not only reduce patients' life quality but also restrict their working capacity tremendously [1].

Ocular reanimation constitutes of static and/or dynamic components. "Static" is defined as techniques involving an insertion of an implant or an intervention, which passively assists in eyelid closure but does not allow for a physiological pathway for restoration of synchronous and coordinated blink. These early static concepts to reduce the height of the palpebral aperture include the palpebral spring in the 1960s inserting a stainless steel wire spring in the upper lid aiming at restoration of proper synergism of eye-

H. J. Klein (✉)
Department of Plastic Surgery and Hand Surgery, University Hospital Zurich, Zurich, Switzerland
e-mail: holger.klein@usz.ch

A. Rodríguez-Lorenzo
Department of Plastic and Maxillofacial Surgery, Uppsala University Hospital, Uppsala, Sweden

Department of Surgical Sciences, Uppsala University, Uppsala, Sweden
e-mail: andres.rodriguez.lorenzo@surgsci.uu.se

C.-H. J. Tzou
Plastic and Reconstructive Surgery, Hospital of Divine Savior (Krankenhaus Goettlicher Heiland), Sigmund Freud University, TZOU MEDICAL, Vienna, Austria

© Springer Nature Switzerland AG 2021
C.-H. J. Tzou, A. Rodríguez-Lorenzo (eds.), *Facial Palsy*, https://doi.org/10.1007/978-3-030-50784-8_25

lid movement, and improved cosmesis while respecting the importance of the tear-film [2]. Similar approaches followed soon after, e.g., by Arion in the 1970s with the *cerclage technique* also addressing the lower lid as well as lid loading techniques as introduced by Jobe [3, 4]. With the advances of microsurgical techniques and instruments and to comply with the essential rule to replace "like with like" several autologous concepts for eye sphincter reconstruction have been described. These "dynamic" concepts involve the creation of active eye closure via nerve and/or muscle transfer and usually apply to long-standing, irreversible facial palsy or congenital absence of the facial nerve or muscles. They can be classified as either regional muscle transposition or free muscle grafts.

25.2 Regional Muscle Transfer

25.2.1 Temporalis Muscle Transposition

The classic temporalis muscle transposition—first described by Gillies and Millard in 1934—is still often considered first choice to achieve dynamic eyelid closure in adults [5, 6]. In the authors' opinion, this approach is not to be used in children as masticatory muscles should not be compromised at a young age as well as to prevent negative effects on the growth of the facial skeleton.

The temporalis muscle is a fan-shaped muscle located in the temporal fossa of the temporal bone. The muscle fibers take origin from the periosteum of the inferior temporal line and from the infratemporal crest of the temporal bone. All the fibers converge towards the tendon, which inserts on the coronoid process of the mandible. Before inserting into the coronoid process, the muscle runs underneath the zygomatic arch. The blood supply of the temporalis muscle is primarily the deep, anterior and posterior temporal arteries of the internal maxillary system, which enter the deep surface of the muscle between the zygoma and the pterygoid muscle. The nerve supply is from the deep, anterior and posterior temporal nerves, branches of the mandibular division of the trigeminal nerve. The temporalis muscle and fascia fuse together with the galea aponeurosis at the superior insertion of the muscle. Inferiorly, the muscle fascia splits into two layers before inserting to the zygomatic arch.

The operative technique described in the following paragraph is based on Gillies and Millard's approach with some modifications introduced by Frey and Giovanoli [1]. The temporalis muscle is exposed by a preauricular skin incision, which is elongated into the hair-bearing temporal area vertically with a bow-like incision towards the hairline. In a complete, irreversible lesion, no care has to be taken with the branches of the facial nerve, and subcutaneous fat tissue is removed onto the lateral orbital rim to prevent a bulging deformity by creating space for the transposed part of the muscle. A 2- to 2.5-cm-wide central strip of the temporalis is mobilized by cutting the temporal fascia and the muscle with two parallel vertical incisions down to the temporal bone (Fig. 25.1). The posterior incision has to be somewhat longer than the anterior incision to keep the transposed muscle fibers under the same resting tension. The anterior fibers have to go a shorter distance than the posterior fibers, and it is very important that the ventrally neighboring temporal fascia is maintained intact. This allows for functioning as a hypomochlion for the muscle fibers of the transposed part. Otherwise, the fibers altering their direction of pull by about 90° will not be effective to the eyelids during contraction. At this point, a 1-cm strip of temporal fascia is taken from its anterior part just next and parallel to the hypomochlion. It is taken in maximal length from the temporal line down to the zygomatic arch, where it separates to the superficial and deep layers of the temporal fascia with some fat tissue in between. This procedure again creates additional space for the muscle to be transposed. The fascial strip is divided into two equal strips about 5 mm wide. The central part of the temporalis is mobilized subperiosteally and divided for 2 cm at the end into equal slips. The two slips of the muscle are elongated with the prepared fascial strips, which are

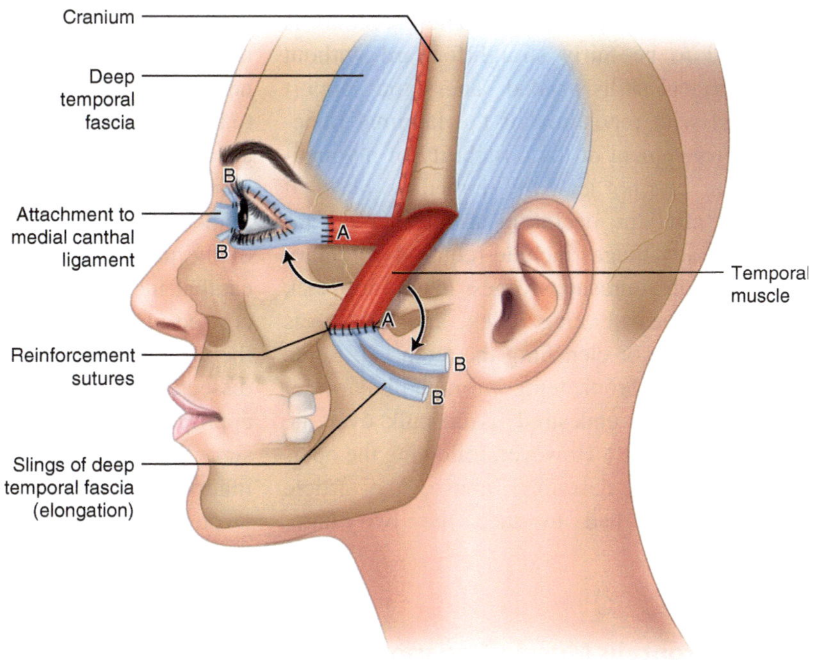

Fig. 25.1 Schematic drawing of the surgical technique of temporalis muscle flap for eye reanimation

sutured to the ends by nonabsorbable 4-0 sutures. Two tunnels are created by blunt dissection. A thread of silk is pulled through each tunnel in the upper and lower eyelids using special scissors with a hole in the tip. The tunnel in the upper eyelid should be made bow-like, with some distance from the lid edge. That way, the lateral pull of the transposed temporal muscle will push down the upper eyelid more efficiently. Complete closure is realistically obtained. In contrast, the tunnel in the lower lid has to be as near to the lid edge as possible to prevent or correct ectropion of the lower lid as much as possible. The anterior crus of the medial palpebral ligament is exposed by a small angled incision of the overlying skin. The elongated muscle slips are pulled through the tunnels. The fascial strips are both brought behind the ligament and sutured carefully to the ligament with nonabsorbable 4-0 sutures. The tension of the two slips of transposed temporalis is of crucial importance. The lower slip needs overcorrection for good lasting support of the lower eyelid, which has a tendency to sag because of gravity. The upper slip is at risk of too much tension, which can cause an asymmetrically narrow lid fissure if it is too tight, or of too little tension, which can cause ineffective sphincter function during contraction of the transposed temporalis. Some fine-tuning of the resting tension is still possible by placing some stabilizing fixation sutures between the rims of the temporal muscle and the fascial strip serving as hypomochlion in the temporal region. This is one of the most crucial part of the operation, as it has a great impact on the functional result. The remaining posterior part of the temporalis is now mobilized, leaving the temporal fascia behind, and the mobilized part of the muscle is used to fill up the depression at the donor site of the transposed part. In that way, a donor-site deformity is prevented. In the majority of patients, temporalis transposition is combined with a cross-face nerve graft during the same operation to prepare for a free gracilis muscle transplant to the cheek for smile reconstruction 8–10 months later.

The basic advantage of this technique is the introduction of a large volume of living and dynamic muscle into the face. The procedure is supposed to be fairly straightforward without microsurgical skills needed. The static support provided with reposition of the lacrimal punctum, enhancement of the possibility of myoneurotization, and not least the immediate onset of function after the operation are further advantages. Disadvantages include required voluntary eyelid closure, unresponsiveness to emotion, lack of spontaneous blinking reflex, and synkinesis when chewing or clenching the teeth [7]. Some authors report chronic temporal-mandibular joint dysfunction and undesired tissue bulk over the zygomatic arch [8]. However, following the operative technique described above, the article authors rarely had to face the two latter problems.

25.2.2 Frontalis Muscle Transposition

In-depth studies of the frontalis muscle as transposed substitute for the eye sphincter introduced by Lee and Terzis in 1984 demonstrated sufficient eye closure with successfully restored coordinated involuntary blink [8, 9]. This procedure should be kept in mind for young facial palsy patients with severe ocular involvement.

The frontalis is a thin, quadrilateral muscle, which adheres to the superficial fascia of the forehead. The frontalis muscle has no bony attachments as it is continuous with the procerus, the corrugator, and the orbicularis oculi muscle. From these attachments the fibers are directed upward and join the galea aponeurotica below the coronal suture. The frontal branch of the facial nerve innervates the frontalis muscle while its dominant blood supply comes from the supraorbital and supratrochlear vessels.

The following operative concept is adopted from Terzis and Karypidis [10]. Transferring the contralateral, unaffected frontalis muscle to the paralyzed orbicularis oculi as a pedicled muscle transfer is performed via a bi-coronal skin incision posterior to the hairline followed by subgaleal dissection to the level of the left and right supraorbital rim. A subcutaneous pocket is developed over the unaffected frontalis muscle. Lateral dissection allows for identification of the frontal nerve branches facilitated by use of electrical nerve stimulation. Once the frontal flap is raised to the supraorbital rim, the supratrochlear vessels are identified. The frontalis muscle dissection is then continued just beyond the midline creating a tunnel over the glabella from the supraorbital rim of the unaffected side to a contralateral medial canthal incision. Subcutaneous tunnels are then created along the upper and lower eyelids from the medial to the lateral canthal areas. Once fully dissected, the frontalis muscle is separated in appropriate medial and lateral segments, making sure that each half remains vascularized and innervated. Each slip of the frontalis is passed through the glabellar tunnel to the medial canthal incision and then each segment is subsequently tunneled across the upper and lower eyelid to the lateral canthal region. The tension is then adjusted so as to reproduce a complete sphincter around the eye. The overlapping ends of the frontalis muscle are finally sutured at the level of the lateral canthal tendon and around a periosteal flap at the lateral orbital rim. The previously placed cross-facial nerve graft allowing for reinnervation of the eye sphincter is then identified and coapted to the frontal nerve of the frontalis muscle using 11-0 nylon sutures. The scalp and orbital incisions are then closed in layers (Fig. 25.2).

This concept describes a fairly straightforward dissection without need of vascular anastomosis achieving sufficient eye closure and coordinated involuntary blink. Donor-site morbidity is acceptable as the "removal" of the unaffected frontalis muscle usually leads to a more symmetrical position of both eyebrows with the option to correct it by static brow elevation in a later step. Careful dissection of the unaffected frontal branch as well as precise microsurgical nerve coaptation to the previously placed cross-face nerve graft is needed.

25.2.3 Orbicularis oculi Transposition

A rather recent approach to ameliorate eye sphincter function was introduced by Sadiq and

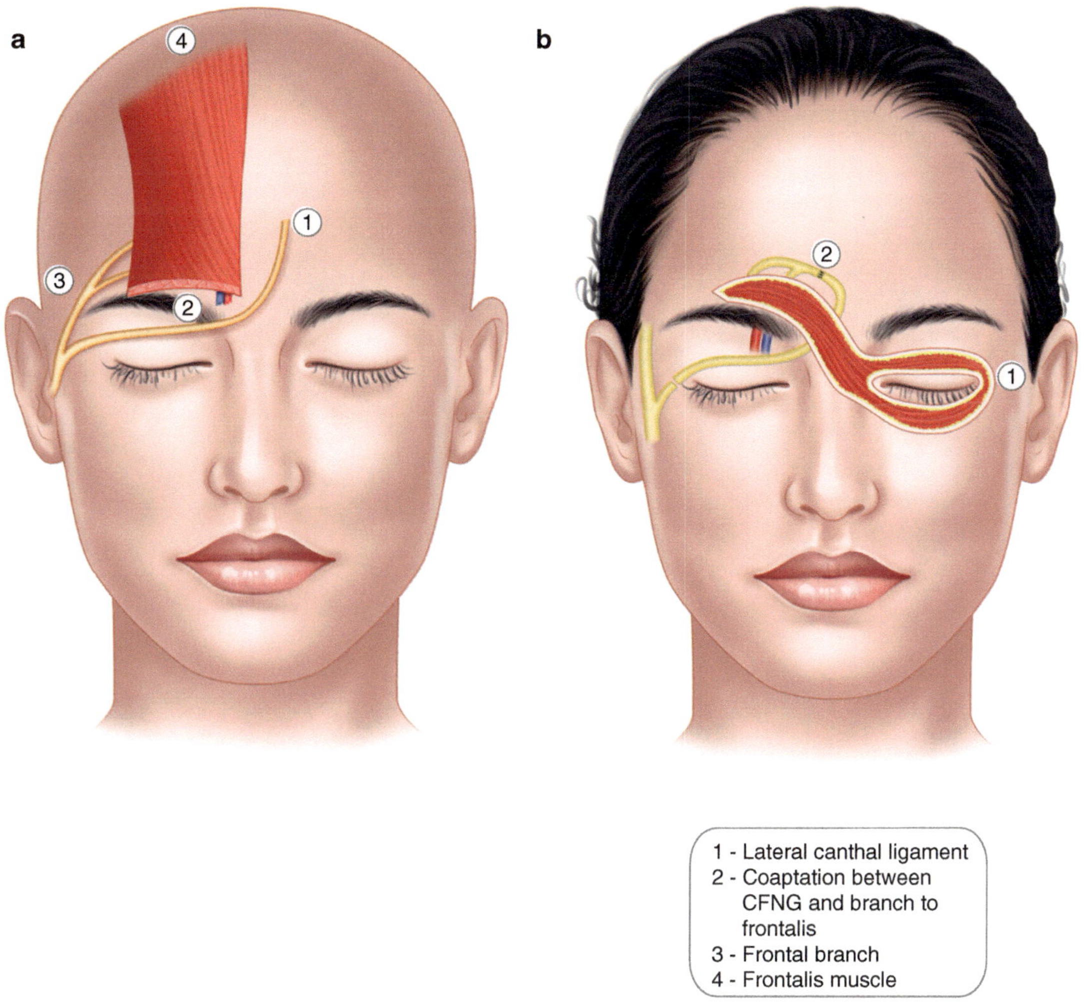

Fig. 25.2 (**a**) First stage of CFNG from frontal branches of the non-paralyzed face to the contralateral eye. (**b**) Transposition of contralateral frontalis muscle based on supratrochlear vessels and nerve anastomosis from the CFNG to the nerve branch of the frontalis muscle

Dharmasena [11]. They propose the transposition of the contralateral orbicularis oculi muscle as potential extension of previously performed muscle transfers aiming at restoration of an involuntary blink and medial eyelid support.

Arising from the nasal part of the frontal bone, from the frontal process of the maxilla, and from the anterior surface of the medial palpebral ligament, the orbicularis oculi muscle directs laterally as a thin layer covering the eye lids, circumference of the orbit as well as spreading over the temple and downward on the cheek. The palpebral part comprises of the preseptal and pretarsal orbicularis muscle which distinction is crucial for the procedure described below. It is innervated by rami zygomatici of the facial nerve and its dominant blood supply comes from small branches arising from the superficial temporal artery.

The following technique described is adopted from Sadiq and Dharmasena [11]. The preseptal orbicularis oculi muscle from the unaffected upper eyelid is exposed via an upper lid skin blepharoplasty. A flap of healthy orbicularis muscle is raised, remaining attached medially via a wide pedicle to spare its nerve and vascular supply (Fig. 25.3). A subcutaneous tunnel just below the glabella is then prepared and the orbi-

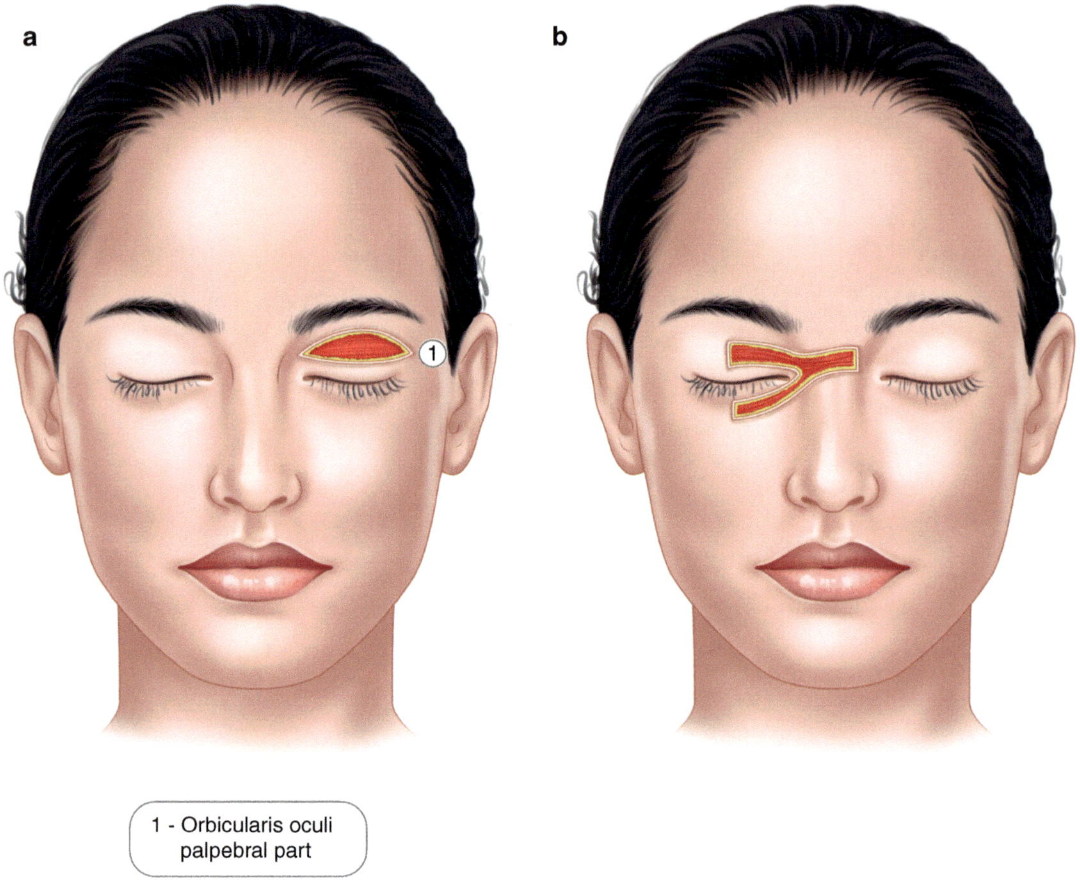

Fig. 25.3 (**a**) Harvesting of the orbicularis oculi, palpebral portion from the non-paralyzed face. (**b**) Transposition and split in two segments for the lower and upper eyelids

cularis flap is passed to the affected side. It is then divided into a superior and inferior slip, which are then sutured into the paralytic orbicularis in the upper (via an upper lid skin crease incision) and lower eye lid (via a subciliary incision). The orbicularis oculi muscle of the affected eyelid is incised about one-third along the eyelid length and the transposed muscle flap sutured into the gap using 6-0 Vicryl sutures. The incisions are closed with 7-0 Vicryl suture.

Sadiq and Dharmasena emphasize that dynamic muscle transfer using the contralateral orbicularis muscle may be considered an adjunct to *improve* the voluntary lid closure and spontaneous blink reflex in patients with complete facial nerve palsy and persistent symptoms of exposure keratopathy who have not benefited from conventional surgical procedures.

25.2.4 Free Functional Muscle Grafts

Free functional muscle grafts constitute another reconstructive entity in long-standing and irreversible facial palsy—combining the benefits of introducing autologous functioning muscle tissue into the paralyzed face with freely adjustable angles and vectors, sufficient excursion, simultaneous multi-level facial reconstruction (e.g., split gracilis for eye closure and smile), allowance for blink restoration, and not least low donor-site morbidity. Presence of an intact donor nerve (e.g., cross-face nerve graft, masseteric nerve) remains a prerequisite. The most commonly transferred muscles for facial reanimation go back to the 1970/1980s and include the gracilis and the pectoralis minor muscle [12, 13]. Further donor muscles for eye sphincter restoration represent the free platysma, occipitalis, extensor digitorum brevis, and a slip of adductor longus transfer [9]. The choice of the flap mainly depends on the physician's preference. For reasons of clarity, the authors will exemplarily describe the principles and operative details of eye sphincter restoration by means of the free functional gracilis transfer followed by the free platysma transfer.

25.2.5 Free Functional Gracilis Transfer

The authors prefer using the free functional gracilis transfer for simultaneous eye sphincter and smile restoration in young patients in order not to compromise the growth of the facial skeleton. In adults, a free gracilis muscle transplant for eye closure is used if the temporalis muscle is no longer available for transposition. The possibility of separating the gracilis muscle into two functional territories goes back to Manktelow and Zuker in 1984 [14]. Muscle transplantation with micro-neurovascular anastomoses is performed 8–10 months after double cross-face nerve grafting between a zygomatic branch and a temporal branch of the facial nerve on the contralateral healthy side and the paralyzed side of the face. Eight to 10 months are necessary for the regenerating facial nerve fibers to reach the distal ends of the cross-face nerve grafts. The Tinel sign is an excellent tool to clinically monitor the progress of nerve regeneration.

Details on gracilis flap harvest can be found in literature, e.g., Chuang [15]. The gracilis muscle is exactly tailored while still in situ and under the original resting tension at the medial thigh. Anesthesia should be carried out without muscle relaxation. After identification of the dominant proximal vascular pedicle and the motor nerve as a branch of the obturatorius nerve, the motor nerve is separated into two fascicles. The territories innervated by the two fascicles are identified by electrostimulation. The degree of overlapping of the two territories of innervation will influence the degree of synkinesis of the muscle parts used for the eye and mouth region. Clearly divided territories will make the movements of both regions independent and only controlled by their own cross-face nerve graft. About two-thirds of the width of the muscle is used for transfer; the length depends on the needs of the recipient site in the face. The greater territory is split distal to the muscle hilus into three strips, which are exactly planned before division according to the face measurements. The shortest strip is used for the corner of the mouth, the midsize strip is used for the upper lip, and the longest strip is used for the lower lip. The other territory is split into two strips, a thin one for the upper lid and a thicker one for the lower eyelid. This should prevent a too strong closure of the upper lid during rest. At the same time, the strip for the lower eyelid should give good support against gravity and prevent ectropion. Documentation of the resting tension by using a stretched silk thread sutured to the surface of the muscle gives the chance to put the muscle transplant under the same resting tension in the recipient area after transfer. The recipient bed in the face has to be prepared before ligation of the vascular pedicle of the gracilis muscle graft. From a preauricular face lift incision, tunnels are dissected towards the upper and lower eyelids. The medial palpebral ligament is exposed by an angular incision, and two long threads are pulled through the tunnels. When the gracilis muscle is transferred to the face, the two muscle strips are carefully pulled through the prepared tunnels in the upper and lower eyelids. The muscle origin is attached at the temporal fascia with 2-0 nonabsorbable sutures. The muscle strips are then positioned behind the palpebral ligament and fixed there with 4-0 nonabsorbable sutures under correct tension. At the end of the operation, slight overcorrection is intended. After fixation of the other muscle parts to the perioral region, the vascular anastomoses are performed on the superficial temporal vessels under the microscope. Finally, the distal ends of the two cross-face nerves are coapted to the two fascicles of the gracilis muscle nerve. Great care has to be taken that the cross-face nerve graft connected to the zygomatic nerve branch at the healthy side is sutured to the correct nerve fascicle supplying the territory used for the eye sphincter reconstruc-

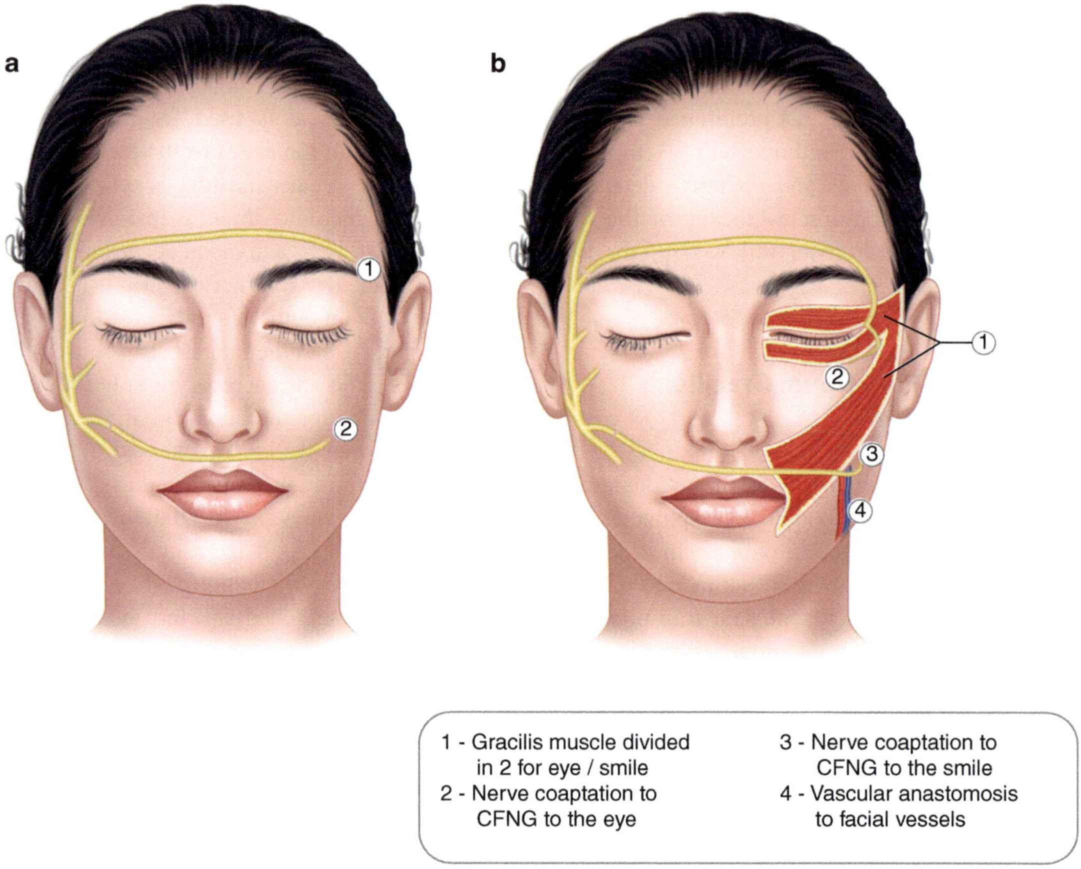

Fig. 25.4 (**a**) First stage with double CFNG to the eye and smile. (**b**) Second stage with free gracilis transfer split in an eye component and smile component with separation of functional units and separate innervation to the CFNG

tion. Marking of one of the fascicles with a 10-0 suture at the donor site is recommended for correct matching later on in the recipient area (Fig. 25.4a, b).

Whereas a regional muscle transposition like the temporalis muscle has its advantage in the onset of immediate function after the operation, the gracilis muscle transplant achieves stronger functional long-term results [1]. Patients with gracilis muscle transplant should expect symptoms of lagophthalmos for up to 1 year. But in the final outcome, however, it is the authors' experience that eye closure is more complete and has a higher amplitude of movement after free gracilis transfer as compared to temporalis muscle transposition. Synkinesis when smiling or blinking after free split gracilis transfer constitutes an unsolved sequela. Although two separate cross-face nerve grafts are usually used for reinnervation of the two territories for the eye as well as the mouth, neuronal overlapping is unpreventable. Sometimes, hyperfunction has to be corrected by surgical myectomy. The authors prefer this small intervention in the case of overcorrection over the risk of a final unsatisfying result caused by undercorrection without the additional possibility of functional improvement.

25.2.6 Free Functional Platysma Transfer

Lee and Terzis et al. first came up with idea to transfer the platysma as a free functional muscle graft for eye closure reanimation in 1984, but the technique was discarded soon after due to technical problems and difficulties. Twenty years later free platysma transfer was again considered an option for eye closure reconstruction of the paralyzed face. To date, only few studies using this approach have been reported [9, 16]. There is only one major series with 24 patients recently published by Guelinckx [17]. The operative technique described in the following paragraph is mainly derived from his publication.

The approach starts with the cross-face nerve grafting (CFNG) procedure (Fig. 25.5), which is performed via a facelift incision with extension in the temporal hair and submandibular crease to fully expose the facial nerve on the healthy side. Tedious dissection is needed for selection of the donor branches to connect the CFNG to. Guelinckx uses one branch for forceful closure of the upper eyelid together with one-half branch of the preseptal portion of the upper eyelid for blink. Intra-operative stimulation is obligatory spearing at least 60% of the branches for normal eye closure and blink on the healthy side. The sural nerve graft is placed supraorbitally in an orthodromic manner with end-to-end or end-to-side coaptation using 11-0 nylon. About 9 months later with Tinel's confirmation of CFNG sprouting, the patient is scheduled for platysma transfer. With the patient in supine position, dissection of the temporal vessels of the paralyzed side is performed via a common facelift incision on the paralyzed side. The plane of the facelift incision is continued to the lateral canthus and then joined with the eyelid incisions.

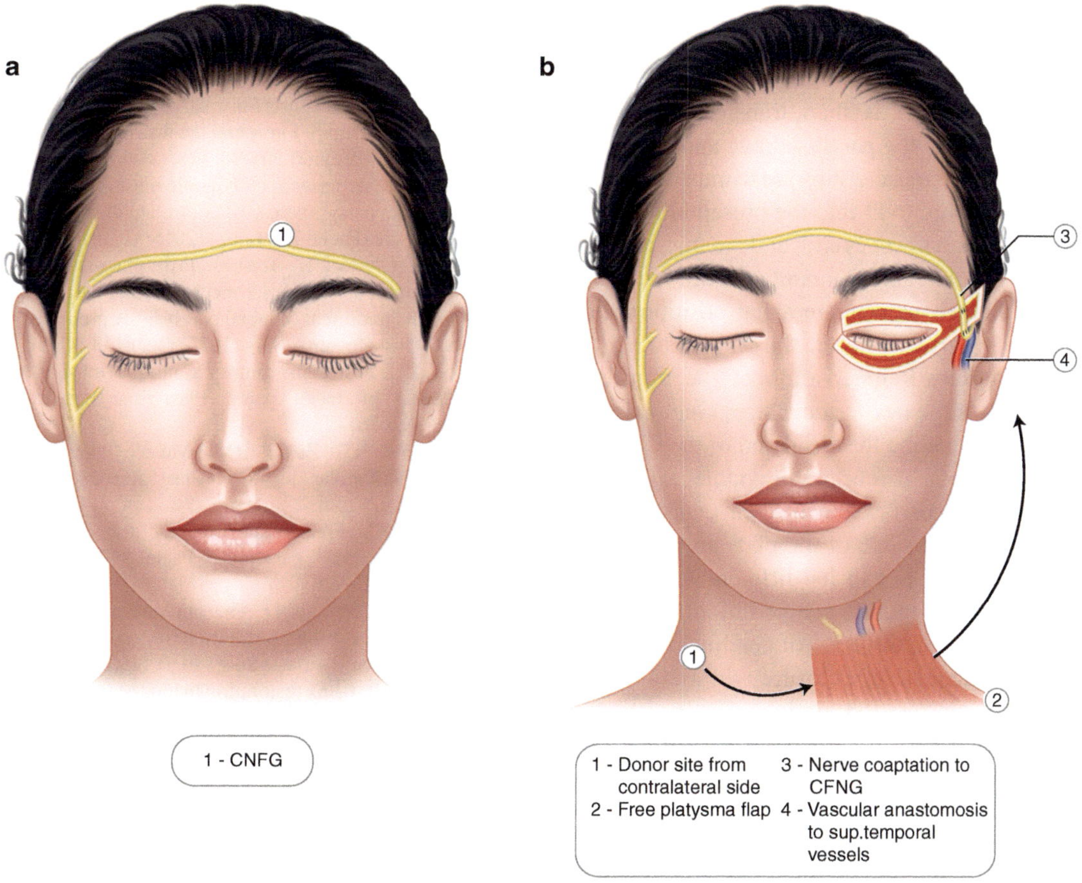

Fig. 25.5 (**a**) First stage with CFNG. (**b**) Free platysma muscle harvest from the contralateral side and insetting and anastomosis to the superficial temporal vessels and the CFNG

On the contralateral side, a 6 cm incision 2 cm below the mandibular border allows for full dissection of the anterior surface of the platysma from the mandible to the clavicle. The distal insertion of the platysma is sharply transected using scissors. Two transfixing sutures may help elevating the thin platysma from the underlying tissues from caudally to cranially. The facial artery and vein are clipped above the mandibular border and followed downwards until the branches to the platysma are identified. There is no need to isolate these perforating vessels to the platysma; the facial vessels are followed towards their origin to lengthen the pedicle. The motor nerve to the platysma is isolated on the lateral border using electrical stimulation. This thin nerve should be dissected up to the marginal mandibular branch of the facial nerve. Before dividing the pedicle, the parallel-fibered architecture of the platysma muscle allows for dividing the muscle into an upper and lower portion without impairing the blood supply or neural input.

The platysma is then transferred from the healthy side to the paralyzed eye and revascularized. The two muscle slips are trimmed down to a width of 9 mm to fit into the preseptal portion of the upper and lower eyelid, and are then anchored to the medial canthal ligament. Care is taken to place the neosphincter in a flat position around the eye to perfectly mimic the original orbicularis oculi muscle. Reinnervation of the transferred platysma is the next critical step; Guelinckx recommends sending the distal end of the CFNG for frozen section to check for viable axons. One adequate nerve fascicle is then coapted to the single nerve fascicle of the platysma; the rest of the CFNG is split in its different fascicles and used for direct muscle neurotization.

After 16 months, 87% of Guelinckx's patients showed adequate eye closure with 62% exhibiting blink restoration, indicating that the free functional platysma transfer is a feasible, satisfactory option for eye closure reanimation. However, more clinical experience and evidence are needed to further establish this renewed approach in the near future.

References

1. Frey M, Giovanoli P, Tzou CH, Kropf N, Friedl S. Dynamic reconstruction of eye closure by muscle transposition or functional muscle transplantation in facial palsy. Plast Reconstr Surg. 2004;114(4):865–75.
2. Morel-Fatio D, Lalardrie JP. Palliative surgical treatment of facial paralysis. The palpebral spring. Plast Reconstr Surg. 1964;33:446–56.
3. Arion HG. Dynamic closure of the lids in paralysis of the orbicularis muscle. Int Surg. 1972;57(1):48–50.
4. Jobe RP. A technique for lid loading in the management of the lagophthalmos of facial palsy. Plast Reconstr Surg. 1974;53(1):29–32.
5. Deutinger M, Freilinger G. Transfer of the temporal muscle for lagophthalmos according to Gillies. Scand J Plast Reconstr Surg Hand Surg. 1991;25(2):151–4.
6. Gillies H. Experiences with fascia lata grafts in the operative treatment of facial paralysis: (section of otology and section of laryngology). Proc R Soc Med. 1934;27(10):1372–82.
7. Salimbeni G. Eyelid reanimation in facial paralysis by temporalis muscle transfer. Oper Tech Plast Reconstr Surg. 1999;6(3):159–62.
8. Terzis JK, Bruno W. Outcomes with eye reanimation microsurgery. Facial Plast Surg. 2002;18(2):101–12.
9. Terzis JK, Karypidis D. Blink restoration in adult facial paralysis. Plast Reconstr Surg. 2010;126(1):126–39.
10. Wei F-C, Mardini S. Flaps and reconstructive surgery. Amsterdam: Elsevier; 2017.
11. Sadiq SA, Dharmasena A. Dynamic muscle transfer in facial nerve palsy: the use of contralateral orbicularis oculi muscle. Facial Plast Surg. 2015;31(2):145–51.
12. Harii K, Ohmori K, Torii S. Free gracilis muscle transplantation, with microneurovascular anastomoses for the treatment of facial paralysis. A preliminary report. Plast Reconstr Surg. 1976;57(2):133–43.
13. Terzis JK. Pectoralis minor: a unique muscle for correction of facial palsy. Plast Reconstr Surg. 1989;83(5):767–76.
14. Manktelow RT, Zuker RM. Muscle transplantation by fascicular territory. Plast Reconstr Surg. 1984;73(5):751–7.
15. Chuang DC. Free tissue transfer for the treatment of facial paralysis. Facial Plast Surg. 2008;24(2):194–203.
16. Terzis JK, Karypidis D. The outcomes of dynamic procedures for blink restoration in pediatric facial paralysis. Plast Reconstr Surg. 2010;125(2):629–44.
17. Guelinckx PJ. Blink restoration in long-standing facial paralysis: use of free neurovascular platysma transfer. Plast Reconstr Surg Glob Open. 2018;6(10):e1939.

26 Corneal Neurotization

Simeon C. Daeschler, Ronald Zuker, Asim Ali, and Gregory H. Borschel

Key Points

- Corneal neurotization describes the surgical transfer of sensory donor nerve fibers to (re-) innervate the anesthetic cornea and thereby provide corneal sensation and improve ocular surface health.
- Direct techniques connect the donor nerve directly to the anesthetic cornea whereas indirect neurotization techniques use nerve grafts to guide the donor axons to the cornea.
- The sural nerve and the great auricular nerve may be used as autologous nerve grafts.
- The supraorbital nerve or the supratrochlear nerves are reliable axon donors.
- *Caveats:* Thoroughly map the facial sensation to define an appropriate donor nerve and fallback options preoperatively, use a surgical microscope approved for ophthalmic procedures to avoid phototoxic retinal damage, avoid nerve (graft) desiccation, gently handle the nerve graft and trim the manipulated nerve ends.

S. C. Daeschler
The Borschel Lab, Neuroscience and Mental Health Program, Hospital for Sick Children (SickKids), Toronto, ON, Canada
e-mail: simeon.daeschler@sickkids.ca

R. Zuker
Division of Plastic and Reconstructive Surgery, Hospital for Sick Children (SickKids), University of Toronto, Toronto, ON, Canada
e-mail: ronald.zuker@sickkids.ca

G. H. Borschel (✉)
Division of Plastic and Reconstructive Surgery, Riley Hospital for Children and Indiana University (SickKids), Indianapolis, IN, USA
e-mail: gregory.borschel@sickkids.ca

A. Ali
Department of Ophthalmology and Vision Sciences, Hospital for Sick Children (SickKids), University of Toronto, Toronto, ON, Canada
e-mail: asim.ali@sickkids.ca

© Springer Nature Switzerland AG 2021
C.-H. J. Tzou, A. Rodríguez-Lorenzo (eds.), *Facial Palsy*,
https://doi.org/10.1007/978-3-030-50784-8_26

26.1 Definition of Corneal Neurotization

Corneal neurotization describes the surgical transfer of sensory donor nerve fibers to (re-) innervate the anesthetic cornea and thereby provide corneal sensation and improve ocular surface health.

26.2 Background

26.2.1 Corneal Nerve Fibers Maintain Ocular Surface Health

Corneal transparency is indispensable for vision. To maintain transparency the corneal epithelium undergoes a continuous renewal process. Apical epithelial cell layers desquamate and are replenished by new epithelial cells that arise from proliferating limbal stem cells located at the corneal limbus. Following corneal injury, these processes of stem cell proliferation and epithelial cell migration are normally upregulated to restore the integrity of the ocular surface, but are impaired when corneal innervation is absent [1].

Physiologically, the cornea is densely innervated by predominantly sensory nerve fibers arising from the ipsilateral ophthalmic branch of the trigeminal nerve. These nerve fibers provide sensibility to the ocular surface, modulate the blinking reflex and govern adequate lacrimation in order to protect the susceptible cornea from injury and desiccation. Patients with significantly impaired or absent corneal innervation develop a degenerative corneal disease termed neurotrophic keratopathy [1]. Although multiple definitions of neurotrophic keratopathy exist, all of them agree on the process of corneal breakdown based on the fundamental lack of corneal innervation. Essentially, two pathological key aspects occur following corneal nerve fiber loss. First, the lack of protective sensation facilitates repetitive and unperceived microtrauma to the ocular surface aggravated by surface desiccation due to insufficient lacrimation. Second, following corneal denervation the efficacy of the physiological epithelial renewal and repair mechanisms in the cornea worsens, resulting in slow and incomplete healing of epithelial defects. Consequently, the affected patients suffer from chronic ulceration that leads to corneal thinning, perforation and scarring, eventually culminating in permanent vision loss.

The etiology of neurotrophic keratopathy is diverse. Congenital disorders like trigeminal hypoplasia, systemic diseases such as diabetes and surgical or nonsurgical nerve trauma due to tumor resection, skull fractures or herpetic infections may cause corneal denervation. Reliable data on incidence and prevalence of neurotrophic keratopathy are scarce. Based on the extrapolation from epidemiological data of its most common causes, neurotrophic keratopathy is classified as an orphan disease with an estimated prevalence of one to five individuals in 10,000 (ORPHA: 137596). However, given the multitude of underlying causes these numbers must be interpreted with care and most likely underestimate the actual prevalence of neurotrophic keratopathy.

Clinically, neurotrophic keratopathy can be classified in three disease stages according to the Mackie classification and based on the extent of corneal surface damage. Mackie stage 1 is characterized by epithelial instability with punctate fluorescein staining as well as impaired lacrimation as indicated by decreased tear breakup time and conjunctival lissamine green/Rose Bengal staining. The presence of corneal epithelial defects without stromal involvement is indicative of Mackie stage 2. Mackie stage 3 is characterized by advanced neurotrophic keratopathy with deep ulceration, stromal melting, and the risk for corneal perforation.

26.2.2 Indications and Contraindications for Corneal Neurotization

Presently, neurotrophic keratopathy in the anesthetic cornea is the main indication for corneal neurotization. Untreated neurotrophic keratopathy can culminate in loss of the affected eye and irreversible blindness [1]. Therefore, adequate management and regular clinical reevaluation of this potentially devastating disease are indispensable.

The conventional ophthalmic management of neurotrophic keratopathy aims to cope with the symptoms and prevent disease progression but does not address the underlying neuropathophysiology. Conventional treatment strategies include the topical application of lubricants, antibiotics, platelet rich plasma, and growth factors as well as therapeutic contact lenses and eyelid closure. For advanced disease stages surgical interventions such as amniotic membrane transplantation and conjunctival flaps may be used. However, none of these approaches address the fundamental lack of corneal innervation.

Corneal neurotization reroutes healthy donor nerve fibers to the anesthetic cornea in order to restore corneal innervation. Consequently, this approach offers a potentially definitive treatment for neurotrophic keratopathy. Therefore, the traditional therapeutic stepladder approach that reaches from topical ointments to more invasive surgical strategies being escalated with increasing disease severity, may not be applicable to corneal neurotization. In our current understanding, early (re-)innervation of the anesthetic cornea reduces the risk for disease progression, corneal ulceration and irreversible stromal scarring, therefore being more likely to salvage vision long term than neurotization in advanced disease. Beyond that, the pre-operative presence of large epithelial defects (Mackie stage 2 and 3) increases the risk for post-surgical eye infection and temporary worsening of the neurotrophic keratopathy and thereby may put the nerve graft and even the eye at risk.

For the selection of appropriate candidates for corneal neurotization, the following criteria may be used:

1. Impaired or absent corneal innervation
2. Presence of neurotrophic keratopathy Mackie stage 1 or better
3. Situations in which recovery of corneal innervation is unlikely based on:
   (a) the cause of corneal denervation i.e., congenital trigeminal hypoplasia, or ophthalmic nerve resection
   (b) a prolonged period of time has passed since the event that caused corneal denervation (at least 1 year)
4. Availability of an appropriate sensory donor nerve
5. Absence of active eye infection (viral, bacterial or mycotic)

Contraindications for corneal neurotization are active eye infections, particularly herpetic keratitis. Relative contraindications include abnormal sensation in the donor nerve dermatome. Also, extensive epithelial defects (Mackie stage 2 and 3) should be healed prior to surgery by conventional means.

26.2.3 History and Recent Developments in Corneal Neurotization

Madjid Samii, an Iranian neurosurgeon based in Germany, described the general principle of corneal neurotization in 1972: a surgical transfer of donor axons to the cornea aiming to restore corneal innervation. He described a greater occipital nerve to ophthalmic nerve transfer using a 17 cm autologous sural nerve graft. To approach the dysfunctional ophthalmic nerve Samii performed a frontal craniotomy, opened the orbital roof and incised the periorbita. He then transected the ophthalmic nerve and coapted the sural nerve graft end-to-end to the distal ophthalmic nerve segment. Although he reported improvements in ocular surface health, the cornea remained anesthetic in Samiis' patients. Owing to its invasiveness and limited success, this early approach for corneal reinnervation did not take hold.

In 2009, Terzis and colleagues described a novel technique to restore corneal innervation through direct nerve transfers to the affected cornea, termed "corneal neurotization" [2]. This approach provided the basis for the currently used techniques and facilitated a broader acceptance among clinicians and patients for neurosurgical treatment strategies for neurotrophic keratopathy. In Terzis' case series, the contralateral supraorbital and the supratrochlear nerve were used as axon donor nerves and approached via bicoronal incisions. The dissected and mobilized nerves were then subcutaneously tunneled to the corneoscleral junction and sutured to the sclera in subconjunctival pockets. Terzis reported improved corneal sensation and cornea clarity as well as enhanced best corrected visual acuity following corneal neurotization with a mean follow up of 16.3 ± 2.42 years. Later, Leyngold and colleagues introduced an endoscopically assisted technique for supraorbital nerve dissection through smaller skin incisions aiming to avoid the long visible scars and reduce perioperative complications [3]. However, the considerable extent of forehead dissection and limited number of suitable donor nerves encouraged further advancements of the direct neurotization techniques.

The interposition of a nerve graft between donor nerve and anesthetic cornea enabled minimally invasive corneal neurotization and was described in 2014 [4]. This technique avoids long bicoronal incisions and overcomes the need for the surgical mobilization of long donor nerve segments in the patients' face. However, it does necessitate a second surgical site to harvest the graft with additional donor site morbidity. One advantage of using nerve grafts for corneal neurotization is their flexibility. The easily adaptable nerve graft length makes a multitude of axon donor nerves available and offers the possibility to reroute a large number of nerve fibers by accessing the donor nerve proximally. Thus, the nerve graft-based corneal neurotization offers a potential treatment for patients with bilateral trigeminal dysfunction with neurotrophic keratopathy. Other patients with donor sensory nerves available on only one side but with bilateral neurotrophic keratopathy cannot be treated with direct nerve transfer alone, but may be treated by nerve grafts in which the unilateral donor sensory nerve source provides fibers to nerve grafts to both corneas. Also, if the donor nerve function is deemed critical, its continuity can be preserved by combining the nerve graft interposition with a side-to-end nerve coaptation [5]. Further, nerve grafting allows the surgeon to select the best sensory donor source and route that to the affected cornea. For example, if the V1 branches are insufficient, one may then choose V2 as the source, and if that is also insufficient, then one may choose the great auricular nerve.

26.2.4 Relevant Anatomy

26.2.4.1 Potential Axon Donor Nerves

Even though a multitude of potential donor nerves for corneal neurotization become available by nerve graft interposition, the basic principles of short regeneration distance and minimized donor site morbidity hold true. Based on these principles, the ipsilateral or contralateral supraorbital and supratrochlear nerves are reliable axon donors for direct as well as indirect corneal neurotization [6]. If these first-choice axon donors are ineligible due to their unfavorable course and/or branching, a small caliber or a functional deficit, the infraorbital or great auricular nerve may be considered as primary fallback options (see Fig. 26.1). The smaller occipital nerve or supraclavicular nerves are feasible axon donors as well, but require increased nerve graft lengths to reach the affected cornea and thereby represent secondary fallback options that to date we have not used in our center.

The supraorbital and supratrochlear nerves arise from the frontal nerve, a branch of the ophthalmic division of the trigeminal nerve. Both nerves provide sensation to the forehead and scalp as well as the upper eyelid and conjunctiva with the supratrochlear nerve usually supplying a smaller, medial portion of the dermatome. This distribution is reflected by the course of both nerves: The supratrochlear nerve runs medially along the orbital roof and exits the orbital cavity through the frontal notch coursing in a cranial direction and piercing the corrugator supercilii muscle around 10–18 mm lateral to the facial midline. The supraorbital nerve exits the orbital cavity usually a few millimeters lateral to the supratrochlear nerve and runs parallel to it in a craniolateral direction through or beneath the corrugator supercilii muscle [6]. For minimally invasive corneal neurotization, the supratrochlear and/or supratrochlear nerve are identified by dissecting through the corrugator supercilii muscle through a subbrow incision. Here, the supraorbital nerve usually provides a good size match to the autologous sural nerve graft, making the supraorbital nerve the axon donor of first choice and the supratrochlear nerve a good alternative when it is of suitable caliber.

26.2.4.2 Nerve Grafts for Corneal Neurotization

Presently, autologous nerve grafts are considered gold standard for nerve gap reconstruction as they provide an excellent regeneration environment and essential growth support for regenerating donor axons. This concept also applies to corneal neurotization when bridging the gap between donor nerve and anesthetic cornea. Autologous nerve grafts are usually harvested from smaller sensory nerves elsewhere in the patient's body,

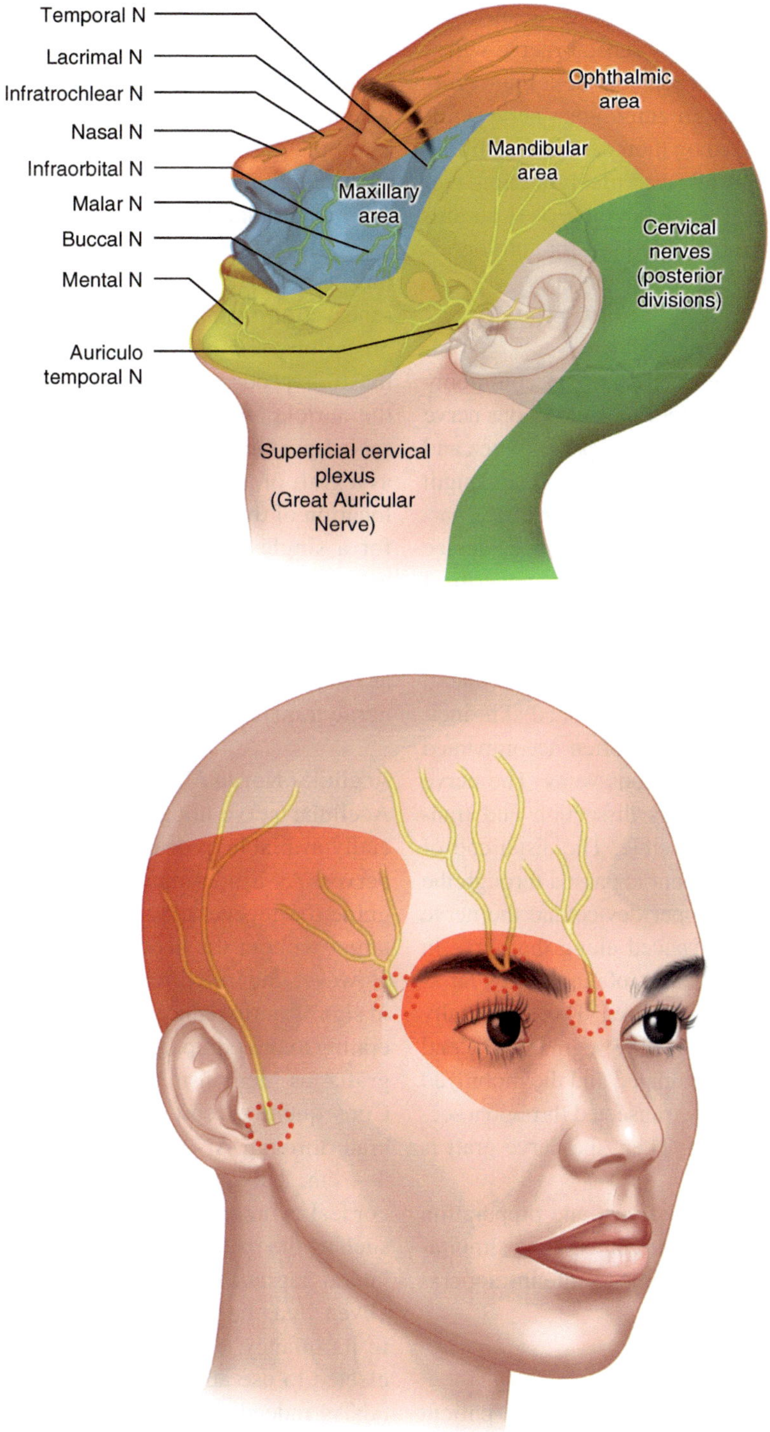

Fig. 26.1 Anatomical drawing visualizing the course of the following donor nerves for corneal neurotization:

- Course of Supraorbital, supratrochlear, infraorbital, great auricular, smaller occipital and supraclavicular nerves (semi-transparent skin),
- Semi-transparent sternocleidomastoid muscle as landmark,
- The dermatomes encircled such as in perspective 1

providing noncritical sensation e.g., in the distal lower leg (sural nerve) or earlobe (great auricular nerve) [5, 7]. Generally, any sensory nerve with a suitable diameter and acceptable donor site morbidity can be used as an autologous nerve graft donor. However, based on their easy accessibility, suitable graft length and noncritical function, two donor sites, the sural nerve, and the great auricular nerve are most frequently used for autologous nerve grafting for facial nerve surgery.

Sural Nerve Grafts

The sural nerve represents the most commonly used graft for nerve transfers and autologous nerve reconstruction. Depending on the patients' sex and body size, sural nerve grafts of up to 30 cm length can be easily harvested. Minimally invasive harvesting techniques using a nerve stripper device are available and usually produce a noncritical sensory deficit on the distal lower leg and lateral aspect of the foot. The sural nerve can be identified 2 cm posterior and 2 cm proximal to the lateral malleolus through a 1–2 cm horizontal skin incision. Here, the sural nerve is often accompanied by one or two small saphenous veins. The nerve is mobilized using scissors dissection and transected as far distal as possible. The distal end of the proximal nerve segment is passed through the orifice of the nerve stripper device and the nerve stripper is carefully advanced along the nerve in cranial direction, with gentle rotation and as far as the nerve graft length is required. There is usually no branching in this sural nerve segment. The end of the nerve stripper is palpated and the mobilized sural nerve is proximally transected through a second, small skin incision. Then, the nerve graft is gently harvested.

The sural nerve graft harvest and preparation of the facial axon donor site can be done simultaneously by two surgical teams to safe intraoperative time.

Great Auricular Nerve Grafts

If the sural nerve is unavailable or the patient requires intact foot sensation for occupation or sports the great auricular nerve (GAN) can be an alternative autograft donor [7]. The GAN is approached via a horizontal skin incision 3 cm caudal and parallel to the mandible. The platysma is carefully dissected to expose the GAN that emerges from the posterior margin of the sternocleidomastoid muscle and courses in rostral and cranial direction toward the mandibular angle. Here the GAN gives rise to two cutaneous branches. The anterior branch provides skin innervation over the parotid gland whereas the posterior branch innervates the skin over the mastoid process and the lower dorsal part of the auricle and earlobe. The GAN can be transected proximal to its bifurcation and harvested as a graft of around 7 cm in length. Whereas the location of the GAN might appear advantageous for a single surgical team, a time saving two-team approach can be challenging due to limited space around the patient's head, and we have avoided its use as a nerve graft (but have used it as a source of sensory fibers in the context of a nerve transfer).

Acellular Nerve Allografts

Acellular nerve allografts (ANAs) are commercially available, processed human cadaver donor nerves. As a non-immunogenic scaffold, ANAs guide the regenerating donor nerve fibers to the target without the need for immunosuppression. However, the lack of viable Schwann cells results in significantly reduced growth support for regenerating axons compared to fresh autologous nerve grafts as demonstrated in laboratory studies. Consequently, regrowing axons reliably regenerate through ANAs only over distances below 3–4 cm. This graft length may be sufficient for corneal neurotization with selected donor nerves such as the ipsilateral, or even mobilized contralateral supraorbital or supratrochlear nerves [8]. Given that the field of corneal neurotization is in its infancy, our group has for the time being elected to use autologous nerve grafts; however, ANAs indeed offer a promising future perspective worthy of study.

26.3 Methods and Technique

26.3.1 Pre-surgical Assessment and Planning

26.3.1.1 Past Medical History

The patients' past medical history may include previous hospital visits, ocular or brain trauma and/or surgery, ophthalmic infections or systemic chronic conditions such as diabetes and therefore often reveal the underlying cause for corneal denervation. Based on the nature of this underlying cause and the time that has passed since the event, the likelihood for spontaneous corneal reinnervation and thereby the need for neurotization can be evaluated.

26.3.1.2 Ophthalmic Examination

The ophthalmic assessment includes the examination of the external eye and cornea. First, the external eye is assessed for eyelid deformities and eyelid closure as well as blink frequency. Next the cornea and conjunctiva are examined. The extent and stage of neurotrophic keratopathy and the presence of active ulceration, stromal melting, extensive neovascularization, infection or scarring are determined. Fluorescein staining shows epithelial defects and tear film stability. Sensory mapping of the corneal surface via Cochet-Bonnet esthesiometry reveals reduced or absent corneal sensation. In unclear cases, in vivo confocal microscopy (IVCM) allows the visual assessment of corneal nerve fibers.

26.3.1.3 Sensory Mapping of the Donor Nerve Dermatomes

To ensure a healthy donor axon population, intact sensation in the donor nerves dermatome is an essential selection criterion for choosing donor nerves. Thus, the patient's face and neck undergo systematic pre-operative sensory mapping to uncover ineligible donor nerves with sensation below normal levels. This includes the assessment of tactile thresholds (Semmes-Weinstein monofilaments), subjective touch perception (Ten-Test), and pain perception (e.g., Pinch Test). We emphasize the importance of normal pain sensation at the donor site especially in congenital corneal anesthesia since normal touch sensation may be combined with trigeminal analgesia in one of both sides of the face.

26.3.2 Surgical Technique

In many cases of corneal anesthesia, direct and indirect corneal neurotization techniques may be applied with a comparable corneal outcome. Both techniques may offer specific advantages in certain cases, however, we prefer the use of nerve grafts for corneal neurotization due to a lesser risk for facial donor site complication, a favorable aesthetic outcome and reliable corneal innervation.

A necessary prerequisite for corneal neurotization is an appropriate surgical microscope. Surgical microscopes are specifically adapted to the needs of the respective surgical specialty. Consequently, microscopes for neurosurgery or plastic and reconstructive surgery differ from those for ophthalmic surgery. The powerful light sources in non-ophthalmic microscopes may cause considerable phototoxic damage to the retina, and as such are not approved for ophthalmic surgery (usually indicated by a warning sticker). A microscope suitable for use with the eye is therefore indispensable for corneal neurotization, and therefore we only use the Ophthalmology microscope to perform nerve coaptations in the periocular region.

26.3.3 Neurotization with Nerve Transfers Alone ("Direct" Neurotization)

These corneal neurotization techniques connect the distal end of the mobilized donor nerve directly to the affected cornea without nerve graft interposition, as described by Terzis [2]. The supraorbital and supratrochlear nerve are the most frequently used axon donors for direct corneal neurotization due to their close proximity to the cornea and often moderate branching at the forehead. The desired donor nerve is approached either via bicoronal skin incision and subsequent open forehead dissection up to the supraorbital rim, or through two smaller skin incisions along the hairline as inlet for the endoscopic donor nerve dissection. The donor nerve is mobilized over at least 6 cm from the orbital rim (longer for contralateral donor nerves) in order to provide sufficient length to reach the affected cornea and allow unrestricted post-surgical eyeball excursion. Next the dissected donor nerve is subcutaneously tunneled to a small skin incision along the lid crease of the upper eyelid and further into the subconjunctival space of the anesthetic eye through a blepharotomy. The subsequent surgical steps are largely similar to the indirect neurotization technique and described below.

26.3.4 Neurotization with Nerve Transfers and Nerve Grafts ("Indirect" Neurotization)

Minimally invasive corneal neurotization (the authors' preferred technique; see Fig. 26.2) can be performed in two teams with one team harvesting the nerve graft and one team preparing the facial donor site simultaneously. This two-team approach saves the operative time necessary for sural nerve harvest (1 h) and reduces overall OR time.

The patient is under general anesthesia and placed in the supine position. Eyes, forehead and nerve graft harvesting site are freely accessible, surgically prepped and draped. The anesthetic eye is prepared with povidone-iodine ophthalmic solution. The unaffected contralateral eye is closed with a single stich tarsorrhaphy for the duration of the surgery.

26.3.4.1 Facial Donor Site Preparation

In cases with normal forehead sensation, the ipsilateral supraorbital nerve is considered as pri-

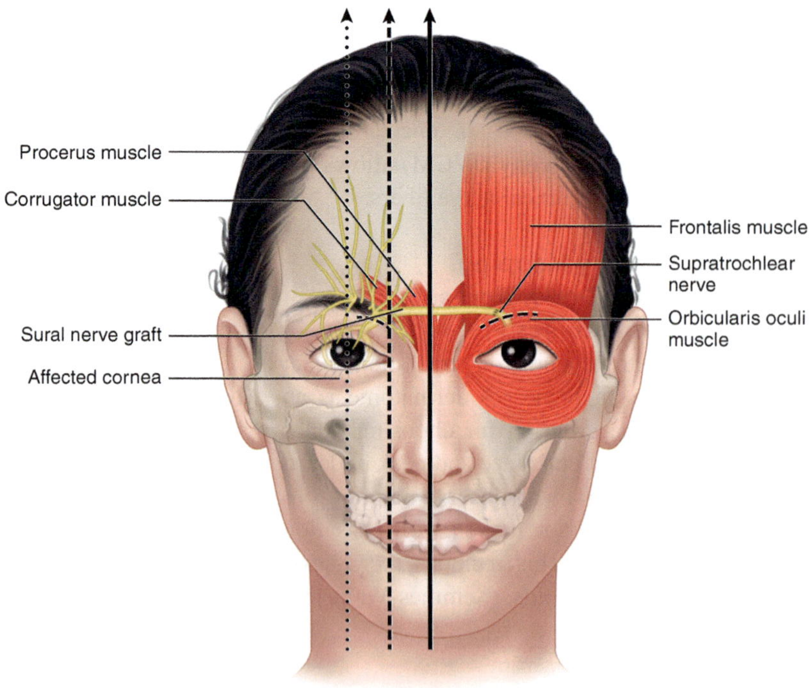

Fig. 26.2 Showing a frontal overview of the patients face and the course of the nerve graft from the supraorbital nerve to the contralateral cornea (a combination of the illustrations below)

mary axon donor with fallback options being the supratrochlear nerve or their respective contralateral counterparts. A 2 cm transverse subbrow skin incision is made, starting 1.5 cm lateral to the facial midline and extending up to the mid-pupillary line. The corrugator supercilii muscle is exposed and dissected to identify the supraorbital and supratrochlear nerves. The supraorbital nerve may be expected 20 mm lateral to the facial midline whereas the supratrochlear nerve usually runs 2–10 mm medial to the supraorbital nerve (10–18 mm lateral to facial midline). Following dissection of both nerves, the most appropriate donor nerve is chosen based on a larger diameter and reasonable size match with the harvested nerve graft. If both nerves are small in diameter, both nerves can be used as donors and connected to one or two nerve grafts.

26.3.4.2 Sural Nerve Harvest and Nerve Graft Design

The diameter of the nerve graft ideally matches the donor nerve diameter. In some cases, when the nerve graft is thin and monofascicular two parallel nerve graft cables can be used instead of one. This needs to be taken into account when defining the length of the nerve graft during harvest. The sural nerve can be identified dorso-proximal to the lateral malleolus and the desired graft length can be harvested with a nerve stripper device. Traction to the graft is avoided to preserve its endoneurial architecture and only the very ends of the nerve graft are grasped and will be resected eventually. The proximal end of the graft is labeled and placed in moist sterile gauze until further use. Skin incisions are closed.

The appropriate nerve graft length can be estimated by placing the graft on the patient's face: one end of the graft is touching the donor nerve at the desired coaptation site and the graft is placed transversal above the nasal rim up to the mid-pupillary line of the affected eye, angling in a caudal direction and coursing caudally up to the top of the nasal ala. As a rule of thumb this distance provides sufficient length for tensionless nerve grafting and permits unrestricted globe excursion following surgery. For ipsilateral corneal neurotization, the ipsilateral top of the nasal ala can be used as a landmark.

26.3.4.3 Tunneling and Corneoscleral Insertion of the Nerve Graft

A reversed graft orientation is used for corneal neurotization. Thus, the formerly distal nerve graft end is coapted to the donor nerve eventually. This reversed orientation ensures that each provided endoneurial tube inside the graft guides the regenerating donor axons to their target and not to a former nerve branch. In the anesthetic eye, a 5 mm conjunctival and Tenon's incision is made parallel to and approximately 5 mm distant to the superonasal corneal limbus. Another incision is created in the superior and medial upper fornix, through which a Wright fascia needle is directed, to create a tunnel from the conjunctival incision to the ipsilateral skin incision below the brow. Then, the nerve graft is loaded into the eyelet and gently passed through the tunnel and then under the Tenon's capsule to the first conjunctival incision.

An epineurectomy of the distal 3–4 cm of the nerve graft is performed to separate the fascicles, grasping only the very end of the fascicle. Depending on the total number of separated fascicles (usually 3–4) the insertion point for each fascicle at the corneoscleral junction is defined. The insertion points are evenly distributed around the whole corneoscleral circumference to aim at an even corneal innervation pattern. Wescott scissors are used for blunt dissection of a tunnel in the subconjunctival plane, extending in a constant 5 mm distance to the corneoscleral junction and up to the limbus at the predefined fascicle insertion points. Auxiliary conjunctival incisions may be used if necessary. Subsequently, the individual fascicles are tunneled to their predefined insertion points. Nerve graft desiccation must be avoided at all times.

Partial-thickness corneoscleral tunnels are established at the individual insertion points in order to minimize the physical barriers for the regenerating donor axons (see Fig. 26.3). A crescent blade creates a scleral tunnel incision 1 mm posterior to the limbus, extending 0.5 mm into clear corneal stroma. Now, the end of the

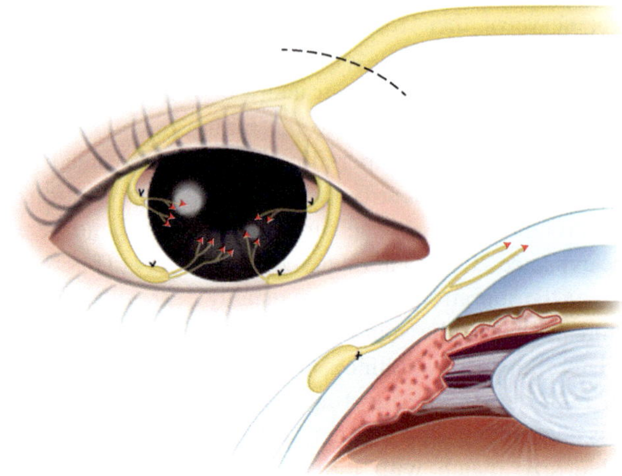

Fig. 26.3 Showing the course of the fascicles below the conjunctiva in higher magnification and the final position of the fascicle ends inside the corneoscleral tunnels (frontal overview and cross-sectional view, adapted from the illustrations below)

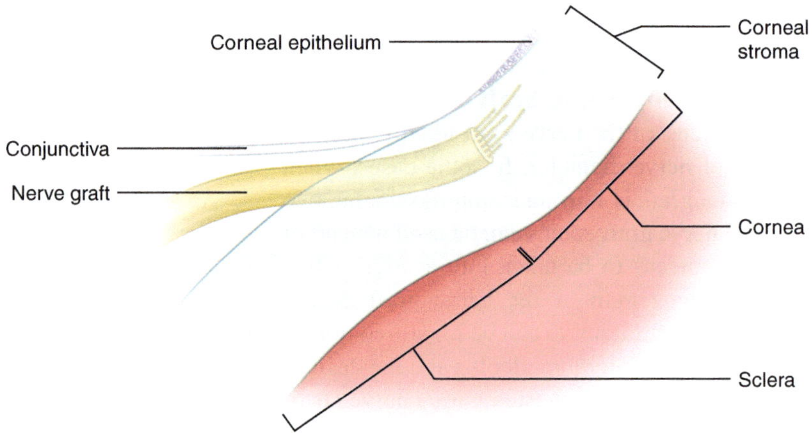

fascicles is trimmed with Vannas scissors to resect the segment that has been grasped by the surgical instruments to ensure a healthy fascicular architecture. The end of the fascicle is carefully inserted into the corneoscleral tunnel. The perineurium of the graft fascicle is sutured to the sclera proximal to the corneoscleral tunnel using a single stich (10-0 absorbable monofilament suture) and taking care not to compress the nerve. Then, all conjunctival incisions are closed with 10-0 absorbable, monofilament suture. If there is severe subconjunctival scarring and therefore tensionless conjunctival closure is not possible, larger conjunctival flaps are mobilized to prevent compression of the subconjunctival nerve graft.

26.3.4.4 Proximal Nerve Coaptation

The mechanical stress at this specific nerve coaptation site is negligible if the patient is compliant and avoids rubbing his eyes following nerve surgery. Therefore, apart from standard epineurial suture repair, fibrin glue can be used to connect the nerve graft to the donor nerve. To do so, the donor nerve is transected and the end of the nerve graft is trimmed. The graft is then coapted to the distal end of the donor nerve with thorough epineurial alignment. The coaptation site is covered with fibrin glue and fibrin aggregation is awaited before proceeding. The skin incision is closed and the operated eye is irrigated with sterile saline. Corticoid-antibiotic-ointment (e.g., Tobradex, Novartis AG, Switzerland) is applied to control postsurgical inflammation and swelling and a temporary tarsorrhaphy is made to protect the operated eye. The tarsorrhaphy of the unaffected eye is removed.

26.3.5 Postsurgical Management and Potential Complications

Usually, minimally invasive corneal neurotization can be done on an outpatient basis. The corticoid-antibiotic-ointment is continued two to three times per day until the protective tarsorrhaphy is removed during the first follow up, 1 week after surgery. As of week 2, lubricant eye drops can be used at the same frequency as prior to corneal neurotization. Any eye manipulation or rubbing must be avoided within the first weeks post-surgery as this potentially results in nerve graft displacement or extrusion.

Usually, follow-up assessments take place 1 week and 1 month after surgery, and then in a 3 months interval or as needed afterwards. On each follow up visit, the operated eye will be checked for complications. Early after surgery these may include general postsurgical complications such as bleeding, hematoma, surgical site infection and wound healing deficit. Beyond that, the eye needs to be examined for extrusion or displacement of the nerve graft. If the patient reports continuous pain, this may be indicative of neuroma development, most likely at the nerve coaptation site or the insertion sites at the corneoscleral junction. Neuromas following minimally invasive corneal neurotization are rare but can be painful and typically occur at physical barriers that potentially impair the axonal regeneration and corneal innervation process. Also, corneal neurotization can result in temporary, or seldom even permanent paresthesia and/or pain at the donor site (e.g., forehead and scalp for supraorbital or supratrochlear donor nerves).

26.3.6 Prognosis

26.3.6.1 Corneal Reinnervation and Recovery of Corneal Sensation

Restoring sensation in the anesthetic cornea is a therapeutic goal of corneal neurotization. Clinical magnetoencephalography, IVCM and in experimental neuronal back-labeling studies demonstrated that following corneal neurotization, axons that arise from the donor nerve (re-) innervate the cornea [9, 10]. The time to corneal innervation following minimally invasive corneal neurotization with nerve graft interposition depends on the length of the graft and individual factors that affect the axonal regeneration rate such as the patient's age. Likewise, the recovery of tactile corneal sensation assessed via esthesiometry depends on these factors and starts to recover approximately 3 months following surgery, when the supraorbital of supratrochlear nerve was used as axon donor [10]. After corneal (re-)innervation, neuronal circuits that have previously been connected to the donor site now process corneal stimuli. As a result, neuronal signals that have been elicited by stimulation of the neurotized cornea will be processed, and initially even perceived, as stimulation of the donor site [5]. Mechanisms of central plasticity may allow re-allocation of the perceived stimulus in a process of sensory relearning.

Approximately 65% of the patients eventually reach normal levels of tactile corneal sensation (Cochet-Bonnet esthesiometry 60 mm) and approximately 90% of the patients reach tactile thresholds above 75% (40 mm) of the normal corneal sensation [10]. The onset of patient reported sensation often precedes the tactile sensation assessed via esthesiometry. Initially, these subjective sensations may include unpleasant paresthesias such as tingling or burning and sometimes even pain. We hypothesize that this might be the result of the corneal innervation process when the regenerating sensory nerve fibers encounter the adverse environment of the defective cornea. Over the time, the refueled corneal repair and healing mechanisms may explain the symptoms' mitigation.

26.3.6.2 Corneal Clarity and Surface Health

In neurotrophic keratopathy, corneal opacity, persistent epithelial defects, and corneal ulceration threaten vision. Therefore, a second treatment objective for corneal neurotization is to restore and maintain ocular surface health. The incidence of persistent epithelial defects can be significantly reduced by corneal neurotization and in many patients the corneal clarity improves by mitigating epitheliopathy [2, 10]. If patients develop deep corneal ulceration before surgery, residual stromal scarring can impair visual acuity even following successful corneal neurotization. To achieve visual rehabilitation in these patients, subsequent corneal transplantation 2–3 years after corneal neurotization may be an option. In early disease stages though, the visual acuity can be, at least in part, recovered by corneal neurotization.

26.3.6.3 Donor Site Sensory Deficit

The surgical transfer of donor nerve fibers implies the (partial) denervation of the donor site. Initially this results in donor site hypo- and/or paresthesia including numbness and sometimes itching or tingling [2]. Over time, sensory nerve fibers of adjacent nerves terminally sprout and reinnervate the donor site. For the most frequently used axon donors, the supraorbital and supratrochlear nerve, patients report a regression of the sensory donor site deficit up to subjectively normal forehead sensation within months after direct and indirect corneal neurotization [2, 5].

26.3.6.4 Necessity of Adjunct Treatment Following Corneal Neurotization

Corneal neurotization may overcome the need for long-term usage of bandage or scleral contact lenses and tarsorrhaphy. However, the lacrimation of the affected eye often remains below normal levels. A potential reason for the insufficient recovery of the tearing reflex is that the sensory donor neuron population is not embedded in the original neuronal circuit that governs the tearing response. As a result, afferent corneal nerve fiber signals may not be translated into efferent signals to the lacrimal glands. Consequently, the patients often need to proceed with lubricants and/or autologous serum drops even after successful corneal neurotization [10]. This needs to be a subject of the preoperative patient discussion.

26.4 Conclusion

Congenital absence or acquired loss of corneal innervation causes neurotrophic keratopathy. The progressive epithelial breakdown and repetitive unperceived corneal trauma can culminate in loss of the affected eye and irreversible blindness. Conventional ophthalmic treatment strategies manage the symptoms yet are unable to address the fundamental lack of corneal nerve fibers. Corneal neurotization reroutes healthy donor nerve fibers to the anesthetic cornea to restore corneal innervation. These rerouted nerve fibers provide the cornea with sensation and thereby protect the cornea from injury. Beyond that, corneal clarity and surface health can be recovered due to corneal (re-)innervation, with a significantly reduced incidence of nonhealing epithelial defects. These results underpin the clinical value of corneal neurotization in the management of neurotrophic keratopathy.

Ideally, corneal neurotization would overcome the need for conservative ophthalmic treatments by addressing the fundamental lack of corneal nerve fibers. However, current surgical strategies fail to completely restore the insufficient lacrimation, which necessitates a continued daily application of lubricant eye drops even following successful corneal neurotization. Therefore, creating a realistic level of expectation in the pre-surgical patient discussion is mandatory to achieve satisfactory results and further the acceptance of this promising treatment.

References

1. Dua HS, Said DG, Messmer EM, Rolando M, Benitez-Del-Castillo JM, Hossain PN, Shortt AJ, Geerling G, Nubile M, Figueiredo FC, Rauz S, Mastropasqua L, Rama P, Baudouin C. Neurotrophic keratopathy. Prog Retin Eye Res. 2018;66:107–31.
2. Terzis JK, Dryer MM, Bodner BI. Corneal neurotization: a novel solution to neurotrophic keratopathy. Plast Reconstr Surg. 2009;123(1):112–20.
3. Leyngold I, Weller C, Leyngold M, Tabor M. Endoscopic corneal neurotization: technique and initial experience. Ophthalmic Plast Reconstr Surg. 2018;34(1):82–5.

4. Elbaz U, Bains R, Zuker RM, Borschel GH, Ali A. Restoration of corneal sensation with regional nerve transfers and nerve grafts: a new approach to a difficult problem. JAMA Ophthalmol. 2014;132(11):1289–95.
5. Bains RD, Elbaz U, Zuker RM, Ali A, Borschel GH. Corneal neurotization from the supratrochlear nerve with sural nerve grafts: a minimally invasive approach. Plast Reconstr Surg. 2015;135(2):397e–400e.
6. Gyori E, Tzou CH, Weninger WJ, Reissig L, Schmidt-Erfurth U, Radtke C, Dunavoelgyi R. Axon numbers and landmarks of trigeminal donor nerves for corneal neurotization. PLoS One. 2018;13(10):e0206642.
7. Benkhatar H, Levy O, Goemaere I, Borderie V, Laroche L, Bouheraoua N. Corneal neurotization with a great auricular nerve graft: effective reinnervation demonstrated by in vivo confocal microscopy. Cornea. 2018;37(5):647–50.
8. Leyngold IM, Yen MT, Tian J, Leyngold MM, Vora GK, Weller C. Minimally invasive corneal neurotization with acellular nerve allograft: surgical technique and clinical outcomes. Ophthalmic Plast Reconstr Surg. 2019;35(2):133–40.
9. Catapano J, Antonyshyn K, Zhang JJ, Gordon T, Borschel GH. Corneal neurotization improves ocular surface health in a novel rat model of neurotrophic keratopathy and corneal neurotization. Invest Ophthalmol Vis Sci. 2018;59(11):4345–54.
10. Catapano J, Fung SSM, Halliday W, Jobst C, Cheyne D, Ho ES, Zuker RM, Borschel GH, Ali A. Treatment of neurotrophic keratopathy with minimally invasive corneal neurotisation: long-term clinical outcomes and evidence of corneal reinnervation. Br J Ophthalmol. 2019;103(12):1724–31.

Part V

Facial Simmetrization

Principles of Symmetrisation Techniques in Facial Palsy

27

Caroline Driessen, Chieh-Han John Tzou, and Andrés Rodríguez-Lorenzo

Key Points

- Ancillary procedures balance between enhancing the happy mimic expression group and attenuating the unhappy mimic expression group.
- Autogenous fascia lata grafts are strong, immune compatible and ample available.
- Ancillary procedures by means of static reinforcement may improve ectropion, epiphora, keratitis, nasal obstruction, oral competence, articulation and aesthetic appearance.
- Static support may be used as a singular operation or in conjunction with dynamic reconstruction.
- Consider botulinum toxin injection in the affected side for both flaccid as non-flaccid facial features and in the non-affected side for hyperkinesis.

Surgical techniques for facial reanimation may be good, but unfortunately, it's not perfect. Also, due to comorbidity or life-expectancy, dynamic reconstruction may be less attractive. Therefore, there is a need of ancillary procedures to improve symmetrisation. Depending on the underlying illness and patients' age and wishes ancillary procedures to the forehead, periocular complex, nose, and lips should be considered to optimize the result. The chapter will introduce the principles that will guide the surgeon through choosing the best symmetrisation techniques in facial palsy.

Each face is different, and even more so after facial reanimation. A thorough study of the face should precede a tailored plan of treatment.

Generally, to achieve symmetry in unilateral facial palsy, the affected side may be enhanced or the unaffected side may be weakened. Some of the facial muscles can roughly be divided into a 'happy' mimic expression group (risorius muscle, zygomaticus major muscle, zygomaticus minor muscle, buccinator muscle, levator labii superioris muscle, levator labii superioris alaeque nasi muscle) and an 'unhappy' mimic expression group (procerus muscle, corrugator supercilli muscle, depressor supercilli muscle, depressor anguli oris muscle, depressor labii inferioris muscle, mentalis muscle, platysma muscle).

Furthermore, it should be evaluated if synkinesis or hyperkinesis is present. They are a symptom of aberrant nerve activity and represent partial recovery. Synkinesis is referred to as

C. Driessen (✉) · A. Rodríguez-Lorenzo
Department of Plastic and Maxillofacial Surgery, Uppsala University Hospital, Uppsala, Sweden
e-mail: andres.rodriguez.lorenzo@surgsci.uu.se

C.-H. J. Tzou
Plastic and Reconstructive Surgery, Department of Surgery, Hospital of Divine Savior (Krankenhaus Goettlicher Heiland), Sigmund Freud University, Vienna, Austria
e-mail: science@tzou.at, science@tzoumedical.com

© Springer Nature Switzerland AG 2021
C.-H. J. Tzou, A. Rodríguez-Lorenzo (eds.), *Facial Palsy*,
https://doi.org/10.1007/978-3-030-50784-8_27

involuntary, synchronous movements of different muscles. The co-contraction may regard agonist muscles, such as the orbicularis oculi muscle with the zygomatic major muscle, or antagonist muscles, such as the depressor anguli oris muscle with the zygomatic major muscle. The antagonist co-contraction will result in an apparent paralysis. Faccid paralyses is associated with a great functional deficit due to the apparent paralysis. Other synkinesis, as well as hyperkinesis, results in a non-flaccid face which may be aesthetically unpleasing. Hyperkinesis may also be present at the unaffected side, as a compensatory change. This results in an asymmetric static and dynamic appearance of the unaffected side.

The face should be structurally evaluated with the subunits as following: 1. forehead, 2. periocular complex, 3. cheek, 4. nose, 5. lips and 6. neck (Fig. 27.1). Photographic, possibly with videographic documentation should be taken and after facial analysis and grading a treatment plan should be developed.

Treatments may be divided into operative and nonoperative treatment modalities. Mime therapy is of great importance as a stand-alone treatment or as an adjunct to other treatment. Botulinum toxin injection is an interesting nonoperative solution to synkinesis as well as contralateral 'hyper' kinesis. Synthetic fillers or lipofilling may be useful to add volume to the affected side or to the nonparalyzed nasolabial fold. Operative ancillary techniques are mainly static using autogenous or alloplastic materials, but may also be dynamic. Most often, they are performed with a delayed timing, but recently there has been an increase in the use of static support simultaneous with the dynamic reconstruction. Note that several approaches may be combined to optimize the result. Most procedures may be done under local anaesthesia depending on the wish of the surgeon and patient. Generally speaking, overcorrection is mandatory to prevent an insufficient long-term result of the tension of the soft tissues is normalized postoperatively.

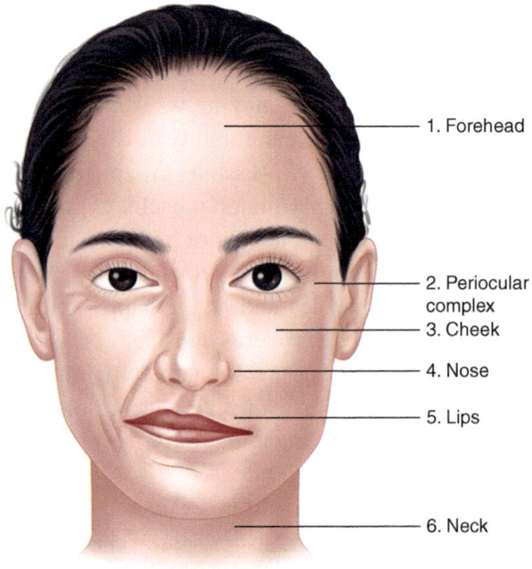

Fig. 27.1 Structural evaluation of the face. Each of the following subunits should be evaluated. 1. Forehead, 2. periocular complex, 3. cheek, 4. nose, 5. lips and 6. neck

Several considerations should be made to develop the treatment plan.

- Is the face flaccid or non-flaccid?
- What is most striking: the deficit, synkinesis or hyperkinesis at the affected side or the activity or hyperkinesis at the unaffected side?
- Would a face benefit from enhancing the happy muscles or attenuating the unhappy muscles?
- Is there a preference for either surgical or non-surgical treatment?

27.1 Botulinum Toxin

Botulinum toxin injection is used increasingly for facial symmetrisation and to counteract synkinesis by means of selective chemo denervation. The toxin is derived from the bacterium Clostridium botulinum and leads to temporary paralyses by blocking pre-synaptic acetylcholine release at the neuromuscular junction. There are two types available, namely A and B which are produced by different strains of the bacterium, of which type A is most powerful and is most commonly used. The clinical effects usually arise in the first 4 days to 2 weeks, and is maximally present 1 month after injection. After 3 months, the effects usually diminish as a resultant of newly sprouted axon terminals that regain synaptic contact with the muscle. Contra-indications for Botox injections are pregnancy, lactation, myasthenia gravis, peripheral motor neuropathies, active infections or illness and previous adverse response. Botox injections may be considered for the affected side in case of a non-flaccid face as well as for the contralateral, healthy side for the flaccid face. They may result in an improved resting and dynamic symmetry. Interestingly, there is even evidence from animal studies that suggests that contralateral Botox injections and thus transient paralysis of the unaffected side, even improves the motion on the affected side [1]. The dose is specific for each individual and different for each muscle group. It should be titrated to achieve the maximum decrease in unintended motion without minimizing intended motion. Since it takes some days to weeks for the effect to appear, it may be useful to ask a patient to make a self-portrait after 1 month so that the dose may be adjusted next time. Possible dosages are listed in Table 27.1 [2]. Several special indications for Botox are gustatory hyperlacrimation also known as crocodile tear syndrome, focal hyperhidrosis in case of Frey's syndrome and pseudoptosis in case of oro-ocular synkinesis.

The evidence for Botox for patients with facial palsy is sparse, although its use in the facial palsy clinics is well established. A review that included three interventional studies, has shown that botulinum toxin injections are well tolerated and effectively improve symmetry [3]. Several objective clinical scores were used including distance measurements of the eye, synkinesis grading scale, the Facial Disability Index, the Clinical score for Facial Palsy and Sunnybrook Score. There was also a subjective improvement in quality of life. Side effects mainly include overuse, which results in functional deficit; e.g., lagopthalmus, blepharoptosis, speech abnormalities, and/ or (rarely) oral incompetence.

In some countries, it is hard to justify these injections since they resemble techniques used in aesthetic surgery. It is important to underline that the patient population is totally different with a need for functional improvement above restoring the facial symmetry and prevention of relapse or worsening. More evidence is arising that these surgical and nonsurgical procedures are an indispensable part of the facial palsy treatment.

Table 27.1 Botulinum toxin dose ranges for synkinesis

Botulinum toxin dose ranges for synkinesis (units, type A)		
	Affected side	Unaffected side
Corrugator supercilii	5–10	–
Frontalis	–	5–10
Orbicularis oculi	2.5–7.5	7.5–10
Levator labii alaeque nasi	–	2.5–7.5
Buccinators	10–20	–
Depressor labii inferior	–	2.5–5
Depressor anguli oris	2.5–10	–
Mentalis	2.5–10	–
Platysma	10–30	–

27.2 Harvest of the Fascia or Tendon

Autogenous material may be preferred over other materials because they are immune compatible, free of cost, have limited donor site morbidity and have a low risk of extrusion and infection. They are strong and maintain its presurgical length. Most commonly, fascia lata grafts or palmaris longus tendon grafts are used as autogenous donor grafts. Harvest is as following.

The fascia lata is the deep fascia of the thigh, which gives rise to three muscular septa dividing the thigh into an anterior, posterior and medial compartment. The strength of the fascia varies, but is greatest at the upper lateral part of the leg. Here it's also reinforced by insertions of the tensor fascia lata muscle and gluteus maximus muscle which together form the iliotibial tract. This is a conjoint tendon of the fascia lata muscle and gluteus maximus muscle and it should be maintained to preserve extension, abduction and lateral rotation of the hip stabilization of the lateral knee. To harvest fascia lata, a longitudinal incision of 3–5 cm is made at the lateral aspect of the upper leg. It should be positioned there where the lateral border of the vastus lateralis muscle is expected (Fig. 27.2). Dissection through the skin and fat will bring you to the fascia lata (Fig. 27.3). The muscle fascia can be spared. There is a small potential for muscle herniation which should be discussed with the patient preoperatively. Alternatively, the posterior fascia of the rectus femoris muscle can be used without the potential of muscle herniation.

To harvest palmaris longus, first of all its presence should be confirmed since it is absent in up to 20% of people. It may also be present only at one side. The assessment is performed with the patient being awake whom is asked to flex the wrist and press the tip of the thumb against the tip of the 5th finger. A small incision is made at proximal wrist flexion crease. Different from all other tendons in the forearm, the palmaris longus tendon is always superficial to the antebrachia fascia. For orientation, palpate the flexor carpi radialis tendon on the lateral side. The more distal you go, the more difficult it is to recognize the tendon since it blends with the palmar fascia. A tendon stripper may be used and the tendon may be pulled out from its muscle without a need to make a second proximal incision. When in doubt, or when having difficulty with advancing the stripper do make a second (or even third incision). The presence and length of the palmaris longus tendon varies, which makes the fascia lata a more reliable choice if several strips are needed.

Alternatives to autogenous material are lyophilized dried cadaveric fascia, acellular dermal grafts, acellular porcine dermis and even Gore-Tex.

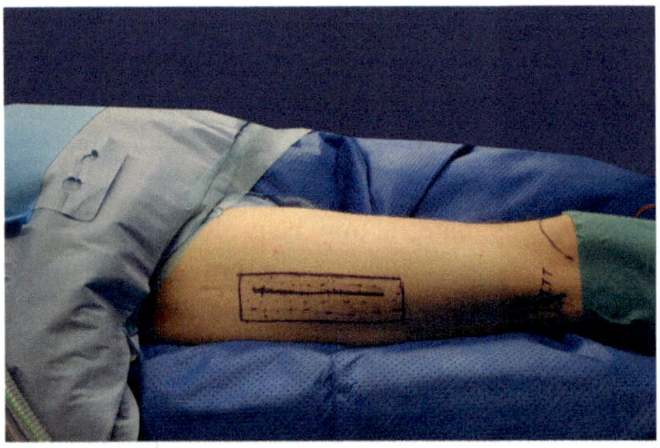

Fig. 27.2 Fascia lata harvest from the right leg of a male patient. Plan a longitudinal incision of 3–5 cm there where the lateral border of the vastus lateralis muscle is expected

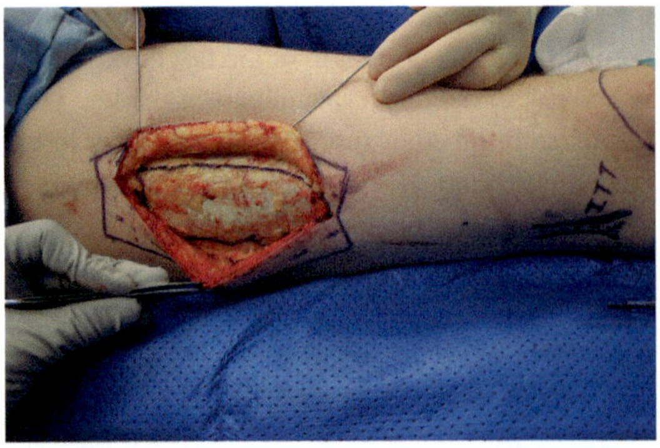

Fig. 27.3 Dissection through the skin and fat will bring you to the fascia lata. The iliotibial tract and the fascia of the vastus lateralis muscle are preserved

27.2.1 The Forehead

Palsy of the forehead will result in ptosis on the affected side and dynamic rhytides on the unaffected side. In the younger patient, with little rhytides and good quality of the skin botulinum toxin injection on the unaffected side may be satisfactory. Operative procedures include unilateral forehead which can be performed endoscopic or open or a direct eyebrow lift. The choice of endoscopic or direct brow lifting depends on the severity of brow ptosis, quality of the skin and the age of the patient. Younger patients and less severe ptosis may be addressed by means of endoscopic eyebrow lifting. Endoscopic is relatively ineffective among elderly patients whose eyebrow ptosis is severe. If these patients agree to a somewhat more visible scar, conventional juxta-brow excision is indicated [4]. Direct brow lifting may include a skin excision only or combined with dermal.

An alternative way is the trans-blepharoplasty approach. In the era of Endotine®, this is a relatively easy technique with a direct effect on the eyebrow position but without the visible scar. It is often combined with upper lid blepharoplasty and is performed through the same incision. Also, the longevity of brow elevation in endoscopic brow lift with Endotine® has been established, some argue that the amount of lifting is limited so that it's indicated in mild to moderate ptosis of the brow [5].

27.2.2 The Periocular Complex

The periocular complex may be affected in different ways that should carefully be evaluated. Closure of the eyelids is of vital importance to protect the eye. Facial palsy may result in paralytic retraction of the eyelid, lagophthalmos, paralytic ectropion, epiphora due to malposition of the lower eyelid punctum and even midface ptosis. The vision may be severely affected, mainly after longstanding paralysis of the temporal branch. Moreover, the orbicularis oculi muscle is a significant contributor of facial expression when smiling. Asymmetry of the aperture of the eyes and the lower eyelid and at the level of the lateral orbit may thus be observed when smiling. Botulinum toxin injection may therefore be needed to weaken the unaffected side. This must be carefully addressed since overuse of botulinum toxin may result in lagophthalmos of the unaffected eye.

Operative procedures include upper eyelid loading with a gold weight or platinum chain, medial and lateral canthoplasty and suspension of the inferior palpebra with allogenous or autogenous unvascularized fascia or tendon. Weight placement typically is the first step. Transposition of a double-belly temporalis flap may be used as a dynamic procedure to enhance closure of the eye. Midfacelifting has been described to address ptosis. A lift of the SOOF or (subperiostal midfacelift) have been described to address a ptotic palpebral-malar sulcus, retraction and lower eyelid and ptosis of the midface [6–9].

Periocular surgery should not be postponed to avoid corneal complications due to lagophthalmos from upper eyelid retraction or lower lid laxity. The ophthalmologists should be involved from the beginning onwards. Little interventions improve eye comfort, safety, and aesthetics.

27.2.3 The Cheek

The nasolabial fold occurs because of connections between upper lip elevators and the dermis. When smiling, the connections contract too and as a result the fold gets deeper. A lack of motion of the midface results in a lack of the nasolabial fold, which may be quite striking. It may be recreated by creating a scar at this location. There are several variations of techniques to deepen the nasolabial fold by attaching fascia transplants from the sub–superficial musculoaponeurotic system plane of the face to the dermis, even without creating a linear scar [10]. The nasolabial incision may also be used for suspension of the nose and lips. A case in whom the nasolabial fold was recreated, as well as the corner of the mouth was lifted, is presented in Figs. 27.4, 27.5, 27.6 and 27.7.

There may be a role for injectables and implants to improve the patient's appearance. Lipofilling is relatively new.

27.2.4 The Nose

The nose may show collapse of the nostril at the affected side due to flaccidity of the lateral nasal wall and inferior medial displacement of the alar base. A lack of tonic muscular support of the alar and transverse nasalis muscles may result in functional deficit which presents as nasal airway obstruction. It is characterized by both internal external nasal valve narrowing and collapse during inspiration. This may be further aggravated by pre-existing external and nasoseptal deformities. Nasal obstruction has a negative influence on the quality of life. It has often been over-

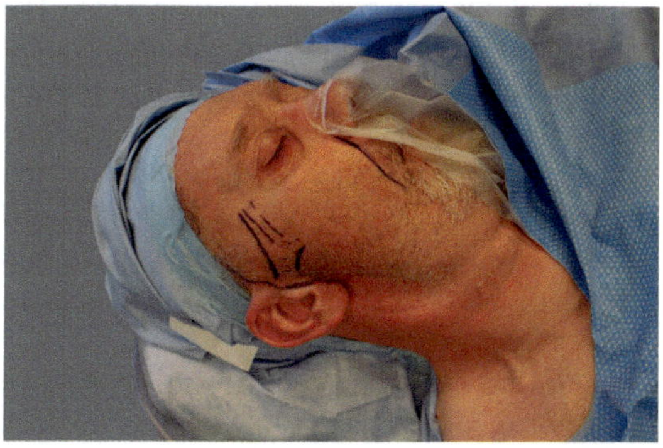

Fig. 27.4 Patient after masseter to facial nerve reconstruction after radical parotidectomy. Good dynamic function but poor static outcome due to flaccid appearance of the face

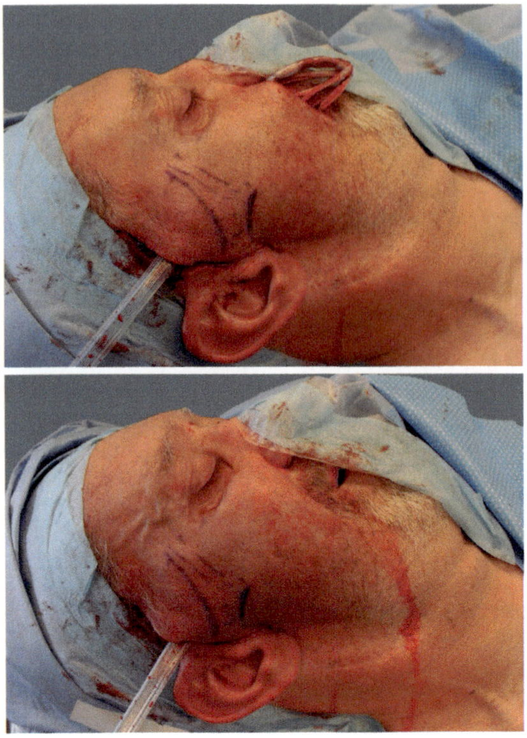

Fig. 27.5 Upper photo: positioning of the fascia lata. Lower photo: suturing the fascia lata to the orbicularis oris muscle; cranially at the floor of the nose; middle at the level of the modiolus and caudally at the level of the lower lip (white circle)

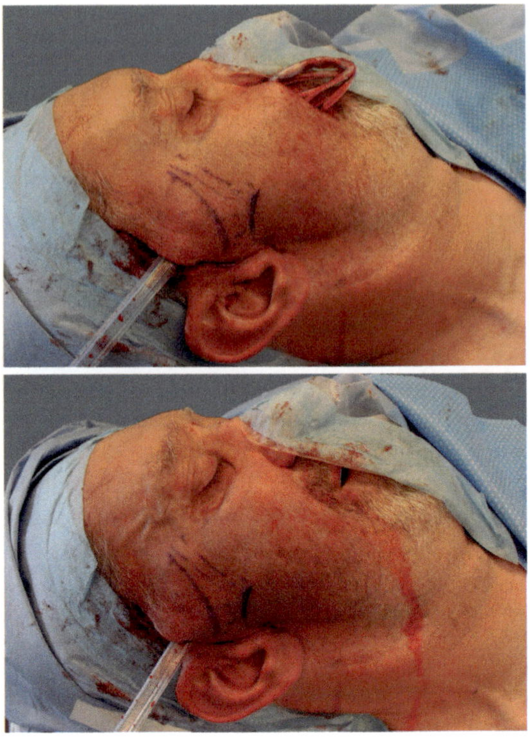

Fig. 27.6 Upper photo: tunnelling the fascia lata using a penrose drain. Lower photo: note the new nasolabial fold. Finish surgery by suturing the fascia lata with a non-resolvable suture to the temporal fascia

looked, although there is a straightforward surgical solution. Suspension of the external valve can be performed operatively by using unvascularized fascia or tendon. Fascia lata sling placement has been proved to result in great improvement in patency of the external nasal valve [11]. The exact vector is chosen at a maximal nasal widening without distortion of nasolabial philtrum. Alternatively, Paniello has described a suture to secure the nasal valve area to the inferior orbital rim periosteum [12]. This may be performed simultaneous with a facial nerve resection and immediate reconstruction or any other kind of delayed reconstruction.

Note that cartilage grafts are ineffective because they do not adequately address the lack of tonic muscular support that displaces the ala and sidewall in patients with facial palsy.

27.2.5 The Lips

Drooping of the mouth corner can be addressed on the side of paralysis or on the healthy side. It is possible to suspend the lips directly using one or multiple strips of unvascularized fascia or tendon and insert them into the superior and inferior part of the paralyzed orbicularis oris muscle (Figs. 27.5, 27.6 and 27.7). The most proximal part is attached to the temporal fascia, the parotid fascia or zygomatic arch and the fascia may be woven through the free muscle transplant if present. It may be sutured or a bone anchor could be used if the fascia is fixated to, or wrapped around the zygoma. The mouth opening is restricted to some extent because the fascia is fixed to an immovable area. Alternatively, fascia could suspend the mouth corner to the mandibular coro-

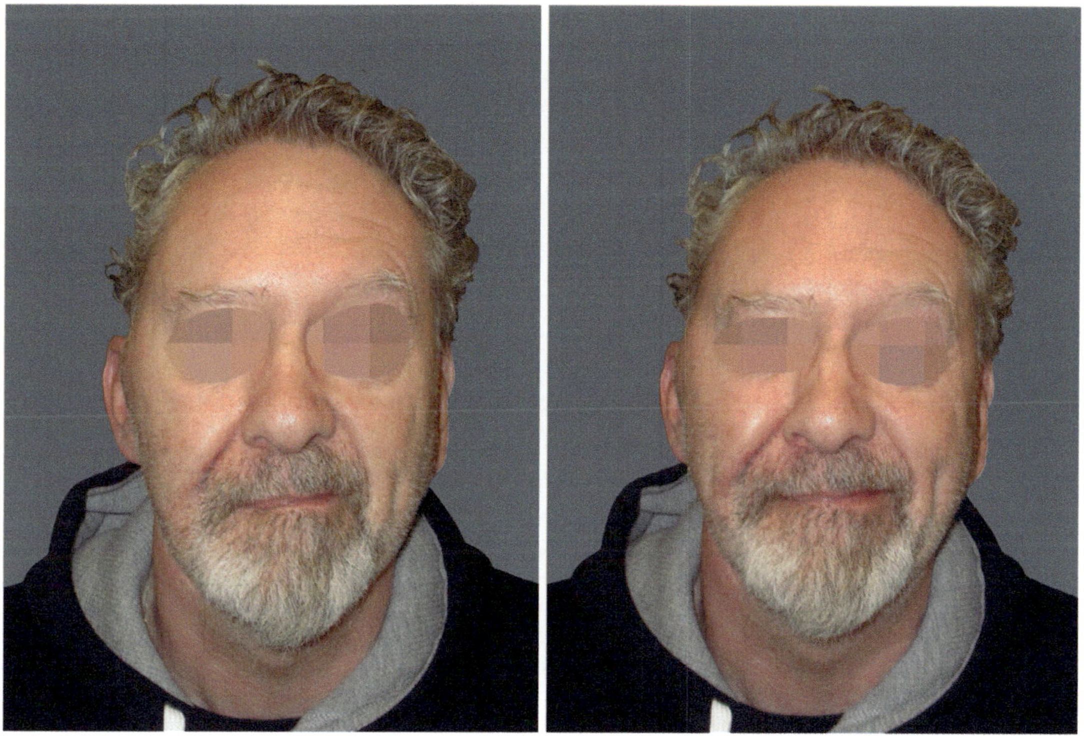

Fig. 27.7 Postoperative result at 6 weeks after surgery. Left in rest. Right while smiling. Patient was very happy. He was advised to restart mime therapy to improve the dynamic function again after this ancillary procedure

noid process to enable a shift of the mouth corner with mouth opening and closure [13]. It has also been described that the strips are inserted into the free muscle transplant proximally, and distally into the orbicularis oris muscle of the upper and lower lip on the nonparalyzed side. This reconstruction makes use of the active and spontaneous muscle contraction of the contralateral side [14]. For the lower lip, suspension of the paralyzed side has the preference. However, it is much easier to denervate the contralateral depressor labii either by means of botulinum toxin injection, neurectomy of the healthy marginal mandibular nerve or myectomy.

27.2.6 The Neck

The cervical branch of the facial nerve has a synergistic function with the marginal branch which innervate the unhappy mimics of the lower face. Inability to use the platysma muscle will alter the.

Depression of the lower lip as well as the aesthetic appearance of the neck are partially dependent on the function of the platysma muscle. Botulinum toxin injection or myectomy of the contralateral platysma muscle may be considered.

27.3 Ancillary Procedures Simultaneously with Dynamic Reconstruction

There is a trend towards using static support to the upper and lower lip in conjunction with dynamic reconstruction. It is a more aggressive approach that contributes to rebalancing the face by using fascia or tendon to function as internal splinting while waiting for re-innervation to occur [14, 15].

Suspension of the mouth using fascia or tendon may function as internal splinting of the muscle that is inactive until re-innervation occurs. With both one-stage or two-stage innervated free muscle transplantation, it takes times for the muscle flap to regain its function. This period may last for several months up to over 1 year and during this time, internal splinting may be useful to improve the oral continence and appearance of the face.

27.4 Outcome of Ancillary Procedures

The benefit of ancillary procedures may be enormous, including an immediate functional improvement in chewing, oral retention, speech articulation, smile symmetry, nasal obstruction and ectropion and aesthetic improvement. As a result, there is a tremendous improvement in quality of life. Several studies have been performed to assess the need for ancillary procedure and its effects [15]. Generally, the improvement of facial architecture was restored at 4–6 weeks after surgery, cq after the operative swelling resolved [16]. Especially scleral show, keratitis [16] and nasal obstruction [11] greatly improve after ancillary procedures. Also, in one study all patients experienced immediate subjective functional improvement in speech, fluid retention, and chewing [16].

Facial rehabilitation is of utmost importance if an ancillary procedure is performed in conjunction to a dynamic reconstruction, or if an ancillary procedure is aimed to function in a dynamic way, such as attaching fascia or tendon to a functional muscle.

Procedure-specific complications include unsatisfactory improvement and visibility of the weight, chain or strip of fascia. It is difficult to properly position the fascia. Often, a slight overcorrection is introduced during surgery to make up for the unavoidable decrease in tone during follow up.

To conclude, there is a scala of possibilities to further improve symmetry simultaneously with or after previous reanimation or as a singular treatment. Generally spoken, these procedures have a low morbidity and result in immediate aesthetic improvement.

References

1. Guntinas-Lichius O, Glowka TR, Angelov DN, Irintchev A, Neiss WF. Improved functional recovery after facial nerve reconstruction by temporary denervation of the contralateral mimic musculature with botulinum toxin in rats. Neurorehabil Neural Repair. 2011;25(1):15–23.
2. Cabin JA, Massry GG, Azizzadeh B. Botulinum toxin in the management of facial paralysis. Curr Opin Otolaryngol Head Neck Surg. 2015;23(4):272–80.
3. Cooper L, Lui M, Nduka C. Botulinum toxin treatment for facial palsy: a systematic review. J Plast Reconstr Aesthet Surg. 2017;70(6):833–41.
4. Takushima A, Harii K, Sugawara Y, Asato H. Anthropometric measurements of the endoscopic eyebrow lift in the treatment of facial paralysis. Plast Reconstr Surg. 2003;111(7):2157–65.
5. Tyers AG. Brow lift via the direct and transblepharoplasty approaches. Orbit. 2006;25(4):261–5.
6. Alford EL. The SOOF lift as an adjunct in rehabilitation of facial paralysis: help or hype? Facial Plast Surg. 2000;16(4):345–9.
7. Fedok FG, Ferraro RE. Restoration of lower eyelid support in facial paralysis. Facial Plast Surg. 2000;16(4):337–43.
8. Ibrahim AM, Rabie AN, Kim PS, Medina M, Upton J, Lee BT, et al. Static treatment modalities in facial paralysis: a review. J Reconstr Microsurg. 2013;29(4):223–32.
9. Olver JM. Raising the suborbicularis oculi fat (SOOF): its role in chronic facial palsy. Br J Ophthalmol. 2000;84(12):1401–6.
10. Faris C, Heiser A, Jowett N, Hadlock T. Minimal nasolabial incision technique for nasolabial fold modification in patients with facial paralysis. JAMA Facial Plast Surg. 2018;20(2):148–53.
11. Lindsay RW, Bhama P, Hohman M, Hadlock TA. Prospective evaluation of quality-of-life improvement after correction of the alar base in the flaccidly paralyzed face. JAMA Facial Plast Surg. 2015;17(2):108–12.
12. Paniello RC. Nasal valve suspension. An effective treatment for nasal valve collapse. Arch Otolaryngol Head Neck Surg. 1996;122(12):1342–6.
13. Yoshimoto S, Sato N, Kuroki T, Rikihisa N, Ichinose M. Static reconstruction of malar region in facial paralysis: a new alternative technique for plasty of

symmetric mouth appearance. J Plast Surg Hand Surg. 2013;47(5):390–3.
14. Horta R, Correia-Sa I, Nascimento R, Silva A, Amarante J. Correction of residual static and dynamic labial deviations in a paralyzed face after free gracilis muscle transplantation. J Craniofac Surg. 2016;27(8):2143–5.
15. Bianchi B, Ferri A, Ferrari S, Leporati M, Ferri T, Sesenna E. Ancillary procedures in facial animation surgery. J Oral Maxillofac Surg. 2014;72(12):2582–90.
16. Rose EH. Autogenous fascia lata grafts: clinical applications in reanimation of the totally or partially paralyzed face. Plast Reconstr Surg. 2005;116(1):20–32; discussion 3–5

28 Aesthetic Consideration and Ancillary Procedures in Facial Paralysis Reanimation

Per Hedén

28.1 Personal Background

Already in the early 1990s the author started to use botulinum toxin for facial paralysis patients and aesthetic indications. He was also part of the introduction of Hyaluronic Acid and has built a large nonsurgical practice within his chain of clinics, Akademikliniken in Scandinavia. Since the early 1980s Dr. Hedén has also had a profound interest in facial paralysis reanimation and worked for more than 30 years with microneurovascular reanimation procedures and added a number of different aesthetic components to the reanimation problem.

28.2 Introduction

A facial paralysis is a difficult reconstructive problem relating to several different factors:

1. The variability of the condition is greatly different related to (a) the functional loss, (b) the aesthetic loss, (c) the patient suffering and (d) the duration of the paralysis. This last point is greatly relevant for the timing of reconstruction and important for final results of a reanimation procedure.
2. Secondly facial paralysis reanimation is technically demanding repairs with a multitude of different techniques and treatment to consider.
3. It is also impossible to achieve as good result as the healthy side of a hemifacial paralysis has or as natural movements as an unaffected face has in a bilateral paralysis. This is due to the great facial animation variability relating to the 35 different mimic muscles present in the face. All these muscles are innervated by the seventh cranial nerve.
4. The fourth factor making facial palsy reanimation difficult is that optimal outcome involves a multitude of different considerations and use of a multitude of different procedures to achieve a good result. Thus, a reconstructive surgeon dealing with facial paralysis has to master many different both aesthetic and reconstructive operations.

When it comes to selection of the reconstructive technique, this relates to

1. Duration of the paralysis.
2. Age of the patient.
3. Complicating diseases.
4. Functional problems.
5. Aesthetic loss and suffering.

The duration of the paralysis greatly affects the reinnervation prognosis, the earlier reinnervation can be performed the better the

P. Hedén (✉)
Department of Plastic Surgery, Akademikliniken, Stockholm, Sweden
e-mail: per.heden@ak.se

© Springer Nature Switzerland AG 2021
C.-H. J. Tzou, A. Rodríguez-Lorenzo (eds.), *Facial Palsy*, https://doi.org/10.1007/978-3-030-50784-8_28

chances are for a good outcome. Over time a paralysis of mimic muscle will gradually result in fibrosis and permanent muscle injury making any reanimation of these muscles impossible. It is not clearly demonstrated how long reanimation can be performed but it is unlikely that any innervation procedure of facial muscles of mimic two years after a paralysis will be effective. Most successful reinnervation procedures of paralyzed muscles are done within a year after the start of the paralysis.

Another important factor when selecting the reconstructive technique is the age of the patient. Young patients have more favorable outcomes of reanimation and adopts better to a reanimation procedure compared to elderly patients. This does not exclude however that reanimation with nerve transplantation and muscle transfer can be achieved even in the more senior patients and successful free muscle reanimations have been performed in complicating diseases such as irradiation after cancer and diabetes mellitus must be considered as these reduce the chances for success with reanimation procedures. Another important factor when it comes to selecting reconstructive technique is the functional loss. Minor functional loss may be disturbing to the patient but may be a week indication for reanimation procedures. However, patients' suffering is of great importance, and the more the patient suffers from the aesthetic and functional loss the stronger the indications are for reanimation attempts.

28.3 Acute and Subacute Facial Paralysis 0–18 Months

Unfortunately most patients and many physicians do not recognize the importance of the duration of a denervation. Considering the fact that no reconstructive procedure never can replace the versatile 17 facial mimic muscles on one facial side or the 35 on both sides it is of great importance not to neglect the possibility of early muscle reinnervation of acute facial paralysis. However, it is widely common practice that patents with an acute facial paralysis are treated with "wait and see" before being referred to a reconstructive facial paralysis surgeon. This is especially true, and can even be considered the best option for Bell's palsy as most of these spontaneous paralysis restore completely. Some of these (6–10%) do however have such a pronounced sequel that they may need advanced microneurovascular muscle transfers. If treated early with e.g., cross-facial nerve grafts this might have been avoidable. There is no consensus on early treatment of Bell's palsy but an active approach to other etiologies to the paralysis (such as trauma or surgical lesions) should definitely be considered. Denervated facial muscles have increased sensitivity for axon sprouting and this has a duration of up to 18 months. If muscles are not reinnervated within this time there is a replacement of collagen and fat, thus fibrosis within the muscle. To avoid these problems early reinnervation of the facial muscles is important if this is possible. Thus some type of primary nerve repair as soon as possible with the help of a direct nerve suture for peripheral injuries and hypoglossal transfer with combination of cross facial nerve grafting may be indicated in more central nerve injuries. Cross-facial nerve grafts can be used to minimize the mass movement seen after hypoglossal transfer. The author has used a complete transection of the hypoglossal nerve with end to end anastomosis of the facial nerve in patients with relatively long duration of the paralysis (12 months) with good outcomes in the reinnervation. To avoid problems from the paralyzed tongue a nerve graft is put end to side to the hypoglossal facial anastomosis and connected to the distal end of the cut hypoglossal nerve in the base of the tongue. For bilateral acute facial paralysis a jump graft from the hypoglossal to the facial nerve is favored to minimize risks for bilateral affection of tongue. For chronic facial paralysis with the duration of more than 18 months dynamic reconstruction is usually favored, regional muscle transposition with temporalis (Labbé) could be considered but for younger individuals the author has favored a two stage free gracilis transfer with cross facial nerve grafting in stage one. In some situations this has been combined with powering of the muscle with an end to side anastomosis of the masseter nerve. Initially the author used pectoralis minor but due to its short vascular stalk more difficulty in harvesting the gracilis muscle has been favored in most cases. In secondary cases a segment of latissimus has also been used as this gives long neurovascular pedicles for anastomosis to more distant vessels. This chapter only deals with aesthetic considerations for these procedures and not the other aspects of free muscle transplant that are covered in other chapters of this book.

28.4 Aesthetic Consideration in Chronic Facial Paralysis (>18 Months Duration) with Free Muscle Transplants

The chronic facial paralysis patient may suffer a multitude of different problems. These are of three different kinds: (a) functional, (b) emotional, (c) aesthetic. Functional loss relates to mainly the mouth and eye. With loss of orbicularis oculi function the blink function of the eye is reduced or lost. This creates dryness, reactive tear flow, and possibly corneal sores. A partially healed facial paresis, e.g., after Bell's palsy, may result in synkinesia when the eye is closed during smiling. Treatment of this is covered below.

The loss of function in perioral muscles mainly zygomaticus major and minor may give the patient problems with food intake and speech. Other for most patients equally or worse suffering in unilateral facial paralysis relates to the aesthetic appearance with exaggerated asymmetry during smile. The emotional suffering, thus loss of normal interpersonal communication is best illustrated in bilateral facial complete facial paralysis. It has been said humans can only speak the language of the sole with the facial nerve intact. Thus complete loss of facial animating muscles also eliminates the normal emotional contact with other human being's. Just imagine a laughing patient with a complete bilateral facial paralysis who cannot express this in any way with a parallel smile. Other persons will not regard this as a happy person even though the patient may feel great happiness inside.

Treatment of chronic facial paralysis involves both aesthetic procedures such as elevation of the eyebrow, corner of the mouth, midface lifting, etc. (covered below) and free muscle transplant with cross facial nerve grafting and/or masseter innervation in more pronounced losses. Even if free muscle transplants with cross facial innervation can be performed in a one stage procedure the author prefers a two stage procedure with cross facial nerve grafting in the first stage. The benefit of this is shorter time to reinnervate and less atrophy and fibrosis of the transplanted muscle. To achieve both a good functional and aesthetic result of a free muscle transplantation, many surgical details have to be taken into consideration and mastered. In this chapter only the aesthetic considerations for a successful free micro neuro vascular muscle transfer will be discussed.

The following points are of importance to consider for successful aesthetic outcome of a free muscle transplant:

1. The incision and exposure.
2. The dissection plane.
3. The fixation points.
4. The fixation techniques.
5. The pulling vectors.
6. The muscle tension.
7. The facial volume.

28.4.1 Incisions

A modified facelift-parotidectomy incision is recommended. If skin closing principles for facelifts are employed the scar is usually very inconspicuous after these types of incisions. Even if a shorter incision without a neck extension has been described it limits the exposure and makes part of the fixation of the muscle more difficult and risky (Fig. 28.1a, b). A nasolabial fold incision can be avoided with a modified facelift-parotidectomy incision, neither is intraoral incisions necessary. During cross facial nerve grafting a small incision is done in the contra lateral intra nasal is used for subcutaneous placement of the sural nervegraft. Mid cheek insicions should be avoided if a scar is not located in this region due to previous trauma or surgery (Fig. 28.2a–c).

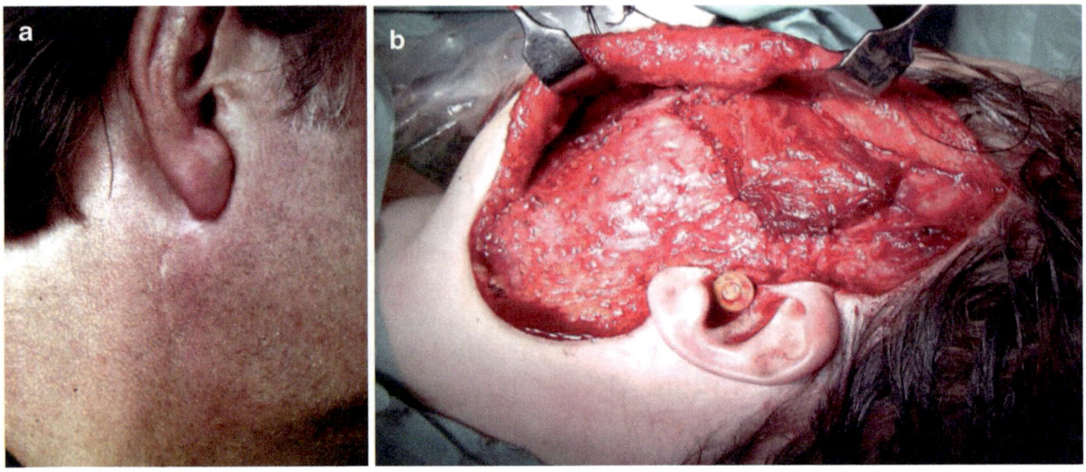

Fig. 28.1 (**a**) An average scar 6 months after a modified facelift-parotidectomy incision and (**b**) the good exposure obtained for muscle insertion and anastomoses

28.4.2 The Dissection Plane

Superficial skin dissection when elevating the flap may result in muscle movements visible through the skin (Fig. 28.3a). Therefore a sub-SMAS supra muscular dissection is favored (Fig. 28.3b). This covers the muscle transplant well and minimizes animation visibility. This dissection plane should be used with caution in the partial facial paresis but experienced facelift surgeons being used to extended high SMAS elevation has no problem with this dissection plane. The author has in a selected cases used a supraperiosteal dissection on top of the zygomatic arch and the zygoma but this advanced dissection plane is not necessary to avoid muscle animation visibility. Supraperiosteal placement of a muscle transplant also makes the insertion of the muscle and the nerve and vessels anastomosis more complicated. In addition to this the position of the parotid duct in relation to the muscle transplant has to be considered.

28.4.3 The Fixation Points

With one free muscle transplant it obviously impossible to mimic all the diverse movements of all of the perioral muscles but by using multiple fixation points a good balanced smile can be achieved. These are the alae nasi, the commissure, the upper and lower lip and the nasolabial fold.

28.4.4 The Fixation Technique

The author has found a transcutaneous suture technique to be more reliable than suturing from only the deep dissection plane the into the desired point of action (Fig. 28.4). The needle (4/0 nylon suture) is placed from the deep dissection point, straight through the skin at the desired point of action and back into the deep dissection plane through the same hole in the skin. This offers a more precise positioning of the muscle and a better control of the movements in this area. Note that when the needle is passed through the skin, the angle going in and out through the hole is different to achieve a good deep dermal bite. Initially small indentations in the skin are noted but these disappear during the first weeks of healing.

28.4.5 The Pulling Vectors

The vectors of tension should parallel the zygomatic major and minor muscle. Thus the dissected facial skin/SMAS flap must reach the lateral part of the orbit, the base of the nose, and the upper and lower lip.

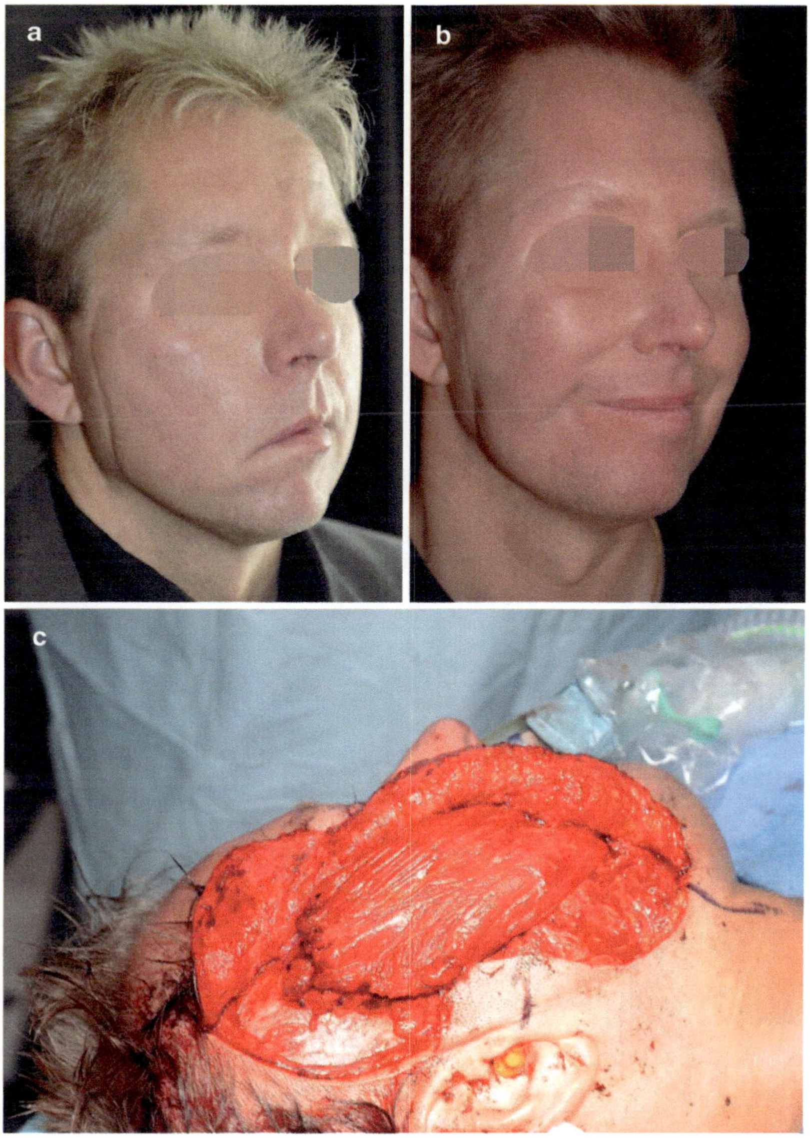

Fig. 28.2 (**a**) After previous unsuccessful free muscle transplantation with a mid-cheek incision by an unknown surgeon. (**b**) After secondary free muscle transplantation with cross-facial and masseter nerve innervation. (**c**) The modified incision for good exposure of operating field

28.4.6 The Muscle Tension

To achieve an adequate muscle tension it is useful to measure and mark (e.g., with small sutures every 1–2 cm along the resting donor muscles surface before it is divided from its donor area. When inserting the muscle the tension should simulate a full smile on the table.

28.4.7 The Facial Volume

As a free muscle transplant adds volume to the paralyzed muscle side there may be volumetric differences with facial asymmetry after a successful free muscle transplant. Therefore a fat transplantation on the healthy side could be considered. Even if this could be done at a later stage

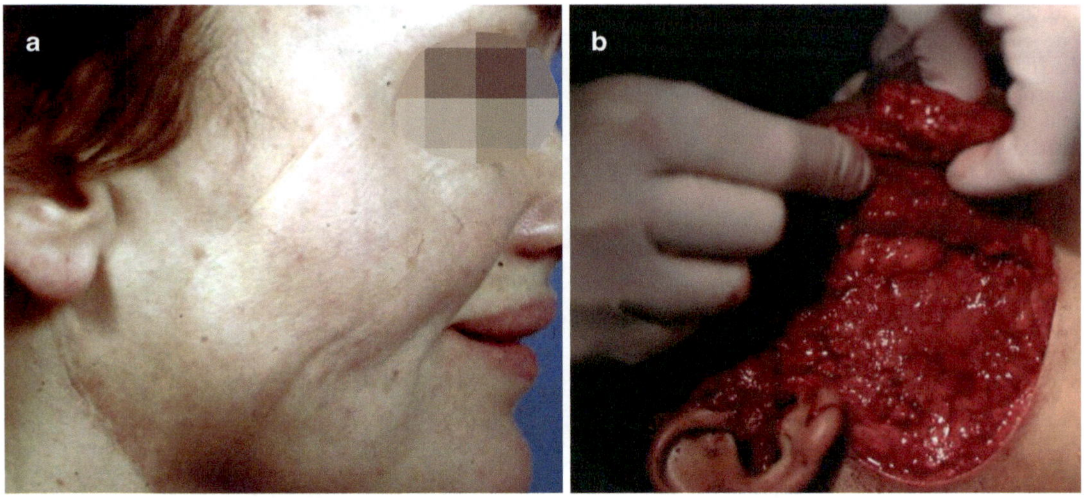

Fig. 28.3 (**a**) Mid-cheek rhytids during smiling after free muscle transplant as a result of a thin skin flap elevation. (**b**) The recommended supramuscular dissection plane including the SMAS/parotid fascia and platysma

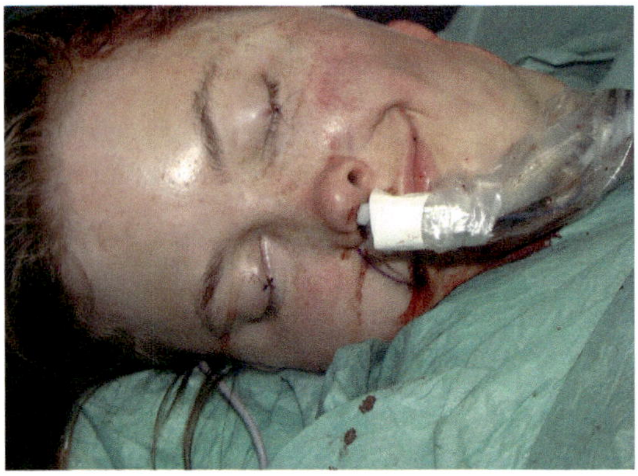

Fig. 28.4 The muscle tension on the table with transcutaneous fixation in the commissure nasolabial fold and alar base

as a complementary secondary procedure it could also be considered at the time of the cross facial nerve grafting where a small segment of fat transplant can be sutured on top of the cross facial nerve graft in a place so it mimics the contralateral muscle transplant done at a later stage. During the free muscle transplant a fat injection can also be done on the contra lateral side and to avoid too much volume during the muscle transplant a careful trimming of the muscle at primary insertion is important. However, extreme care not to over trim the muscle is recommended as a successful but weak transferred muscle makes the procedure partly unsuccessful. Bircha's fat pad removal on the paralyzed side during the muscle transplantation can also be considered to balance facial volumetric differences.

28.5 Aesthetic Considerations and Ancillary Procedures in Facial Paralysis Reanimation

In chronic facial paresis with a partial restitution and limited loss of function, free muscle transplantation is seldomly indicated, neither is regional muscle transplants. This is in spite of the fact that the patient may suffer greatly from the paresis. Much of this suffering is aesthetic but also functional problems from the eye are common. Even if free muscle transplant from the platysma and frontalis has been used by the author to reanimate the eye the indications and success of these procedures makes the indication very week for such advanced surgery. Regional muscle transplant from the temporalis muscle may be indicated but in most cases eye closure is better achieved by local procedures such as tarsoraphy, canthopexy, and possibly gold weight loading to the upper lid. These more functional procedures will not be covered in this chapter which mainly deals with the aesthetic aspects of facial paralysis reanimation. Considering the great aesthetic suffering patients with facial paralysis suffer from it is surprisingly little written about ancillary aesthetic procedures for this group of patients [1]. Most publications refer to the use of botulinum toxin and hyaluronic acids injections [2–5].

There are a number of ancillary procedures that should be mastered and considered in facial paralysis patients. These include:

1. Botulinum neuro toxin A injection
2. Hyaluronic acid injections
3. Fat grafting procedures
4. Lip lifting procedures
5. Forehead lifting procedures
6. Blepharoplasties
7. Canthopexy's
8. Midface and facelifting procedures

28.6 Botulinum Toxin (BoNt)

Botulinum toxin (BoNt) is probably the most important tool for all muscular imbalances and this is something that any physician dealing with facial paresis patients should learn and master. In many situations injectables are the only alternatives to treat a patient; this is especially true in minor muscular imbalances where botulinum toxin is the work horse (Fig. 28.5a–d). It is also an invaluable drug for refinements of more advanced free muscle transplant procedures where it is impossible to achieve exactly the same situation as on the contra lateral healthy side. An example of this is the inability to give a good depressor muscle activity during free muscle transplants. Therefore BoNt treatment of the depressor labii inferior muscles on the healthy side should be considered in many of these patients. When treating a patient with BoNt, it is of great importance to underline for the patient that this is a highly individualized treatment. Patients must be aware of the fact that it takes one to three follow-ups to find out the exact needed dose and that the duration of this is highly variable. Most facial paralysis patients need injections three to four times per year to maintain a good balanced facial situation.

Planning and performing the BoNt injection involves a detailed information to the patient about goals of the treatment and expected results. Patients should also be informed about the fact that if they don't like the treatment or if a slightly too high dose is injected in one area this problem will disappear within a couple of months. They should also understand that one or several follow-ups with a complementary injection usually is needed for fine tune the injection strategy for the future. A meticulous analysis of the facial movements involving careful photography, preferably also with video documentation, and communication related to these pictures with the patient is important before the first injection. Injections

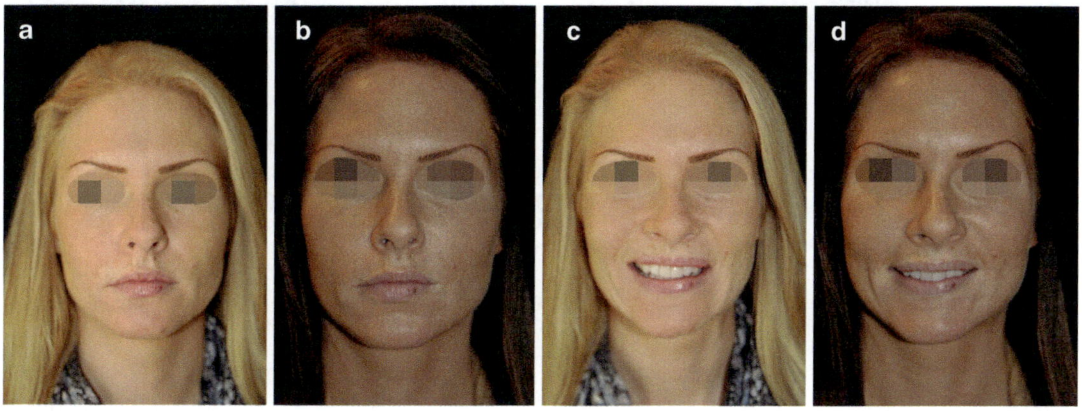

Fig. 28.5 (**a**) The sequel after Bell's palsy may be very subtle at rest but apparent (**c**) during a smile. After BoNt treatment (**b**) at rest and (**d**) smiling

involve both muscles on the contra lateral healthy and the affected paralyzed side. On the paralyzed side most common injections involves a synkinesia of the eye where injections in the upper eyelid into the pretarsal muscle are carefully tittered out. Usually 0.5 units of Botox®, if this product is used, is given in the lateral part of the pretarsal muscle over the tarsus and in the most medial part of the tarsus. Also, a similar dose in the center of the lower lid below the rim is usually given. Even if the orbicularis occuli is slighty week but has synkinesia during e.g., smiling this dose seldom create lagophtalmos problems with dry eye symptoms and more commonly the dose carefully have to be increased at follow-up. The paralyzed side can also benefit from treatment of the depressor angulis oris muscle and the platysma muscle if these have increased tonus. The contra lateral healthy side is injected to balance the paralyzed side and usually this involves the frontalis, nasalis, zygomaticus major and minor, the depressor labia inferior and the risorius muscles. Also platysma muscle and depressor angulis oris may be considered for injection and also the orbicularis oris. Many patients express that they experience increased movements on the paralyzed side when the healthy side has been injected. This may be due to the fact that reduced activity on the healthy side increases the patients' subconscious willingness to activate facial activity affecting both sides in a positive way.

Remember that BoNt treatment is like a tug of war, if we weaken one end of the rope the tug of war will move in the opposite direction. Therefore the synergistic and antagonistic effect of different muscle and also gravitational forces should be considered when planning and performing botulinum toxin injections. When it comes to the doses of BoNt this should, as mentioned above, be highly individualized and depends on the age of the patient, the sex (usually men need higher doses than women), the skin type where thick skin may need a slightly higher dose but mainly the muscle volume and the strength of the muscle. Also a great interindividual variability exists. Sometimes, even extremely small doses of botulinum toxin have profound effects for the patient.

The carefully titrated dose of BoNt should be recorded onto a facial schedule which would be the regime to follow for later injections. At follow-up, usually approximately 14 days after the first injection a new series of photos are taken and possibly also video documentation. (Fig. 28.6a, b).

The patient's satisfaction with the injections is recorded. If needed touch-up injections are given with a new follow-up 2 weeks later. When the patient is happy and the aesthetic outcome is as improved as it can be by a BoNt treatment the patient is told to wait 5 months before the follow-up and to carefully record when the imbalance reoccurs. This will help to define the ideal

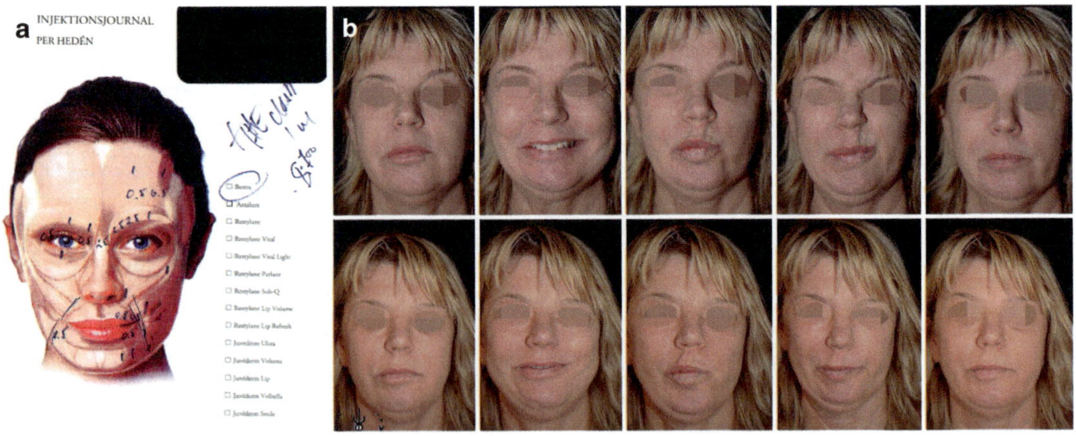

Fig. 28.6 (**a**) Example of an anatomy chart and the treatments with HA and BoNt given and (**b**) The result and examples of a series of pictures taken before and at the first follow-up after the treatment

interval between two treatments. Patients are recommended to have their re-treatments before a full recovery of the facial muscles activity. BoNt treated facial paralysis patients usually are highly satisfied and has big confidence in the physician that know and regularly treat the patient and it is often difficult to delegate this type of treatment to others. As these patients usually need injections three to four times a year, these tend to become a high burden on the outpatient clinics. For a busy surgeon it can be difficult to find time for these clinics as the number of patients rapidly increases. To master this problem and to increase the productivity during these clinics without losing quality a dedicated injections clinic is recommended where other types of outpatient follow-ups are avoided. This is a considerable time saver where several toxin vials are diluted into a larger container and syringes are prefilled by nurses. Usually 0.3 and 0.1 insulin syringes (BD®insulin syringe) are used. During these clinics HA products should also be available if needed for the reasons mentioned below. If possible patients should be treated by one physician in up to three (even four for a fast physician) different rooms with three assisting nurses who are responsible for taking patients into the treatment room, be well educated in photography and take the before and after pictures (if needed but obviously not to be done during every injection session), put the patient in the treatment chair, remove EMLA cream if used, and wipe the face clean with alcohol. The nurses are also responsible for tidying up after the injection, applying ice pack, cleaning the face, and applying moisturizing cream and take the patient out to the reception area. The nurses should also help to book the next appointment. Very important to be effective in these clinics is also to have a good documentation on a facial anatomy chart. On this the exact localization and dose of BoNt is recorded. This chart should be placed in the lap of the patient when the physician arrives to the treatment room. A new schedule is made only when the dose is changed which may be indicated after years of treatment. This is especially true for certain areas e.g., synkinesia of the eye (see below).

Even if botulinum toxin has a well-recognized duration of between 2 and 6 month in facial muscles also much longer effects have been observed. Exemplifying this is a number of patients with a partially healed Bell's palsy treated by the author with BoNt for synkinesia with eye closure. Usually the eye closure occurs during smile or other type of facial movements e.g., pursing of lips, nasalis activation, etc. The treatment for these symptoms is pretarsal low dose BoNt injection to minimize the spastic tendency of the orbicularis oculi muscle. These treatments have been able to permanently cure the synkinesia for many patients. The mechanism for these findings is not fully known but as we know that the effect of BoNt always is reversible it is likely that these long-term effects related not to direct drug effect but rather to the plasticity of the brain plasticity. (Fig. 28.7a–c) Thus, repeated BoNt injections modified long-term brain signaling. It is difficult to find other explanations for these interesting findings.

28.7 Hyaluronic Acid Injection

With the introduction of the first botulinum toxin A (Botox®) in the early 1990s a very important tool for dealing with facial paresis patients became available. In 1996 The Q-MED company introduced the first synthetic Hyaluronic acid filler (HA) on the market (Restylane®). Since then a large number of different neurotoxins and fillers has been introduced to the market and preferences for products depends on the physicians experience but also the characteristics of different products. This chapter will not deal with these matters but rather just conclude that the use of botulinum toxin and HA fillers can act in a synergistic way to improve the outcome of injectables during facial paresis treatments (Figs. 28.8a, b, and 28.9).

Hyaluronic acid is a naturally occurring sugar in the body and its effect on attracting water makes it an ideal as a commercially available filler. Permanent fillers are avoided for these groups of patients as they will come for regular botulinum toxin treatments. There are also many

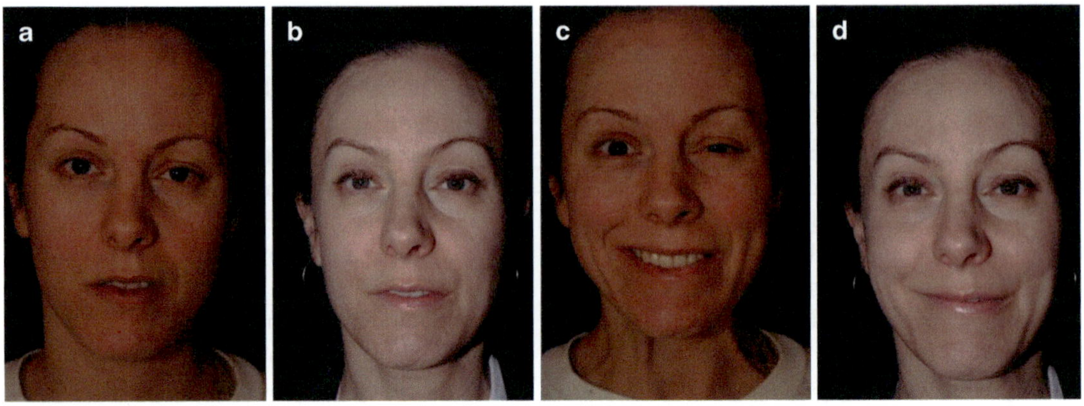

Fig. 28.7 (**a**) and (**c**) Relaxed and smiling 2 years after a Bell's palsy. (**b**) and (**d**) Nine years later after regular BoNt treatments. Note the absence of synkinesia in the left eye in spite of the fact that treatments in the orbicularis occuli have not been given for 6 years. It is likely that the initial 3 years of orbicularis occuli treatment retrained the brain not to send out signals of eye closure during a smile

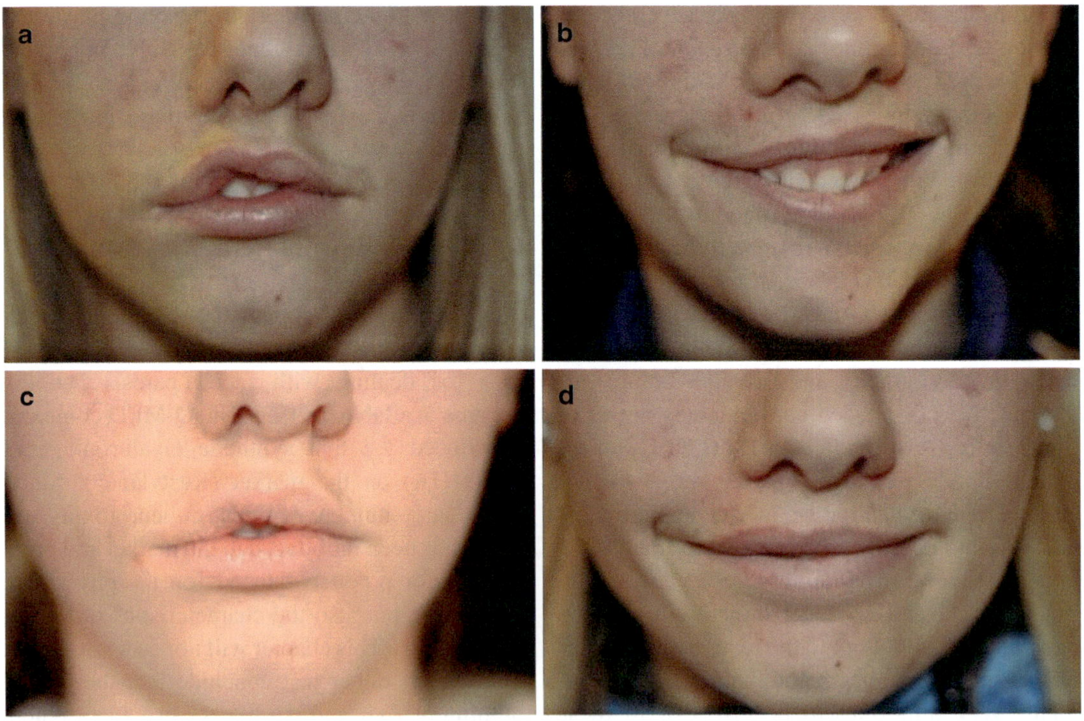

Fig. 28.8 (**a**) and (**b**) A patient referred from another country for free muscle transplant before treatment with HA injection in the lips and global facial BoNt treatment (**c**) and (**d**) after injections (no surgical intervention needed)

other reasons to avoid permanent fillers e.g., the risk for development of granulomas. These can be very difficult to remove whereas HA fillers can easily be removed by injection of the hyaluronidase enzyme. A partially healed facial paresis may have a deepened nasolabial fold on the partly paralyzed side due to increased tonus of the facial muscles and this is usually successfully treated with HA injections. Also, rhytids on the cheek after free muscle transplants can be treated with these injectables as can be imbalances in peri oral rhytids. It has also been noted that

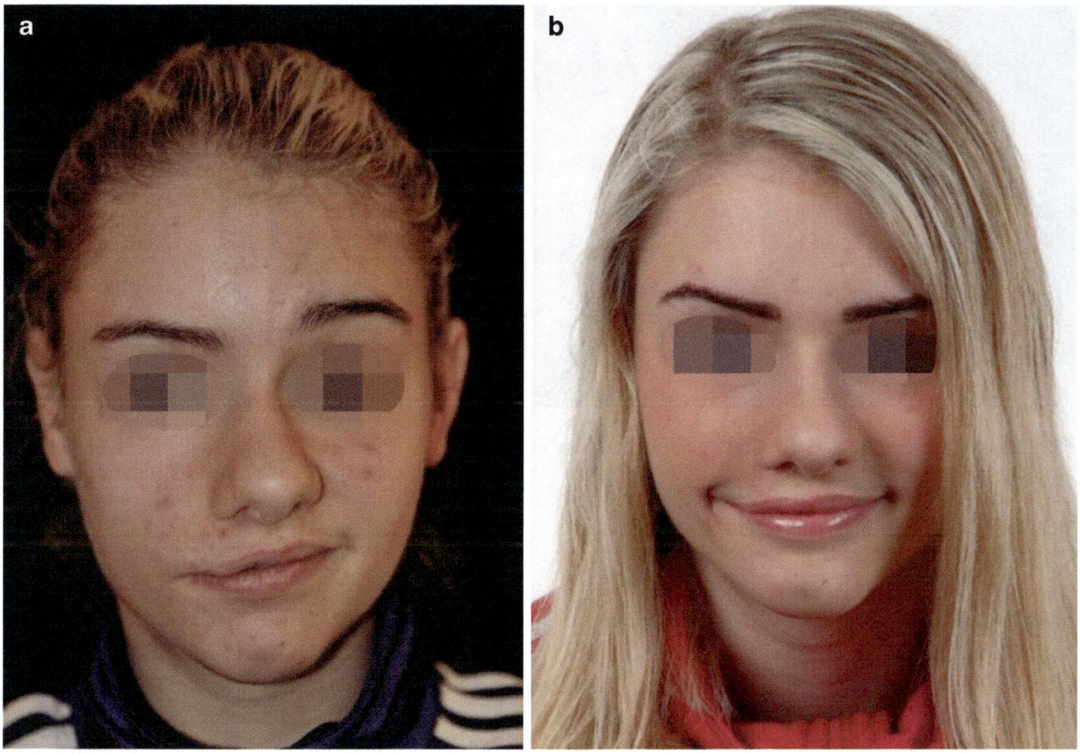

Fig. 28.9 The same patient as in Fig. 28.8 (**a**) before and after (**b**) after adjustment and fine tuning of the right dose of BoNt and volume of HA. This is a good illustration to how these relatively simple and highly cost-effective procedures can give a greatly improved quality of life

Hyaluronic acid injections alone without neurotoxins has animation effects, probably acting like a underwire in a brassiere stretching of cloth of the bra. Similarly when injecting e.g., in the lip contour it minimizes the animation rhytids in the upper lip caused by activation of the orbicularis oris muscle . HA fillers are also excellent to volumize the face and after reconstructive procedures with free muscle transplantation as mentioned above there could be volumetric differences between the two facial sides. Injecting a volumizing filler can compensate for these volumetric imbalances. These injectable can also have a soft facial lifting effect if injected in a proper way. Accidental injections into arteries my create necrosis and even blindness. To avoid unintended intravascular injections of HA fillers blunt cannulas are recommended for use in the sub cutaneous layer. For lip contour injections, intradermal injections or augmentations on the bone needles are however favored .Obviously good knowledge of facial anatomy is of great importance when using injectables.

BoNt and HA injections is like playing a violin: Anybody with a basic training in medicine can give these type of injectable as anybody can pick up a violin and produce a sound, but this does not mean that the result will be good. As for the violin the injection treatments has to be fine-tuned. Thus follow-up and analysis of results are necessary. The violin player also needs experience, interest, training, and good knowledge and the same if true for the injector of these substances to achieve an optimal outcome.

28.8 Fat Grafting

As mentioned above fat grafting should be considered to balance the face for volumetric imbalances that could be the result of a successful free muscle transplant. There are however also many

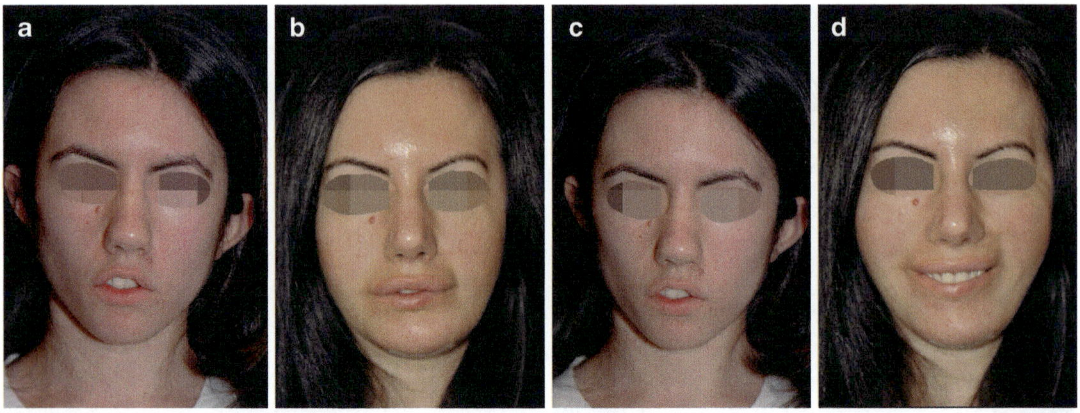

Fig. 28.10 (**a**) relaxed and (**c**) full facial animation; Moebius syndrome with complete bilateral facial paralysis. (**b**) Relaxed and (**d**) smiling after bilateral free gracilis muscle transplantation with masseter innervation. Secondary V-Y mucosal advancement lip lengthening and segmental fat transplantation (Resitu®) to the lips to aid with lip closure (a rhinoplasty was also performed)

other indications for fat grafting to the face after a facial paralysis [6]. This may involve a lip imbalance where the paralysis of the orbicularis muscle on one side may reduce lip volume and indicate fat grafting. Injections of fat with the Coleman [7] technique or micro fat according to Tonnard [8] frequently produce insufficient volume in the lips. The reason for poor fat survival in the lips is unclear but the author has found that segmental fat transplant where a piece of fat is implanted into the lip has much better fat survival. Thus segmental fat grafting is favored in the lips and a simplified instrument for harvesting and implantation of such fat has been invented and patented by the author (Resitu® technique) (Fig. 28.10a–d).

When it comes to peri oral rhytids SNIF (sharp needle intradermal fatgrafting according) can be useful to balance the perioral area as can injections into the nasolabial fold and the chin area. It is important to analyze the whole face when planning for fat grafting and frequently both the midface, periorbit, and lips are treated. Fat grafting in the eyelid region usually has very good survival but the risk for irregularities under the thin eyelid skin is higher. Thus the technique for injection of fat in the periorbit is of importance. Injections should preferably be done with microfat, thus prepared not to contain larger fat lobules. The injection is done with thin cannulas 0.7 or 0.9 mm ø and a large number of rapid passes are recommended to implant 1 ml of fat. Placement should be deep on the supraperiosteal layer.

Many harvesting and preparation techniques have been used and fat survival is greatly variable between individuals and in different regions. Fat injections can be done with a multitude of different techniques and it goes beyond the scope of this book to detail different cleaning procedures and injection techniques. Instead the reader is referred to textbooks and articles on this subject. It is however important to underline that fat grafting is an important tool also in facial paralysis reanimation.

28.9 Lip Lifting Procedures

With a facial paralysis effecting the mouth different types of lifting procedures can be indicated both after free muscle transplant but also after partial paresis such as after Bell's palsy. This may result in a slightly lowered commissure of the mouth on the paralyzed side. A lip corner [9] can create the illusion of a balanced and more smiling corner even if the movement is not improved. If the whole lip is hanging an extension of the corner lift can be done with an excision of skin along and above the lip contour close to the cupids bow.

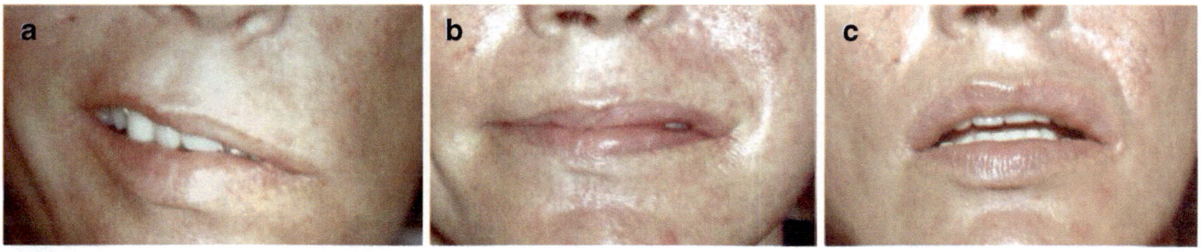

Fig. 28.11 (**a**) Before and (**b**) after free muscle transplantation of a left sided facial paralysis with remaining lip asymmetry. (**c**) after secondary lip contour elevation (R side), mucosal resection (L commissure), mucusal V-Y advancement (L side). Segmental fat transplantation (RESITU® technique) upper and lower lips

The excision should not include the cupids bow but stop lateral to it. To achieve good volume on the paralyzed side also mucosal advancement with multiple V-Y mucosal advancement flap could be considered. Frequently the best volumetric improvement is achieved with a combination of V-Y mucosal advancement and segmental fat transplantation (Fig. 28.11a–c).

28.10 Forehead Lifting

A very common sequelae after facial paralysis is ptosis of the eyebrow. This is probably due to the fact that the frontalis muscle is a thin and relatively weak muscle with a small volume and thus, probably more sensitivity to denervation. Even after healing of a Bell's palsy the eyebrow elevation frequently is weaker than on the contralateral side. When making aesthetic evaluation of a paralyzed face it is important to analyze the position of the brow. Contra lateral BoNt injection may lower a high brow on the healthy side but more frequently it is indicated to lift the brow. This can be done as coronal exposure and lifting or endoscopic approach with release of the corrugator muscles or lateral forehead lifting alone [10, 11]. Today lateral lifting [12] is more common as aesthetic procedures and especially in the younger paralyzed patients a unilateral treatment sometimes in combination with BoNt treatments are relatively common. In the middle-aged patients it is commonly indicated to do a bilateral treatment. In the elderly patient a local eyebrow lifting with an oval excision of skin exactly at the margin of the eyebrow is favored [13].

Many different techniques for lateral eyebrow lifting has been described but usually the eyebrow in mobilized from a temporal incision in the hair-bearing area and fixation with cortical bone tunnel screws or Endotine® plates are common. The author has favored a direct approach with a temporal incision, dissection and release of the lateral brow and transcutaneous sutures passed through the eyebrow under the elevated forehead scalp skin and then externalized and tied over foam bolsters during 14 days. This gives a very strong lift to the lateral brow at the desired point of action in the brow where the transcutaneous sutures are passed in and out through the skin (Fig. 28.12a–d). Other fixation techniques have the fixation point relatively far away from the desired point of action.

28.11 Blepharoplasty

Even if much of the upper eyelid skin excess may be related to ptosis of the eyebrow there are sometimes indications for blepharoplasty's which even may be indicated bilaterally for good symmetry. When evaluating the indication for an upper blepharoplasty it is very important to analyze the brow position and frontalis function. Carefully also examine if lid ptosis with an age related extension of the levator aponeurosis is present. In a facial paralysis this in not uncommonly unilateral and affects the healthy side in older individuals. Ptosis correction with shortening of the levator aponeurosis should be done simultaneously with the blepharoplasty if needed attempt to correct lateral brow ptosis with aggressive resection of eyelid skin should never be

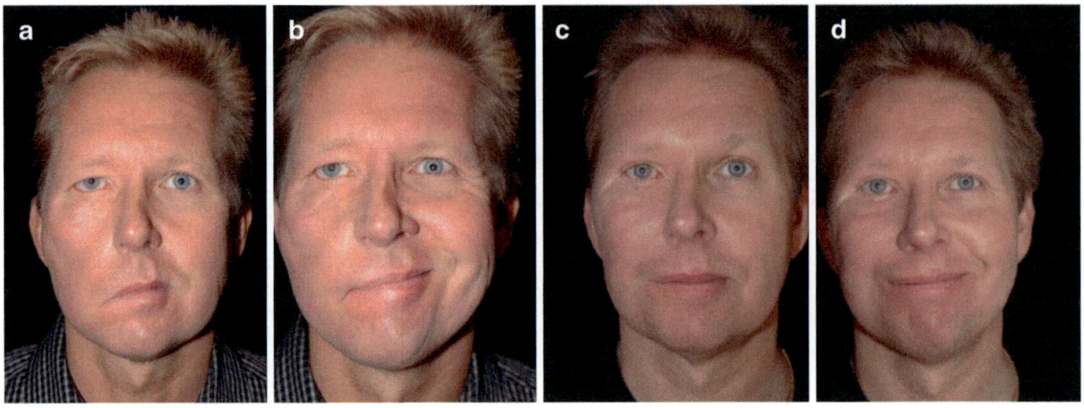

Fig. 28.12 (**a**) Relaxed and (**b**) smiling before secondary free muscle transplantation. (**c**) Relaxed and (**d**) smiling after secondary free muscle transplantation with cross facial and masseter nerve innervation. Also an eyebrow-elevation, upper blepharoplasty, and canthopexy was done on the right eye

done. This will destroy the normal anatomy of the upper lids and make a later eyebrow repositioning impossible for the lack of eyelid skin. When marking the skin excision, the lower incision should be marked 8 mm above the eyelashes and a minimum of 15 mm of upper eyelid skin should be left to the border of the brow above the upper excision. A small strip of orbicularis muscle is resected above the lower incision line to improve the fold if this is poorly defined. Only clear excess of fat, usually medially in the elderly patients, is resected, also considering fat grafting in the orbital rim in the hollow upper eyelid. This is done with a thin 0.7 or 0.9 blunt cannula to avoid problems. Obviously an upper blepharoplasty can also be combined with a gold weight implantation positioned on the upper tarsal border in patients suffering from lagopthalmos. However, it is common that patients treated with gold weight implantation for functional improvement of the eye closure regard this an aesthetic worsening of the appearance. To minimize gold weight visibly, reduce the risk for exposure and extrusion and to improve the aesthetic appearance the author developed a technique of covering the gold weight with a small piece of temporal fascia.

28.12 Canthopexy

Even if a canthopexy may be indicated for functional reasons there are also aesthetic reasons to consider a canthopexy. If the orbicularis occuli is weak or paralyzed the tonus of the lower lid is reduced and scleral show is common. Even if this does not cause the patient functional problems it may result in a wider and rounder looking eye. A canthopexy may improve both the aesthetic and functional problems related to scleral show. If a lower lid blepharoplasty is considered for aesthetic reasons it is also of paramount importance to examine the tonus of the lower lid. This can be done with a snap test when the lid is pulled down form the globe and the released. If the lid does not return to the globe within 2 s the tonus is reduced. Remember that the patient cannot blink during this maneuver, is she/he does the test must be redone. In the paralyzed eye the tonus, especially in the aged patient is frequently so poor that a bone fixation during canthopexy is recommended. This can be performed via a small upper lateral eyelid incision and exposure of the bone at the Whytham's tubercle. Two drill holes are made and a 4–0 nylon suture is passed to the lower eyelid grasping the lateral tarsus and the inferior retinaculum of the cantal ligament. Frequently a canthotomy and possibly also shortening of the lower lid may be combined with the canthopexy. The sutures are passed under the lateral elevated skin and orbicularis muscle and up to the drill hole. The suture is tied so the knot comes on the inside of the orbital rim, giving a very stable fixation of the lower lid. This procedures balance the appearance of the lower lids but also helps the patient with closure and minimizes the eyes sensitivity for wind. If a true ectropion is present the canthopexy may be combined with a midfacelift (as described below) for maximal support of the lower lid.

28.13 Midface and Face Lifting

A midface lift can be performed in different ways [14, 15] but the author favors a transoral sub periosteal route. This is especially indicated after previous free muscle transplant where avoiding dissection into the plane of the muscle transplant do not jeopardize the microneurovascular supply to the transplanted muscle. (Fig. 28.13a–c). An approximately 2.5 cm long L-shaped mucosal incision is made intra orally at the third upper tooth and via direct visualization of the midfacial bone a subperiosteal release is done of the whole zygoma and the zygomatic arch. The masseter tendon and upper part of the masseter is exposed and the infraorbital rim released including the orbicularis retaining ligament and the arcus marginalis. The infra orbital nerve is visualized and preserved and the dissection is carried out up to the lateral orbital rim where the temporal zygomaticofacial sensory nerve is visualized and preserved. An oblique incision is done in the hair above the ear and the deep temporal fascia is exposed down to the orbital rim and communicated to the intraoral dissection plane. An Endotine® midface plate is placed in the SOOF (suborbicularis fat pad) midface fat and sutured to the deep temporal fascia giving very strong elevation of the midface. These types of midface lifts do not only rejuvenate the midface but also achieve lower lid support and rejuvenation. Usually a lower lid blepharoplasty with fat transposition is avoided at this stage and recommended to do at the second stage if needed. Sometimes midface lifts are performed bilaterally for best balance of the face but in many situations a unilateral treatment is also indicated.

Facelift with high SMAS elevation has certain indications in the elderly facial paralysis patients but the indication for this procedure is less strong than midface lifts according to the technique described above. When performing a high SMAS elevation a good face lifting effect is achieved and improvement of the corner of the mouth can also be seen. This could be very beneficial for a patient with a partial facial paralysis. Details on how to perform this procedure in the optimal way

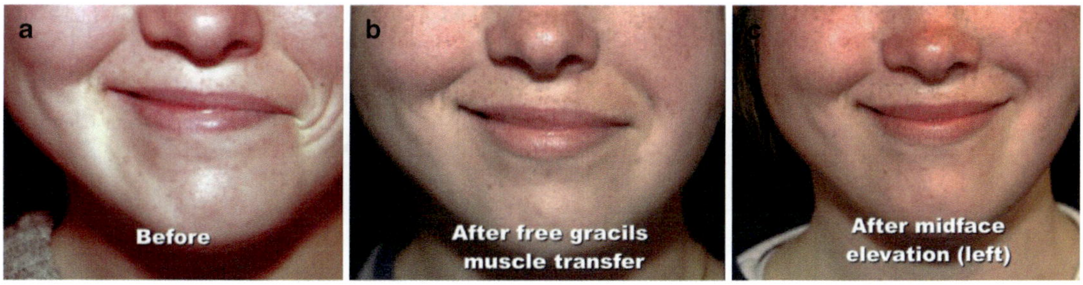

Fig. 28.13 Smiling (**a**) before and (**b**) after free muscle transplantation with cross-facial innervation. (**c**) Smiling after subperiosteal midfacelift to balance the position of the commissure and the free muscle transplant. A corner-lift of the mouth [9] was also performed

goes beyond the scope of this chapter and referral to a text book on this chapter is recommended instead.

28.14 Summary

Facial paralyses are usually difficult reconstructive problems and a large number of different treatment options must be considered. The treatment selection depends on the patients suffering, the aesthetic and functional loss but also the patient age and complicating diseases must be considered. It is of utmost importance that the patient has realistic expectations of the outcome and understanding that it is impossible to achieve as good result as on the healthy contra lateral side in a unilateral facial paralysis. Reconstructive surgeons performing facial reanimation procedures must not only master advanced reconstructive free muscle transplants but also must consider a number of aesthetic procedures such as fat grafting, midface and forehead lifting, etc. Facial paralysis is probably the best illustration to how intimately reconstructive and aesthetic surgery is connected. A reconstructive surgeon must have good knowledge of aesthetic procedures to achieve optimal outcomes for facial paralysis patients and reversely an aesthetic physician without training in reconstructive surgery should preferably refer patients with these problems to physicians who deal with both aesthetic and reconstructive parts of these difficult problems.

References

1. Bianchi B, Ferri A, Ferrari S, Leporati M, Ferri T, Sesenna E. Ancillary procedures in facial animation surgery. J Oral Maxillofac Surg. 2014;72(12):2582–90.
2. Clark RP, Berris CE. Botulinum toxin: a treatment for facial asymmetry caused by facial nerve paralysis. Plast Reconstr Surg. 2005;115:573–4.
3. Clark RP, Berris CE. Botulinum toxin: a treatment for facial asymmetry caused by facial nerve paralysis. Plast Reconstr Surg. 1989;84:353–5.
4. Mancini R, Taban M, Lowinger A, et al. Use of hyaluronic acid gel in the management of paralytic lagophthalmos: the hyaluronic acid gel "Gold Weight". Ophthal Plast Reconstr Surg. 2009;25(1):23–6.
5. Salles AG, da Costa EF, Ferreira MC, Remigio AF, Moraes LB, Gemperli R. Epidemiologic overview of synkinesis in 353 patients with longstanding facial paralysis under treatment with botulinum toxin for 11 years. Plast Reconstr Surg. 2015;136(6):1289–98.
6. Siah WF, Litwin AS, Nduka C, Malhotra R. Periorbital autologous fat grafting in facial nerve palsy. Ophthalmic Plast Reconstr Surg. 2017;33(3):202–8.
7. Coleman SR, Katzel EB. Fat grafting for facial filling and regeneration. Clin Plast Surg. 2015;42(3):289–300.
8. Lindenblatt N, van Hulle A, Verpaele AM, Tonnard PL. The role of microfat grafting in facial contouring. Aesthet Surg J. 2015;35(7):763–71.
9. Austin HW, Weston GW. Rejuvenation of the aging mouth. Clin Plast Surg. 1992;19(2):511–24.
10. Holtmann L, Büchsenschütz K, Eckstein A, Schlüter A, Lang S, Mattheis S. Endoscopic browlift via endotine forehead device in patients with facial palsy. Laryngorhinootologie. 2017;96(10):691–7.
11. Takushima A, Harii K, Sugawara Y, Asato H. Anthropometric measurements of the endoscopic eyebrow lift in the treatment of facial paralysis. Plast Reconstr Surg. 2003;111(7):2157–65.
12. Fogli AL. Temporal lift by galapexy: a review of 270 cases. Aesthet Plast Surg. 2003;27(3):159–65.
13. Lewis JR Jr. A method of direct eyebrow lift. Ann Plast Surg. 1983;10(2):115–9.
14. Gordon NA, Adam SI 3rd. Deep plane face lifting for midface rejuvenation. Clin Plast Surg. 2015;42(1):129–42.
15. Le Louarn C. Specificity of facelift surgery, including mid facelift, in case of facial palsy. Ann Chir Plast Esthet. 2015;60(5):454–61.

Reconstructing Facial Contour Deformities with Vascularized Flaps in Facial Reanimation Surgery

29

Goo-Hyun Mun and Kyeong-Tae Lee

Key Points

- Free tissue transfer has served as the gold standard for correction of major facial contour deformity. Adipofascial flap can be considered primarily.
- Simultaneous reconstruction of facial paralysis and contour deformity requires two different flap components; one of the functional muscle segment for smile reconstruction and additional flap for contour correction.
- A chimeric flap in which two flaps are combined with a common pedicle is a viable option for reconstruction of complex facial paralysis.
- The latissimus dorsi muscle donor site has enormous strengths of designing chimeric flap.
- Diligent secondary correction with lipoinjection and/or liposuction should be accompanied to enhance final aesthetic results.

29.1 Introduction

The etiology of facial contour deformity is diverse, ranging from congenital anomalies such as craniofacial macrosomia, degenerative diseases such as progressive hemifacial atrophy, to acquired causes including trauma and defects following oncologic ablative surgery or craniofacial operations. If the extent of contour deformity is not severe or extensive, lipoinjection can be a good treatment method in most cases, although repetitive procedures are often required due to unpredictable absorption and survival of the grafted fat. However, a major contour deformity often involves multiple tissues, ranging from skin and subcutaneous tissue to muscle and even bony structures, and requires substantial tissue volume for reconstruction, for which lipoinjection alone would not suffice and tissue transfer is favored. A pedicled flap can be considered, but its use may be very limited in facial region due to insufficient volume of adjacent tissue and donor site morbidity. Free tissue transfer from remote places has served as the gold standard for the reconstruction of a major contour deformity. Distinct strengths of this method include the availability of abundant well-vascularized tissue, acceptable donor morbidity, and reliable, natural-appearing, and long-lasting final outcomes. Various kinds of workhorse free flaps including a radial forearm flap, anterolateral thigh flap, and a groin flap, and

G.-H. Mun (✉) · K.-T. Lee
Department of Plastic Surgery, Samsung Medical Center, Sungkyunkwan University School of Medicine, Seoul, South Korea

© Springer Nature Switzerland AG 2021
C.-H. J. Tzou, A. Rodríguez-Lorenzo (eds.), *Facial Palsy*,
https://doi.org/10.1007/978-3-030-50784-8_29

a thoracodorsal artery perforator flap, have been commonly used.

Meanwhile, some of the diseases that cause facial contour deformity can be related to dysfunction of the facial nerve and result in facial paralysis as well. Oncologic resection of a parotid gland tumor or schwannoma is representative condition that can cause facial contour deformity accompanied by facial nerve paralysis. Since the causes of acquired facial paralysis are diverse, a patient can present with various facial contour deformities with iatrogenic, pathologic, or traumatic origins. Congenital facial paralysis associated with craniofacial microsomia can also have varying degrees of atrophy on the affected side of the face. Reconstruction of complex facial paralysis, consisting of facial paralysis and concomitant contour deformity, presents an added challenge to the reconstructive microsurgeon. Achieving both functional and aesthetic reconstruction simultaneously can be a treatment goal in this situation. Smile reconstruction is a priority in the planning and execution of reconstructive procedures; however, without appropriate correction of a facial contour deformity, the value of reanimation surgery can fade, resulting in overall suboptimal results. Functional muscle transfer, with or without cross-facial nerve grafting, has been a main modality for the treatment of established facial paralysis. Thus, simultaneous reconstruction of facial paralysis and major contour deformity requires two flap components: a functioning muscle flap to reanimate the paralyzed face and a vascularized flap, such as an adipofascial flap or muscle flap, to replace the tissue deficit in contour deformity [1, 2].

Adversely, a functional muscle flap for dynamic smile reconstruction can itself generate a contour deformity, such as bulkiness. To avoid this situation, insetting a functional muscle flap with adequate size and thickness in the cheek is desired. Primary debulking of the muscle segment and/or adipose tissue in the cheek pocket can be performed intraoperatively when excessive bulkiness is anticipated. Secondary revision by debulking of cheek fat or an implanted muscle segment is also a viable solution to this problem.

29.2 Surgical Considerations for Simultaneous Reconstruction of Complex Facial Paralysis

29.2.1 Chimeric Flap Design Combining a Functional Muscle Segment with Vascularized Tissue for Contour Correction

Usually, the location requiring contour correction is different from that of optimal inset of a functional muscle flap for smile reconstruction. Therefore, two flaps that can be inset with spatial independence are usually required. Ideally, two flaps share the donor incision and should leave minimal donor morbidity. A chimeric flap in which a functional muscle segment for smile reconstruction and additional vascularized tissue for contour correction are combined with a common pedicle is an excellent option for reconstruction of complex defects [3] (Fig. 29.1). Use of the chimeric flap enables obtaining different tissue flap types from a common donor site. This economic use of donor site tissue can reduce donor site morbidity. Moreover, as both flaps are connected with a common pedicle in the chimeric flap, only one recipient vessel is needed (Fig. 29.2).

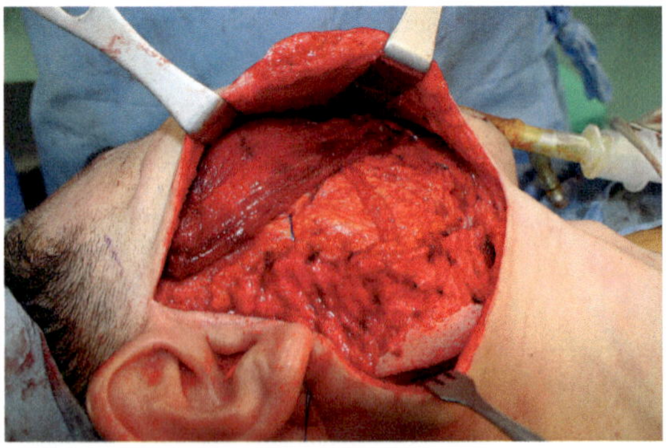

Fig. 29.1 Intraoperative image of the inset chimeric flap. A functional latissimus dorsi muscle flap and an adipofascial flap in retromandibular region are inset independently into locations as required

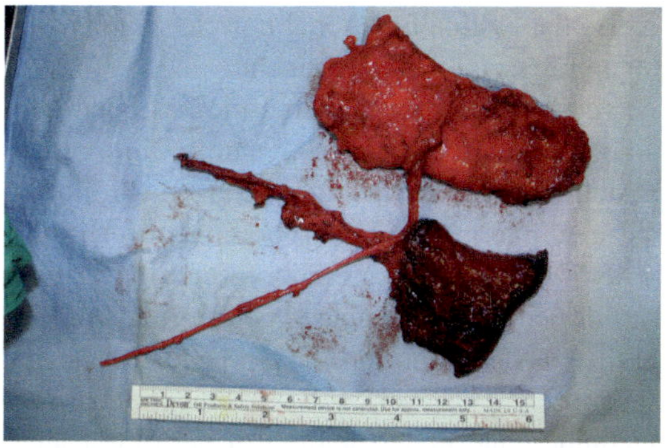

Fig. 29.2 Appearance of a harvested chimeric flap. A thoracodorsal artery perforator flap-chimeric functional latissimus dorsi muscle flap with a long thoracodorsal nerve stalk is harvested. The flap has Y-shaped pedicle configuration composed of common pedicle and pedicles for each flap component, which facilitate independent inset of each flap component

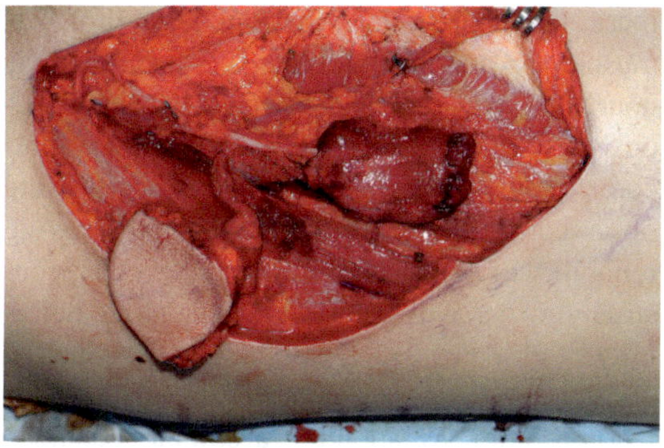

Fig. 29.3 Intraoperative photos of flap harvesting. A thoracodorsal artery perforator flap is designed and elevated based on sizable perforators that were targeted preoperatively. Meticulous intramuscular dissection proceeds to the main branch of the thoracodorsal artery, which is usually the descending branch. The branch is dissected to follow its course in a proximal-to-distal direction for sufficient distance to flap inset, and a muscle segment is harvested. Dissection of common pedicle and a thoracodorsal nerve proceeded as usual

To obtain adequate mobility of flap components for inset at the appropriate position, the chimeric flap should have sufficient pedicle length for each flap from the confluence point of the pedicles as well as from the common pedicle [4] (Fig. 29.3). This can be achieved with detailed preoperative planning with regard to perforator anatomy and course in the main pedicle, and by meticulous intramuscular dissection of the perforator pedicle.

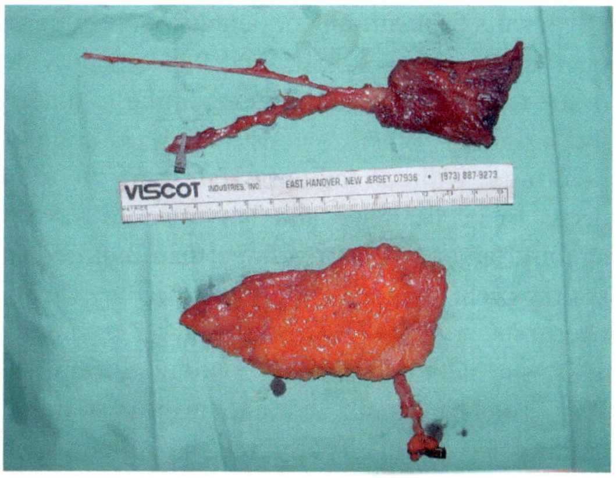

Fig. 29.4 When the anatomy is not suitable for harvesting a chimeric flap, elevating two separate flaps with each pedicle can be considered. A functional latissimus dorsi muscle flap for dynamic reconstruction (above) and a thoracodorsal artery perforator for contour correction (below) are harvested

However, harvesting a chimeric flap is not possible in every situation. When location of the contour deformity is far from the inset position of a functional muscle flap or when adequately sized perforators are not identified near the functional muscle flap to be harvested, reconstruction with the chimeric flap is not possible. In such cases, two separate flaps for each pedicle can be used: one functional muscle flap for smile reconstruction and another flap for contour deformity correction (Fig. 29.4). Spatial freedom while insetting the separate flaps can be acquired. However, the need for two recipient vessels is a limitation of the two flap method.

29.2.2 Tissue Component for Contour Deformity Correction

Various kinds of additional tissue flaps can be used for reconstruction of a contour deformity, including adipofascial, adipose, dermal-adipose, or segmental muscle flaps. Of those options, an adipofascial/adipose flap is highly favored over the muscle segment flap as the former shows better retention of flap volume and less atrophy during the postoperative period. Moreover, considering that a facial contour deformity usually results from atrophy or deficits of subcutaneous fat tissue, the adipofascial flap can provide tissue with texture and firmness similar to that of the original. When reconstructing a contour deformity with an adipofascial flap, the flap needs to be designed and harvested to have a slightly larger size and volume than required in the recipient site, as the flap volume may shrink over time.

Tissue deficits in facial contour deformities vary widely in depth and size, even in a single contiguous defect. Therefore, the adipofascial flap may need to be designed in a stereoscopic fashion with varying thickness according to the defect to achieve fine outcomes of contour restoration [5]. Considering the extent of tissue deficits in the recipient site, the thickness of an adipofascial flap can be adjusted by controlling the thickness of the adipose tissue and/or including other kinds of tissue, such as dermis. This stereoscopic designing of an adipofascial flap can reduce donor morbidity by minimizing harvesting of unnecessary tissue from the donor site.

A small ellipse of skin paddle can be attached to an adipofascial flap for convenient monitoring of flap circulation. This monitoring skin paddle can be removed after determining that flap circulation has been stabilized. In cases lacking suitable nearby perforators to nourish adipofascial/adipose tissue, a separate muscle segment can be harvested for contour correction in addition to a functional muscle segment for smile reconstruction. In this case, significant volume atrophy and increased donor site morbidity should be anticipated.

29.2.3 Donor Sites

Several body regions can be candidates for harvesting two kinds of flaps for simultaneous reconstruction of facial palsy and facial contour deformity. Popular donor sites for harvesting functional muscle flaps are the medial thigh region for a gracilis muscle flap, back region for a latissimus dorsi muscle flap, and anterior chest for pectoralis minor muscle. Thus, these regions can be primarily considered for harvesting a chimeric flap with a functional muscle segment and an adipofascial flap component.

A functioning gracilis muscle has been considered a main option for dynamic smile reconstruction [6]. Cross-facial nerve grafting followed by a chimeric flap incorporating a functional gracilis muscle and an adipofascial flap can be performed. There has been a concern about reliability of perfusion in the skin paddle overlying the muscle. However, with refinement of surgical technique and understanding of perforator anatomy, outcomes have steadily improved. Chuang et al. presented outcomes of reconstruction using a free proximal gracilis muscle and skin paddle compound flap transplantation in eight patients with complex facial paralysis including combined facial paralysis and contour deformity [2]. After performing a cross-facial nerve graft, a chimeric flap consisting of the functional proximal muscle flap and the overlying skin paddle that is nourished by septocutaneous or musculocutaneous perforators is transferred. Satisfactory outcomes both aesthetically and functionally were observed in the majority of patients, showing reliability of this method for simultaneous reconstruction of facial paralysis and contour deformity. Subsequently, Lykoudis et al. reported excellent outcomes in complex facial paralysis reconstruction by adopting a similar technique with the use of a medial circumflex femoral artery perforator-chimeric functional gracilis muscle flap following cross-facial nerve grafting. In their series, a single musculocutaneous perforator was skeletonized over the gracilis muscle flap, not preserving the intermuscular septum as reported by Chuang et al., thereby increasing freedom in insetting the adipofascial flap [7].

Since its introduction in the late 1990s [8], use of the latissimus dorsi muscle has emerged as an important option for dynamic smile reconstruction. This allows for one-staged reconstruction by co-harvesting a long thoracodorsal nerve stalk within the flap and can achieve reliable and acceptable outcomes, showing a spontaneous and synchronous smile with low donor morbidity. With regard to harvesting a chimeric flap for simultaneous reconstruction of facial palsy and contour deformity, the latissimus dorsi muscle has enormous advantages [1]. Several sizable perforators that can be the source vessel for the adipofascial component are distributed in the back [9]. The multiplicity of perforators can provide versatility in designing adipofascial flaps (Fig. 29.5). Occasional difficulty in finding reliable perforators due to relatively variable perforator anatomy and tedious perforator dissection has been considered the main drawbacks of thoracodorsal artery perforator flaps. However, this can be overcome with detailed planning using preoperative computed tomography angiography, intraoperative perforator mapping with Doppler, and meticulous surgical technique. Another strength of this donor site is that sufficient pedicle length for both components in the chimeric flap can be easily obtained, which can enable efficient placement of each flap component without risk of pedicle tethering. Perforators derived from a different major branch of the thoracodorsal vessel are usually favored for a flap pedicle to obtain sufficient spatial freedom during flap insetting (Figs. 29.6 and 29.7). Surgeons should be able to adapt to intraoperative anatomy of sizable perforators in the surgical field. In cases with lack of sizable perforators from the descending and transverse branches of thoracodorsal vessels, for instance, perforators derived from other branches, such as the branch to the serratus anterior muscle, can be identified and captured as a pedicle for the adipofascial flap. In addition, the back region is very generous when harvesting a large adipofascial flap. For flaps with widths up to 12 cm, all donor sites can allow for primary closure without difficulty. With regard to donor site morbidity, harvesting a thoracodorsal artery perforator-chimeric latissimus dorsi muscle flap is safe and leaves as little dysfunction in the shoulder joint as harvesting a simple thoracodorsal artery perforator flap [10].

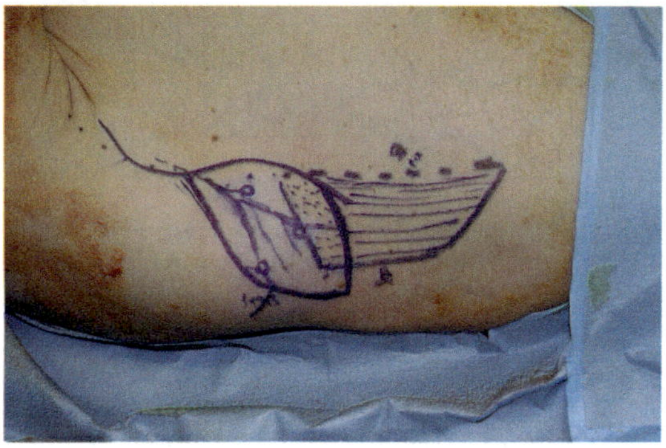

Fig. 29.5 A chimeric flap design for simultaneous reconstruction of complex facial palsy. A thoracodorsal artery perforator adipofascial flap-chimeric functional latissimus dorsi muscle flap is designed

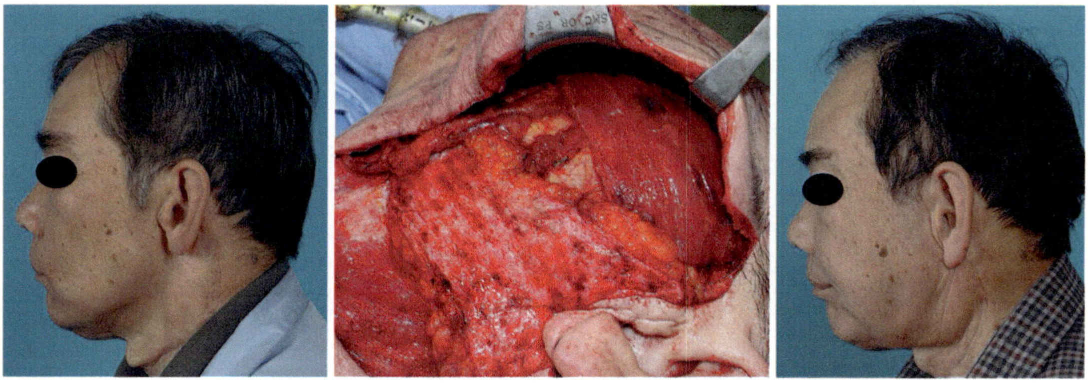

Fig. 29.6 A 62-year-old man presented with left hemifacial paralysis following ablative surgery for treating the parotid gland tumor. He developed a focal depression contour deformity on left retromandibular area due to oncologic resection and adjuvant radiotherapy. (Left) Lateral view of preoperative appearance (Center) He was treated with a thoracodorsal artery perforator adipofascial-chimeric functional latissimus dorsi muscle transfer. Intraoperative image of the inset chimeric flap. (Right) At postoperative 55 months, the depression deformity of his retromandibular area resolved and symmetric contour was observed

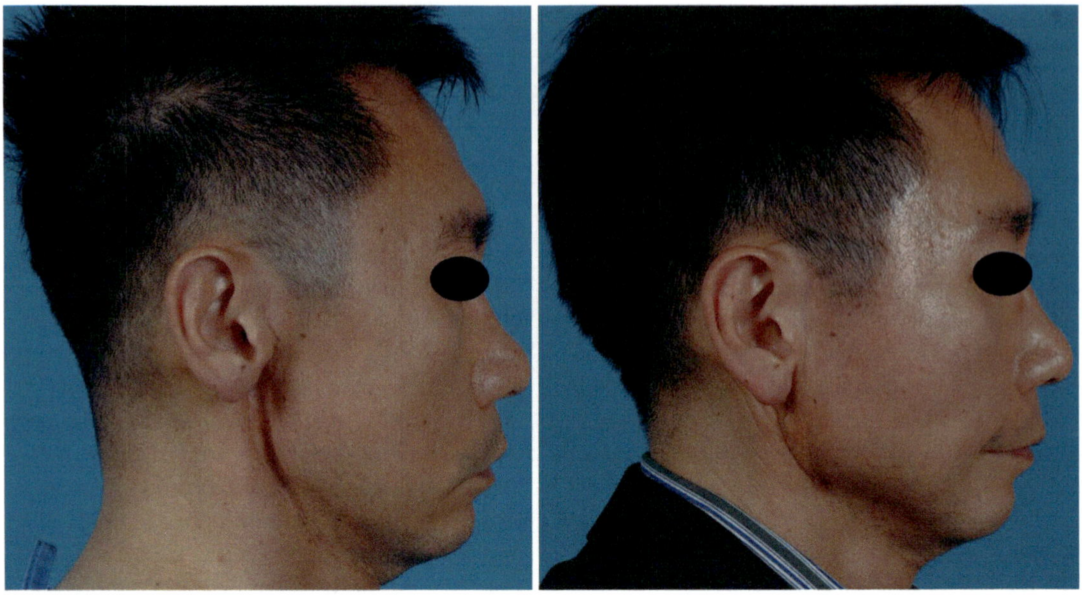

Fig. 29.7 A 46-year-old man had right facial paralysis with focal depression on retromandibular area, which developed following parotidectomy for treating recurrent pleomorphic adenoma. (Left) Preoperative appearance. (Right) A thoracodorsal artery perforator adipofascial-chimeric functional latissimus dorsi muscle transfer was performed. A photograph at postoperative 11 months

29.3 Secondary Revision

Secondary revision can be considered to improve outcomes of facial contour correction when indicated. Fat grafting or liposuction can be a good option for correcting a minor residual contour deformity following vascularized tissue transfer, and can be combined with revision for reanimation. Judicious practical planning of the degree and extent of initial contour correction surgery may be desired, as subsequent secondary revision can effectively resolve remaining problems and enhance the aesthetic results.

Financial Disclosure None.

References

1. Takushima A, Harii K, Asato H, Yamada A. Neurovascular free-muscle transfer to treat facial paralysis associated with hemifacial microsomia. Plast Reconstr Surg. 2002;109(4):1219–27.
2. Chuang DC, Mardini S, Lin SH, Chen HC. Free proximal gracilis muscle and its skin paddle compound flap transplantation for complex facial paralysis. Plast Reconstr Surg. 2004;113(1):126–32; discussion 33–5
3. Hallock GG. Simultaneous transposition of anterior thigh muscle and fascia flaps: an introduction to the chimera flap principle. Ann Plast Surg. 1991;27(2):126–31.
4. Lee KT, Wiraatmadja ES, Mun GH. Free latissimus dorsi muscle-chimeric thoracodorsal artery perforator flaps for reconstruction of complicated defects: does muscle still have a place in the domain of perforator flaps? Ann Plast Surg. 2015;74(5):565–72.
5. Kim EJ, Lee KT, Lim SY, Pyon JK, Bang SI, Oh KS, et al. Reconstructing facial contour deformities using stereoscopic thoracodorsal artery perforator adipofascial flaps. Microsurgery. 2017;37(4):300–6.
6. O'Brien BM, Pederson WC, Khazanchi RK, Morrison WA, MacLeod AM, Kumar V. Results of management of facial palsy with microvascular free-muscle transfer. Plast Reconstr Surg. 1990;86(1):12–22; discussion 3–4
7. Lykoudis EG, Spyropoulou G-AC, Vlastou CC. The conjoint medial circumflex femoral perforator and gracilis muscle free flap: anatomical study and clinical use for complex facial paralysis reconstruction. Plast Reconstr Surg. 2005;116(6):1589–95.

8. Harii K, Asato H, Yoshimura K, Sugawara Y, Nakatsuka T, Ueda K. One-stage transfer of the latissimus dorsi muscle for reanimation of a paralyzed face: a new alternative. Plast Reconstr Surg. 1998;102(4):941–51.
9. Mun GH, Lee SJ, Jeon BJ. Perforator topography of the thoracodorsal artery perforator flap. Plast Reconstr Surg. 2008;121(2):497–504.
10. Lee KT, Kim A, Mun GH. Comprehensive analysis of donor-site morbidity following free thoracodorsal artery perforator flap harvest. Plast Reconstr Surg. 2016;138(4):899–909.

Myectomies and Neurectomies in the Management of Hyperkinetic Asymmetries and Synkinesis in Facial Palsy

30

Eleonora O. F. Dimovska and David Jensson

Key Points

- Severe or refractory hyperspastic conditions such as synkinesis can benefit from surgical intervention to treat resulting asymmetries.
- Myectomies are commonly performed for lower lip asymmetries, but are gaining popularity for synkinesis of the eyelids and neck.
- Neurectomies can be used separately or in combination with myectomies to ensure surgical success and prevent recurrence of symptoms.
- Selective neurectomies have been developed in order to target-specific synkinetic muscles.
- Botulinum toxin continues to play an important role as a primary treatment option and can also form an adjunct to surgical patients with recurrent symptoms.

30.1 Introduction

Facial nerve dysfunction can be encountered following e.g., trauma, infection or malignancy. The most common cause of a resolving facial palsy is Bell's Palsy; in fact a diagnosis of exclusion following thorough evaluation of other treatable causes. Facial nerve dysfunction is characterized by several abnormal hypo- and/or hyperactive nerve responses that result in different asymmetric phenotypic phenomena, in animation and/or repose. Common dysfunctional facial nerve responses include hemifacial spasms and synkinesis. Synkinesis should be distinguished from hemifacial spasm. Compared to synkinesis, hyperspasm is a chronic, non-resolving disease of the facial nerve characterized by mass contraction of the entire hemiface, rather than distinct muscle groups. Up to 30% of patients with Bell's palsy experience synkinesis and about 6% experience severe symptoms, either unresponsive to Botox or recurring after surgical treatment. These can involve a single nerve branch, a combination of nerve branches or the entire hemiface.

Synkinesis, derived from the Greek words "*syn*" (meaning "together with") and "*kinesis*" (meaning "movement"), is a complex phenomenon characterized by spontaneous co-contraction of unwanted muscle groups, unrelated to a desired movement. It is a relatively common post-palsy sequalae believed to occur due to an aberrant regenerative pathway of nerve axons in

E. O. F. Dimovska (✉) · D. Jensson
Department of Plastic and Maxillofacial Surgery, Uppsala University Hospital, Uppsala, Sweden
e-mail: david.jensson@akademiska.se

© Springer Nature Switzerland AG 2021
C.-H. J. Tzou, A. Rodríguez-Lorenzo (eds.), *Facial Palsy*,
https://doi.org/10.1007/978-3-030-50784-8_30

a resolving facial palsy. However, the occurrence is a sign of poor chance to full facial nerve recovery. A damaged axon will sprout in its attempt to regrow and in doing so potentially risk innervating several different facial muscles as it grows down different endoneurial tubules. For example, axons that originally innervated the zygomaticus major muscle choose a different regenerating pathway and end up innervating the orbicularis oculi muscle instead. This then gives rise to involuntary unintended contractions of the eye during an attempted smile. Chuang et al. define the process of synkinesis as a co-contraction between a triggering muscle and a synkinetic muscle [1]. Beurskens et al. found the most common combination of these to be the oral-ocular synkinesis, where a voluntary oral action such as a smile or puckering of the lips results in a synkinetic ocular action e.g., contraction of the orbicularis occuli and closure of the eye [2]. A voluntary smile could be also coupled with synkinetic spasms of mentalis and/or platysma, occasionally leading to a frozen appearance with no elevation of the commissure possible due to the two muscles are working synchronously and antagonistically.

Indications for surgical treatment are severe, unresponsive or refractory synkinesis. Functionally, these severe situations can lead to inability to communicate (loss of normal facial expressions) and even pain due to severe and chronic spasms. Aesthetically, ageing can occur asymmetrically. The chronic spasms are said to lead to slower ageing signs on the skin due to constant tonicity and less facial soft tissue descent [3]. The affected flaccid side of the face has more soft tissue laxity and thus patients on occasion seek rejuvenation treatments for this reason. Psychological, facial palsy and is post-paralytic sequalae can lead to massive repercussions on quality of life. Bell's palsy commonly occurs in younger/middle-aged patients, resulting in the risk for many years of lost quality of life.

30.2 Upper Zone of the Face

30.2.1 Forehead and Eyebrows

30.2.1.1 Anatomy

The forehead and Eyebrows are controlled by several muscle groups [4]. Elevation of the eyebrows, and thereby wrinkling of the forehead, is actioned by a co-contraction of the frontalis and occipitalis, joined through the galea apponeurotica. The antagonist group of muscles in charge of depression of the brows and forehead, thereby frowning are the corrugator supercilii, depressor supercilii, procerus, and the medial part of the orbicularis occuli. The nervous supply of the frontalis is singlehandedly supplied by the frontal branch. The nervous supply of the depressor is more complex. The corrugator supercilii is in fact supplied by the frontal branch to its transverse head and a zygomatico-buccal branch to its oblique head [5]. The temporal branch enters the muscle from its superolateral portion. The zygomatico-buccal branch courses from the medial canthus to firstly supply procerus from its inferomedial aspect and then continue cephalad to supply corrugator inferiorly form its superficial aspect [6].

An important aspect to note and be aware of, particularly during endoscopic procedures in this region, is the relationship of the supraorbital nerve to the corrugator supercilii. The anatomy of the supratrochlear nerve is more familiar as it is known to exit just lateral to the origin of the corrugator, enter the muscle and within it divide in to several branches before moving more cephalad to enter the frontalis and finally penetrate it to become more superficial. Before division, the common stem exits through the supraorbital notch, but in about 10% exits through a foramen that could be located up to 1.5 cm superior to the orbital rim. Immediately after exiting the orbit, the corrugator divides into a superficial and deep portion. This branching pattern of the supraorbital nerve was studied in detail by Janis et al. and found to have several branching patterns and relationships to the corrugator [7]. In a cadaveric study the authors found 40% of specimens to have only the deep division to run on the undersurface of the corrugator, with no branches of from the superficial division. 34% of specimens had branches from both the superficial and deep divisions within the muscle. 4% had a few divisions of the superficial division only and no branches from the deep division. 22% had all branches from the superficial division occur cephalad to, and fully away from, the corrugator.

30.2.1.2 Evaluation

Hypoactive dysfunction affecting the frontal branch of the facial nerve, results in patients presenting with complete paralysis of the ipsilateral forehead and eyebrow due to both depressors and elevators being affected. Asymmetry is in part caused by this unilateral flaccidity, however, it is often exaggerated by compensatory hyperactivity on the non-affected site. The forehead or eyebrows can also be involved in a synkinetic dysfunction. Hyperactivity of the frontalis will result in horizontal rhytides. Horizontal rhytides in the glabellar region are due to hyperactivity of the procerus, whereas vertical rhytides are due to corrugator supercilii hyperactivity. The corrugator in combination with the orbicularis are often involved in an oro-ocular synkinesis. The forehead can also occasionally be involved where voluntary lip action produces a brow lift.

30.2.1.3 Surgical Management

The presence of facial asymmetry from synkynesis, hypoactivity, or contralateral compensatory hyperactivity can all be treated surgically with single or a combination of procedures. Flaccid paralysis of the forehead and eyebrow is commonly treated with a browlift. Techniques are varied and include direct excision lift, open lift via a limited hairline incision, open lift via a coronal incision or endoscopic. The chosen technique depends on the severity of brow ptosis, location, and depth/severity of rhytides. A unilateral asymmetry would commonly be treated with more limited and less morbid procedure, such as the direct browlift or a limited open approach. When performed for aesthetic indications, it is imperative that the most powerful of depressor muscles, the corrugator, is completely transected in the procedure. This is indeed true in paralytic indications as well, especially since the corrugator has double innervation from both the zygomatic and temporal nerve branches, and thus could still activate and thus create further asymmetry. In addition, the orbital ligament can be divided to achieve maximal elevation.

In cases of non-flaccid paralysis, i.e., spasmic contractions in synkinesis or contralateral compensatory hyperactivity, the focus is firstly on deactivating the spasmic muscles. This can be done either through a myectomy or neurectomy, or in some cases both. It is often combined with a browlift in order to obtain a satisfactory static position of the eyebrow. This combination of techniques can be performed open, but since the endoscopic technique was introduced by Isse in 1992, it is often preferred [8]. In a study comparing the different surgical exposures, the endoscopic technique was found superior in visualizing the depressor complex and thus achieving complete resection of both the oblique and transverse heads of the corrugator, as well the procerus and depressor supercilii [5]. In addition to the myectomy and browlift, a neurectomy can performed to further limit the risk of recurrence. This has also been shown to be more precise and less morbid in endoscopic versus open techniques, since it enables direct visualization of the nerve branches and muscle fibers through minimum access.

The access through the endoscopic technique normally requires three incisions, one central and two temporal, but this can be altered depending on the surgical goals. The access points are commonly made in the hairline, but this risks alopecia. In a modification of the technique, Vasconez et al. advocate the use of "pre-hairline" incisions with excellent healing and limited scarring due to hiding the scar in present rhytids [9]. Following blunt subperiostal dissection with an elevator through the central access to about mid-forehead, the endoscopic camera is advanced. A dissector and grasper is introduced through the temporal access points. Advancement is made beneath the temporo-parietal fascia to about 1 cm superior to the zygomatic arch and medially to the temporal crest. At the temporal crest, the periosteum is incised and elevated and the temporal and central access points meet. The lower point of this dissection reaches the zygomatico-frontal suture, the lateral orbital rim and the presence of the sentinel vein [10]. This forms an important landmark, as the branching of the frontotemporal facial nerve occurs about 2–9 mm cephalad to it [11]. Once the connection between the temporal and central access points has been made and the supraorbital nerve is identified. This is done from lateral to medial. The periosteum is then incised from the lateral orbital rim and across the supraorbital rim. This fully exposes the depressor complex and enables transection. It is important not to resect portions of the corrugator as this would not only risk nerve injury, but also risk a visible concave contour deformity in the eyebrow area. Transection of the corrugator is preferably done both at its medial origin and lateral insertion [5]. At this point, a selective neurectomy can also be performed. The temporal branch to the corrugator can be found entering the muscle form its lateral and superficial aspect. A zygomatico-buccal branch can be found on the inferior and medial aspect of the corrugator. Procerus is also innervated by this nerve on its distal aspect, and can be included in the neurectomy.

30.2.2 The Eye

30.2.2.1 Anatomy

The orbicularis occuli is the prime constrictor of the eyelids. It is composed of different muscular regions; an inner-most pre-tarsal component is surrounded by pre-septal and finally orbital muscular fibers. The pre-tarsal orbicularis is involved in providing lower lid tone, involuntary blinking and lacrimal gland pumping mechanism. The pre-septal fibers assist with blinking. The outermost orbicularis fibers are in charge of forceful eyelid closure, animated eyelid movements and also provide depression of the most lateral and medial aspect of the eyebrow. The orbicularis interdigitates with the frontalis muscle and the corrugator supercilii. The nerve supply comes from a dense interconnecting plexus from the temporal, zygomatic, and buccal facial nerve branches, which reach the orbicularis from its inferior surface [12].

30.2.2.2 Evaluation

Ocular synkinesis is the most common form of facial synkinesis. Myectomy or neurectomy procedures have not become mainstream treatment options in most centers and the majority of patients are treated with botulinum toxin injections and physiotherapy. In selective cases, refractory synkinesis despite botulinum toxin injections or severe synkinesis, surgical intervention with myectomy or neurectomy can to be a suitable treatment option. As with all patients planed for myectomy or neurectomy procedure, patient selection is crucial. Involuntary eye closure can be observed as strong to very strong in patients with severe synkinesis. This is however not necessarily the case during voluntary eye closure. Myectomy on a patient with strong synkinesis with weak voluntary closure can result in postoperative lagopthalmus and the strength of the voluntary eye closure should therefore be thoroughly examined and discussed with the patient.

30.2.2.3 Surgical Management

Myectomy of the orbicularis oculi muscle is a rare procedure and better known in spasmatic conditions resulting in blepharospasm. Rarely, it can also be performed for aesthetic indications, primarily in cases of upper eyelid-fold disparities and mild lid ptosis. Blepharospasm can involve more or less of the periocular musculature, from the orbicularis to the entire eyebrow depressor complex. Myectomies and neurectomies as single or combined procedures have been described for the treatment of periocular spasmic conditions.

Myectomy

Several different techniques have been described with resection of different parts of the orbicularis, depending on the surgical goals and the area of spasm one wishes to relieve. Both upper lid and lower lid myectomies have been described. In addition, both peripheral and more central orbicularis fibers have been targeted for myectomies. The exact part of the orbicularis involved in the post-palsy synkinesis has not been described, but is believed to originate in the pre-septal portion of the orbicularis [13]. In surgical procedures aiming for myectomy-only relief of spasm, resection of the upper or lower lid pre-septal orbicularis (or on occasion both), managed to relieve the patient of periocular spasms without impairing eye closure. This procedure can be done through upper and lower blepharoplasty incision.

Neuromyectomy

In order to prevent recurrence of muscular tonicity, a myectomy can be combined with a neurectomy. Yoshioka described the processes of simultaneously excising muscle and nerve, en-bloc [14]. With this technique, a portion of the peripheral orbicularis in the lower lid is excised. A subciliary access exposes the undersurface of the muscle, as the access proceeds submuscularly to dissect the muscle off the orbital septum until the peripheral margin of the orbicularis is reached. At this point, a nerve stimulator is used to identify the temporo-zygomatico nerves one wish to eliminate. An approximately 1-cm-wide strip of orbicularis with accompanying nerves is then resected from its most lateral aspect going medially, in order to protect the angular vessels and the medial nerve branches going to the medial orbicularis, procerus and corrugator. During closure the muscle-skin flap is trimmed and sutured to the periosteum of the lateral orbital rim.

30.2.3 Selective Neurectomy

In hyperkinesis, specific to the glabellar and medial eyebrow portion, selective neurectomy can be performed to the zygomatico-buccal branch innervating the procerus, medial orbicularis occuli and medial portion of the corrugator. Nemoto et al. describe a triangular area in the inferomedial aspect of the peri-orbital area, outlined medially by the levator labii superioris alaeque nasi, laterally by the zygomaticus minor and superiorly by the inferior margin of the orbicularis occuli. The superficial and deep buccal branches are identified traversing superficial to the levator labii superioris, which forms the floor of the triangle. The superficial buccal branches can at this point be specifically transected to target the medial ocular and partially also eyebrow synkinesis. The deep branches can be transected to partially target the orbicularis.

When desiring a selective neurectomy to the larger portion of the orbicularis, the branches could be identified via an open face-lift approach, identified with a nerve stimulator, and resected. This approach can be effective, but unpredictable. Hohman et al. described an advanced technique of this selective neurectomy, using a two-stage approach [15]. A primary exploratory operative procedure under general anesthesia identifies the nerve fibers, which in a secondary procedure with the patient awake are sequentially divided to achieve the desired deneurotization. The operative procedure is performed via open access. The approach follows the subSMAS face-lift plane past the anterior border of the parotic gland. At this point, the branches to the orbicularis oculi are identified using a nerve stimulator. The nerve branches to the lateral and lower part of the orbicularis oculi are dissected and secured with vessel loupes and pulled out through stab incisions in the skin. The neurectomy is then performed in the outpatient clinic, giving the surgeon better control during the nerve resection while observing the synkinetic relieve on the patient. Van Veen et al. reviewed the outcomes of this procedure and unfortunately found synkinesis to return after a short period of regression. However, they did found previous botox non-responders to become sensitive to the treatment again [15].

30.3 Lower Zone of the Face

30.3.1 Lower Lip

30.3.1.1 Anatomy

The lower lip musculature is organized in layers and composed of several important lip depressors. The depressor anguli oris (DAO) is the most superficial muscle originating from the parasympheseal area of the mandible and inserting into the modiolus of the lip. It also has musculofibrous attachments to the nasolabial fold, emphasizing its depth. The depressor labii inferioris (DLI) muscle takes origin from the parasympheseal area deep to the DAO and just inferior to the mental foramen. Its muscle fibers are orientated cranially and medially, fuse with the fibers of the orbicularis oris and inserts into the subcutaneous area of the lower lip vermillion. The mental nerve fibers are found deep to the surface of the DLI. The nerve supply to the depressor complex of the tower lip (DLI, DAO and to a lesser degree platysma and mentalis) is by the marginal mandibular branch of the facial nerve. The mentalis muscle is also considered a weak depressor, but also raises the lower lip and the skin of the chin and causing protrusion. The orbicularis oris acts as the antagonist muscle, and is innervated by the buccal branch of the facial nerve.

30.3.2 Evaluation

30.3.2.1 Marginal Mandibular Lip Deformity

Unilateral paralysis of the marginal mandibular branch results in lower lip asymmetry characterized by a unilateral inability to depress, evert, and lateralize the lower lip. This creates a lower lip asymmetry in both animation and repose as there is a visible ipsilateral elevated appearance of the lip on the affected side, with impaired smiling and a lack of exposed teeth. In some cases, compensatory hyperactivity of the contraleral lower lip depressors can occur in response to the flaccid paralysis on the affected side, further worsening the asymmetry. This can be observed in repose, but also during facial animation in sadness, anger or while speaking and eating. A myectomy or neurectomy of the contralateral functioning depressor labii muscle aims to restore balance to the lower lip by decreasing the downward pull on the lip on the non-affected side. Depressor labii inferioris (DLI) myectomy is typically done under local anesthesia in the outpatient clinic and is arguably one of the more commonly performed myectomy procedures in patients with facial paralysis. Likewise, a myectomy of the depressor anguli oris can be performed to augment oral commissure elevation.

30.3.3 Surgical Management

30.3.3.1 Myectomy of the Lower Lip Depressors

Pre-operatively the DLI and the DAO muscles are marked on the patients' skin. Palpation of their borders are facilitated by asking the patient to depress and evert the lower lip (showing their teeth). Following a mental nerve block, one or two sutures are placed through the lower lip for traction and eversion. A mucosal incision is made about 0.5 cm above the buccal sulcus and a gentle dissection exposes the mental nerve branches. The nerve branches are protected by vessel loops and retracted to the side. The DLI is identified by the direction of the muscle fibers, which are oblique to the orbicularis oris muscle [16]. The medial and lateral boarders of the muscle are dissected in order to delineate the extent if its width. A central horizontal portion of the muscle is then resected, rather than simply transected, preferably from mid-length of the muscle. The same is performed with the DAO. Patients receiving preoperative chemodenervation to the DLI can practice their operative results and thus limit unexpected outcomes. Alternatively, local anesthetic can be injected in to the muscle preoperatively, inducing a short trial paralysis. The recurrence rate of the depressor function after myectomy has been reported as high as 30% and patients occasionally require reresection of the muscle. Fatty tissue surrounding the depressor muscles can make the border of the muscle hard to outline. Locating the boarders of the muscle is thus crucial to ensure complete resection. Performing a resection of a strip of muscle of at least 1 cm, rather than a simple transection is preferred to prevent inadequate results.

Case 1. Lower Lip Myectomy (Figs. A–F)

Intraoperative photos showing the surgical sequence. Outline of the lower lip depressors (A). Incise the mucosa and continue the intra-oral dissection until the mental nerve is reached, normally positioned anterior to the first pre-molar tooth. Protect the nerve with vessel loops (B). Resect the DLI and DAO (C). Wound closure with Vicryl (D).

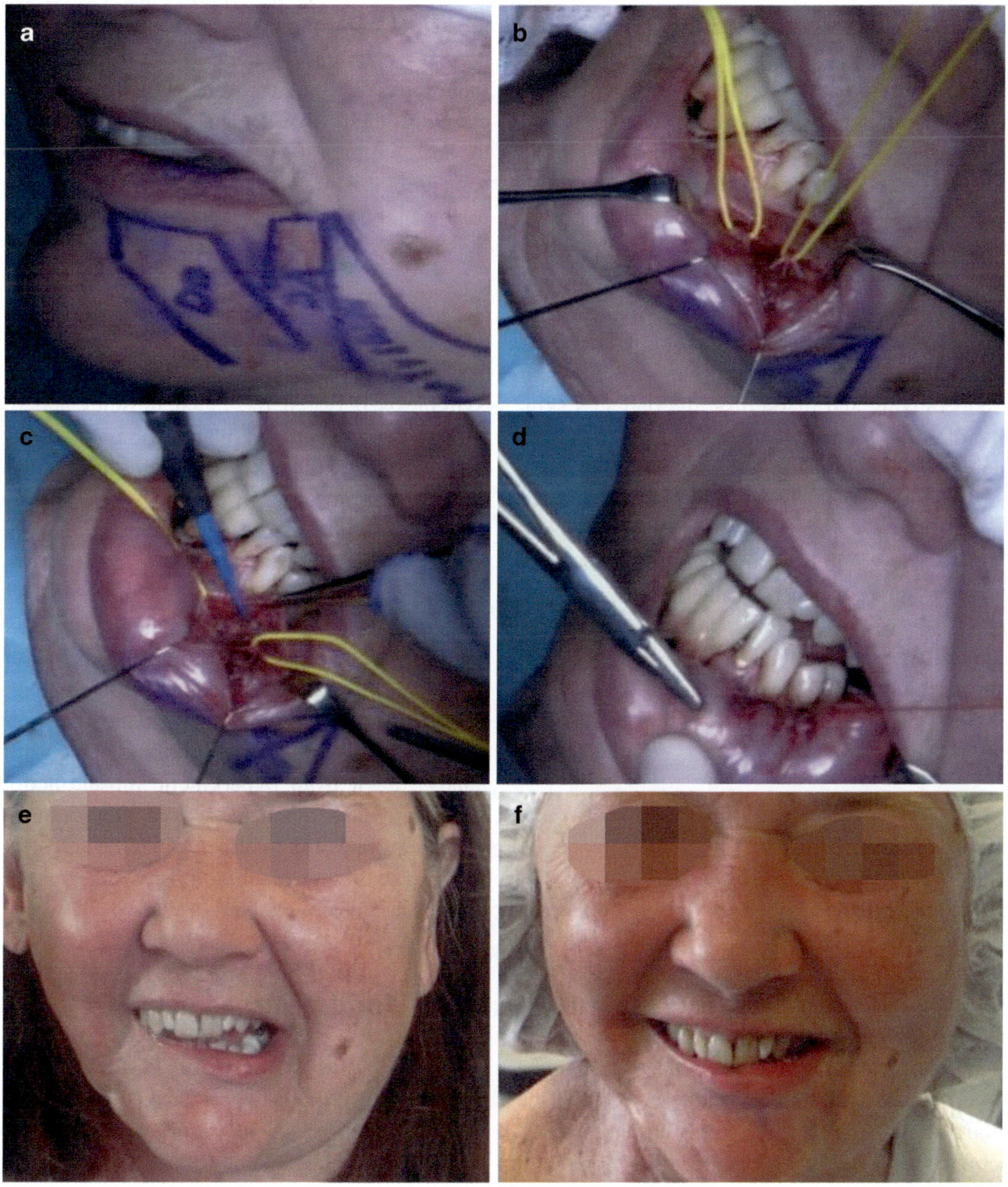

A 65 years-old woman with right-sided marginal mandibular nerve palsy after mandible reconstruction with free fibula flap for a right-sided mandibular osteoradionecrosis, before left lower lip depressors myectomy (E) and after myectomy (F), showing better position of the lower lip without exposure of the lower teeth in full smile.

30.3.3.2 Selective Marginal Mandibular Neurectomy

Selective marginal mandibular branch neurectomy has shown good results. The surgery is however more time consuming and technically complex. In cases where cross facial nerve graft is planned, selective neurectomy might be a good treatment option, addressing the lower lip asymmetry in an selective group of patients undergoing smile reconstruction.

The operative procedure is similar to the myectomy. The depressor muscles are identified preoperatively and marked on the patient's skin. The incision is through an extended preauricular incision allowing good visual access. Using a nerve stimulator, nerve branches to the Depressor Labii Inferioris muscle (alternatively also the Depressor Anguli Oris muscle) are identified. Through micro dissection the nerves are then selectively resected with 2 cm segments. Only branches innervating the lower lip depressors are resected thus minimizing the risk of denervation of the Orbicularis Oris muscle and potential subsequent oral incontinence.

30.4 Neck

30.4.1 Anatomy

The platysma originates from the fascia of the pectoralis and deltoid muscles and runs cephalad and medially to end in a broad insertion on the mandible, skin, and subcutaneous tissue of the lower face and muscles around the corner of the mouth and lower lip [17]. It has an antagonistic action to the zygomaticus major muscle, in that it is a week lower lip depressor. Therefore, involuntary contraction in the muscle can exaggerate a "frozen smile" appearance in patients with partial paralysis. The platysma is innervated by the cervical branch of the facial nerve distally, and gets co-innervation by the marginal mandibular nerve proximally [18]. The marginal mandibular and the cervical branch arise from the lower division of the facial nerve. Their common branch runs posterior to the ramus of the mandible before dividing. The division point can be reliably located at approximately 1 cm below a perpendicular line from the angle of the mandible to a line drawn from the mentum to the mastoid process with the neck extended and the head turned to the contralateral side. The nerve then curves to run parallel, 3–4 cm caudal to the mandible, deep to the platysma muscle and at the level of the hyoid fans out into its terminal branches.

30.4.2 Evaluation

Synkinesis between the facial muscles and the platysma is a frequent observation in patients with facial synkinesis. Involuntary chronic muscle contraction and subsequent hypertrophy of the platysma muscle is often accompanied with a feeling of tightness or pain in the neck and the lower face. Beurskens et al. found the platysma to be a common synkinetic muscle in all facial movements, both ocular and oral [2]. The patient examination is pertinent to deciding the management required patients with abundant subcutaneous fatty tissue will have less prominent platysmal bands shown from hyperkinetic muscle action, but could have much pain from the condition. Similarly, the botox treatment could be less effective in necks with much adiposity, thus surgical options could provide better relief.

30.4.3 Surgical Management

30.4.3.1 Platysmectomy

Preoperatively, the patient is asked to provoke the platysmal synkinesis in order to delineate the border of the platysma and its contracted bands, which are marked. The access line is marked in an existing neck crease on the mid portion of the muscle belly. The incision goes down to the superficial fascia of the platysma muscle. The dissection is extended in this plane, raising skin flaps to expose the whole width of the muscle. The muscle is then penetrated and the deep plane is developed. The myectomy is then performed removing 2–3 cm segments of the length of the muscle from the medial to lateral border. If the operation is done under local anesthesia, the patient can then be asked to provoke the platysmal synkinesis and the discontinuation of the muscle can be assessed. The skin is then closed in a standard manner. Postoperative results have shown significant improvements in tension, spams and pain both in the neck and facial region [19]. Loss of platysma function is well tolerated by patients and the scar is usually well hidden within a natural neck crease.

30.4.3.2 Neurectomy of the Cervical Branch

Neurectomy of the cervical branch is an interesting treatment option for patients with platysmal synkinesis. Anatomical studies have offered landmarks for accurately locating the cervical branch and introduced its potential in reconstructive and esthetic surgery [18]. The skin incision can be made 4 cm caudal and parallel to the mandible. The platysma is then penetrated and the submuscular plane is developed. Using a nerve stimulator, the cervical branch can be located. The ascending branch innervating the facial portion of the platysma muscle can be resected or spared dependent on the patient symptoms. A neurectomy can be combined with a platysmectomy, and the surgical procedure is similar.

Case 2 Combined Platysmectomy and Neurectomy of the Cervical Branch (Figs. A–F)

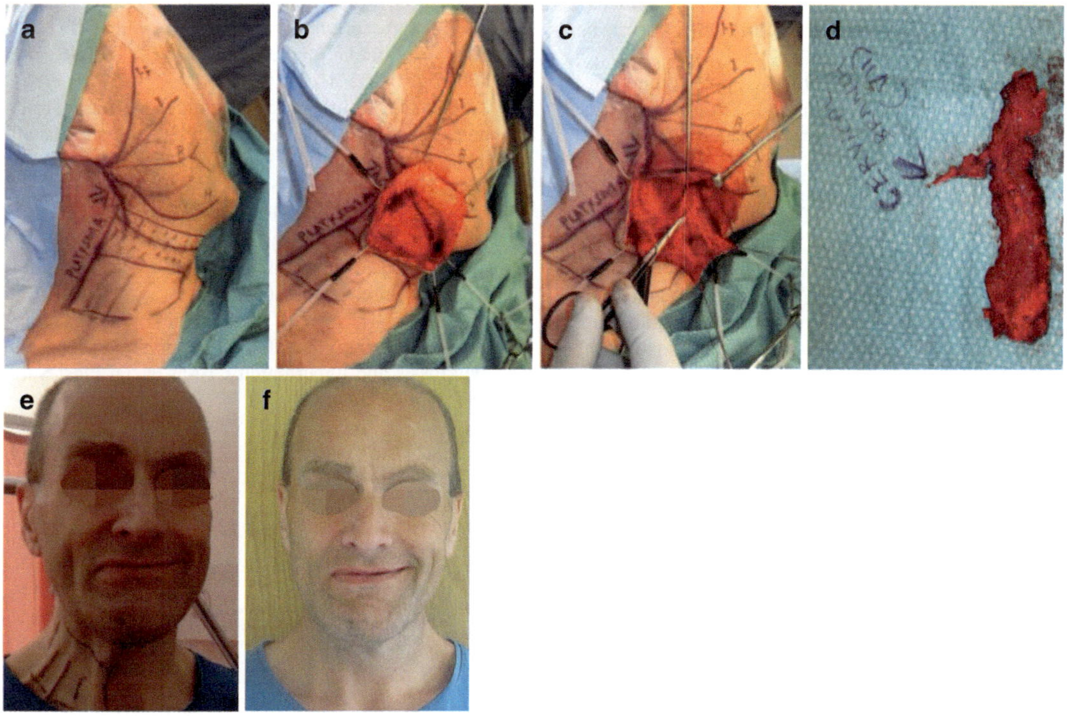

Intraoperative picture showing the surgical sequence. Surgical markings demonstrating the platysma and facial nerve branches (A). Undermining of skin over platysma (B) followed by dissection of platysma and identification of platysma motor nerve i.e., the cervical branch (C). Platysma and nerve resected en-bloc (D).

Pre and postop appearance of a 49-year-old man with severe synkinesis of the right hemiface after Bell's Palsy. Picture (E) demonstrates his appearance before having a combined neuromyectomy of the platysma, and picture (F) after.

References

1. Chuang DCC, Chang TNJ, Lu JCY. Postparalysis facial synkinesis: clinical classification and surgical strategies. Plast Reconstr Surg Glob Open. 2015;3(3):1–14.
2. Beurskens CHG, Oosterhof J, Nijhuis-Van Der Sanden MWG. Frequency and location of synkineses in patients with peripheral facial nerve paresis. Otol Neurotol. 2010;31(4):671–5.
3. Markey JD, Loyo M. Latest advances in the management of facial synkinesis. Curr Opin Otolaryngol Head Neck Surg. 2017;25(4):265–72.
4. Warren Richard J. Forehead rejuvenation Warren Richard J Peter & Neligan editors. in Plastic Surgery. Aesthetic Surgery. Philadelphia. Saunders. 2012;2(3):93–107.
5. Janis JE, Ghavami A, Lemmon JA, Leedy JE, Guyuron B. Anatomy of the corrugator supercilii muscle: part I. Corrugator topography. Plast Reconstr Surg. 2007;120(6):1647–53.
6. Caminer DM, Newman MI, Boyd JB. Angular nerve: new insights on innervation of the corrugator supercilii and procerus muscles. J Plast Reconstr Aesthet Surg. 2006;59(4):366–72.
7. Janis JE, Ghavami A, Lemmon JA, Leedy JE, Guyuron B. The anatomy of the corrugator supercilii muscle: part II. Supraorbital nerve branching patterns. Plast Reconstr Surg. 2008;121(1):233–40.
8. Withey S, Witherow H, Waterhouse N. One hundred cases of endoscopic brow lift. Br J Plast Surg. 2002;55:20–4.
9. Vásconez LO, De La Torre JI. Fine-tuning the endoscopic brow lift. Aesthet Surg J. 2002;22(1):69–71.
10. Mackay GJ, Nahai F. The endoscopic forehead lift. Oper Tech Plast Reconstr Surg. 1995;2(2):137–44.
11. Moody F, Losken A, Bostwick J, Trinei F, Eaves F. Endoscopic frontal branch neurectomy, corrugator myectomy, and brow lift for forehead asymmetry after facial nerve palsy. Plast Reconstr Surg. 2001;108(1):218–23.
12. Nemoto Y, Sekino Y, Kaneko H. Facial nerve anatomy in eyelids and periorbit. Jpn J Ophthalmol. 2001;45(5):445–52.
13. Lai CS, Lu SR, Yang SF, Teh LS, Lee SS. Surgical treatment of the synkinetic eyelid closure in marinamat syndrome. Ann Plast Surg. 2011;67(5):498–501.
14. Yoshioka N. Selective orbicularis neuromyectomy for postparetic periocular synkinesis. J Plast Reconstr Aesthet Surg. 2015;68(11):1510–5. https://doi.org/10.1016/j.bjps.2015.06.015.
15. van Veen MM, Dusseldorp JR, Hadlock TA. Long-term outcome of selective neurectomy for refractory periocular synkinesis. Laryngoscope. 2018;128(10):1–5.
16. Hussain G, Manktelow R, Tomat L. Depressor labii inferioris resection: an effective treatment for marginal mandibular nerve paralysis. Br J Plast Surg. 2004;57(6):502–10.
17. Laskawi R, Rohrbach S, Roumldel R. Surgical and nonsurgical treatment options in patients with movement disorders of the platysma. J Oral Maxillofac Surg. 2002;60(2):157–62.
18. Chowdhry S, Yoder E, Cooperman R, Yoder V, Wilhelmi B. Locating the cervical motor branch of the facial nerve: anatomy and clinical application. Plast Reconstr Surg. 2010;126(3):875–9.
19. Henstrom D, Malo J, Cheney M, Hadlock T. Platysmectomy: an effective intervention for facial synkinesis and hypertonicity. Arch Facial Plast Surg. 2011;13(4):239–43.

Management of Synkinesia

31

Andrés Rodríguez-Lorenzo
and Chieh-Han John Tzou

Key Points

- Synkinetic movements are involuntary movements during the voluntary movement of a different muscle (group).
- Moderate to Severe Synkinesias are present in 6 to 7% of patients with Bells Palsy.
- Facial synkinesia occurs with voluntary facial movements but can also be associated with the blink reflex.
- There are two types of facial synkinesia: post-facial palsy synkinesia and post-facial reanimation synkinesia. The first occurs after spontaneous regeneration of the facial nerve and the second is a side effect of facial reanimation surgery.
- Treatment of facial synkinesia in facial palsy patients includes physiotherapy, denervation using Botulinum toxin injections, and surgical options like myectomy and selective denervation.

31.1 Facial Synkinesia

Facial synkinesia is defined as involuntary movements of facial muscles during the voluntary movement of a different facial muscle group [1]. Symmetrical facial synkinesia has no burden of disease as it occurs naturally during facial movements. Pathological synkinetic movements are defined as asymmetrical movements with greater amplitude of motion on the affected side, that can be triggered by either voluntary facial movements or the blink reflex [2].

The terminology for most types of facial synkinesia involves the trigger movement and the synkinetic movement, for example "oculo-oral synkinesia" describes the synkinetic movement of the mouth during eyelid closure [3].

Synkinesia is a common and distressing sequela of facial paralysis, which affects 15–20% to more than 50% of patients, depending on the case series [4]. Moderate to severe synkinesias are present in 6,6% of patients with Bells Palsy at twelve months after onset of the paralysis [5].

A. Rodríguez-Lorenzo (✉)
Department of Plastic and Maxillofacial Surgery, Uppsala University Hospital, Uppsala, Sweden

Department of Surgical Sciences, Uppsala University, Uppsala, Sweden
e-mail: andres.rodriguez.lorenzo@surgsci.uu.se

C.-H. J. Tzou
Plastic and Reconstructive Surgery, Hospital of Divine Savior (Krankenhaus Goettlicher Heiland), Sigmund Freud University, TZOU MEDICAL, Vienna, Austria

Facial Palsy and Lymphedema Center Vienna, Vienna, Austria
e-mail: science@tzoumedical.com

© Springer Nature Switzerland AG 2021
C.-H. J. Tzou, A. Rodríguez-Lorenzo (eds.), *Facial Palsy*,
https://doi.org/10.1007/978-3-030-50784-8_31

Facial palsy patients described synkinetic movements as one of the emotionally most straining sequelae of the paralysis. In quality of life assessments, synkinesia was found to impair social interaction and reduce the productivity of patients [6]. In severe cases, synkinesia can be associated with pain and spasms of facial muscles, and may cause contractions of facial muscles. In unilateral facial palsy, the movement on the healthy side of the face can be impaired as patients try to avoid synkinetic movements by reducing their facial expression altogether [4].

31.2 Etiology of Synkinetic Facial Movements

The mechanisms leading to facial synkinesia in facial palsy patients are multifactorial and the pathophysiological mechanisms (Table 31.1) are still not fully established.

Generally, facial synkinesia can occur after spontaneous regeneration of facial nerve function ("postparalysis facial synkinesia") and after facial reanimation surgery [7]. The incidence of facial synkinesia is higher after severe injuries to the facial nerve. The most widely recognized pathophysiological mechanism leading to facial synkinesia is aberrant nerve regeneration, where outgrowing axons of regenerating neurons innervate new muscle targets, which were previously not innervated by them. This can be caused by collateral or terminal axonal sprouting [1].

A different mechanism leading to synkinetic movements is ephaptic transmission, which describes non-synaptic electrical transmission between two adjacent axons after injury of the myelin sheet. Experimental studies demonstrated that the somatotopic organization of the facial nucleus is disturbed after injury, which may contribute to the development of synkinesia. The excitation level of the facial nucleus was found to be increased after regeneration of the facial nerve, which is thought to contribute to the development of synkinesia [2].

Table 31.1 Pathophysiological mechanisms leading to facial synkinesia

Pathophysiological mechanisms of facial synkinesia
• Aberrant nerve regeneration. • Increased excitability of the facial nucleus. • Alteration of the somatotopic organization of the facial nucleus. • Ephaptic, non-synaptic electrical transmission after injury to the myelin sheet.

31.3 Postparalysis and Post-facial Reanimation Synkinesia

Synkinetic facial movements can occur after spontaneous regeneration of facial nerve function, which is described as postparalysis synkinesia [7]. Facial synkinesia can also occur after surgical reanimation of the paralyzed face, which is termed postoperative or post-facial reanimation synkinesia [4, 7].

The potential for spontaneous recovery of facial nerve function depends on the severity of facial nerve impairment and the underlying etiology. In traumatic or iatrogenic cases where the proximal nerve stump is severe d, spontaneous recovery and thus the development of synkinetic movements cannot be expected. In idiopathic cases of facial palsy, recovery rates of 70–90% have been reported. In large case series of patients suffering from idiopathic facial palsy, 16% of patients subsequently developed moderate-to-severe sequelae like dyskinesia (blepharospasm and hemifacial spasm) and synkinesia. Spontaneous recovery rates of 89% were reported for infectious etiologies causing facial palsy. Fewer data is available on facial palsy due to traumatic or iatrogenic causes. Reported recovery rates for traumatic etiologies were approximately 57%. About 30% of patients undergoing parotidectomies were found to develop postoperative facial palsy. The facial nerve function recovered completely in 68% of these patients within 6 months. Time to recovery indicated the severity of facial nerve injury. It was found that more severe facial nerve injuries result in higher incidences of facial synkinesia upon recovery [3]. Patients with idiopathic, traumatic, and infectious causes of facial palsy showed the highest percentage of postparalysis facial synkinesia of around 15% [4, 7]. The time until the onset of postparalysis facial synkinesia has been described to range from around 3.5 to 6 months [3].

There is very limited data available on the incidence of post-facial reanimation synkinesia, which can develop after dynamic reanimation of the paralyzed face. In a large series, around 50% of patients undergoing dynamic facial reanimation developed mild-to-moderate facial synkinesia, while severe synkinesia was only reported in 1% of cases [4]. The highest incidences of post-facial reanimation synkinesia were reported for territorially differentiated gracilis muscle transplantation innervated by two cross-facial nerve grafts, which was attributed to the in some cases overlapping innervation of the two territories of the gracilis muscle, which are used to innervate the eye and mouth region, respectively. In cases where cross-face nerve grafts were used to innervate the denervated facial muscles directly, 25% of patients developed postoperative facial synkinesia [4]. The time until post-facial reanimation synkinesia develops is not sufficiently explored. Onset times of approximately 12 months after facial reanimation have been reported, but onset times are expected to vary highly depending on the type of dynamic facial reanimation, the source of innervation and the regeneration distance.

31.4 Types of Facial Synkinesia and Associated Symptoms

The type of synkinesia is determined by the trigger movement and the synkinetic movement (Table 31.2).

Any facial region can be affected by synkinesia (Fig. 31.1). Moran and Neely found that facial synkinesia occurs in a nonrandom pattern and some forms of synkinetic movements are found more frequently [2]. The most common type is the oculo-oral synkinesia, the involuntary movement of the mouth during eyelid closure. VanSwearingen and Brach introduced the expression "multiway synkinesis," which describes synkinesia triggered by more than one voluntary facial movement [8]. There are also complex cases where more than one synkinetic muscle group is triggered during a voluntary movement.

Table 31.2 Types of facial synkinesia

Type of facial synkinesia	Symptoms
Oculo-oral synkinesia	Movement of the mouth during eyelid closure
Oro-ocular synkinesia	Eyelid closure during movement of the mouth
Levator labii superioris synkinesia	Deepened nasolabial fold
Synkinesia of the frontalis muscle	Brow elevation, raised brow position at rest
Sykinesia of the depressors	Lower lip depression or reduced craniolateral smile excursion
Synkinesia of the mentalis muscle	Chin dimpling, lower lip depression
Synkinesia of the platysma	Platysmal cords
Blink reflex triggered synkinesia	Most commonly oral synkinesia during the blink reflex, but other muscle groups can also be affected
Multiway synkinesia	More than one trigger movement for synkinetic movement

Synkinetic movements have also been classified as synergistic and paradox types of movements. Synergistic synkinetic movements resembled those of the healthy hemiface, whereas paradox synkinesia were movements in inappropriate directions [2]. The synkinetic movement is not necessarily reciprocal. Patients with oculo-oral synkinetic movements, where the mouth corner is raised during eyelid closure, are in most cases not affected by oro-ocular synkinesia, even though they can suffer from both types.

Rare forms include oculo-stapedial synkinesia, which describes a clicking sound during eyelid closure. Non-motor axons of the facial nerve can also be misdirected and lead to the gusto-lacrimal reflex, which is also describes as "crocodile-tears." Rare cases of aberrant nerve regeneration connecting two different cranial nerves were reported. Examples include: synki-

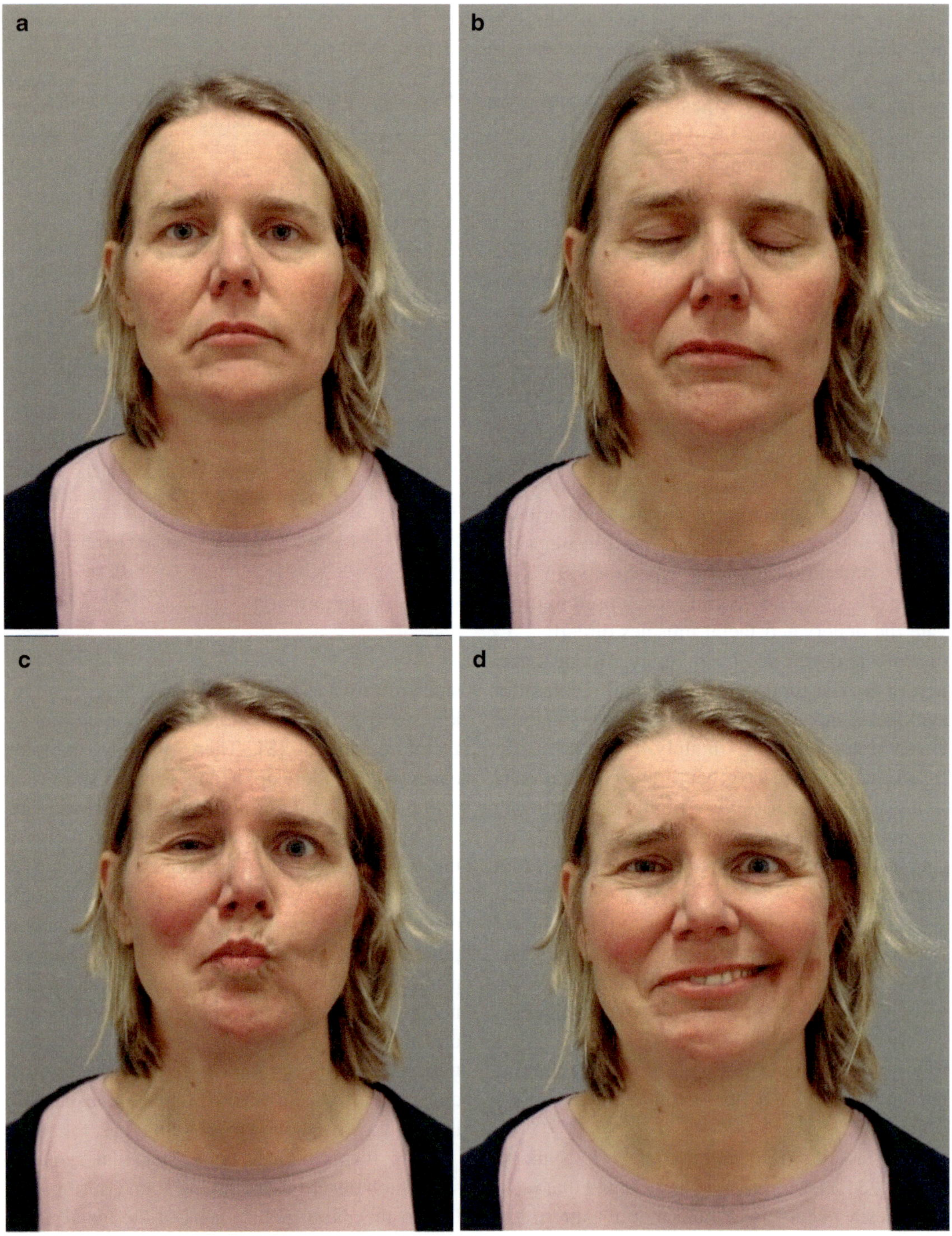

Fig. 31.1 Photographs of a 47-year-old woman with right facial synkinesias after Bell's palsy. (**a**) In rest (**b**) Oculo-oral synkinesia (**c**) Oro-ocular synkinesia (**d**) Synkinesia of depressors with reduction of smile excursion on the right side and synkinesia of mentalis muscle

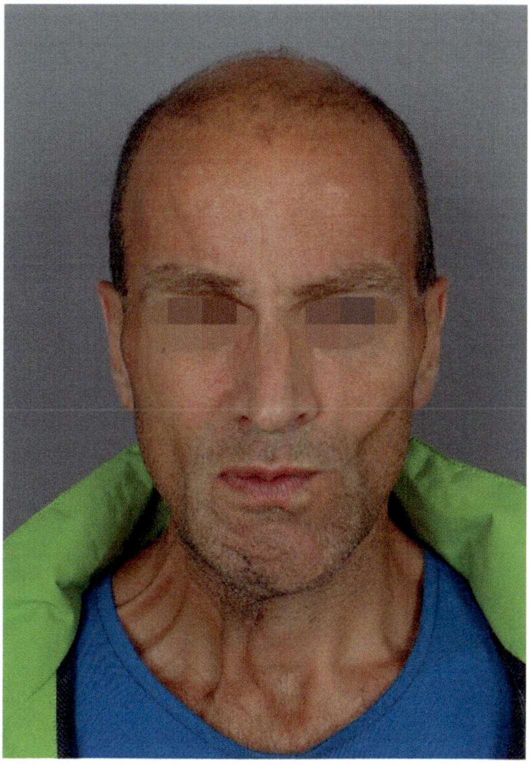

Fig. 31.2 Platysmal strands and synkinesia of the mentalis muscle as sequalae of Bell's palsy

nesia of the facial and the trigeminal nerve, synkinesia of the facial and oculomotor nerve [2].

Longstanding severe facial synkinesia can lead to contractures and asymmetry of the resting face. Patients can suffer from deepened nasiolabial folds and chin dimpling at rest [7]. Untreated platysmal synkinesia can lead to platysmal strands at rest and during facial movements (Fig. 31.2).

The type of synkinetic movement influences its clinical significance along with the severity of the synkinesia. Mild forms of synkinesia or synkinesia triggered by movements that the patient rarely applies during daily activities carry less burden of disease than for example, synkinesia associated with the blink reflex.

31.5 Diagnosis of Synkinetic Facial Movements

Different diagnostic tools and grading systems for facial synkinesia are available. Subjective gradings are either patient-based or observer-based. Most grading systems are developed for general assessment of facial function in facial palsy patients and include a section for synkinetic movements. Well established observer-based grading systems include the Regional House-Brackmann Facial Nerve Grading System [9], the Sunnybrook Facial Grading System [10], the Sydney Facial Grading System [10] and the Chang Gung Memorial Hospital PPFS Examination Sheet [7] (Table 31.3).

Several patient-based questionnaires assessing synkinesia were introduced, like the Synkinesis Assessment Questionnaire [11] or the FaCE Scale Instrument [12], however, many reports in the literature applied non-validated "ad-hoc" questionnaires.

Clinically, most groups adapted the grading system of facial introduced by Ross et al. [13]

Table 31.3 Observer-based and patient-based gradings of synkinesia

Subjective grading systems of facial synkinesia
• Observer-based gradings: – Sunnybrook Facial Grading System [13]. – Regional House-Brackmann Facial Nerve Grading System [9]. – Sydney Facial Grading System [10]. – Chang Gung Memorial Hospital PPFS Examination Sheet [7]. • Patient-based gradings: – Synkinesis Assessment Questionnaire [11]. – FaCE Scale Instrument [12].

Table 31.4 Subjective grading of facial synkinesia after Ross et al. [13]

Grade of synkinesia	Facial movement
None	No synkinetic facial movement
Mild	Slight synkinesia
Moderate	Obvious but not disfiguring synkinesia
Severe	Disturbing synkinesia; gross mass movement of several muscles

(Table 31.4). Synkinetic movements are graded by the observer from none to severe. This offers an easily applicable way for gross grading of the different types of synkinesia, which this scale can be applied to. Interobserver variability needs to be considered with any subjective grading.

Synkinetic movements can also be analyzed with objective facial grading systems like the Neely-Cheung Facial Analysis Computerized Evaluation system, the maximal static response assay (MSRA) of facial nerve function, the Peak Motus Motion Measurement System, the Automated Facial Image Analysis, or the Three-Dimensional Video Analysis of Facial Movement [4]. Studies found that objective tools diagnosed synkinesia more frequently than subjective gradings. Among objective analysis systems, three-dimensional assessment of facial movements should be preferred, as it was demonstrated that two-dimensional analysis of facial movements underestimated three-dimensional amplitudes by as much as 43% [14].

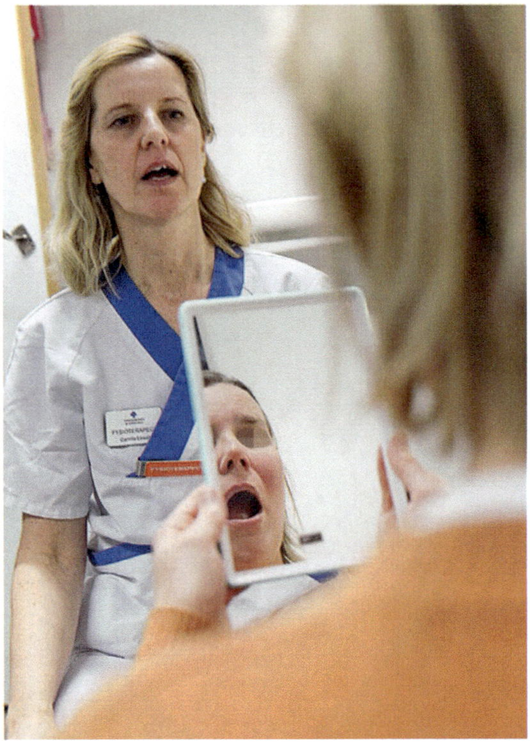

Fig. 31.4 Imaging of mirror training with physiotherapist guidance

31.6 Treatment of Synkinetic Facial Movements

For successful treatment of facial synkinesia, the patients need to be informed about the underlying causes of the condition. It is the responsibility of the treating facial plastic surgeon to raise awareness for synkinetic movements and to establish a treatment plan that takes the severity and type of synkinesia into consideration. Conservative treatment options include physical therapy, mirror training, biofeedback rehabilitation that applies electromyographic feedback and neuromuscular reeducation (Figs. 31.3 and 31.4). Brach et al. showed that oral synkinesia is significantly reduced by facial neuromuscular retraining, a facial exercise program in combination with electromyographic biofeedback [15]. Facial neuromuscular reeducation led to alternated muscle recruitment in patients with facial palsy, who suffered from moderate-to-severe synkinesia or mild-to-moderate multiway synkinesia. The study showed that neuromuscular reeducation improved voluntary facial movements and decreased synkinesia [8].

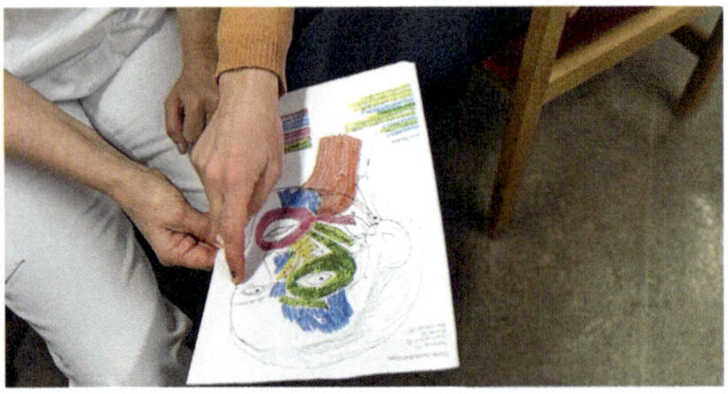

Fig. 31.3 Image that illustrates patient education during physiotherapy training in synkinesias. Understanding of the different facial muscles and the involuntary facial movements increases patient engagement in the treatment

Botulinum toxin injections are commonly used in the treatment of facial synkinesia [7]. Increased resting tone of synkinetic muscle groups can be improved. The treatment effect is, however, temporary and repeated applications are required. It is advisable to systematic docu-

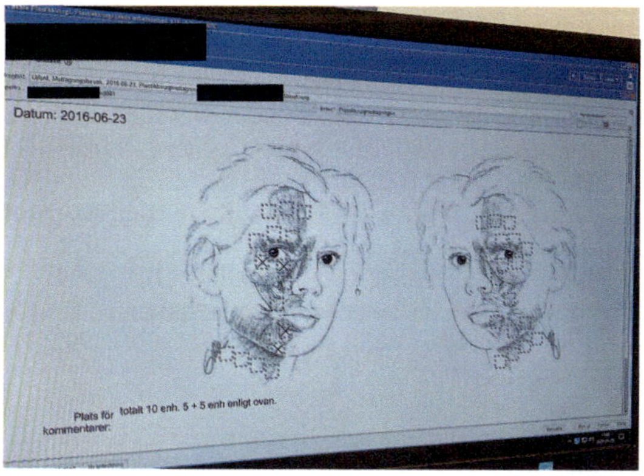

Fig. 31.5 Chart documentation of Botulinum toxin treatment in facial synkinesias at the Facial Palsy Clinic, Uppsala University Hospital

ment the location and dose of injections (Fig. 31.5). The affected patients need to be counseled regarding the indications, possible side effects and limitations of Botulinum toxin injections.

Chuang et al. developed a severity and pattern directed treatment algorithm for facial synkinesia [7]. The treatment goal of facial synkinesia is not the mere suppression of unintentional movement, but the improvement of facial function and symmetry. Mild cases of facial synkinesia can be managed with physical therapy and Botulinum toxin injections. Botulinum toxin injections are also used to improve static asymmetries like chin dimpling and deepened nasolabial folds or platysmal strands. In severe cases, the trigger and the synkinetic muscles need to be addressed [7]. Surgical treatment concepts of facial synkinesia need to consider the severity and type of synkinesia in context of the patients' facial function [4]. Surgical interventions range from small corrective surgeries, like blepharoplasty or fat grafting to extensive procedures that include denervation of the affected part of the face with myectomy of synkinetic muscles, followed by facial reanimation with alternate sources of innervation and free muscle transplantation [7].

Static corrections to improve facial symmetry include brow lift, fat grafting to improve nasolabial fold and chin, lip revision, blepharoplasty, tensor fasciae lata sling, or fat grafts [7]. Myectomy of synkinetic muscle groups are well established for the corrugator muscle, the depressor and mentalis muscles, as well as the platysma. Myectomy of parts of the orbicularis oculi has been reported, but the eyelid closure needs to be preserved.

In severe cases of facial synkinesia, radical myectomy and two-stage reconstruction with cross-face nerve grafts and a free gracilis muscle transplant can be performed. Alternatively, one-stage procedures can be performed with alternative donor nerves like the spinal accessory nerve, or the masseter nerve [7]. The patient needs to be carefully counseled about the complexity of the reconstruction and possible complications.

Given the complexity of the treatment of facial synkinesia, patient education and research focusing on the causes and prevention of synkinesia are important.

Acknowledgment Co-Author Eva Gyoeri, M.D. withdrew from this chapter upon her request in May 2020.

References

1. Crumley R. Mechanisms of synkinesis. Laryngoscope. 1979;89(11):1847–54.
2. Moran C, Neely J. Patterns of facial nerve synkinesis. Laryngoscope. 1996;106(12 Pt 1):1491–6.
3. Husseman J, Mehta RP. Management of synkinesis. Facial Plast Surg. 2008;24(2):242–9.
4. Placheta E, et al. Facial synkinesia before and after surgical reanimation of the paralyzed face. Plast Reconstr Surg. 2014;133(6):842e–51e.
5. Bylund N, Jensson D, Enghag S, Berg T, Marsk E, Hultcrantz M, Hadziosmanovic N, Rodriguez A, Jonsson L. Synkinesis in Bell's palsy in a randomized controlled trial. Clin Otolaryngol. 2016;42(3):673–80.
6. Coulson SE, et al. Expression of emotion and quality of life after facial nerve paralysis. Otol Neurotol. 2004;25(6):1014–9.
7. Chuang DC, Chang TN, Lu JC. Postparalysis facial synkinesis: clinical classification and surgical strategies. Plast Reconstr Surg Glob Open. 2015;3(3):e320.
8. VanSwearingen J, Brach J. Changes in facial movement and synkinesis with facial neuromuscular reeducation. Plast Reconstr Surg. 2003;111(7):2370–5.

9. Yen T, Driscoll C, Lalwani A. Significance of House-Brackmann facial nerve grading global score in the setting of differential facial nerve function. Otol Neurotol. 2003;24(1):118–22.
10. Coulson S, et al. Reliability of the "Sydney," "Sunnybrook," and "House Brackmann" facial grading systems to assess voluntary movement and synkinesis after facial nerve paralysis. Otolaryngol Head Neck Surg. 2005;132(4):543–9.
11. Mehta R, WernickRobinson M, Hadlock T. Validation of the synkinesis assessment questionnaire. Laryngoscope. 2007;117(5):923–6.
12. Kahn J, et al. Validation of a patient-graded instrument for facial nerve paralysis: the FaCE scale. Laryngoscope. 2001;111(3):387–98.
13. Ross B, Fradet G, Nedzelski J. Development of a sensitive clinical facial grading system. Otolaryngol Head Neck Surg. 1996;114(3):380–6.
14. Gross M, Trotman C, Moffatt K. A comparison of three-dimensional and two-dimensional analyses of facial motion. Angle Orthod. 1996;66(3):189–94.
15. Brach J, et al. Facial neuromuscular retraining for oral synkinesis. Plast Reconstr Surg. 1997;99(7):1922–31; discussion 1932–3

Part VI

Innovations and New Frontiers

32 Frontiers and Innovations in Facial Palsy

Caroline Driessen, Andrés Rodríguez-Lorenzo, and Chieh-Han John Tzou

Key Points

- Direct neuronization of transplanted muscle grafts may be useful in reanimation of the periocular complex.
- Reanimation of the nose was neglected too long and should be considered in every facial palsy patient.
- Synkinesis surgery moves from botulinum toxin injections alone to myectomy, neurectomy, nerve transfers, and combinations. The challenge is to remain sufficient motor activity.
- Endoscopic approaches should be considered in every facial palsy related operation with the benefit of less skin and soft tissue injury, better aesthetic result and even preserved nerve integrity due to a smaller wound.
- Ideally, bionic reanimation uses electrical stimulation by the non-affected side to activate the paralyzed muscles or vascularized muscle flap of the affected side. If it will be clinically feasible in the future, it may create spontaneity and it would make surgery and a cross-facial nerve graft unnecessary.

This book has outlined the variable options that are currently available to reanimate the face after facial palsy. There are numerous unsolved problems and there are ongoing projects to finetune the current solutions. This search includes direct neurotization, novel use of expandable donor nerves, different adaptations of the commonly used donor nerves, different muscle transfers and static procedures but also changes in indications and the use of medical technologies. This chapter will introduce the hot topics among the exploration of new solutions in facial palsy. The treatment of facial palsy highly depends on organization and research.

Regarding organization, facial palsy is registered in the 'National organisation of rare disorders' in the United States. This organization

C. Driessen · A. Rodríguez-Lorenzo (✉)
Department of Plastic and Maxillofacial Surgery, Uppsala University Hospital, Uppsala, Sweden
e-mail: andres.rodriguez.lorenzo@surgsci.uu.se

C.-H. J. Tzou
Plastic and Reconstructive Surgery, Department of Surgery, Hospital of Divine Savior Vienna (Krankenhaus Goettlicher Heiland Wien), Vienna, Austria

Sigmund Freud University Vienna, TZOU MEDICAL, Vienna, Austria

Facial Palsy and Lymphedema Center Vienna, Vienna, Austria
e-mail: science@tzoumedical.com

© Springer Nature Switzerland AG 2021
C.-H. J. Tzou, A. Rodríguez-Lorenzo (eds.), *Facial Palsy*,
https://doi.org/10.1007/978-3-030-50784-8_32

coordinates patient information but is also facilitates connections with colleagues, the possibilities to apply for grants and research collaboration. Similarly, in Europe, there are European Reference Networks (ERN). They are virtual networks involving healthcare providers across Europe. The aim is to tackle complex or rare diseases for which specialized treatment is required. A virtual expertise team of medical specialists across different disciplines may advise in the treatment of patients with a specific rare disease without the need for the patient to travel. The concentration of knowledge and resources may improve the clinical outcome. It's for the first time in healthcare that this voluntary collaboration between healthcare providers is created in a formal structure. They are supported by the European Commission. Facial palsy is included in the ERN that covers Rare craniofacial anomalies and ENT disorders (cranio). This ERN mainly embraces a congenital population. The collaboration is a great example of how knowledge is shared, which hopefully results in better care and facilitates research.

Research may be facilitated by these networks. To draw widely applicable conclusions, standard outcome parameters are of utmost importance. Dr. Hadlock has published a detailed and thorough proposition [1]. She emphasizes that not only outcomes, but also the expected timeframe should be included when setting up the planning of outcome measurement. It should still be agreed on which objective measure are most precise and relevant. Computer-based analyses, such as the MATLAB-based image analysis software tool which is used in the Facial Assessment by Computer Evaluation (FACE) program, may contribute to objective outcome measurements [2]. Like for many diseases, facial palsy research should also include patient reported outcomes measures (PROMs). Although several questionnaires are available to analyze the face, there are little that focus on facial palsy in specific. Quality of life is often derived from general health related questionnaires such as PROMIS global health/physical and symptom-specific questions such as the FACE Q and FACE Q kids [3]. For pediatric facial palsy, the International Consortium for Health Outcomes Measurement (ICHOM) has developed a standard set of patient reported endpoints (Table 32.1) [4]. Also for adults, these items could be studied to get to an as complete as possible patients' judgment. It is difficult to get all healthcare providers on board so this will be an important challenge for the future.

Table 32.1 International Consortium for Health Outcomes Measurement (ICHOM) standard set of endpoints for pediatric facial palsy

		Evaluation
Burden of care to patients	Major complications from interventions	• Registration
Degree of health	Facial appearance and movement	• eFace • Face Q kids
	Oral continence	• Questions about eating and drinking
	Speech	• Speech questions
	Facial discomfort	• Visual Analogue Scale
	Vision and ocular symptoms	• Snellen chart and ocular symptoms questions
	Health related quality of life	• PROMIS paediatric global health
	Social health	• PROMIS peer relationship

32.1 Surgical Advances

32.1.1 Top-Down State of the Art

Using the top-down approach, the following advances are ongoing.

32.1.1.1 Reanimation of the Forehead

The forehead is often considered to be less relevant with regards to functional deficits and emotional expression. Although both the healthy and affected side may be treated in facial palsy, not so many enhancements have been made to the use of botox and suspension techniques respectively. The biggest improvement in the last period of time has been the introduction of endoscopic surgery which will be addressed later.

32.1.1.2 Reanimation of the Periocular Complex

Paralysis of the orbicularis oculi muscle results in decreased lacrimation, lagophthalmos and the inability to spontaneously blink. If left untreated they can compromise the cornea and vision. Also, a smile is incomplete without moving the eye. To compensate for these deficits, there is an ongoing search for solutions. Static procedures may protect the eye but only dynamic procedures can restore the pathway for blinking and voluntary or even spontaneous movements of the eye. Most advances are in the field of dynamic reconstructions.

Initially it should be decided if the orbicularis oculi muscle is still viable, for example in acute cases of facial palsy, or if another distant muscle transplantation or a static procedure is needed as a substitution. Reinnervation could be achieved by several ways as described by Terzis [5]. Sometimes one of these reinnervation methods is used as an adjunct to another. A cross-facial nerve graft may be used from the contralateral, unaffected side with direct micro-coaptations to eye sphincter branches. This procedure may be combined with a mini hypoglossus nerve transfer to a facial nerve branch may also be used. For each donor nerve, it may be considered to use direct nerve to muscle neurotization. In the latter, any interposition nerve graft is positioned directly in the muscle. The donor nerve is split in one end for the upper part of the orbicularis muscle and one end for the lower part of the orbicularis muscle. In each half, separate fascicles are dissected and divided.

One of the less commonly used, locally available donor nerves is the deep temporal nerve [6], which most often is a branch of the mandibular nerve. The deep temporal nerve further branches into an anterior, posterior and sometimes middle branch, of which the anterior branch is most suitable for transposition and direct neuronization of the orbicularis oculi muscle considering its diameter, size, and length.

If the paralysis has been present for longer over 2 years, or if for another reason it is expected that the native orbicularis muscle cannot be reinnervated anymore, it may be considered to transplant pieces of muscle to the eye. For replacing the orbicularis oculi, the frontal, occipital, platysma, gracilis, extensor digitorum brevis, and adductor longus have been described [5]. From an embryologic point of view, frontal muscle, occipital muscle and platysma muscle are all alike with orbicularis oculi muscle. If the muscle is kept as thin as orbicularis oculi muscle, it has been postulated that it could even take as an unvascularized graft without anastomosing the neurovascular bundle. This innovation was explored first by Thompson and Gustavson in the early 1970s who used the extensor brevis muscle as a free unvascularized graft for eye closure. In those days, the muscle was transplanted to the unaffected side to allow for direct neuronization, with the tendons attached to the affected side to allow for eye closure. In partial paralyses, the hypothesis was that the remaining facial nerve branches would innervate the newly placed muscle. Later, they explored the inclusion of the motor nerve and anastomosing it to nerve branches at the contralateral side. These concepts are currently reused.

Unvascularized platysma transplants in combination with a cross-facial nerve graft have been described by Biglioli [7]. He uses a cross-facial nerve graft from the unaffected facial nerve branches to the orbicularis oculi muscle. These are used to innervate a non-vascularized platysma graft. Simultaneously, he performs a fascia lata string suspension of the lower lid. This combined approach results in 37% decrease in opening of the lids when the eyes are closed. Of course, it is unsure which part of the procedure has the biggest effect on the eye opening.

Vascularized platysma transplants were published first by Terzis, and recently by Guelinckx [8]. The latter did a two-step approach with first a cross-facial nerve graft and nine months later a transfer of a piece of platysma on its neurovascular pedicle (Fig. 32.1). The anastomosis was to the cross-facial nerve graft and the temporal vessels. His reported that his results are very worthy with 88% of good to excellent function. The mean age of his population was 30 years old and he believes that best results may be achieved in patients younger than 40. He believes that trans-

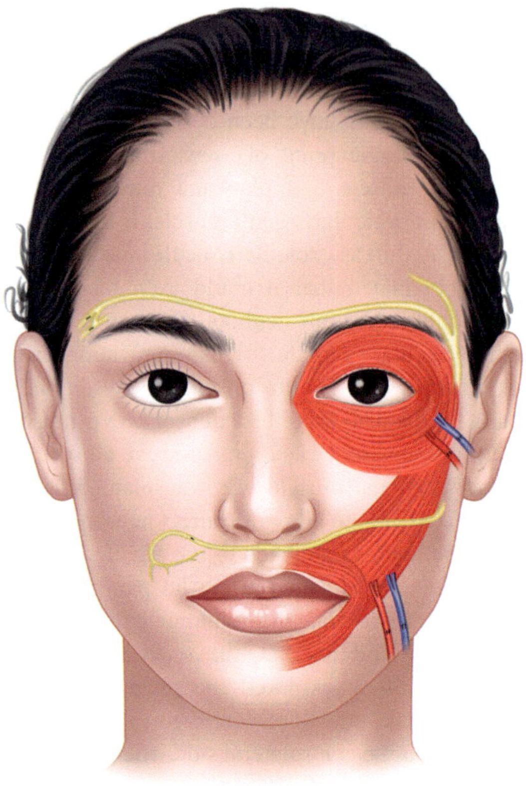

Fig. 32.1 Neurovascular platysma muscle transplant to cross-facial nerve graft based on the work of Guelinckx [8]

plants >1 g need micro-neurovascular repair. In three failed cases (13%), the problem was found to be a lack of reinnervation and not a lack of revascularization.

The future may bring the clinical application of different stimuli to activate the eye, including a mechanical cornea reflex (trigeminus nerve), an electrical supra-orbital sensory nerve reflex and also acoustic or visual stimuli.

32.1.1.3 Reanimation of the Nose

Deviation of the nose with esthetic and functional symptoms is probably the most neglected area in the field facial palsy. Although nasal obstruction due to facial palsy was already reported in the seventies, not much innovation has been going on in addition to the static suspension procedures. As addressed in Chap. 5.1, improvement of the external valve patency results in a significantly better disease-specific quality of life. Nasal signs should be looked for, surgical treatment should be considered and future studies should be done to further optimize results. We suggest, when performing nerve transfers for smile reanimation, to carefully select the facial nerve branches that also innervate the nose.

32.1.1.4 Reanimation of the Lower Lip

Most reconstructions for lower lip palsy focus on paralyzing the contralateral normal lip or providing static support on the affected side. The depressors however are important for all perioral expressions including speech, oral competence and smiling, especially for people with a so called 'full denture smile'. Also, weakening the unaffected side may cause further deprivation of the function of the lower lip. It would therefore be of great benefit if the function of the affected lower lip could be dynamically restored, including depression and eversion. Several techniques have been reported varying from anterior digastric and platysma muscle transfers in addition to direct muscle neurotization and cross-facial nerve grafts [9]. There should be a distinction between patients with short-standing paralysis (up to 6 months) in whom there is muscle viability on EMG, intermediate paralysis (6–24 months) with viable depressor muscles on EMG or long-standing paralysis [9]. Innovation in the short-standing paralysis group includes novel use of donor nerves, including the platysma motor nerve transfer [10] (Fig. 32.2). This nerve is only available in selected cases but should be considered whenever the marginal mandibular brand is specifically injured. In the intermediate paralyses group, a babysitter mini hypoglossus nerve transfer can be used together with a cross-facial nerve graft, in which 40% of the very potent ipsilateral hypoglossus is used to quickly reinnervate the depressor, while waiting for the cross-facial nerve graft to regenerate. An alternative to the hypoglossus nerve is the masseter nerve, accessory nerve or the anterior division of the C7 root. For long-standing paralyses, a functional muscle is required. The platysma muscle can be transposed as a one-stage operation if the vascularization by the submental artery and the innervation

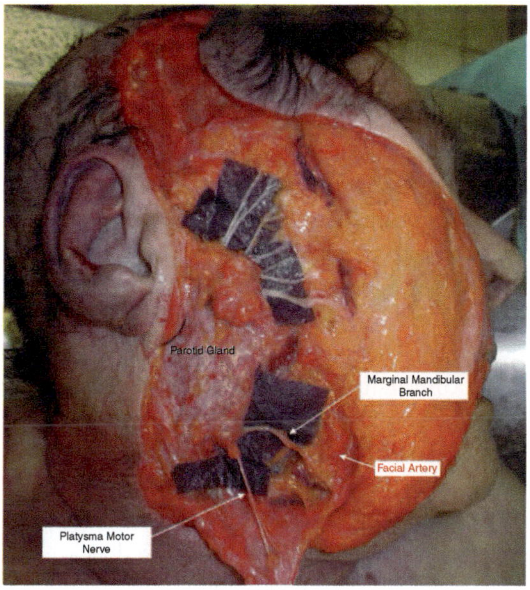

Fig. 32.2 Platysma motor nerve transposition to reinforce the lower lip depressors [10]

by the cervical branch of the facial nerve are preserved. Alternatively, the anterior belly of the digastric muscle has been described. In conclusion, reanimation of the paralyzed face is incomplete without restoration of the lower lip depressors. Dynamic improvements should be enhanced top optimize speech, oral competence, and smiling.

32.2 Surgery for Synkinesis

Although there is no consensus about the best therapy for synkinesis, many patients are currently treated by denervation with botulinum toxin injections or biofeedback training. Surgery may be very useful as an alternative or an adjunct, since persistent or returning synkinesis have a major negative impact on facial asymmetry and resultant quality of life. Surgical results are more stable, but tend to be underutilized which may be explained by a lack of surgical experience with regards to the microsurgery of the smallest facial nerve branches. Moreover, it is difficult to predict the consistency of the results since there are many anastomoses between several facial nerve branches. Several surgical applications are listed and vary from myectomy to neurectomy to nerve transfers and combinations. Probably, the best treatment is a balance of restoring the coordinated movement and decreasing the undesired synkinesis movements. The downside is that paralyzing the muscle will not only decrease the synkinesis, but also weaken its function. To avoid this, many surgeons are less aggressive when operating but therefore also achieve a less satisfying result. The challenge is to remain sufficient motor activity and the side-effect of selective neurectomy is that total paralyses of the target muscle may occur. The choice of which treatment is best, depends on the severity of symptoms and surgeon's and patients' preference.

Generally speaking, the more severe the more severe the synkinesis, the more aggressive the treatment. Terzis et al. distinguish three different steps in the surgical treatment of synkinesis: (1) Cross-facial nerve graft with secondary microcoaptations to break the circle of synkinesis by adding an additional strong stimulus from the contralateral side; (2) Direct cross-facial nerve neuronization; (3) Botulinum toxin injection [11]. Other surgical treatments include myectomy of the affected muscles of which the orbicularis oculi muscle (superior and inferior), corrugator muscle, depressors of the lip and platysma muscle are well known [12]. For the synkinesis of eyelid closure with smiling or vice versa, a neuromyectomy of an inferior, lateral strip of the orbicularis oculi muscle with its nerve could be a solution. It has been reported to be effective in all 11 patients with one case of ectropion [13]. Last but not least, also the free gracilis muscle transplant has been described for the surgical treatment of synkinesis. It could be used as a one-stage procedure to the masseter nerve or accessory nerve or as a two-stage procedure with a cross-facial nerve graft. The free muscle transplant will supply the motor that is needed. This may be preceded by a thorough myectomy on the affected side. Chuang et al. explain their approach as treating a scar for which sometimes a radical excision and resurfacing is required. It is then necessary to remove both the trigger (neurectomy) and synkinetic muscles (myectomy) and supply a new and healthy innervated muscle. All patients with moderate to severe synkinesis ((17 + 34) 51) improved after one or two-stage surgery [12]. No additional botulinum toxin injections were needed.

In case of incomplete facial palsy, a less radical approach by only adapting the innervation may be sufficient. Selective neurectomy of a tiny facial nerve branch to the orbicularis oculi muscle may be considered if eyelid spasm is present. A highly selective neurectomy was performed by Hadlock et al. [14]. The team found a significant change in the palpebral fissure width while smiling, but the results were not sustainable and most needed Botulinum toxin injections after a symptom-free interval. Simultaneous with neurectomy, a cross-facial nerve graft may be performed as well as a masseter nerve to zygomatic facial nerve branch neurorraphy. The authors explain their results by a separation of the neural stimulus of the orbicularis oculi (residual facial nerve function) from that of the zygomatic muscular complex (dual innervation by the masseter nerve and cross-facial nerve graft) [15]. This work is the continuation of the previous thoughts by Terzis and Karypidis, who use secondary micro-coaptations along with botulinum toxin injections and biofeedback to treat synkinesis [11].

32.3 Technical Advances

With the increasing use of multimedia, it is expected that computer-based analyses of surgical results and also training will be more and more available. Nowadays, you can already find mobile phone applications with physiotherapy for facial rehabilitation. These applications could be expanded to personal log books to grade effects after botox injections or holding track of a patient's progress in utilizing a dynamic reconstruction.

Other technical advances include:

32.3.1 Multidimensional Training Models

Two- and three-dimensional models have an important role in the rehabilitation, and the outcome of facial palsy treatment is directly linked to the rehabilitation path. A two-dimensional photo with many landmarks is processed into a three-dimensional image and an extra dimension may provide extra accuracy [16]. Of course, there is a sample error which may affect the procession but it's a promising adjunct to the current rehabilitation programs.

The superlative of these static three-dimensional images is a fourth dimension, being dynamics. The Visual Computing Group (VCG) at the University of Portsmouth is working on the development of refined four-dimensional geometric models may be used to further improve facial palsy treatment. It is claimed that it combines mirror therapy with a facial sensing technology, resulting in a real-time feedback. This may improve the rehabilitation, but also creates an important database of values which can be used for outcome assessments.

32.3.1.1 Endoscopic Surgery

Endoscopic approaches have dramatically increased among different surgical fields with the benefit of less skin and soft tissue injury, better aesthetic result and even preserved nerve integrity due to a smaller wound. Also, for facial palsy there are several applications of endoscopic surgery.

First of all, it is feasible to endoscopically harvest the sural nerve in both the pediatric and adult patient population. The nerve can be harvested through a single incision as small as 12 mm and nerve dissection is performed from proximal to distal to minimize damage to the nerve when side branches are encountered. A nerve stripper is used, which contains a small notch through which the nerve is dissected. An air-inflated balloon may be used to enlarge the endoscopic cavity. Endoscopic harvest greatly reduces the scars on the lower extremity which are quite visible and stigmatizing.

Secondly, endoscopy has been used for several applications in the face. Minimally invasive inset of the gracilis muscle has been reported by Klebuc [17], with a small incision anterior to the ear and endoscopic dissection of the subcutaneously plane to inset the muscle.

Thirdly, ancillary procedures such as brow or forehead lifts are performed endoscopically. There are several techniques with bone anchors and periosteal sutures of which the biodegradable Endotine® has been previously mentioned. It may be introduced by small incisions in the hair-bearing scalp for forehead lifting, or through a trans-blepharic approach for brow lifting. It may be visible and palpable at first, but the device resorbs within a year. There is increasing evidence in a general population for its use in general, with a patient satisfaction as great as 95.3% and the pleased by the lift achieved and felt the device was easy to use [18]. There is only one German case series with nine facial palsy patients [19]. They found it to be a successful tool and reported relapse in one case.

32.3.1.2 Bionic Reanimation

The applications of medical technology expand quickly. Since the vast majority of facial palsy is unilateral, electrical stimulation by the non-affected side may be considered as a reconstructive option. Bionic reanimation includes the design of a device to detect movements on a non-affected side, and activate paralyzed muscles of an affected side. It was previously used to restore the function in upper and lower limbs, bladder, bowel and respiratory function after spinal cord or brain injury. The principles have been established in these patient populations to achieve a safe and reliable activation. Ideally, it creates spontaneity, it makes surgery and the use of a cross-facial nerve graft unnecessary and it may be used for areas of the face wherefore a nerve graft is sometimes not considered such as the eye or forehead [20]. Electrodes can be placed there where it stimulates the underlying muscle on its best [21]. This location should be tested separately. Ultimately, these are placed intramuscular or integrated in electroactive polymer artificial muscle and connected to the healthy nerve at the contralateral side which supplies the impulse whenever a patient spontaneously smiles or blinks. Alternatively, the stimulants can come separately from an external source in case it is expected that there will be a functional recovery of the affected nerve within a few months, for example to treat lagophthalmos in case of Bell's palsy or Lyme's disease. The devices may be able to record and process the signals needed for a certain movement, so that this train of signals is given off whenever a certain motion is needed. It has been studied for stimulating the frontal muscle, blink of the eye and smile, but there are several problems to overcome before a clinical application is successful. The signal shouldn't be too strong to avoid pain [21]. In addition to tolerability, it's not yet feasible to apply all these technical steps in a clinical situation. For the best result, there shouldn't be any delay from the initiating signal to the process to the motion and this is difficult. Once it is successfully implicated, it may need to be adjusted over time to account for small changes that people go through when getting older or when a certain degree of recovery is achieved. It's an exciting and promising technique to closely follow up on in the future.

References

1. Hadlock T. Standard outcome measures in facial paralysis: getting on the same page. JAMA Facial Plast Surg. 2016;18(2):85–6.
2. Hadlock TA, Urban LS. Toward a universal, automated facial measurement tool in facial reanimation. Arch Facial Plast Surg. 2012;14(4):277–82.
3. Klassen AF, Cano SJ, Scott A, Snell L, Pusic AL. Measuring patient-reported outcomes in facial aesthetic patients: development of the FACE-Q. Facial Plast Surg. 2010;26(4):303–9.
4. Butler DP, De la Torre A, Borschel GH, Hadlock TA, Beurskens C, Bogart K, Cárdenas Mejía A, Coombs C, Copeland J, Diels J, González-Otero T, Graham L, Ishii L, Malhotra R, Martinez A, McKinley L, Robinson MW, Suominen S, Takushima A, Vazquez Curiel E, Wachs FL, Grobbelaar AO. An international collaborative standardizing patient-centered outcome measures in pediatric facial palsy. JAMA Facial Plast Surg. 2019;21(5):351–58. https://doi.org/10.1001/jamafacial.2019.0224. PMID: 31070677; PMCID: PMC6512270.
5. Terzis JK, Karypidis D. Blink restoration in adult facial paralysis. Plast Reconstr Surg. 2010;126(1):126–39.
6. Karagoz H, Ozturk S, Malkoc I, Diyarbakir S, Demirkan F. Anatomy of the anterior deep temporal nerve: implications for neurotization in blinking restoration in facial paralysis. Ann Plast Surg. 2015;75(3):316–8.

7. Biglioli F, Zago M, Allevi F, Ciprandi D, Dell'Aversana Orabona G, Pucciarelli V, et al. Reanimation of the paralyzed lids by cross-face nerve graft and platysma transfer. J Craniomaxillofac Surg. 2018;46(3):521–6.
8. P.J. G. Blink restoration in long-standing facial paralysis: use of free neurovascular platysma transfer. Plast Reconstr Surg Glob Open. 2018;6(10).
9. Bassilios Habre S, Googe BJ, Depew JB, Wallace RD, Konofaos P. Depressor reanimation after facial nerve paralysis. Ann Plast Surg. 2019;82(5):582–90.
10. Rodriguez-Lorenzo A, Jensson D, Weninger WJ, Schmid M, Meng S, Tzou CH. Platysma motor nerve transfer for restoring marginal mandibular nerve function. Plast Reconstr Surg Glob Open. 2016;4(12):e1164.
11. Terzis JK, Karypidis D. Therapeutic strategies in post-facial paralysis synkinesis in adult patients. Plast Reconstr Surg. 2012;129(6):925e–39e.
12. Chuang DC, Chang TN, Lu JC. Postparalysis facial synkinesis: clinical classification and surgical strategies. Plast Reconstr Surg Glob Open. 2015;3(3):e320.
13. Yoshioka N. Selective orbicularis neuromyectomy for postparetic periocular synkinesis. J Plast Reconstr Aesthet Surg. 2015;68(11):1510–5.
14. van Veen MM, Dusseldorp JR, Hadlock TA. Long-term outcome of selective neurectomy for refractory periocular synkinesis. Laryngoscope. 2018;128(10):2291–5.
15. Biglioli F, Kutanovaite O, Rabbiosi D, Colletti G, Mohammed MAS, Saibene AM, et al. Surgical treatment of synkinesis between smiling and eyelid closure. J Craniomaxillofac Surg. 2017;45(12):1996–2001.
16. Storey G, Jiang R, Bouridane A. Role for 2D image generated 3D face models in the rehabilitation of facial palsy. Healthc Technol Lett. 2017;4(4):145–8.
17. Facial nerve reconstruction—expert commentary; editor: Hanasono R, Skoracki and Yu Eds, Thieme, page 163–67.
18. Chowdhury S, Malhotra R, Smith R, Arnstein P. Patient and surgeon experience with the endotine forehead device for brow and forehead lift. Ophthalmic Plast Reconstr Surg. 2007;23(5):358–62.
19. Holtmann L, Buchsenschutz K, Eckstein A, Schluter A, Lang S, Mattheis S. Endoscopic browlift via endotine forehead device in patients with facial palsy. Laryngorhinootologie. 2017;96(10):691–7.
20. Kurita M, Takushima A, Muraoka Y, Shiraishi T, Harii K. Feasibility of bionic reanimation of a paralyzed face: a preliminary study of functional electrical stimulation of a paralyzed facial muscle controlled with the electromyography of the contralateral healthy hemiface. Plast Reconstr Surg. 2010;126(2):81e–3e.
21. Frigerio A, Heaton JT, Cavallari P, Knox C, Hohman MH, Hadlock TA. Electrical stimulation of eye blink in individuals with acute facial palsy: progress toward a bionic blink. Plast Reconstr Surg. 2015;136(4):515e–23e.

33 Endoscopic-Assisted Free Muscle Flaps for Facial Reanimation

Michael J. Klebuc and Andres F. Doval

Key Points

- Endoscopic assistance can enhance cosmesis in free muscle flap facial reanimation. The procedure is performed via a limited preauricular incision, avoiding a submandibular scar.
- Endoscopic visualization can be utilized to verify proper suture anchoring in the perioral region, avoiding lateral muscle displacement.
- The superficial temporal artery and vein are the preferred recipient vessels.
- The microsurgical nerve repair is performed prior to the vascular anastomosis to accommodate for the reduced exposure.
- Fascial extensions of the free muscle flap can be delivered into the upper and lower lips to enhance lip symmetry and upper dental show.

The introduction of endoscopic technique has produced a paradigm shift in intercavitary surgery yielding a series of benefits including, decreased postoperative pain, reduced wound infection rates, shorter hospitalizations, and more a rapid return to work [1]. Endoscopic and robotic surgical techniques are also making significant inroads in the field of plastic and reconstructive surgery. They have been successfully utilized to perform both cosmetic and reconstructive procedures including, brow lifts, rhytidectomies, craniosynostosis management, nerve decompression and flap harvest via limited access incisions [2–8]. Endoscopic surgical techniques can also be utilized in an effort to enhance the cosmetic results in facial reanimation surgery. With the aid of endoscopic assistance, free neurovascular muscle flap smile restoration can be successfully performed via a limited preauricular incision, avoiding the traditional, submandibular extension.

M. J. Klebuc (✉)
Director of the Center for Facial Paralysis Surgery and Functional Restoration, Houston Methodist Hospital, Houston, TX, USA

Associate Professor of Clinical Plastic and Reconstructive Surgery, Weill Cornell Medical College, New York, NY, USA

Associate Clinical Professor of Neurosurgery, Houston Methodist Hospital, Houston, TX, USA

A. F. Doval
Research Fellow Institute for Reconstructive Surgery, Houston Methodist Hospital, Houston, TX, USA

© Springer Nature Switzerland AG 2021
C.-H. J. Tzou, A. Rodríguez-Lorenzo (eds.), *Facial Palsy*,
https://doi.org/10.1007/978-3-030-50784-8_33

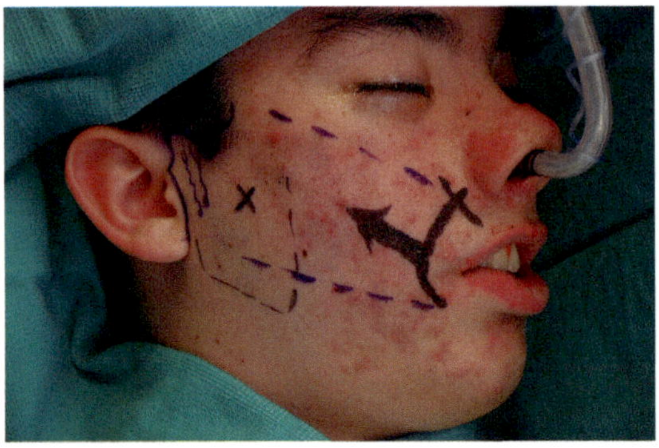

Fig. 33.1 Smile vector, preauricular incision and topographic location of the masseter nerve marked (X)

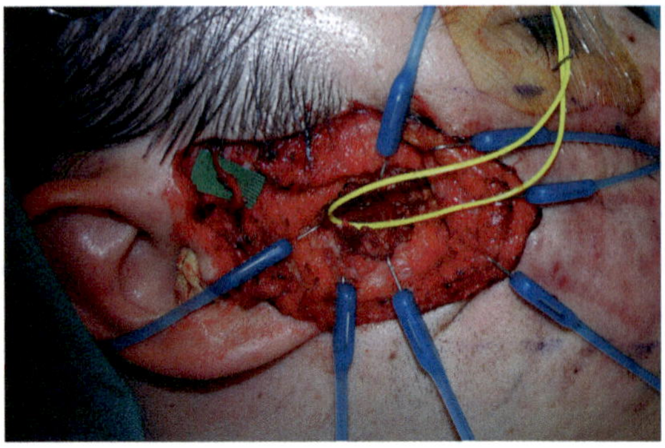

Fig. 33.2 Isolated superficial temporal vessels and descending branch of masseter nerve

33.1 Surgical Technique

Preoperatively the smile vectors and nasolabial folds are marked in the upright, sitting position. If a cross face nerve graft has been previously placed then the site of the Tinel's sign is also marked. The patient is then placed supine on the operating table and sequential compression devices are applied to the lower extremities. General naso-tracheal anesthesia is induced and the nasal RAE tube is sutured to the nasal columella and further secured to the hair-bearing scalp with foam, silk tape and staples to prevent pressure on the nasal alae. A preauricular incision extending into the sideburn is marked as are the borders of the planned cheek flap and the location of the selected motor nerve. If the motor nerve to masseter will be utilized a point 3 cm in front of the tragus and 1 cm below the zygomatic arch is marked to denote its position (Fig. 33.1) [9]. If the ipsilateral facial nerve will be utilized then the general location of the facial nerve branch to the zygomaticus major (Zuker's point) is marked at the midway point on a line drawn from the root of the helix to the lateral commissure [10, 11]. The location of the cross face nerve graft is best identified preoperatively utilizing the Tinel's sign. Sutures (5–0 Proline) are placed to reinforce the nasolabial fold markings and the buccal and perioral region are infiltrated with a solution containing 1:100,000 epinephrine. Injection of the vasoconstrictive solution is avoided in the preauricular region to prevent spasm of the superficial temporal artery and vein. The preauricular incision is created and a thick, skin, and subcutaneous flap is elevated directly above the SMAS with the aid of bipolar cautery. If a cross face nerve graft has been previously placed then it is identified and its course is carefully dissected. After elevating the skin flap in the parotid region the SMAS is incised and the superficial temporal artery and vein are identified to verify their presence and adequacy for microvascular anastomosis. The vessels are then left undissected at this juncture to prevent inadvertent injury. Scissor dissection is now employed in the buccal and perioral regions to elevate a generous skin flap taking care to avoid dermal exposure that could produce adhesions between the free muscle flap and overlying skin. The operating microscope along with electrical stimulation is now utilized to identify the motor nerve of choice (masseter, facial nerve, CFNG). The nerves are selectively transected and marked with a suture to facilitate later identification and the superficial temporal artery and vein are skeletonized (Fig. 33.2). If these vessels are not available then a limited submandibular incision can be created to access the facial vessels reducing the cosmetic advantage of the approach. A 30° browlift endoscope (4 mm diameter, 18 cm length) with an attached optical retractor (Karl Storz SE & Co., Dr.-Karl-Storz-StraBe34, Tuttlingen, Germany) are now utilized to visualize the lateral border of the orbicularis oris (Fig. 33.3). Once the optical window is established, graspers are utilized to secure a series of 2-0 polydioxanone sutures (Figs. 33.4 and 33.5). The sutures are adjusted until gentle traction produces a pleasing facsimile of a smile. Vertical incisions can now be created in the vermilion of the upper and lower lips to facilitate

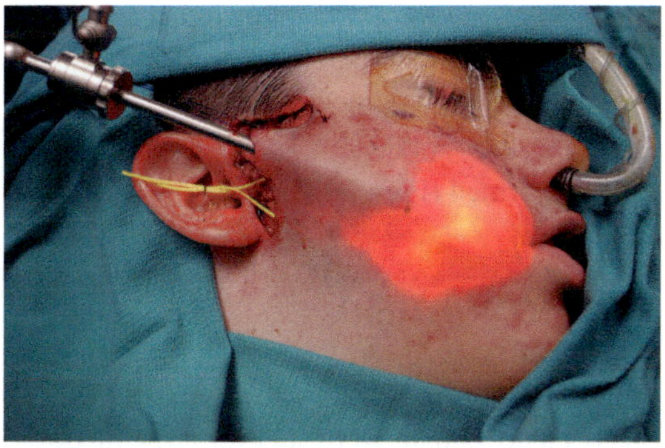

Fig. 33.3 Optical window created with 30° browlift endoscope with attached optical retractor (Karl Storz SE & Co.)

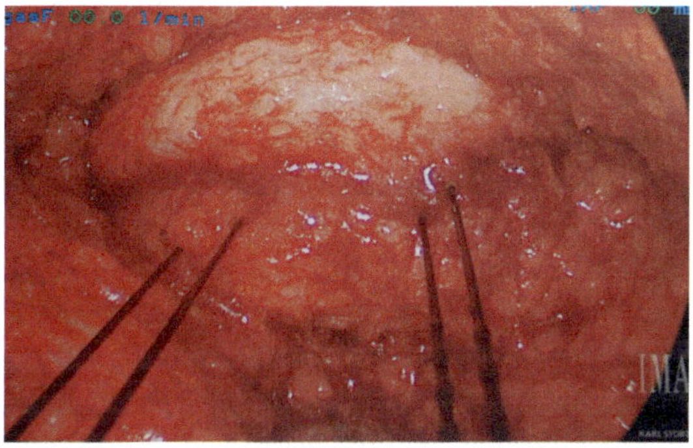

Fig. 33.4 2-0 polydioxanone anchoring sutures secured to the orbicularis oris with endoscopic assistance

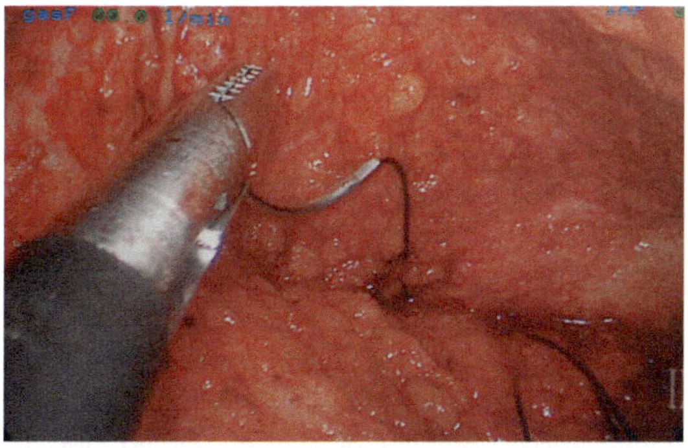

Fig. 33.5 Traction placed on anchoring sutures to simulate a smile

delivery of the free muscle flap's fascial extensions if desired. Fascial extensions are frequently employed as they facilitate the creation of upper dental show and resist lateral displacement of the muscle flap into the check (lateral drift deformity). A new set of instruments are then utilized

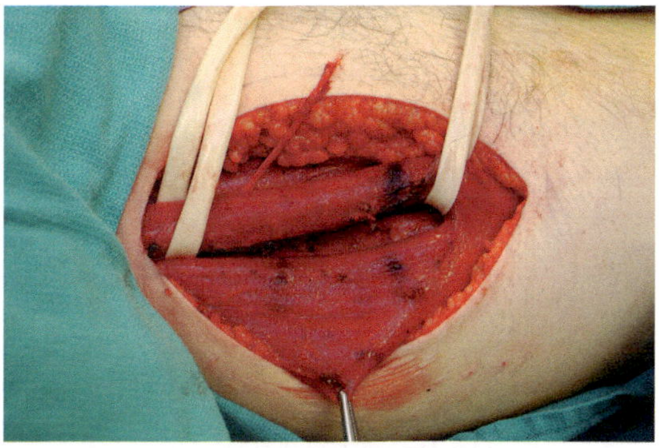

Fig. 33.6 Anterior third of the gracilis muscle incorporated into the flap design

to harvest a contralateral free gracilis muscle flap via a limited incision in the upper, inner, thigh. The anterior third of the muscle is typically incorporated into the flap design, however, the neurovascular hilum is visualized prior to tailoring to rule out a central variant (Fig. 33.6). If the neurovascular pedicle enters the muscle in a central location then the flap design is shifted and fashioned around the posterior segment of the gracilis muscle. The entire length of the obturator nerve and vascular pedicle are harvested to enhance flexibility at the time of muscle inset. Electrical stimulation is frequently utilized during the flap harvest to verify the presence of active contraction. The flap length is determined by measuring the distance from the commissure to the temporal region and adding an additional centimeter to accommodate for anchoring sutures. Proximal fascial extensions can be included in the flap design if desired. Heavy, braided polyglactin sutures are placed in a horizontal mattress fashion at the cut ends of the muscle to prevent later dislodgment of the anchoring sutures. The flap is now delivered to the head and neck region and anchored to the lateral orbicularis oris utilizing the previously placed sutures (Fig. 33.7). Gracilis tendon or fascia lata can be incorporated deep to the flap for additional static support if required. The inset is performed via the limited preauricular incision and is greatly facilitated by utilizing the endoscope in conjunction with an endoscopic knot pusher. After securing the flap in the perioral region the endoscope is again utilized to verify

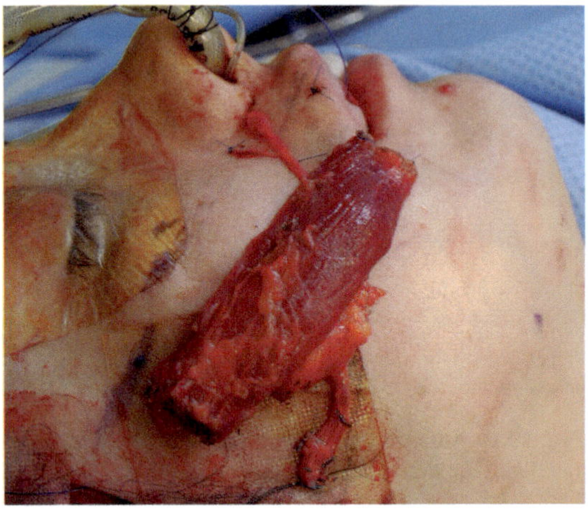

Fig. 33.7 Heavily tailored free gracilis muscle flap prior to inset

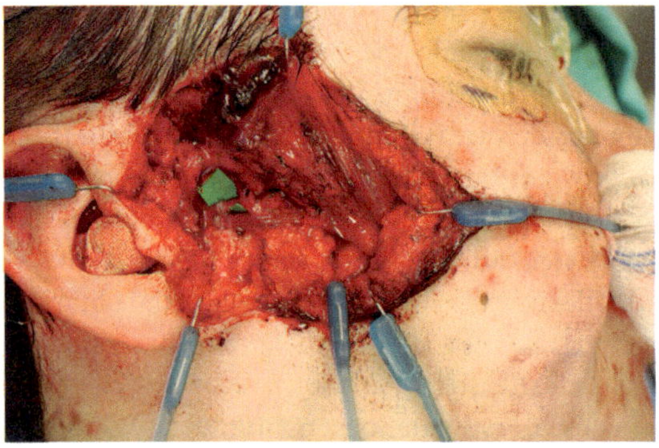

Fig. 33.8 Microsurgical never repair (masseter-obturator) performed prior to vascular anastomosis to compensate for reduced exposure

that the anchoring sutures have only captured the desired distal end of the muscle flap and have not inadvertently incorporated more proximal segments of muscle. The lateral muscle flap border is now temporarily anchored to the temporal fascia and the obturator nerve is stimulated verifying the proper muscle tension and vector have been obtained. The temporal anchoring sutures are now released and the muscle is reflected medially. The microsurgical nerve repair is now performed to accommodate for the limited exposure. Once the nerve repair is completed the muscle is re-anchored to the temporal fascia with 2-0 polydioxanone suture and the microvascular anastomosis is performed (Fig. 33.8). The incision is then repaired over a 10-F closed suction drain placed along the inferior border of the cheek dissection and the cutaneous Doppler signal is marked. A deep, atraumatic, extubation is then performed (Figs. 33.9a–f and 33.10a–h).

33.2 Discussion

Advanced proficiency in reconstructive surgery has been accompanied by an ever growing desire for improved cosmesis as surgeons strive to restore both function and form. To that end, endoscopic assistance has facilitated the performance of numerous reconstructive surgical procedures via limited access incisions. Minimally invasive surgical techniques have been employed in the treatment of the paralyzed face in an effort to improve both donor site and facial aesthetics. Contreras-Garcia and associates have described performing lengthening temporalis myoplasties with endoscopic assistance via limited temporal and intraoral access incisions [12]. Endoscopic techniques have also been utilized in the performance of static procedures including minimally invasive fascia lata graft harvest and insertion for midfacial suspension [6, 12]. Additionally, numerous endoscopic assisted midface lift and brow lift procedures have been described for both cosmetic and reconstructive purposes [7, 13]. Endoscopic vein harvesting equipment has been successfully utilized to procure long segments of sural nerve via a single limited access incision significantly improving the aesthetics of the nerve graft donor site [14]. Endoscopic assistance has also been employed with free muscle flap facial reanimation. Takushima and associates describe a single stage facial reanimation utilizing a free latissimus dorsi muscle flap. The donor facial nerve branches on the unaffected side are explored via two limited access incisions in the preauricular region. The nerve repair between the thoracodorsal and fascia nerve is performed utilizing a single stab incision in the buccal region. Efforts have also been made to harvest free muscle flaps endoscopically. Lin and Wei describe their experience with endoscopic assisted harvesting of 16 free gracilis muscle flaps. Utilizingw

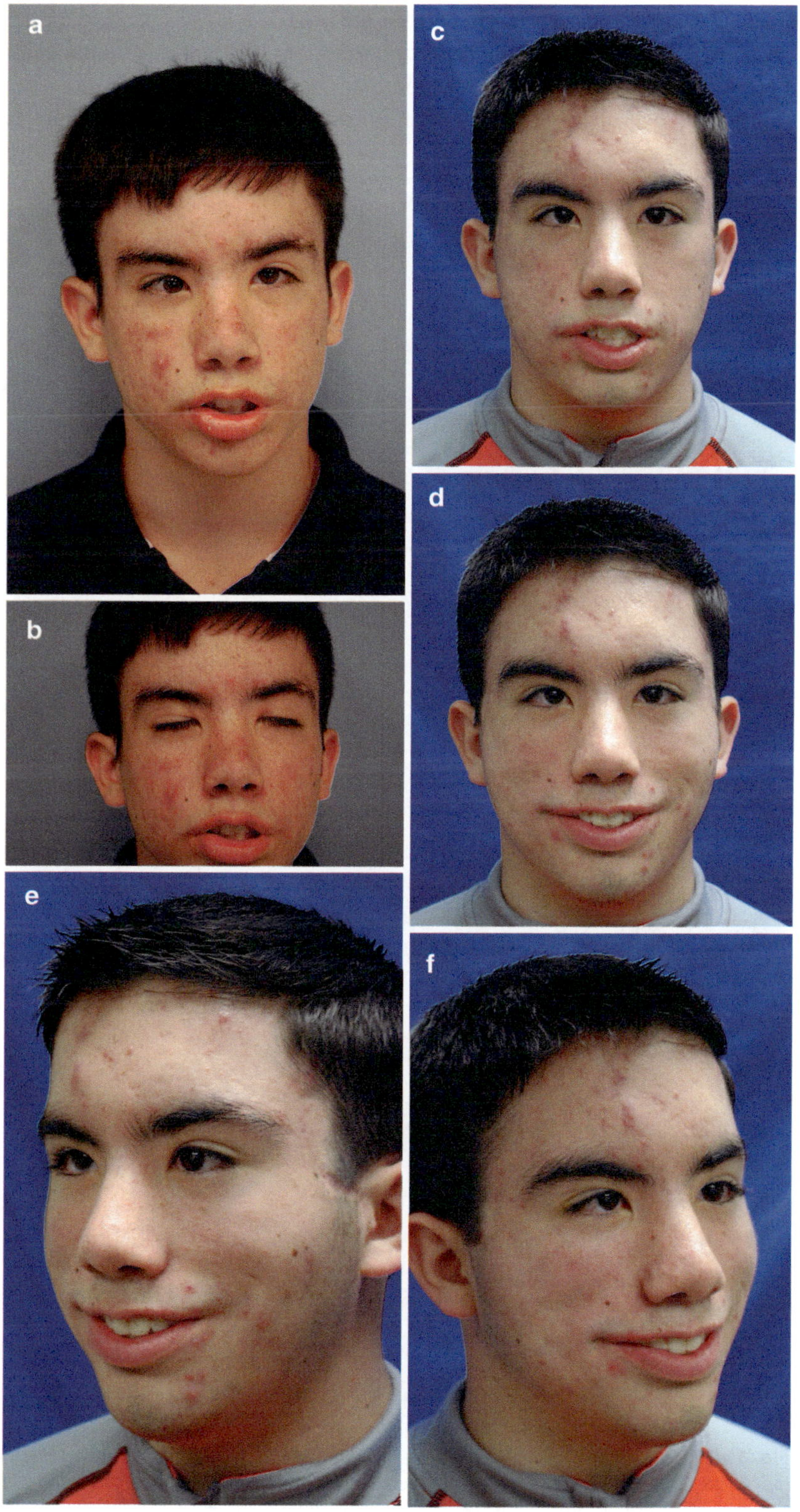

Fig. 33.9 (**a**) A 14-year-old male with bilateral Moebius Syndrome, preoperative at rest. (**b**) Preoperative with maximal smile effort and retained eye closure. (**c**) Postoperative in repose. (**d**) Postoperative smiling. (**e**) Postoperative right lateral smiling. (**f**) Postoperative left lateral smiling

this approach they were able to decrease the average length of the medial thigh incision to 6.5 cm as compared to 15.5 cm in the conventional harvest group. Over the past decade, there has been a steady push to enhance the facial aesthetics of free muscle flap facial reanimation [15].

Extensive tailoring of free gracilis muscle flaps has also been employed for reduction of midface

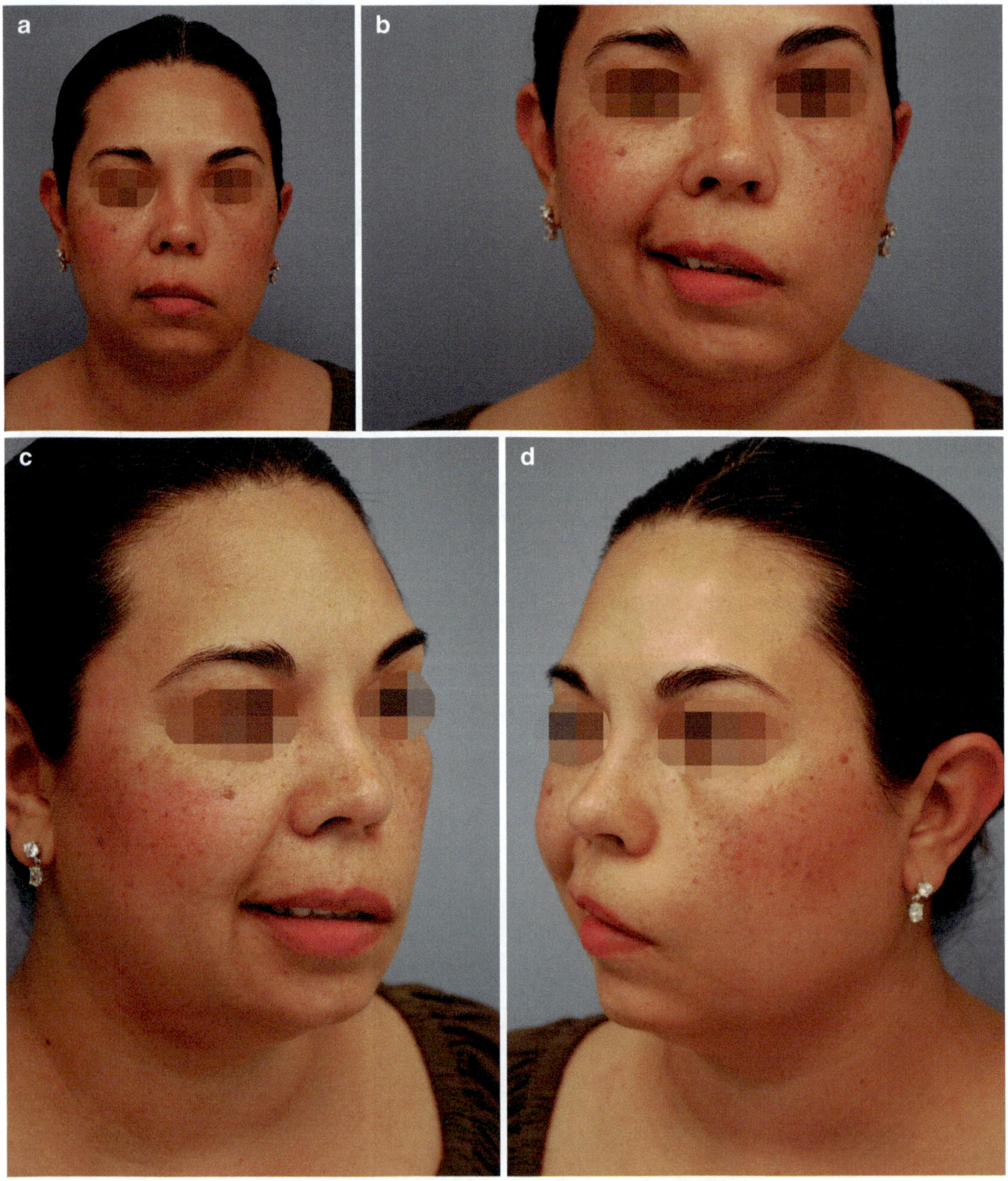

Fig. 33.10 (**a**) A 42-year-old female with 26 months of facial paresis as a result of pseudotumor cerebri, preoperative at rest. (**b**) Preoperative smile. (**c**) Preoperative smile, right lateral. (**d**) Preoperative smile, left lateral. (**e**) 8 months postoperative after free gracilis muscle flap innervated by the masseter nerve in conjunction with a V–VII nerve transfer in repose. (**f**) Postoperative smile, anterior. (**g**) Postoperative smile, right lateral. (**h**) Postoperative smile, left lateral

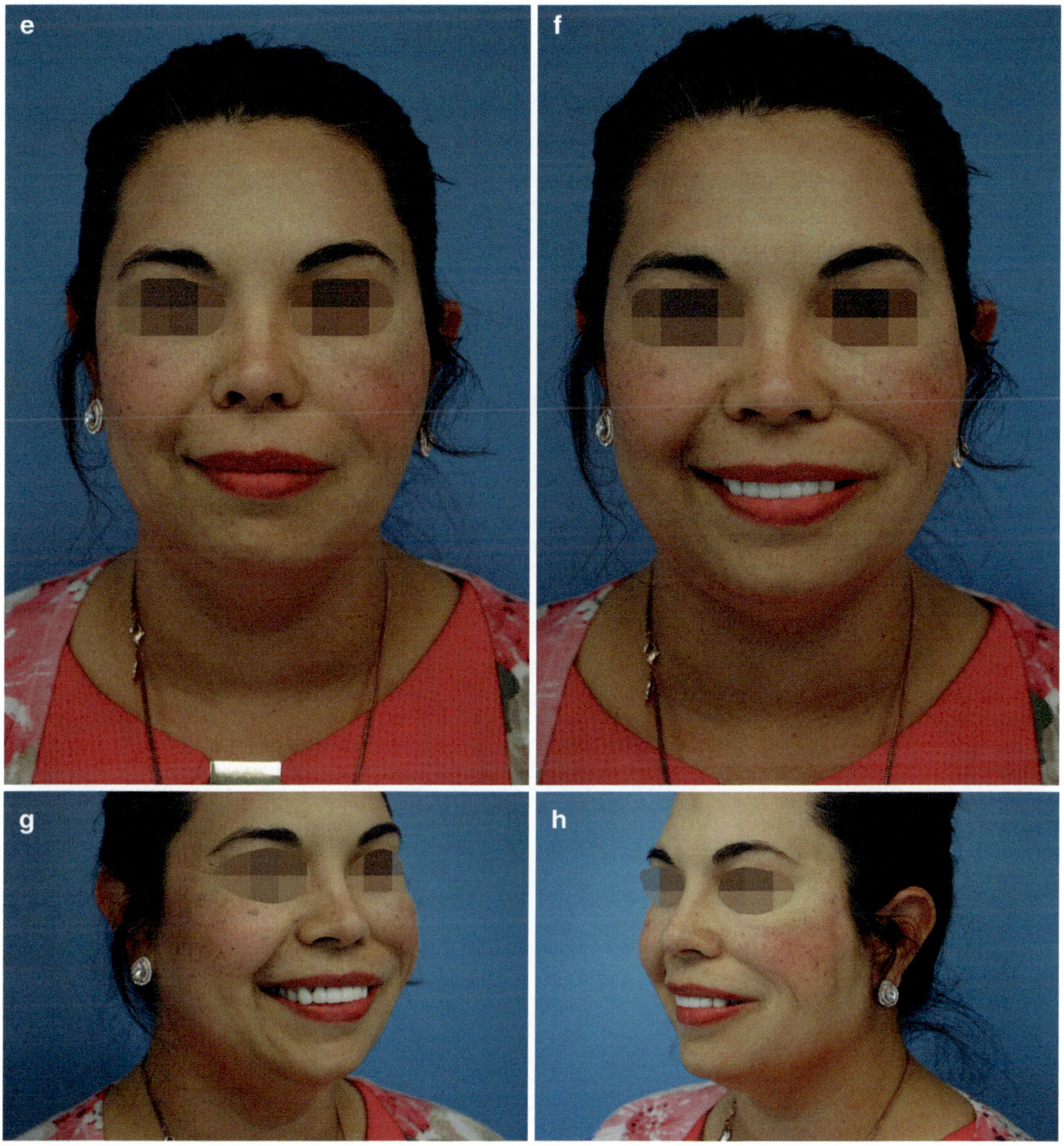

Fig. 33.10 (continued)

bulk with many surgeons incorporating only one quarter to one-third of muscle's diameter in the flap design. Partial excision of the buccal fat pad has also been employed to reduce midfacial fullness. The use of endoscopic assisted free muscle flap inset in facial reanimation surgery is another step in the effort to enhance the aesthetics of a procedure that is both functional and cosmetic in nature. Endoscopic assistance allows the surgery to be performed through a preauricular incision with a concealed sideburn extension. This limited exposure avoids a potentially unsightly elongation of the incision into the neck and reduces the potential for hypertrophic scar formation in this cosmetically sensitive region. The ability to visualize proper perioral suture fixation and avoid lateral muscle displacement is another significant benefit of the endoscopic assisted technique.

33.3 Conclusion

Endoscopic assistance can be utilized to improve the cosmetic results of free muscle flap, smile restoration surgery. The technique allows the surgery to be performed via a limited preauricular approach avoiding the traditional submandibular-cervical incision. Enhanced visualization also facilitates proper suture anchoring of the muscle flap to the orbicularis oris, avoiding unwanted lateral displacement and a malpositioned nasolabial fold. The superficial temporal artery and vein are the preferred recipient vessels. The microsurgical nerve repair is frequently performed before the microvascular anastomosis to accommodate for the reduced exposure.

References

1. Tanigawa N. Advantages and problems with endoscopic surgery. JMAJ. 2009;52(5):330–4.
2. Jimenez DF, McGinity MJ, Barone CM. Endoscopy-assisted early correction of single-suture metopic craniosynostosis: a 19 year experience. J Neurosurg Pediatr. 2018;1:1–14.
3. Seify H, Jones G, Bostwick J, et al. Endoscopic-assisted face lift: review of 200 cases. Ann Plast Surg. 2004;52(3):234–9.
4. Takushima A, Harii K, Asato H. Endoscopic dissection of recipient facial nerve for vascularized muscle transfer in the treatment of facial paralysis. Br J Plast Surg. 2003;56:110–3.
5. Hallock GG. Minimally invasive harvest of the gracilis muscle. Plast Reconstr Surg. 1999;104(3):801–5.
6. Wong GB, Stokes RB, Stevenson TR, et al. Endoscopically assisted facial suspension for treatment of facial palsy. Plast Reconstr Surg. 1999;103(3):970–1.
7. Burnett CD, Rabinowitz S, Rauscher GE. Endoscopic-assisted midface lift utilizing retrograde dissection. Ann Plast Surg. 1996;36(5):449–52.
8. Marchioni D, Soloperto D, Rubini A, et al. Endoscopic facial nerve surgery. Otolaryngol Clin N Am. 2016;49(5):1173–87.
9. Borschel GH, Kawamura DH, Kasukurthi R, et al. The motor nerve to the master muscle: an anatomic and histomorphometric study to facilitate facial reanimation. J Plast Reconstr Aesthet Surg. 2012;65:363–6.
10. Dorafshar AH, Borsuk DE, Bojovic B, et al. Surface anatomy of the middle division of the facial nerve: Zuker's point. Plast Reconstr Surg. 2013;131:253–7.
11. Gur E, Zuker R, Zaretski A, et al. Incomplete facial paralysis: the use of the ipsilateral residual facial nerve as a donor nerve for facial reanimation. Plast Reconstr Surg. 2018;142(1):202–14.
12. Rea PM, Welsh EB, Morley S. Endoscopic access to fascia lata for use in static facial reanimation: a cadaveric and clinical study. Eur J Plast Surg. 2013;36:673–8.
13. Moody FP, Losken A, Bostwick J, et al. Endoscopic frontal branch neurectomy, corregator myectomy, and brow lift for forehead asymmetry after facial nerve palsy. Plast Reconstr Surg. 2001;108(1):218–23.
14. Takushima A, Harii K, Asato H, et al. Fifteen-year survey of one-stage latissimus dorsi muscle transfer for treatment of longstanding facial paralysis. J Plast Reconstr Aesthet Surg. 2013;66(1):29–36.
15. Lin CH, Wei FC, Lin YT. Conventional versus endoscopic free gracilis muscle harvest. Plast Reconstr Surg. 2000;105(1):89–93.

34 Free Muscle Transfer in Partial Facial Palsy

Eyal Gur, Daniel J. Kedar, and Ehud Fliss

34.1 Introduction

Facial paralysis ranges from complete to varying degrees of incomplete paralysis [1]. Patients with incomplete paralysis are characterized by some degree of facial mimetic function in the affected hemiface and can be subdivided according to etiology, duration of paralysis, anatomical distribution and the degree of atrophy and synkinesis [1–3]. Bell's palsy remains the most common cause for acquired facial paralysis and in approximately 10–30% results in incomplete unilateral facial paralysis [4–6].

The main goals of facial paralysis reanimation procedures are to improve static and/or dynamic symmetry and function, specifically in the midface zone thus enhancing the symmetry of the smile [7, 8]. Spontaneity of facial mimetic function is a highly important aspect of the reconstruction goal.

The main risk in performing dynamic reanimation in incomplete paralysis cannot be stressed enough as it can result in damaging the existing facial mimetic function on the affected side [3, 4, 7–9]. The clinically evident facial movement in the incompletely paretic hemiface indicates some active facial nerve axons and the presence of viable facial muscle. Surgical manipulation of these anatomical structures may lead to worsening of the paralysis by injuring facial nerve branches and/or facial musculature. With that said, it has been reported that cross-face nerve grafting (CFNG) with end-to-end coaptation to the paretic facial nerve may be performed with minimal damage to the existing motor function [4]. A distal end-to-side coaptation was also presented in order to address this issue exactly with good results [7]. A one-stage mini-latissimus dorsi free muscle transfer with neural coaptation to a contralateral facial nerve branch has also been reported [8].

We have recently published our experience with a one-stage free gracilis muscle transfer that involves neural coaptation to an ipsilateral buccozygomatic residual branch of the paretic facial nerve [9]. According to this series of patients we recommend to consider using this method in patients with incomplete facial paralysis that present with any degree, even if minimal, of preoperative spontaneous ipsilateral mimetic function in the buccozygomatic region.

34.2 Etiology and Epidemiology

Etiologies for incomplete facial paralysis are mainly acquired. The causes include idiopathic causes, infection, trauma, iatrogenic injury, and neoplasms.

E. Gur (✉) · D. J. Kedar · E. Fliss
Department of Plastic and Reconstructive Surgery, Tel-Aviv Sourasky Medical Center, Tel-Aviv, Israel
e-mail: eyalgur@netvision.net.il

© Springer Nature Switzerland AG 2021
C.-H. J. Tzou, A. Rodríguez-Lorenzo (eds.), *Facial Palsy*,
https://doi.org/10.1007/978-3-030-50784-8_34

Bell's palsy remains the most common cause for acquired facial paralysis. Approximately one half of all acquired cases qualify for the diagnosis of "Bell's palsy." The annual incidence rate of Bell's palsy is between 13 and 34 cases per 100,000 population. There is no race, geographic, or gender predilection, but the risk is three times greater during pregnancy, especially in the third trimester or in the first postpartum week. Diabetes is present in about 5–10% of patients. On presentation approximately one-third have an incomplete paralysis, and two-thirds have complete paralysis. The prognosis of Bell's palsy is related to the severity of the lesion. A simple rule is that clinically incomplete lesions tend to recover: with regard to the House-Brackmann grading system, grades I and II have good outcomes, grades III and IV characterize moderate dysfunction, and grades V and VI portend a poor result. Approximately 10–30% results in incomplete unilateral facial paralysis.

Several other disorders should be considered in the differential diagnosis of incomplete acquired facial nerve palsy. Cholesteatoma or a neoplasm should be suspected if the onset of facial palsy is gradual. Neoplasms can either compress or invade the facial nerve along its course from the cerebellopontine angle to the parotid gland. The Melkersson–Rosenthal syndrome is characterized by facial paralysis, episodic facial swelling, and a fissured tongue, typically beginning in adolescence but with recurrent episodes of facial palsy. Sarcoidosis should be considered, especially in patients with bilateral facial palsy. Severe systemic hypertension has been linked to unilateral primary facial nerve palsy in children and adolescents and rarely in adults. Hypertension should be suspected in a pediatric patient, if facial palsy is associated with headache, altered level of consciousness, vomiting, convulsions, or focal central nervous system deficit.

Congenital incomplete facial paralysis is rare. It may be isolated with the involvement of the facial nerve and its musculature only, or it may be part of a syndrome. It may be the result of developmental defects or of traumatic etiology (mainly forceps delivery). It is estimated that facial paralysis occurs in 2% of live births. In distinguishing developmental from traumatic facial palsies in the perinatal period, some or complete recovery of function favors traumatic lesions.

34.3 Diagnosis and Patient Presentation

Incomplete facial paralysis is defined as a state of facial paralysis that involves any degree of voluntary and/or spontaneous movement of the affected hemiface [3, 9]. This movement may be secondary to native axons that were uninjured in the previous facial nerve insult or may represent partial and unorganized axonal regeneration that takes place in the recovery of the injured facial nerve. Patients with incomplete facial paralysis are usually characterized by fair static symmetry and tone however with obvious dynamic asymmetry and in some patients, synkinesis and facial spasms (Fig. 34.1a, b) [6, 7, 8, 10]. Pattern and extent of dynamic asymmetry is determined by the etiology and mechanism of facial nerve injury as well as duration of paralysis and many other factors. Thus the clinical presentation is highly variable.

A thorough medical interview and physical examination is performed. Age, general medical condition and comorbidities, etiology of paralysis and duration, specific facial paralysis complaints (i.e., dry eye symptoms or epiphora, difficulty in mastication and intra-oral food propulsion, drooling, etc.) all have a roll in the reconstructive decision-making. Patient's chief complaint and expectations are discussed. Physical examination involves assessment of the five divisions of the paretic facial nerve as well as the muscles of mastication and possible donor muscles. At physical assessment one should notice is there is a major hypertonicity or hyper spasticity in the affected side a phenomena that may impair the reconstructive end point.

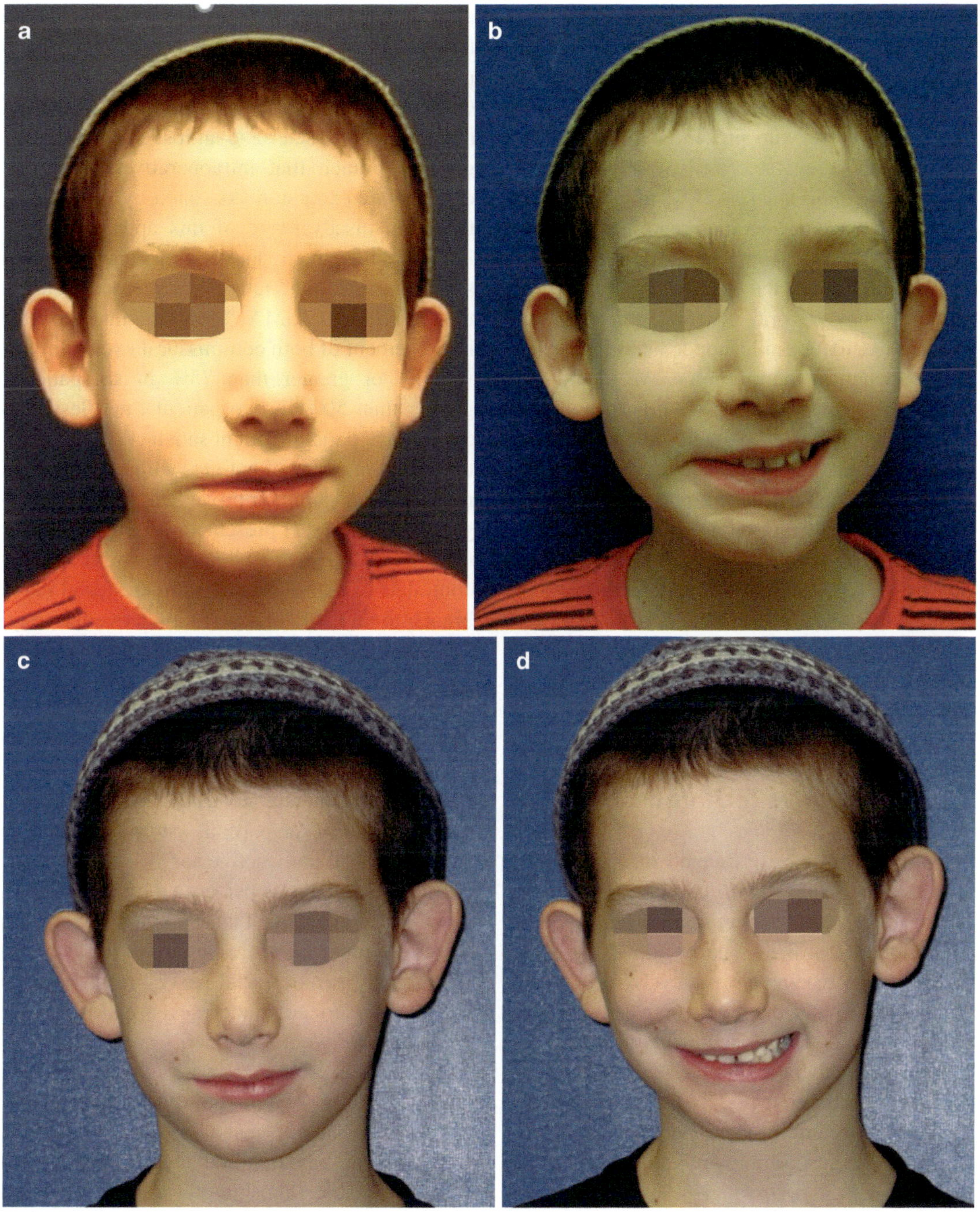

Fig. 34.1 4 year-old male patient with congenital right incomplete facial paralysis. Note fair symmetry at rest (**a**) and mild ipsilateral nasolabial fold and lateral lip elevation on attempt to smile (**b**). The ipsilateral facial nerve branch responsible for this residual movement (**a**, **b**) was used and coapted to the gracilis motor nerve. Note improved symmetry at rest and while smiling (**c**, **d**)

34.4 Patient Selection

Patients suitable for reanimation using the ipsilateral buccozygomatic residual facial nerve branch are those who present with incomplete facial paralysis characterized by any degree of *spontaneous movement*, even if minimal, in the ipsilateral buccozygomatic region. This may include mild nasolabial fold motion, movement of the muscle over the zygomatic arch with no motion of any perioral structure, minimal commissure excursion, mild upper lateral lip elevation or twitch of the modiolus. We hypothesize that this movement is due to the presence of some active native axons of the facial nerve and active facial muscle/s. The movement they produce may be clinically ineffective, probably due to unorganized and partial regeneration and the fact that they innervate small and atrophic motor units. Spastic or hypertonic incomplete facial paralysis patients may benefit from this procedure as well as long as adjunct procedures are performed such as botulinum toxin injections and/or selective neurectomy or myomectomy.

34.5 Operative Techniques

Various authors have presented their experience with treating patients with complete and incomplete paralysis that were treated as a single cohort. Thus there are many publications in which patients with incomplete paralysis were treated with the wide range of reconstructive options used for treating complete facial paralysis. These include static procedures as well as dynamic reanimation procedures including temporalis muscle transfer, masseteric-to-facial and hypoglossal-to-facial nerve transposition and autogeneous fascia lata transfer [5, 6, 9, 11, 12]. Cross-face nerve grafting, with or without the use of a free muscle transfer, has been reported as a safe and reliable method for facial reanimation in incomplete facial paralysis [3, 4, 7, 9, 10, 13–15].

Several authors have addressed the subgroup of patients with incomplete facial paralysis only with the intention to produce specialized procedures for these patients. Hontanilla et al. [6] assessed the efficacy of masseteric to facial nerve transposition in patients with incomplete facial paralysis. A series of nine patients is presented. Coaptation in all cases was performed between the nerve to masseter and an ipsilateral buccozygomatic branch that intraoperatively produced commissure excursion. As stated by the authors, the main disadvantage of this approach is the issue of movement dissociation and lack of a spontaneous smile. Outcome was assessed using the FACIAL CLIMA software that showed improvement of both commissural excursion and velocity of greater than 75% in six patients, greater than 50% in two patients, and less than 50% in one patient. Patient satisfaction was positive in the majority of patients while two patients reported no apparent improvement following surgery. Frey et al. [7] presented their approach for treating incomplete facial paralysis by coapting a contralateral active buccozygomatic facial nerve branch to an ipsilateral partially active buccozygomatic facial nerve branch using a sural CFNG. This approach does not involve a free muscle transfer. The nerve graft is coapted end-to-end on the healthy side and end-to-side on the paretic side via an epineural window. Axons are thought to regenerate along the CFNG and enter the distal part of the partially paretic facial nerve branch. The partially active nerve's axons are left intact as coaptation is performed by an epineural window. Spontaneous facial mimetic function is therefore enhanced while damage of the axons on the partially paretic facial nerve branch is minimized. The series included seven patients; three of them underwent 3D video symmetry assessment and are presented in the chapter. Results showed improved static and dynamic symmetry with what the authors call a functional upgrade of facial mimetic function in the incompletely paralyzed hemiface. Takushima et al. [8] reported a one-stage free mini-latissimus dorsi muscle transfer with neural coaptation to a contralateral facial nerve branch in patients with incomplete paralysis. Ipsilateral facial nerve branches are left untouched in order to avoid damage to the existing motion. The authors present a series of 96 patients. Mild worsening of the paralysis was noted in three cases, all of which resolved back to baseline within several months. Clinical outcome was assessed using a local grading scale that includes subjective symmetry score combined with EMG results. The authors present good postoperative symmetry scores (grades 4 or 5 in the local evaluation criteria used) in the majority of patients of the cohort. There were no cases of long-term worsening of paralysis. Advantages of this method include that it is a one-stage procedure, low complication and revision rate and its use of a free muscle transfer that provides a muscle source for modiolus pull. Of note, the authors do not mention any input regarding spontaneity of movement.

We have recently published our experience with a novel facial reanimation approach designed for patients with incomplete facial paralysis that present with residual ineffective movement in the midface zone of the paralyzed hemiface [9]. This includes using an ipsilateral minimally active buccozygomatic facial nerve branch as the donor nerve in a one-stage free gracilis muscle transfer (Fig. 34.2). The gracilis muscle is harvested with its neurovascular pedicle through a longitudinal incision in the medial thigh. Approximately one-third of the muscle width is used. Length and bulk of the muscle is determined intraoperatively according to the patient's size and proportions. Simultaneously, a preauricular face-lift incision is performed in the partially paralyzed hemiface. Dissection is performed in the supra-SMAS plane and deepens to the masseter fascia at the anterior border of the parotid gland, directed medially until facial nerve branches are identified emerging from the gland under the masseter fascia. At this stage, a meticulous functional mapping of the ipsilateral FN branches is performed using a nerve stimulator. The buccozygomatic branches responsible for the preoperative movement are identified. It is critical to identify the branches that create the exact movement that was evident clinically to activate the gracilis flap that eventually will create a spontaneous smile.

It is important to stress that in many times the muscle excursion that will be created by a nerve stimulator will be stronger than clinically evident at pre op clinical assessment. There are usually

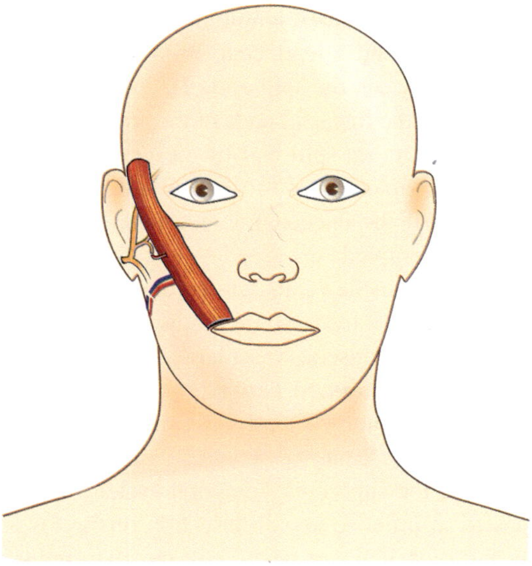

Fig. 34.2 Illustration of the one-stage free gracilis muscle transfer with neural coaptation to an ipsilateral residual buccozygomatic facial nerve branch in right sided incomplete facial paralysis. One of the residual branches is utilized leaving at least one branch intact. The gracilis's vascular pedicle is preferably anastomosed to the superficial temporal artery and vein. Used with permission from Wolters Kluwer Health, Inc.: Gur E, Zuker RM, Zaretski A, Leshem D, Barnea Y, Arad E, Yanko R, Meilik B, Kedar DJ, Fliss E. Incomplete facial paralysis: The use of the ipsilateral residual facial nerve as a donor nerve for facial reanimation. *Plast Reconstr Surg*, 2018 Jul;142(1):202-214. doi: https://doi.org/10.1097/PRS.0000000000004536

more than one such buccozygomatic branch thus elimination of the original motion is avoided when one of these branches is chosen to become the donor nerve for the gracilis flap and is divided. This branch will undergo neural coaptation to the gracilis motor nerve.

It is of utmost importance to make all efforts in order to identify more than one residual buccozygomatic branch in order to leave at least one intact branch thus the chance of worsening the preoperative residual function is minimized. In cases when only one residual buccozygomatic branch is identified, efforts are made to preserve its function on the native facial musculature by splitting it longitudinally and one half will be used as a donor nerve for the gracilis flap. The reminder of the fascicles is left uninterrupted in the native nerve sheath. In this case, the gracilis motor nerve is incised longitudinally leaving two split ends. End-to-end coaptation is then performed between the split end of the donor nerve and one of the free split ends of the gracilis motor nerve. The other split end of the gracilis motor nerve is coapted by end-to-side to the remaining fascicles of the buccozygomatic nerve that was left uninterrupted.

The gracilis flap is inset according to the standard procedure from the modiolus to the superficial temporal fascia. Vascular anastomoses are preferably performed between the flap pedicle and the ipsilateral superficial temporal vessels however the facial vessels may also be used. Chosing the superficial temporal system is suggested in order to avoid dissection of the lower facial zone if it not necessary and thus reduce buccal or marginal mandibular nerve injury (if still present). The face-lift incision is sutured and a penrose drain is left, the donor area is closed and a drain is left. Elastic bandage is placed on the donor leg. Postoperative care includes avoiding pressure on the operated cheek from the bed or pillow or from staff or patient manipulation by placing a curved hard splint from the oral commissure to the temporal scalp, pain management, regular hydration and diet, early mobilization, and respiratory physiotherapy. The penrose drain is removed prior to discharge and the thigh drain is removed according to amount of discharge. First follow-up visit is set to 1 week following discharge where the cheek splint is removed.

34.6 Outcome and Complications

We have published our experience with the above-described method in a series of 16 patients [9]. Our cohort included a majority of women with a mean age of 26.2 years (range 5–59 years). Patients were heterogeneous regarding the etiology of paralysis with the most common cause being iatrogenic paralysis following resection of head and neck tumors or other facial surgery. Mean interval between palsy onset and surgery was 11.2 years (range 1–49 years) and patients were followed for a mean period of 88.3 months (range 16–132 months). Following surgery, mean interval to first muscle flap motion was documented in seven patients and was 2.8 months (range 1–6 months).

In order to assess the procedures efficacy, we have conducted a subjective analysis of static and dynamic symmetry following surgery in 11 of the 16 patients of the cohort. This included a group of 21 reviewers who gave symmetry scores for three facial zones (eye region, nasolabial fold region, mouth region) at rest and while smiling and another score for global symmetry of the face while smiling. The former were assessed according to still photos and the latter according to videos of the patients smiling. All scores were given for pre- and postoperative photos and videos. These scores were later subtracted (postoperative score–preoperative score) in order to produce a *delta* value that represents the clinical change following surgery for the various anatomical zones at rest and while smiling. Statistically significant results demonstrated that in the majority of observations, no clinical apparent change was seen following surgery in the eye region at rest and while smiling and in the nasolabial fold region at rest. Improved symmetry was noted in the majority of observations in the nasolabial fold while smiling and in the mouth region at rest and while smiling. These findings demonstrate that this procedure positively affects the midface zone while not harming other facial zones (Figs. 34.1, 34.3 and 34.4). Global symmetry of the face on dynamic video assessment was also improved in the majority of patients (Table 34.1).

There were a minority of observations that demonstrated downgrading of symmetry following surgery. After reviewing the photos and videos of the cases we concluded that symmetry was interrupted mainly at rest but also in a small percentage of dynamic assessments. It seems this is mainly secondary to the gracilis flap's presence in the affected hemiface which may produce an abnormal appearing bulkiness. Moreover, in some cases the pulling vector of the gracilis flap produced some lateral movement that may by itself impair dynamic symmetry at the midface. These findings can be improved with secondary static procedures.

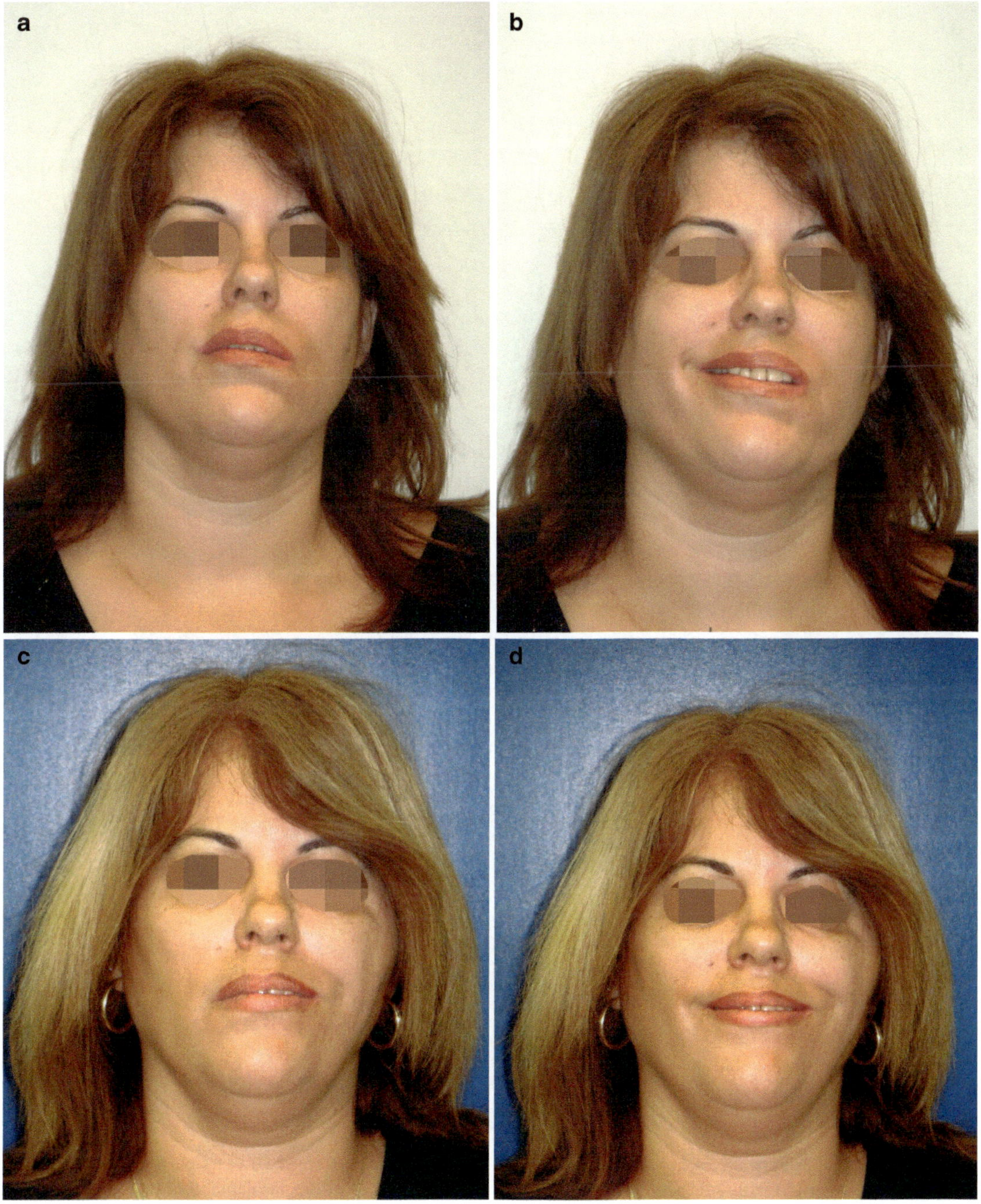

Fig. 34.3 Pre- and postoperative photos at rest and while smiling of a 43 year-old patient who presented with incomplete left facial paralysis secondary to Bell's palsy (**a**, **b**). Surgery was performed 25 years following palsy onset. Note mild upward and lateral movement of the ipsilateral lateral lip on attempt to smile (**c**, **d**). Used with permission from Wolters Kluwer Health, Inc.: Gur E, Zuker RM, Zaretski A, Leshem D, Barnea Y, Arad E, Yanko R, Meilik B, Kedar DJ, Fliss E. Incomplete facial paralysis: The use of the ipsilateral residual facial nerve as a donor nerve for facial reanimation. *Plast Reconstr Surg*, 2018 Jul;142(1):202-214. https://doi.org/10.1097/PRS.0000000000004536

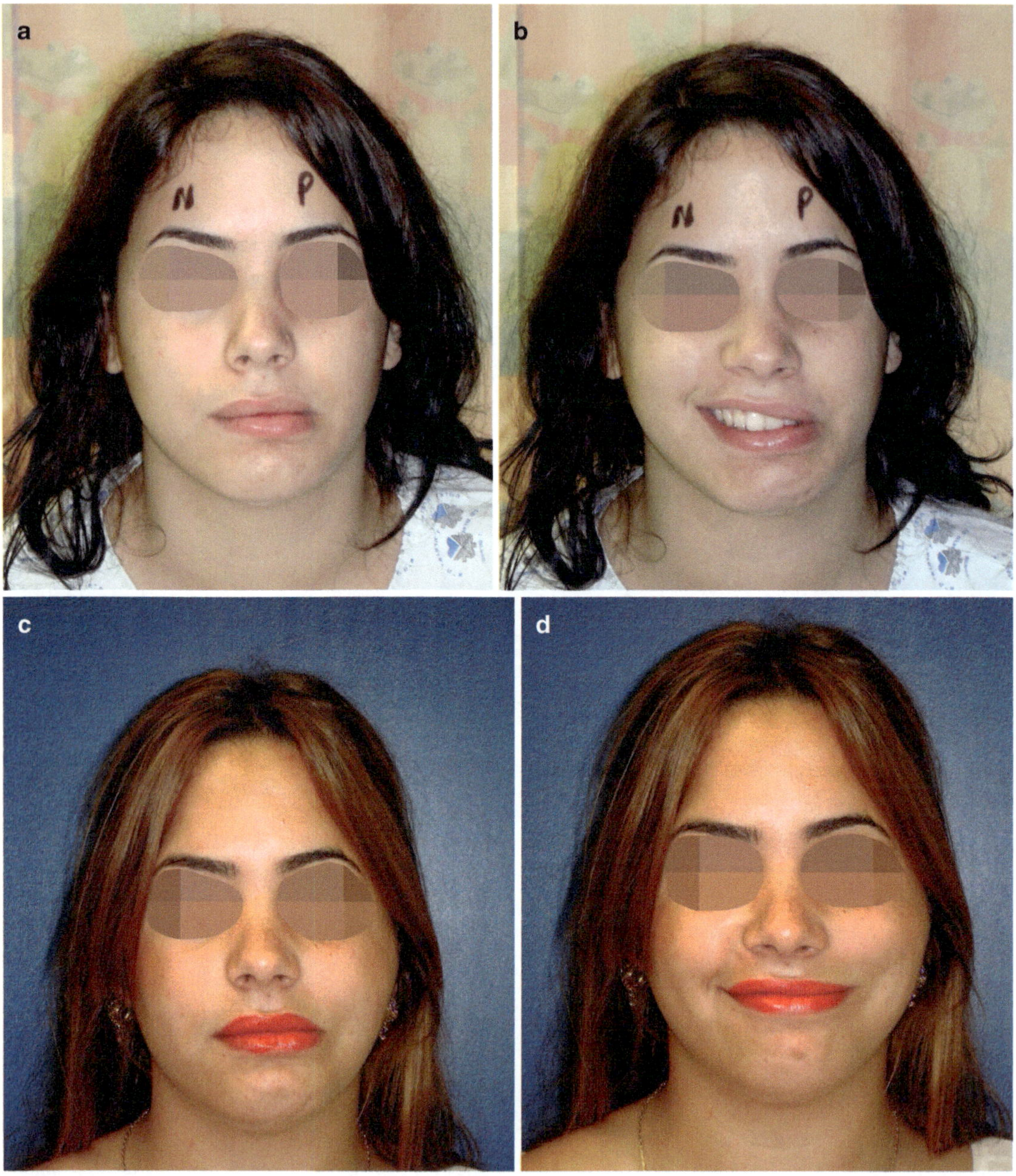

Fig. 34.4 Pre- and postoperative photos at rest and while smiling of a 19 year-old with left incomplete right facial paralysis secondary to traumatic injury at early childhood. Surgery was performed 16 years palsy onset. Note minimal movement of the nasolabial fold on attempt to smile (**b**)

In our series, there were no cases of major complications (partial or complete flap necrosis, flap loss, flap congestion, hemorrhage, or any complication requiring urgent revision surgery). In four patients, minor complications were noted (mild surgical site infection with mild wound dehiscence), all of which resolved with conservative measures. There were no cases of marginal mandibular nerve injury. Ten patients (62%) underwent secondary static procedures for fine-tuning of the aesthetic result. These included scar revision, fat injection, fat suction, adhesiolysis,

Table 34.1 Comparison of mean pre- and postoperative facial symmetry scores for all observations, according to media category and anatomical zone[a]

	Preoperative mean facial symmetry score (± Std. deviation)	Postoperative mean facial symmetry score (± Std. deviation)	*P* value	Mean delta (post-op to pre-op)
Static symmetry, eye At rest	4.02 (±0.96)	4.27 (±0.77)	< 0.001	+0.24
Static symmetry, NLF[b] At rest	3.32 (±1.03)	3.77 (±0.88)	< 0.001	+0.44
Static symmetry, mouth At rest	2.78 (±1.13)	3.90 (±0.92)	< 0.001	+1.12
Static symmetry, eye While smiling	3.42 (±1.22)	3.93 (±0.91)	< 0.001	+0.51
Static symmetry, NLF[b] While smiling	2.90 (±0.86)	3.68 (0.82)	< 0.001	+0.78
Static symmetry, mouth While smiling	2.13 (±0.80)	3.73 (±0.84)	< 0.001	+1.60
Dynamic symmetry While smiling	1.93 (±0.78)	3.61 (±0.85)	< 0.001	+1.68

Used with permission from Wolters Kluwer Health, Inc.: Gur E, Zuker RM, Zaretski A, Leshem D, Barnea Y, Arad E, Yanko R, Meilik B, Kedar DJ, Fliss E. Incomplete facial paralysis: The use of the ipsilateral residual facial nerve as a donor nerve for facial reanimation. *Plast Reconstr Surg*, 2018;142(1):202-214. doi: https://doi.org/10.1097/PRS.0000000000004536

[a]Static symmetry refers to still photograph assessment; Dynamic symmetry refers to video assessment
[b]NLF—Nasolabial fold

and gracilis flap re-anchoring. One patient (6%) showed mainly static improvement of facial symmetry with only minimal dynamic improvement after 14 months of follow-up. On clinical examination, the gracilis flap did contract however the facial movement it produced was weak and non-significant. Revision surgery was decided upon and during surgery the gracilis flap seemed viable however its motor nerve underwent atrophy. After retrospective inspection of the case, we could not find the reason for this course. During surgery, cross-face nerve grafting was performed with direct neurotization of the gracilis flap.

34.7 Conclusions and Future Study

Incomplete facial paralysis is the common form of facial paralysis. It includes a wide range of facial static and dynamic abnormalities with a highly heterogeneous clinical picture. According to current literature, incomplete paralysis is generally treated with the same treatment algorithm as complete facial paralysis. Several publications however did address this entity with the aim of refining the reconstructive approach. Here we present our experience with a one stage procedure designed specifically for patients with incomplete facial paralysis who present with any degree of spontaneous movement in the midface. This involves a one-stage free gracilis muscle transfer with neural coaptation to an ipsilateral, residually, partially active buccozygomatic branch of the paretic facial nerve. It is under debate whether the facial motion weakness is to be attributed to defective facial nerve growth or to facial muscle weakness and atrophy. The suggested procedure overcomes those two options by using the remaining normal facial nerve axons to stimulate a whole new and strong muscle that is transferred to the paralyzed face. Advantages of this procedure are that it is a safe and effective one-stage procedure, coaptation to an ipsilateral facial nerve branch allows for a spontaneous smile, using the gracilis flap provides a strong source for commissure excursion and in case no movement is identified postoperatively, salvage procedures are still possible with cross-face nerve grafting. Results in our cohort are promising and the procedure has proved to be safe and efficacious in this specific sub-group of patients.

34.8 Pearls and Pitfalls

- Contraindications.
  - Non-spontaneous–*only intentional* facial motion or residual smile production.
  - Severely spastic incomplete facial paralysis.
  - Recent progression of the paresis or a history of a recent gradual onset of facial paralysis.
  - Incomplete resection of a brain tumor (as cause of paralysis), with an evidence of slow progression of the tumor.
  - Medical status not permitting long anesthesia.
  - Major depression and/or doubt that the patient understands the nature of the procedure and its targets.
  - Unrealistic expectations.
- Special preoperative considerations
  - Be sure that there is a residual facial motion that is spontaneous (not an eye closure motion).
  - Assess whether there is synkinesis or hypertonicity on the affected side.
  - Assure that the patient understands the nature of those long procedures and the long time lag until the final result shows. Assure reasonable expectations of the final results.
- Special intraoperative considerations:
- Assure that the selected branch does not play a major role in orbicularis oculi action.
- Identify more than one residual buccozygomatic branch in order to leave at least one intact branch thus the chance of worsening the preoperative residual function is minimized.
- In cases when only one residual buccozygomatic branch is identified, the nerve is not divided but first dissected longitudinally, split and followed by partial transection leaving a free end that includes part of the nerve fascicles. The reminder of the fascicles is left uninterrupted in the native nerve sheath. The gracilis motor nerve is also split and an end-to-end coaptation is performed between the split end of the donor nerve and one of the free split ends of the gracilis motor nerve. The other split end of the gracilis motor nerve is coapted by end-to-side coaptation to the remaining fascicles of the buccozygomatic nerve that were left uninterrupted.
- Regarding the gracilis muscle—treat the muscle gently and preserve its epimysium. Tailor the muscle to be transferred, to make it as thin, gentle, and long as possible and needed, while not compromising the neurovascular pedicle that penetrates it. Verify muscle contraction after nerve transection, by nerve stimulation on the side table.
- Place the muscle obliquely from the modiolus to the superficial temporal fascia superior to the auricle.
- Vascular anastomoses are preferably performed between the flap pedicle and the ipsilateral superficial temporal vessels. This is in order to avoid dissection of the lower facial zone and thus reduce other residual nerves injury.
- Special postoperative considerations:
  - Immediate extubation, de-catheterization, and operated cheek stenting for protection.
  - Admit the patient to a step down unit for 24 h after surgery.
  - Protect the operated cheek by attaching worning sticker to the cheek and place the designated splint.
  - When motion starts, several months after the procedure, the patient should practice daily, in front of a mirror, to strengthen the muscle action and create more symmetry with the healthy side smile.

References

1. Zuker RM. Facial paralysis and the role of free muscle transplantation. Ann Chir Plast Esthet. 2015;60(5):420–9. https://doi.org/10.1016/j.anplas.2015.06.001.
2. Fattah A, Borschel GH, Zuker RM. Reconstruction of facial nerve injuries in children. J Craniofac Surg. 2011;22:782–8.
3. Fattah A, Borschel GH, Manktelow RT, Bezuhly M, Zuker RM. Facial palsy and reconstruction. Plast Reconstr Surg. 2012;129(2):340e–52e.
4. Hontanilla B, Marre D, Cabello A. Cross-face nerve grafting for reanimation of incomplete facial paralysis: quantitative outcomes using the facial clima system and patient satisfaction. J Reconstr Microsurg. 2014;30(1):25–30.
5. Hohman MH, Hadlock TA. Etiology, diagnosis, and management of facial palsy: 2000 patients at a facial nerve center. Laryngoscope. 2014; 124(7):E283–93.
6. Hontanilla B, Marre D. Masseteric-facial nerve transposition for reanimation of the smile in incomplete facial paralysis. Br J Oral Maxillofac Surg. 2015;53(10):943–8.
7. Frey M, Giovanoli P, Michaelidou M. Functional upgrading of partially recovered facial palsy by cross-face nerve grafting with distal end-to-side neurorrhaphy. Plast Reconstr Surg. 2006;117(2):597–608.
8. Takushima A, Harii K, Okazaki M, Ohura N, Asato H. Availability of latissimus dorsi minigraft in smile reconstruction for incomplete facial paralysis: quantitative assessment based on the optical flow method. Plast Reconstr Surg. 2009;123(4):1198–208.
9. Gur E, Zuker RM, Zaretski A, Leshem D, Barnea Y, Arad E, Yanko R, Meilik B, Kedar DJ, Fliss E. Incomplete facial paralysis: the use of the ipsilateral residual facial nerve as a donor nerve for facial reanimation. Plast Reconstr Surg. 2018;142(1):202–14. https://doi.org/10.1097/PRS.0000000000004536.
10. Lindsay RW, Bhama P, Weinberg J, Hadlock TA. The success of free gracilis muscle transfer to restore smile in patients with nonflaccid facial paralysis. Ann Plast Surg. 2014;73(2):177–82.
11. Wan H, Zhang L, Li D, et al. Hypoglossal-facial nerve "side"-to-side neurorrhaphy for persistent incomplete facial palsy. J Neurosurg. 2014;120(1):263–72.
12. Yoshioka N. Masseteric nerve as "baby sitter" procedure in incomplete facial paralysis. Plast Reconstr Surg Glob Open. 2016;4(4):e669.
13. Gur E, Stahl S, Barnea Y, et al. Comprehensive approach in surgical reconstruction of facial nerve paralysis: a 10-year perspective. J Reconstr Microsurg. 2010;26(3):171–804.
14. Jowett N, Hadlock TA. A contemporary approach to facial reanimation. JAMA Facial Plast Surg. 2015;17(4):293–300.
15. Terzis JK, Noah ME. Analysis of 100 cases of free-muscle transplantation for facial paralysis. Plast Reconstr Surg. 1997;99(7):1905–21.

35 Gracilis Insetting Under SMAS in Smile Reanimation

Tae suk Oh and Min Ji Kim

Key Points

- Facial palsy affected side has unique soft tissue characteristic, seems like aging appearance.
- Dynamic rejuvenation is a functional free muscle transfer (FFMT) with superficial muscoloaponeurotic system (SMAS) utilization in facial reanimation surgery.
- This can make up some limitation in powerful FFMT and could get good aesthetic advantage.
- A mirrored nasolabial fold reset from healthy side to affected side is the key procedure in harvested gracilis flap insetting.
- A starting from dissecting an extended SMAS flap elevation, gracilis passing through tunnel under SMAS toward nasolabial fold then finally do SMAS fixation suprolaterally has same effect with facelift.

35.1 Introduction

Facial reanimation surgery with free flap has been a mainstream in this field. Various techniques that include various neurorraphy techniques and various donor motor nerve harvest techniques recently developed and this area had remarkable activities. We expected developing nerve regeneration through nerve and muscle harvest which can progressly acquire smiling in facial palsy patients. Motor neuron regeneration and axonal guidance are the main source in surgical facial reanimation [1]. However, even though powerful FFMT has shown improved facial smile excursion compared to previous trials, we couldn't get same degree of muscle power with healthy side [2]. Even successful facial reanimation surgery what we can call "spontaneous smile," does not represent that exact same degree of smiling in both oral commissure. We must concede that this is true inevitability.

To obtain objectively same smiling in FFMT against remaining weakness in symmetry, we need to focus "Facial rejuvenation" concept. In unilateral facial palsy patients, we could find some unique characteristics in affected side; Brow decent, facial soft tissue decent, absent of nasolabial fold and deep jowl formation [3]. The uni-face morphology resembles aging result in mid age. What I suggest the concept of "dynamic rejuvenation" is the more advanced definition that ranges over FFMT with facelift. Aesthetic approach

T. s. Oh (✉) · M. J. Kim
Plastic and Reconstructive Surgery, Seoul Asan Medical Center, Seoul, South Korea
e-mail: tasuko@amc.seoul.kr

© Springer Nature Switzerland AG 2021
C.-H. J. Tzou, A. Rodríguez-Lorenzo (eds.), *Facial Palsy*,
https://doi.org/10.1007/978-3-030-50784-8_35

through SMAS utilization in facial reanimation is the key to obtain symmetrical soft tissue smiling. Biglioli et al. reported his experience: all of the patients in the group who had deep plane lift with free flap surgery in facial reanimation surgery has showed immediate symmetry in rest, compared to the patients who underwent only free flap surgery. In 24 months later follow up, they showed 44.5% patients who has Terzis and Noah grade 5 result which is excellent that has symmetrical smile with teeth showing, compared to the other group has only 28.6% [4]. This dynamic rejuvenation concept helps to improve the final static result with more dynamic facial reanimation.

35.2 Advantage of Dynamic Rejuvenation

Application of facial rejuvenation in facial reanimation is starting from harvest flap inset under SMAS. SMAS flap elevation is the anatomical safe area in dissection for experienced surgeon. We could minimize destroying normal structure even in paralyzed side. In case of incomplete facial palsy, we need to be careful to not avoid remnant facial nerve injury and this technique is a much safer approach than timid subcutaneous dissection. The greatest thing in SMAS flap elevation is restoring more surrounding tissue; it could get to minimize its risk at edema or hematoma. This advantage let patients get early recovery after long time free flap reanimation operation. Regarding how to manage SMAS flap, we could get effectively facelift aesthetic outcome as well. This acquiring soft tissue lifting technique can solve limitation in powerful FFMT that suggested so far (Fig. 35.1).

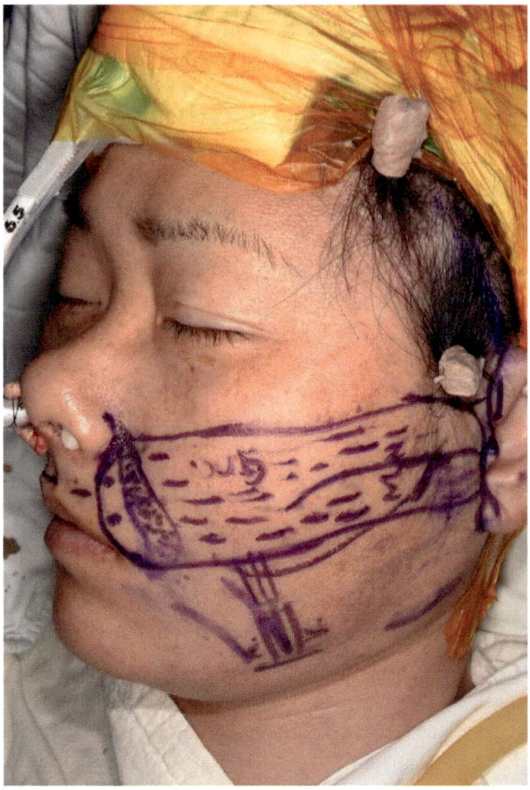

Fig. 35.1 Preoperative flap design. Identification of recipient vessel with hand held Doppler and semicircular design of new nasolabial fold and measure how we need to harvest muscle

35.3 Vectors of Facial Symmetry in Smile Reanimation with SMAS

Understanding of SMAS vector influence in facial symmetry is important. This is the mechanical property of SMAS flap that repositioning can affect postoperative facial contouring with symmetry in facial reanimation. Vertical vector repositioning provides larger amount of fat enhancement toward malar eminence and also it is possible to deepen cervicomental legion. It makes patients to be more tapered and have thinner appearance. In paralyzed side often present as bulky, loosened soft tissue in lower cheek, shallow malar lesion thus this vector can be effectively corrected. Oblique vector repositioning makes relatively lesser volume in malar lesion but larger volume in submalar lesion. In some patients who have buccal fat lacking, this vector can be helpful.

35.4 Operative Procedure

35.4.1 Skin Flap Elevation

I prefer to dissect an extended SMAS flap. Rather than using subcutaneous undermining, we need to precise dissection with leaving proper amount fat in above side of SMAS flap. Lack of fat tissue in elevated flap makes difficult dissection and tear. Acquired facial contouring can be managed through manipulation of SMAS elevation and fixation. Adding to effectiveness of nerve regeneration using free gracilis flap, this aesthetic outcome helps in providing a more sustainable appearance (Fig. 35.2) [5].

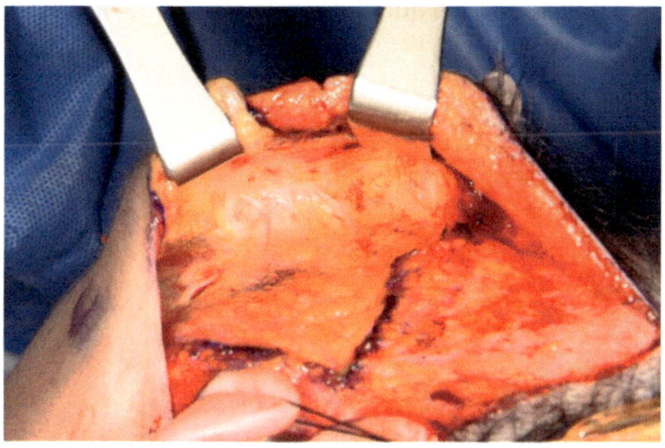

Fig. 35.2 Intraoperative SMAS excision design. An incision begins from 1 cm inferior to the zygomatic arch and proceeded superiorly 3–4 cm toward the lateral canthus and inferiorly at 90° angle toward nasolabial fold

35.4.2 SMAS Elevation

An incision begins from 1 cm inferior to the zygomatic arch to ensure frontal branch preservation. In horizontal perspective, incision is continued to the area where zygomatic arch became zygoma body. Then proceeded superiorly 3–4 cm toward the lateral canthus. When sensate reaching lateral orbit, the incision changes the way inferiorly at 90° angle toward nasolabial fold. In vertical perspective, incision is continued along the passing way preauricular to plastysma to a point 5–6 cm below the mandibular border (Fig. 35.3).

35.4.3 Nasolabial Fold Reset

An affected palsy side has characteristics of soft tissue drooping and decreased muscle tone. Gracilis flap inset and nerve coaptation can effectively recovery of facial reanimation. However, for obtaining more effective powerful muscle action, we need to manage soft tissue. The one

Fig. 35.3 Illustration 1

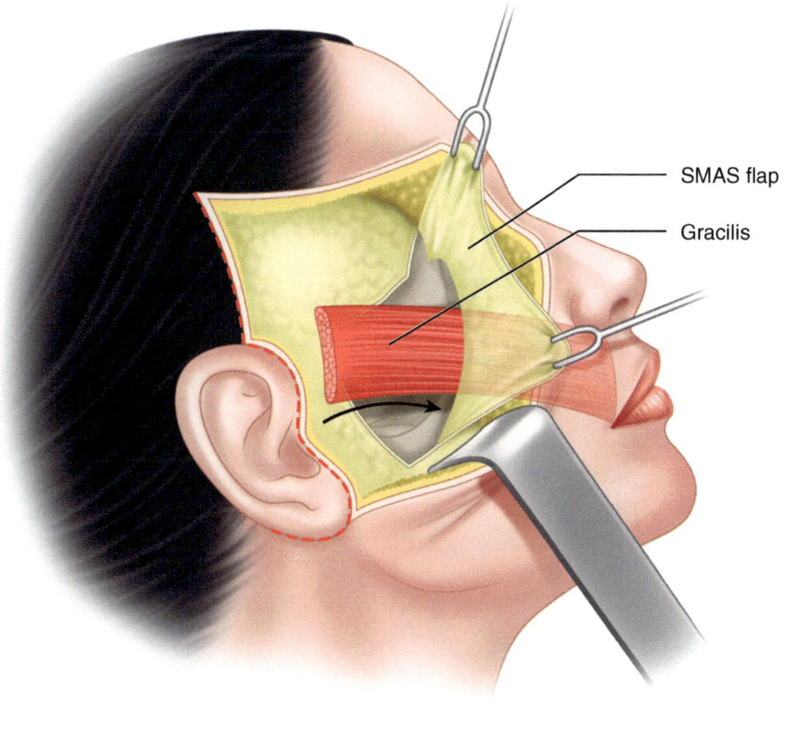

way I prefer is make new nasolabial fold in affected side. Before general anesthesia induction, we can flip over against healthy side nasolabial fold into affected side over using bendable slender wire in sitting position. After marking this mirrored nasolabial fold in resting face, mid cheek soft tissue can be lifted up then put down by hand. Then we can additional marking for new nasolabial fold as smile face. This semicircular shape design is proceeded with de-epithelization. Then incision was made from the lateral side and then dissect into medial side. Then this elevated dermal flap can be mobilized therefore this flap can be hanged toward up/lateral side. After closure of dermal flap, we could find there is visualized as new nasolabial fold medially in affected side and repositioned laterally lay soft tissue looks more bulky and upward lifting. A newly made nasolabial fold can help to being a more natural and spontaneous smile (Fig. 35.4).

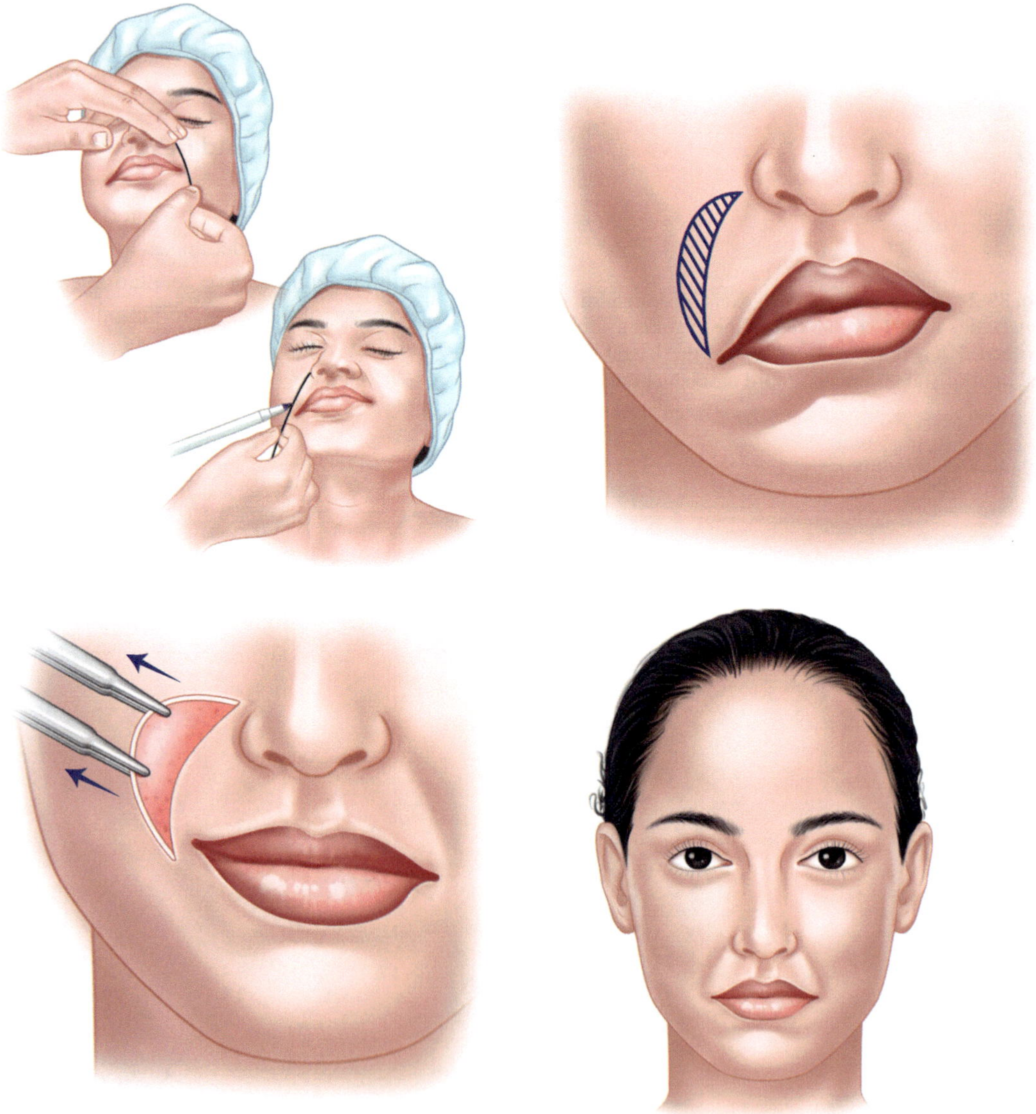

Fig. 35.4 Illustration 2

35.4.4 Tunnelling Under SMAS

What I mentioned above making new nasolabial fold, after elevating semicircular dermal flap, the face lift incision can be extended toward this incision. Then there can be made tunnelling through lateral ear helix to new nasolabial fold. This tunnelling dissection should be made under SMAS flap.

35.4.5 Gracilis Insetting

An initially harvested gracilis can be split and anterior part of the muscle is used. Depending on patient's requiring amount of muscle, it can be manipulated once confirm the way of vascular pedicle. This gracilis passes through tunnel under SMAS toward nasolabial fold. Finally, lateral portion of the gracilis muscle was fixed at the periosteum of the lateral zygomatic bone then medial end to be placing of the modiolus about lip. An each connecting junction is sutured with mattress suture. Attaching around lip part, we need to carefully inset proper position that each muscle fiber should be laid over paralyzed orbicularis oris and below the oral commissure and along the lip. I prefer insetting muscle first then vessel anastomosis later and nerve coaptation finally (Fig. 35.5).

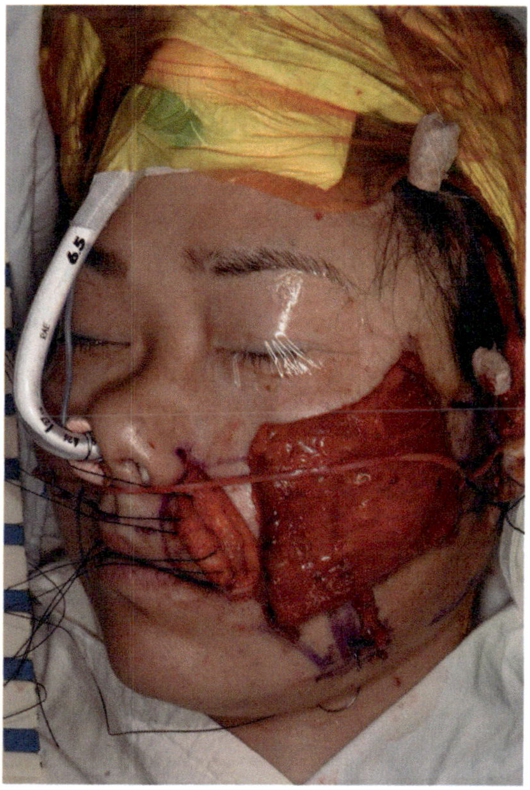

Fig. 35.5 Intraoperative photography. Elevated nasolabial fold dermal flap is readymade for lifting and harvested gracilis muscle and there seen overlying sural nerve for cross face nerve graft

35.4.6 SMAS Fixation

An elevated SMAS flap is repositioned superiorly, laterally, and perpendicular to the mandibular border. Medial direction of SMAS lifting makes newly deepend nasolabial fold. Rotated SMAS can be secured with multiple interrupted sutures. After proper setting of SMAS flap, follow trimming will be needed for resuspension to avoid irregularity or skin dimpling. Then SMAS overlying in preauricular region can be incised then transpositioned behind the ear. This can help restoring mandible border to mental region contouring (Fig. 35.6).

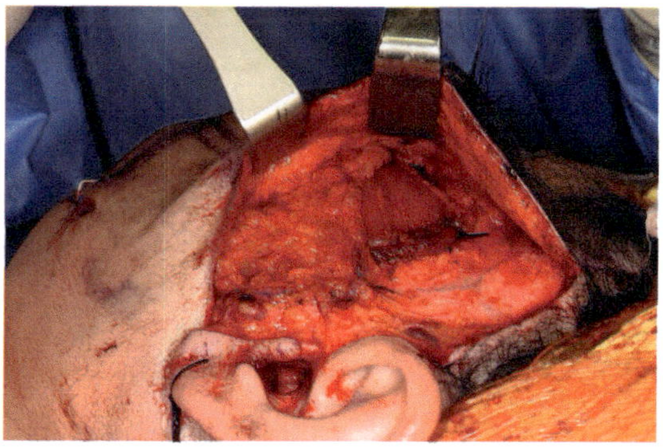

Fig. 35.6 Intraoperative photography. This is the immediate completion of SMAS plication, there shown gracilis insetted status under SMAS tunnelling. Newly made nasolabial fold can be seen symmetrically and inset gracilis and SMAS plication make lift mid cheek

35.5 One-Stage Surgery with Double Innervated FFMT

My preference is double innervated FFMT with gracilis. With standard method, average 10 × 5 cm sized muscle flap harvested with enough length of obturator nerve, medial femoral circumflex artery and vein. Facial artery and vein should be prepared as recipient vessel before muscle separation. A massector nerve can be found in the masseter muscle below the zygomatic arch. The harvest obturator nerve can connected to massector nerve in end-to-end fashion. For more powerful spontaneous smiling, we need to one more motor source from healthy side. Incision is made at Zuker's point in unaffected side, then buccal branch of facial nerve can be found with clue as zygomaticus activity using nerve stimulation. Harvested sural nerve over than usually 18cmm coapted one side with healthy buccal branch with end-to-end fashion. The other side of sural nerve is overlying toward affected side then coapted with harvested obturator nerve from gracilis muscle in end-to-side fashion (Figs. 35.7 and 35.8).

Fig. 35.7 Illustration 8

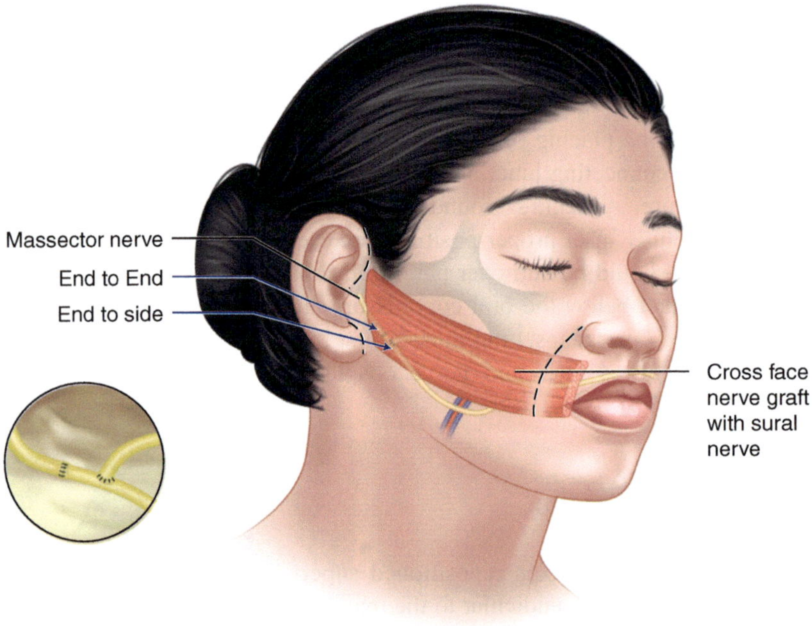

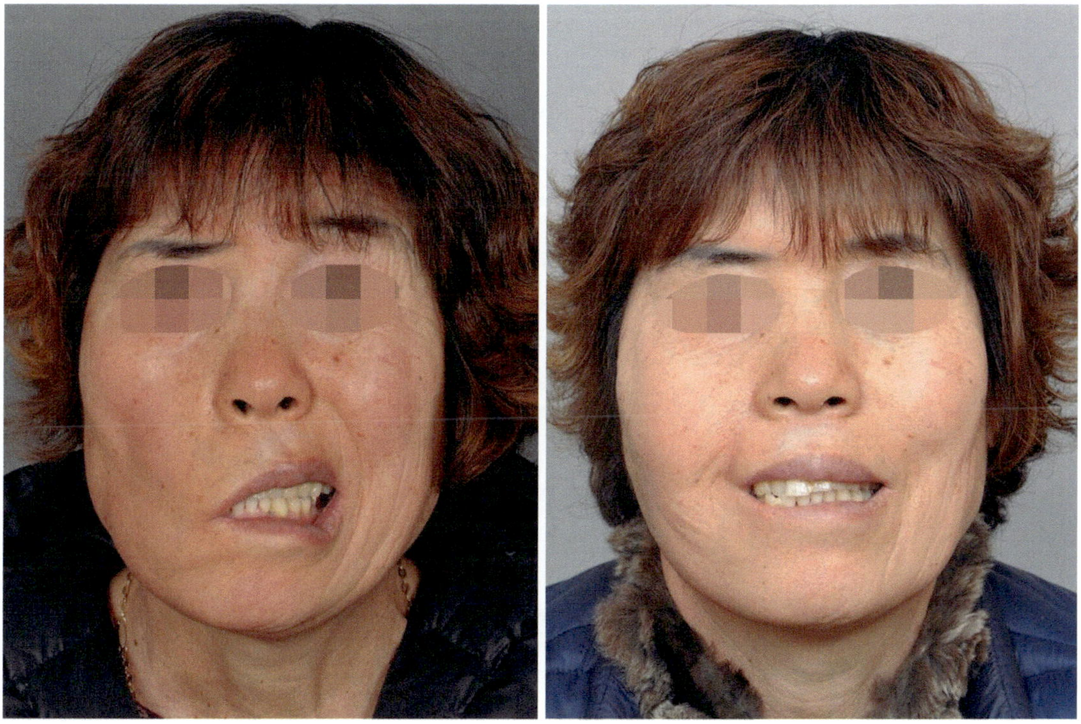

Fig. 35.8 A 53-year-old patient, abruptly gets right incomplete bell's palsy 23 years ago. She underwent double powered functional gracilis muscle transfer with nasolabial fold formation. (Left) Preoperative photography in smile position and (Right) Postoperative photography in smile position in 1 year. Good symmetry smile rest and smile

References

1. Langhals Nicholas B, et al. Update in facial nerve paralysis: tissue engineering and new technologies. Curr Opin Otolaryngol Head Neck Surg. 2014;22(4):291.
2. Akihiko T, et al. Revisional operations improve results of neurovascular free muscle transfer for treatment of facial paralysis. Plast Reconstr Surg. 2005;116(2):371–80.
3. Stuzin JM, Baker TJ, Baker TM. Refinements in face lifting: enhanced facial contour using vicryl mesh incorporated into SMAS fixation. Plast Reconstr Surg. 2000;105(1):290–301.
4. Federico B, et al. Deep-planes lift associated with free flap surgery for facial reanimation. J Cranio-Maxillofac Surg. 2011;39:475–81.
5. Rubin LR, Simpson RL. The new deep plane face lift dissections versus the old superficial techniques: a comparison of neurologic complications. Plast Reconstr Surg. 1996;97(7):1461–5.

Fascicular Turnover Flap for Facial Nerve Gaps and Nerve Transfer for Trigeminal Palsy

36

Isao Koshima, Shuhei Yoshida, Ayano Sasaki, Shogo Nagamatsu, Kazunori Yokota, Haruki Mizuta, Mitsunobu Harima, Jyunsuke Tashiro, and Shuji Yamashita

Key Points

A new method "fascicular turnover method" using vascularized fascicular flap is used for repairing nerve gaps. The advantages are: no need for sacrificing a normal donor nerve and short-time operation. Digital nerve gaps can be repaired under a local anesthesia. Fascicular flap is a vascularized nerve flap and can be expected excellent nerve regeneration even in cases with longer nerve gap and scarred recipient bed. It is a simple and short-time operation compared to free nonvascularized and vascularized nerve graftings. In addition, there is no functional loss resulted from sacrificed fascicle in the operated area. The disadvantage is a need for supramicrosurgical technique using 50 µm needle.

This work was presented in part at the 240th Local Meeting of Tokyo Area in the Japanese Society of Plastic and Reconstructive Surgery, in Tokyo, on December 4, 2004, the invited lecture in the 2005 Annual Meeting of the Americal Society of Reconstructive Microsurgery in Pueru Trico, on January 15, 2005, the 9th International Course on Perforator Flaps, on September 7, 2005, the 34th Annual Meeting of the Japanese Society of Reconstructive microsurgery, in Fukushima City, on October 19, 2007, the invited lectures in the MD Anderson Cancer Center in Houston, on January 16, 2008; and in the 16th International Course on Plastic and Esthetic Surgery of Clinica Planas, in Barcelona, on May 8, 2008.

I. Koshima (✉) · S. Yoshida
International Center for Lymphedema, Hiroshima University Hospital, Hiroshima, Japan

A. Sasaki · S. Nagamatsu · K. Yokota
Plastic and Reconstructive Surgery, Hiroshima University Hospital, Hiroshima, Japan
e-mail: ooyanagi@hiroshima-u.ac.jp

H. Mizuta · M. Harima · J. Tashiro · S. Yamashita
Department of Plastic and Reconstructive Surgery, Graduate School of Medicine, The University of Tokyo, Tokyo, Japan
e-mail: gmd15097@s.okadai.jp

Nerve gaps are usually repaired with nonvascularized nerve graft. However, the postoperative results are in limited level. Meanwhile, it is documented that vascularized nerve grafts have a potential of rapid axonal sprouting of regenerating axons even in cases with poorly vascularized beds and long nerve gaps [1–11]. In the peripheral nerve, it is well documented that fascicles have rich microvascular vessels [12]. Recent supermicrosurgical techniques made an accurate coaptation of single nerve fascicle possible with a 50 µm needle. Therefore, vascularized single fascicular flap to reconnect a nerve gap can be expected to have an excellent nerve recovery as in an island vascularized skin flap for skin defect.

With the introduction of these concepts on micro-vascularization and fascicular suture, we developed a new method for repairing nerve

© Springer Nature Switzerland AG 2021
C.-H. J. Tzou, A. Rodríguez-Lorenzo (eds.), *Facial Palsy*,
https://doi.org/10.1007/978-3-030-50784-8_36

gaps: "fascicular flap turn over method." In this paper, we describe two cases using this method for digital and facial nerve gaps.

36.1 Operative Techniques

Under an operating microscope, a nerve gap is confirmed and the proximal and distal neuromas are resected. Thereafter, using a sharp and small knife or microscissors, a single fascicle is split from the other fascicles of the proximal or the distal nerve trunks. Anatomically, it is well established that a nerve trunk has a micro-plexiform structure composed with fascicles: Each fascicle is connected with many tiny communicating branches through which nerve sprouting could be possible (Fig. 36.1). Therefore, the nearest communicating branches to the gap are preserved to accept sprouting axons and pass distally toward the nerve endings after surgery. The splitted single fascicle is turned over the nerve gap to reach the contralateral nerve end without tension. Suture of the fascicular flap and contralateral nerve end is achieved with four to six stitches using 11-0 or 12-0 nylon with 80 or 50 μm needle.

Nerve gaps less than 20 mm could be connected with a fascicular turn over flap from either side of the proximal or distal stump of the gap. Nerve gaps over 20 mm can be bridged with bilateral turn over flaps from both the proximal and distal nerve stumps and sutured to join the middle portion of the gap (Fig. 36.1).

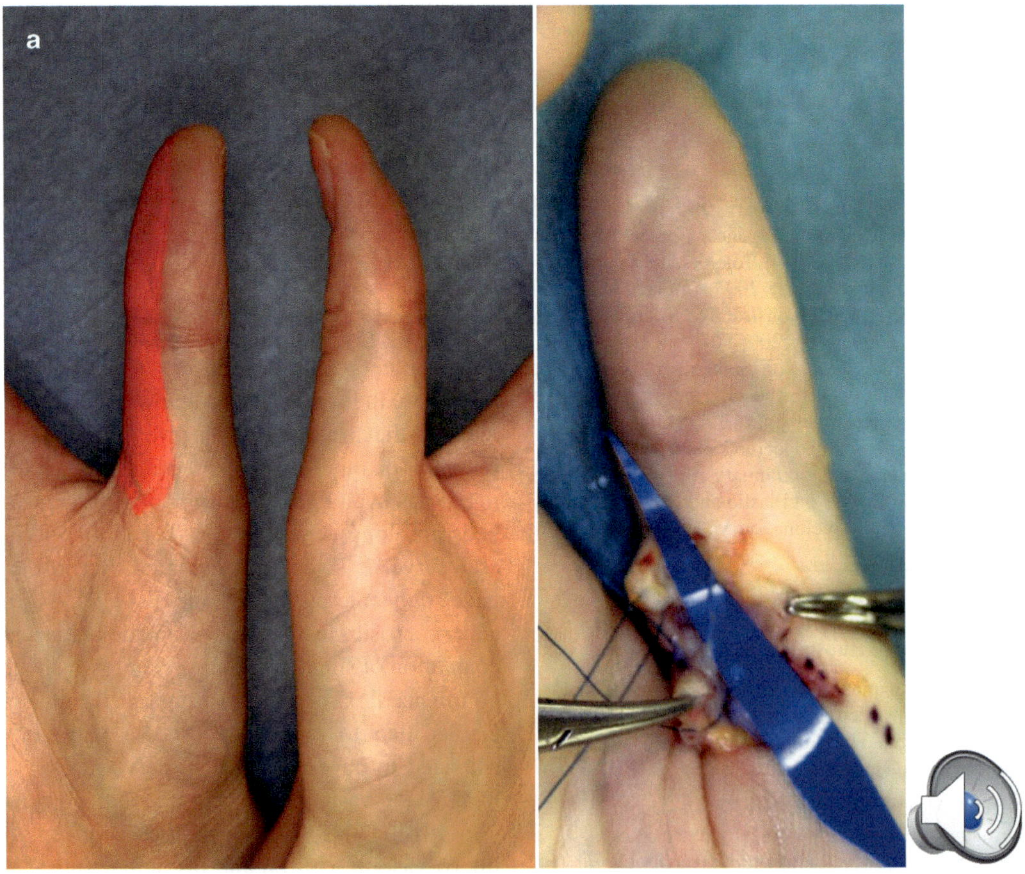

Fig. 36.1 (**a**) Case 3. A 30-year-old woman lost sensation on the ulnar side of the right thumb after injury. (**b**) Left, Bilateral turnover flaps were joined at the middle portion of the defect of 20 mm; Center, Schema of nerve repair; Right, Nerve anastomosis with 12-0 (50 μm) needle; (**c**) Postoperative sensory recovery at 6 months (left, Tinel's sign was in the proximal phalanx), 10 weeks (center, Tinel is at the tip, SW value was 3.61, m2PD was 7 mm), and 4 months (right, SW was 3.61, m2PD was 5 mm) after surgery (Koshima I, Narushima M, Mihara M, Uchida G, Nakagawa M. Fascicular turnover flap for nerve gaps. J Plast Reconstr Aesthet Surg. 63(6):1008–14, 2010)

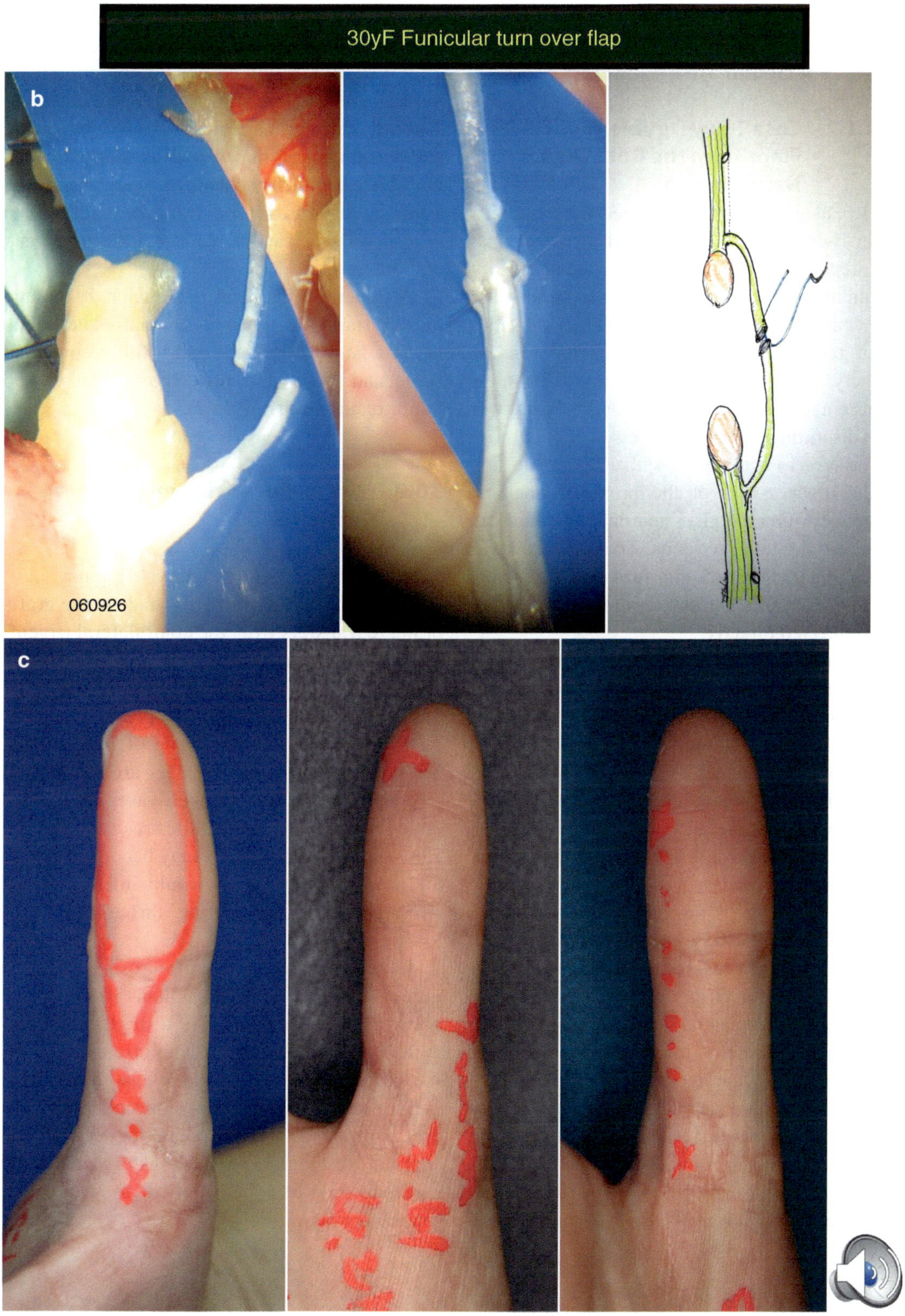

6w 10w 4M 5mm 3.61

Fig. 36.1 (continued)

36.2 Case Reports

36.2.1 Fascicular Turnover Flap

36.2.1.1 Case 1 30y Double Fascicular Flaps from the Both Digital Nerve Stump

A 30-year-old woman had injured the ulnar side of her right thumb at the base of proximal phalanx. Ten months later, she complained of sensory loss on ulnar side of the thumb, severe tenderness with which she could not grasp an object, disability of removing a bottle cap, and no sensory recovery after injury. Preoperative Semmes-Weinstein (SW) value was 4.17, and moving two-point discrimination (m2PD) was over 30 mm.

The surgery was started with a zigzag incision on the ulnar aspect of the proximal phalanx. There were ulnar digital neuromas at the both transected digital nerve ends. The nerve gap was 20 mm in length. Fascicular turn over flaps were elevated from the both the digital nerve stumps, and connected directly.

Postoperatively, the sensory recovery was smooth, the Tinel's sign was in the proximal phalanx at 6 weeks, and it was at the tip at 10 weeks (SW value was 3.61, m2PD was 7 mm). Four months after surgery, SW was 3.61, m2PD was 5 mm. Six months later, the SW value on the distal pulp was 3.22, and the m2PD was 6 mm. The patient could remove a bottle cap without any tenderness (Fig. 36.1).

36.2.1.2 Case 2 65y Fascicular Turn Over Flap for Facial Nerve Gap

A 65-year-old woman had a large parotid tumor, pleomorphic adenoma, for 20 years. During the tumor resection, main feeding arteries from both the left facial and superficial temporal artery were ligated to transect. As the parotid duct and buccal branches were widely involved in the tumor, the buccal branches were sacrificed from just distal from their proximal division of facial nerve. As a result, only the zygomatic and marginal mandibular branches were preserved. Therefore, the distal portion of the superficial musculoaponeurotic fascia was lifted up to decrease a gap of main buccal branch. The nerve gap was finally 30 mm. The distal portion of the main buccal branch had three fascicles. Therefore, a fascicular turn over flap from the distal buccal branch was elevated to reconnect the nerve gap without tension.

Postoperatively, paralyzed major zygomatic muscle started to move at 3 months later. Nine months later, the patient had a full recovery of smile, and now 3 years after surgery, there was no tumor recurrence (Fig. 36.2).

36.3 Cross-Face Trigeminal Nerve Transfer

Patients with trigeminal nerve II palsy have many serious problems. Cross-face nerve grafts or nerve transfers from the contralateral trigeminal nerve to the affected nerve can facilitate trigeminal palsy reconstructions. Our survey of the literature has revealed no previous reports on reconstruction of this type of nerve palsy. We believe that nerve transfers are superior to free nerve grafts because well-vascularized fascicles and only one suture site are used [1–3, 7]. However, the nerve grafts may become necrotic and double-suture scars would interrupt post-operative axonal sprouting through a nerve graft.

In addition, recent supermicrosurgical techniques using needles less than 80 μm wide allow accurate coaptation of a single nerve fascicle [9, 13]. Therefore, single fascicular transfer to connect a nerve could results in excellent nerve recovery. These new concepts and techniques propose a new paradigm for supermicrosurgical fascicular nerve transfer where the methodology can be applied to trigeminal branch II palsy.

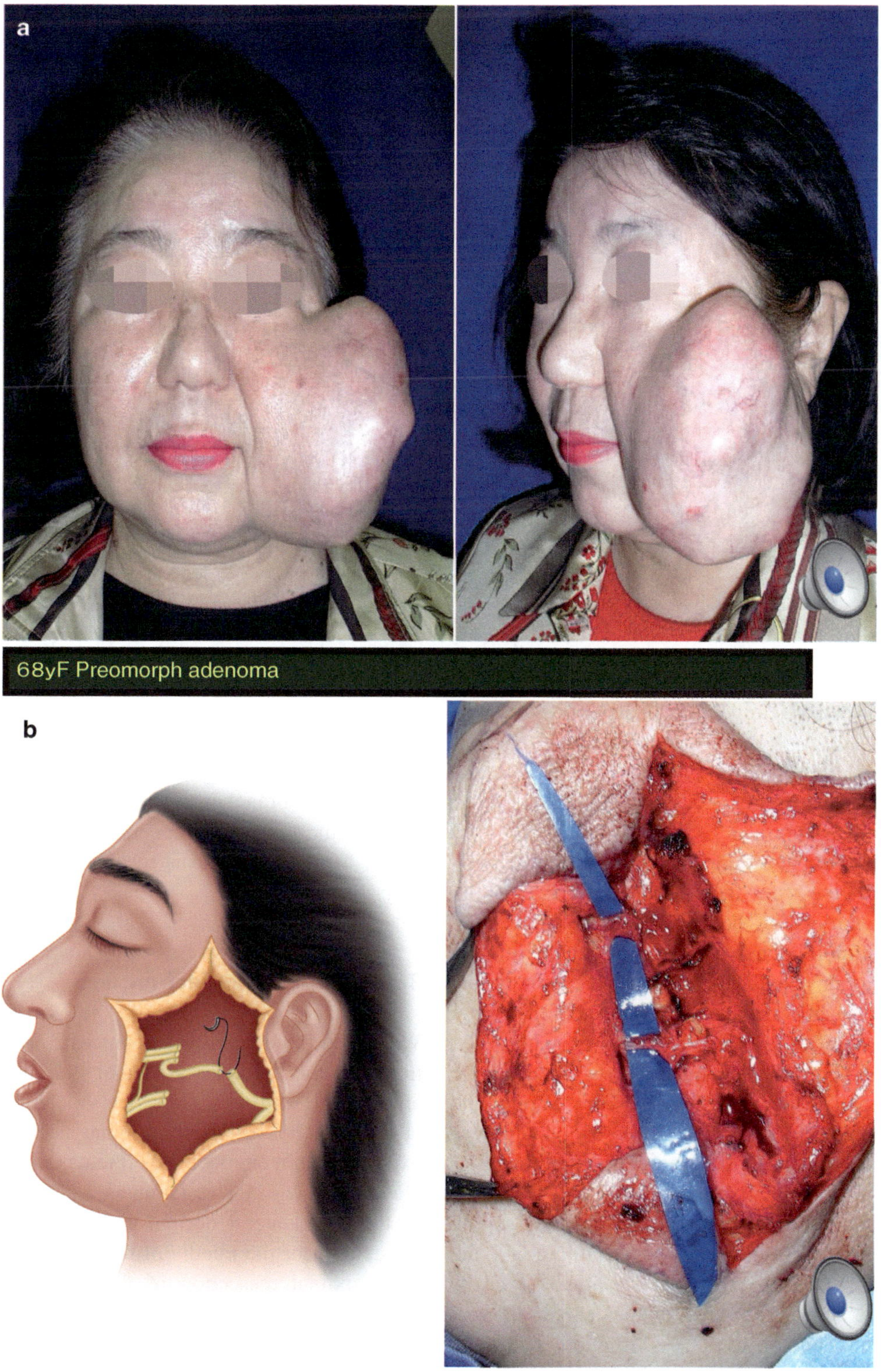

Fig. 36.2 (**a**) Case 2. A 65-year-old woman had a huge parotid tumor for 20 years. (**b**) The defects (30 mm) of buccal branches were repaired with fascicular turn over flaps. (**c**) Postoperative recovery of facial reanimation at 2 (left) and 4 months (center), and 1 year and 8 months later (right) (Koshima I, Narushima M, Mihara M, Uchida G, Nakagawa M. Fascicular turnover flap for nerve gaps. J Plast Reconstr Aesthet Surg. 63(6):1008–14, 2010)

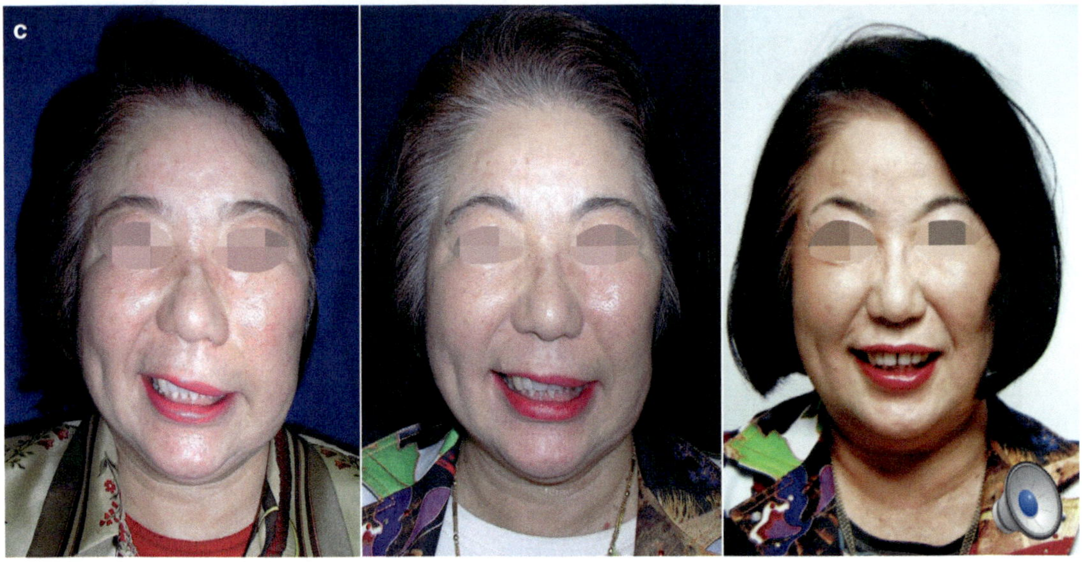

Fig. 36.2 (continued)

In this paper, we report on a new method of intraoral cross-face trigeminal nerve transfer for established trigeminal nerve palsy.

36.3.1 Anatomy

The role of the infraorbital nerve carries sensory information from the lower eyelid, lateral ala, anterior aspect of the face, and upper labial area. The infraorbital nerve passes through the infraorbital foramen and connect to the facial branches. These facial branches are composed of the palpebral, nasal, and superior labial branches. The palpebral branches then pass upward beneath the palpebral orbicularis muscle. They supply the skin and conjunctiva of the lower eyelid with sensation, joining with the facial nerve at the outer edge of the orbital.

The nasal branches pass inward: they supply the skin on the side of the nose and join with the nasal branch of the trigeminal ophthalmic nerve.

The superior labial branches are the largest and most numerous. They descend beneath the levator labii superioris and are distributed to the skin of the upper lip, the mucous membrane of the mouth, and the labial glands. The superior labial branches penetrate the superior labial muscle and orbicular oris muscle, ultimately innervating the subcutaneous layer of the upper lip.

All these branches are joined, immediately beneath the orbit, by filaments from the facial nerve, forming the plexus of infra-orbital nerve (Fig. 36.3a).

36.3.2 Operative Techniques

With an intraoral approach, a mucosal incision is made on the posterior aspect of the upper lip. Under an operating microscope, bilateral upper labial branches of the trigeminal nerve II are exposed within or above the orbicularis oris muscle layer. One of the distal upper labial branches of the contralateral normal trigeminal nerve is dissected near the middle of the upper lip. After the proximal dissection of the affected nerve trunk, using a small sharp knife or microscissors, the denervated nerve trunk is transected at the proximal side near the infraorbital foramen. Then the proximal end of the denervated nerve is

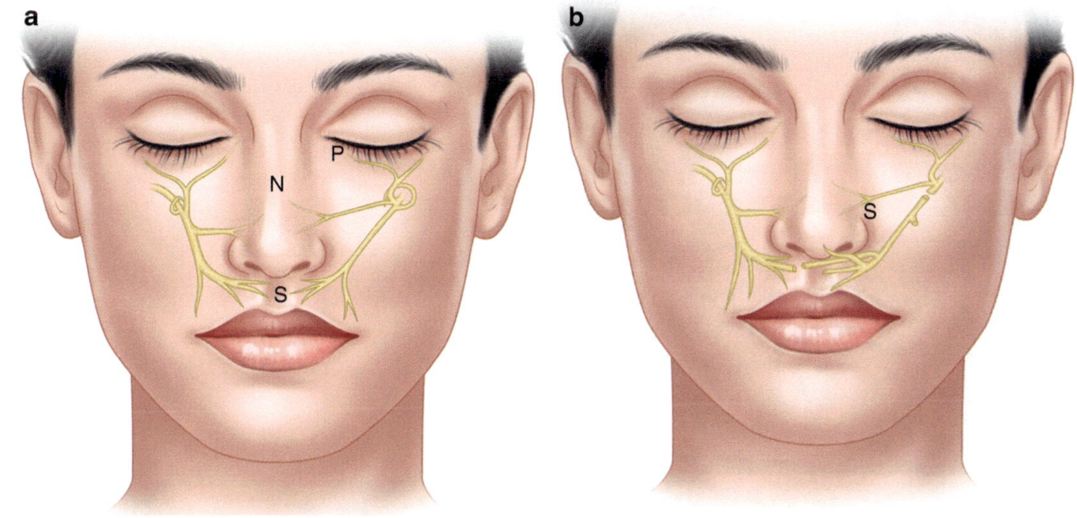

Fig. 36.3 (**a**) Normal anatomy of the infraorbital nerve. The infraorbital nerve is composed of the palpebral (P), nasal (N), and superior labial branches (S). The superior labial branches are the largest and are distributed to the upper lip. (**b**) Schematic drawing of cross-face trigeminal nerve transfer. The proximal side of the left affected nerve was transferred to the distal side of the right normal nerve (superior labial branch) (Koshima I, Narushima M, Mihara M, Uchida G, Nakagawa M. Cross-face nerve transfer for established trigeminal branch II palsy. Ann Plast Surg. 63(6):621–3, 2009)

turned for transfer to the middle portion of the upper lip to connect the contralateral normal labial branch without tension. It is important to dissect enough length of affected nerve trunk to reduce the tension at the suture point. Supermicrosurgical fascicular suture of the upper labial branch and affected nerve is achieved with four to six stitches using 11-0 or 12-0 nylon with an 80- or 50 μm needle. There is no possibility of donor site sensory loss because the normal labial branch sacrificed is distal-level and only one among several branches (Fig. 36.3a, b).

36.4 Case Report

36.4.1 Case 3

A 56-year-old woman, who had suffered a facial bone fracture 10 years ago, complained of left trigeminal nerve II palsy. We performed trigeminal nerve transfer under general anesthesia. We could not follow the patient postoperatively because of the patient's family problems. Nine months after surgery the value measured by Semmes-Weinstein test was 2.41 (contralateral upper lip: 1.65) and moving two-point discrimination was 25 mm (contralateral upper lip: 15 mm). One and half years after surgery, these values were 1.65 and 15 mm (completely normal recovery). The patient felt sensation on the affected side, not at the contralateral donor site. There was no postoperative bleeding, donor site sensory loss around the upper lip, facial paralysis, or no abnormal facial pain (Fig. 36.4).

36.4.2 Case 4

A 46-year-old woman had a recurrent adenoid cystic carcinoma originating from the left orbital cavity and invading the anterior skull base. With an anterior skull-base approach, wide resection including the left orbital cavity and trigeminal nerve was performed. The resulting defect was repaired with a free rectus abdominis

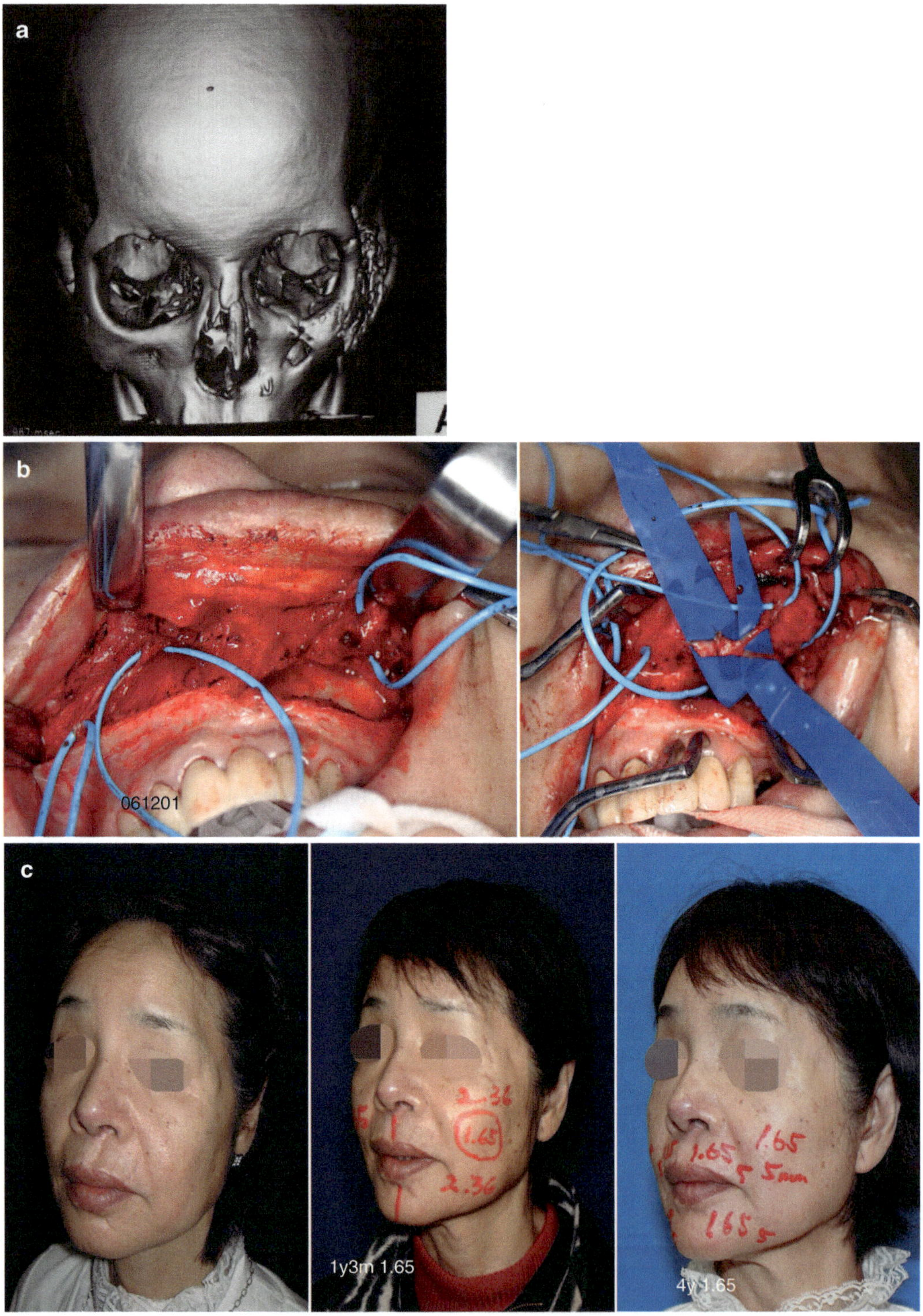

Fig. 36.4 (**a**) Case 5. A 56-year-old woman lost left trigeminal nerve II sensation due to facial bone fracture 10 years previously. Three-dimensional CT shows calvarial bone graft on the left zygomatic bone. (**b**) Left: Bilateral trigeminal nerves were exposed. Arrow head indicates the right normal labial branch. Right: Nerve suture (arrow head) was established. *T* affected trigeminal nerve. (**c**) Postoperative sensory recovery. Left, preope.; SW value and moving 2-PD were 1.65 and 5 mm (normal:1.65) at 1 year and 3 months (Center) and 4 years (Right). (Koshima I, Narushima M, Mihara M, Uchida G, Nakagawa M. Cross-face nerve transfer for established trigeminal branch II palsy. Ann Plast Surg. 63(6):621–3, 2009)

musculocutaneous flap. Six months after the primary surgery, the patient desired a reconstruction and trigeminal nerve transfer was performed from the right upper labial branch to the left trigeminal nerve.

Three months after surgery, sensation emerged in the left upper lip (Semmes-Weinstein value 4.17). Five months and one year after surgery, Semmes-Weinstein value was 2.44 (contralateral upper lip: 1.65) and moving two-point discrimination was 30 mm (contralateral upper lip: 15 mm). In addition, she felt sensation on the affected side, not at the contralateral donor site. The patient did not any complications, such as donor site sensory loss, around the upper lip (Fig. 36.5).

36.5 Discussion

36.5.1 Vascular System Within Peripheral Nerve and Nerve Flap Concept

The supermicrosurgical techniques have made s single fascicular suturing method possible using 11-0 or 12-0 suture material with 80 or 50 μm needle. Meanwhile, the microvascular rich circulations within the fascicle had been well known [12] and their importance have been emphasized in the reports on vascularized nerve flap, because the vascularization of nerve grafts suppress the fibrosis within the nerve grafts [1–11] (Fig. 36.6).

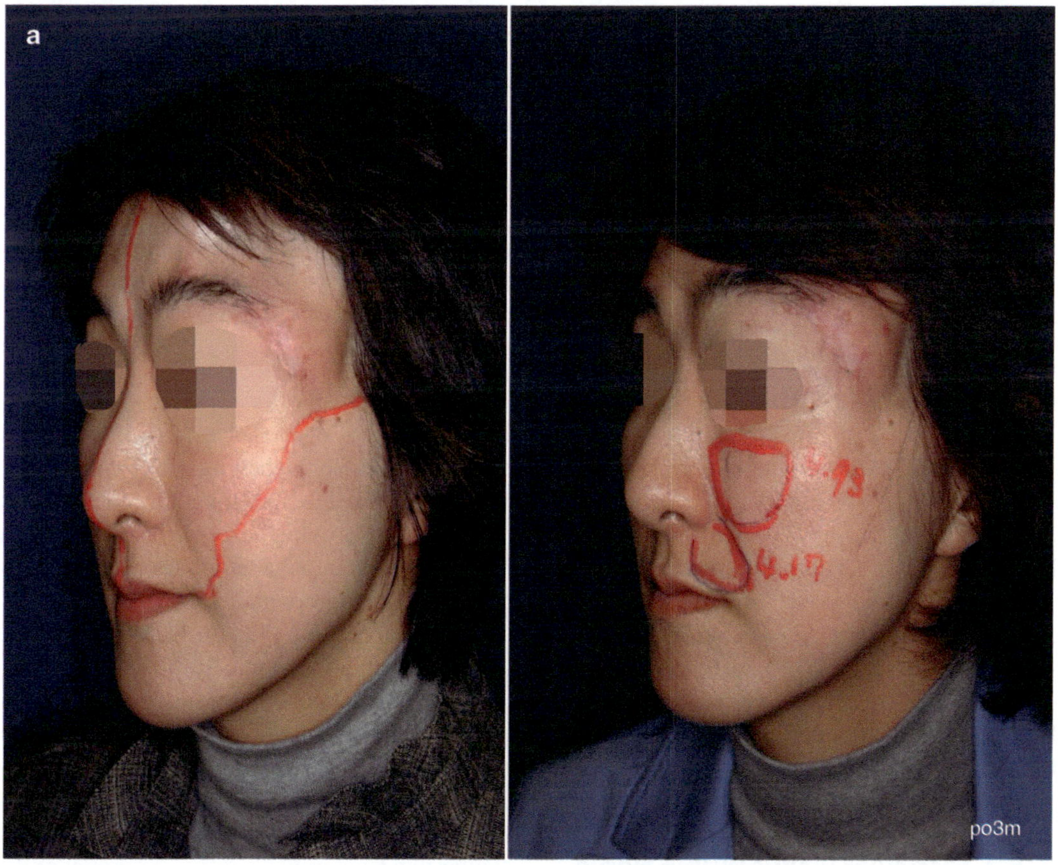

Fig. 36.5 (**a**) Case 4. A 46-year-old woman without left trigeminal nerve I & II resulting from the left skull-base cancer resection. Left, The defect was repaired with free rectus abdominis MC flap. The area circumscribed by red marker lost sensation; Right, 3 months after trigeminal nerve transfer. SW value was 4.17; (**b**) Left, SW 3.22 at 4 months; right, SW 2.44 and m2PD 30 mm at 5 months; (Koshima I, Narushima M, Mihara M, Uchida G, Nakagawa M. Cross-face nerve transfer for established trigeminal branch II palsy. Ann Plast Surg. 63(6):621–3, 2009)

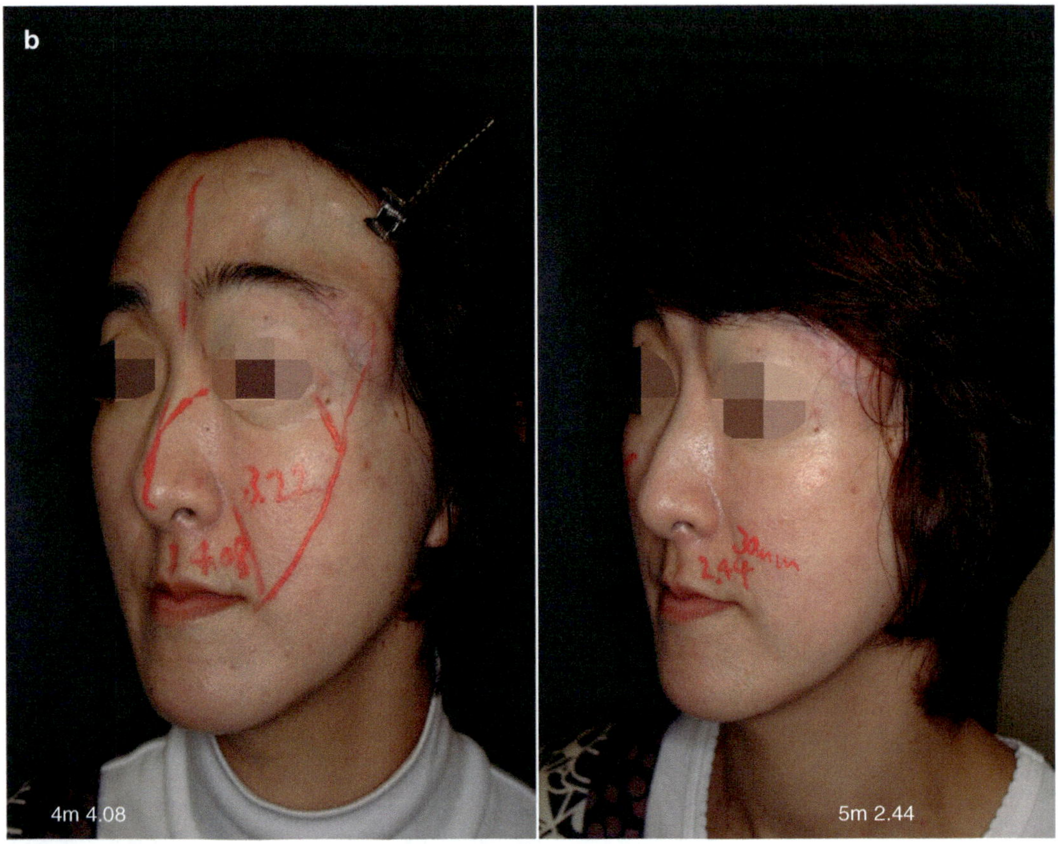

Fig. 36.5 (continued)

Based on our experimental works on microanatomical studies on peripheral nerves, fascicles can maintain its blood circulation even when the fascicle is separated as a pedicle flap or island flap [2, 3]. This fascicular flap concept in nerve surgery is the same as that in skin flap. Developments of these supermicrosurgical technique and microanatomy on nerves have created a new surgical method, "fascicular turn over flap," in nerve reconstruction surgery as well as development of perforator flap surgery.

36.5.2 Fascicular Plexus Within Nerve Trunk

Regarding the routes of axonal sprouting from the proximal to the distal nerve trunks, it is well established that there are bypass routes through the communicating branches between each fascicle. With these branches, turn over method does not prevent axonal sprouting toward the distal direction; i.e., proximal axons from the proximal fascicles sprout into the turned fascicular flap and pass through the communication branches into the distal nerve trunk (Fig. 36.1). Therefore, with this fain techniques, smooth axonal sprouting through a vascularized fascicular flap is theoretically possible with an accurate fascicular anastomosis and less fibrosis due to well vascularization of the fascicular flap.

In cases with longer nerve gaps, a longer fascicular flap from only the either (proximal or distal) side for is difficult because the distal end of the flap shows poor vascularization and strong tension is unavoidable on the anastomosed site. We believe in cases with digital nerve gap less than 20 mm in length, fascicular turnover flap

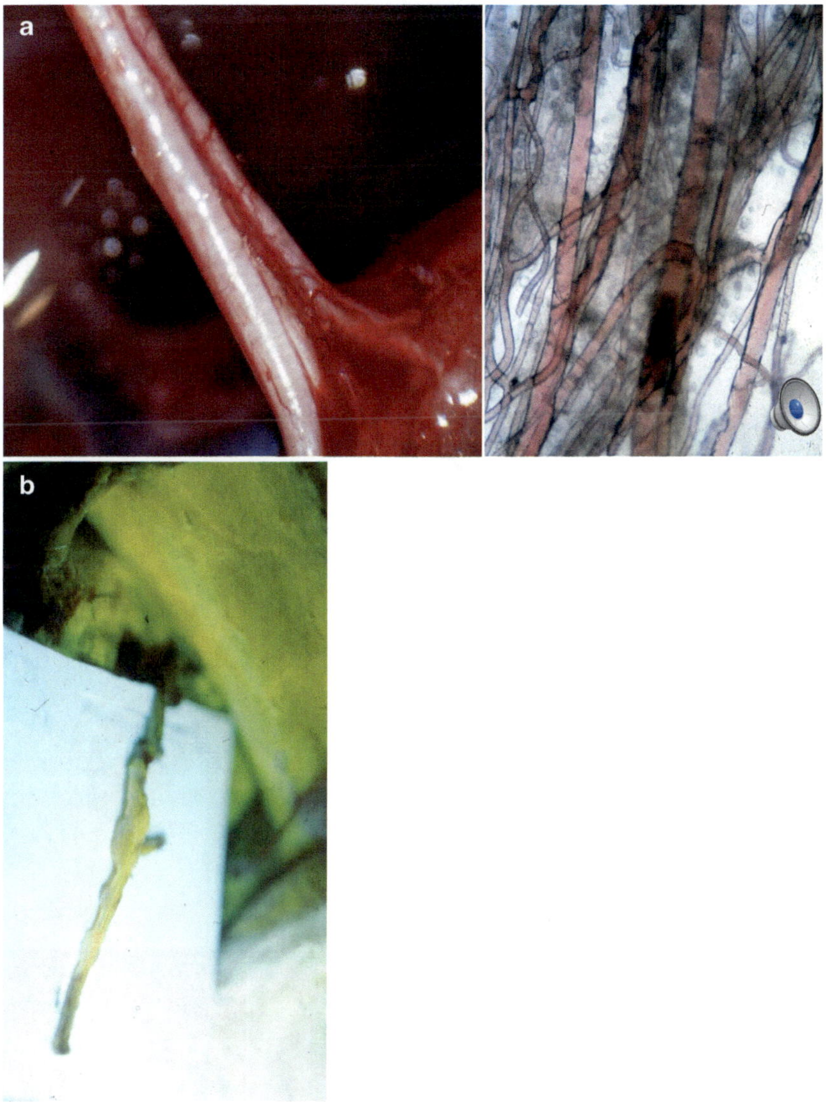

Fig. 36.6 (**a**) Left, Vascular system of rat sciatic nerve; Right, Intraneural vascular system after alkali dissolution for embalmed specimen with colored resin; (Koshima I, Harii K. Experimental study on vascularized nerve grafts: Part I. The pattern of blood circulation in the rat sciatic nerve and the method of obtaining a vascularized sciatic nerve graft in the rat. Jap J Plast Surg. 2: 811–16, 1982). (**b**) Fluorescein staining of island rat sciatic nerve pedicled with muscle perforator from the femoral artery (Koshima I, Harii K. Experimental study on vascularized nerve grafts: Part I. The pattern of blood circulation in the rat sciatic nerve and the method of obtaining a vascularized sciatic nerve graft in the rat. Jap J Plast Surg. 2: 811–16, 1982). (**c**) Schematic drawing of experimental work on vascularized nerve flap. Free sciatic nerve flap was transferred to the contralateral sciatic nerve gap (Ref. 2. Koshima I, Harii K. Experimental study of vascularized nerve grafts: multifactorial analyses of axonal regeneration of nerves transplanted into an acute burn wound. J Hand Surg Am. 10: 64–72, 1985). (**d**) Nerve flap using rat sciatic nerve. Left, Island flap in posterior thigh; Right, contralateral free sciatic nerve flap (N) anastomosed with femoral vessels (P) (Koshima I, Harii K. Experimental study on vascularized nerve grafts: Part I. The pattern of blood circulation in the rat sciatic nerve and the method of obtaining a vascularized sciatic nerve graft in the rat. Jap J Plast Surg. 2: 811–16, 1982); (**e**) Two months after transfer. Left, nerve flap; Right, nerve graft (small strand); (Ref. 3. Koshima I, Harii K. Experimental study of vascularized nerve grafts: Morphometric study of axonal regeneration of nerves transplanted into silicone tubes. Ann Plast Surg. 14:235–243, 1985). (**f**) Histological observation at 2 months. Left, nerve flap with well myelinated axons; Right, nerve graft without myelinated axons; (Ref. 3. Koshima I, Harii K. Experimental study of vascularized nerve grafts: Morphometric study of axonal regeneration of nerves transplanted into silicone tubes. Ann Plast Surg. 14:235–243, 1985)

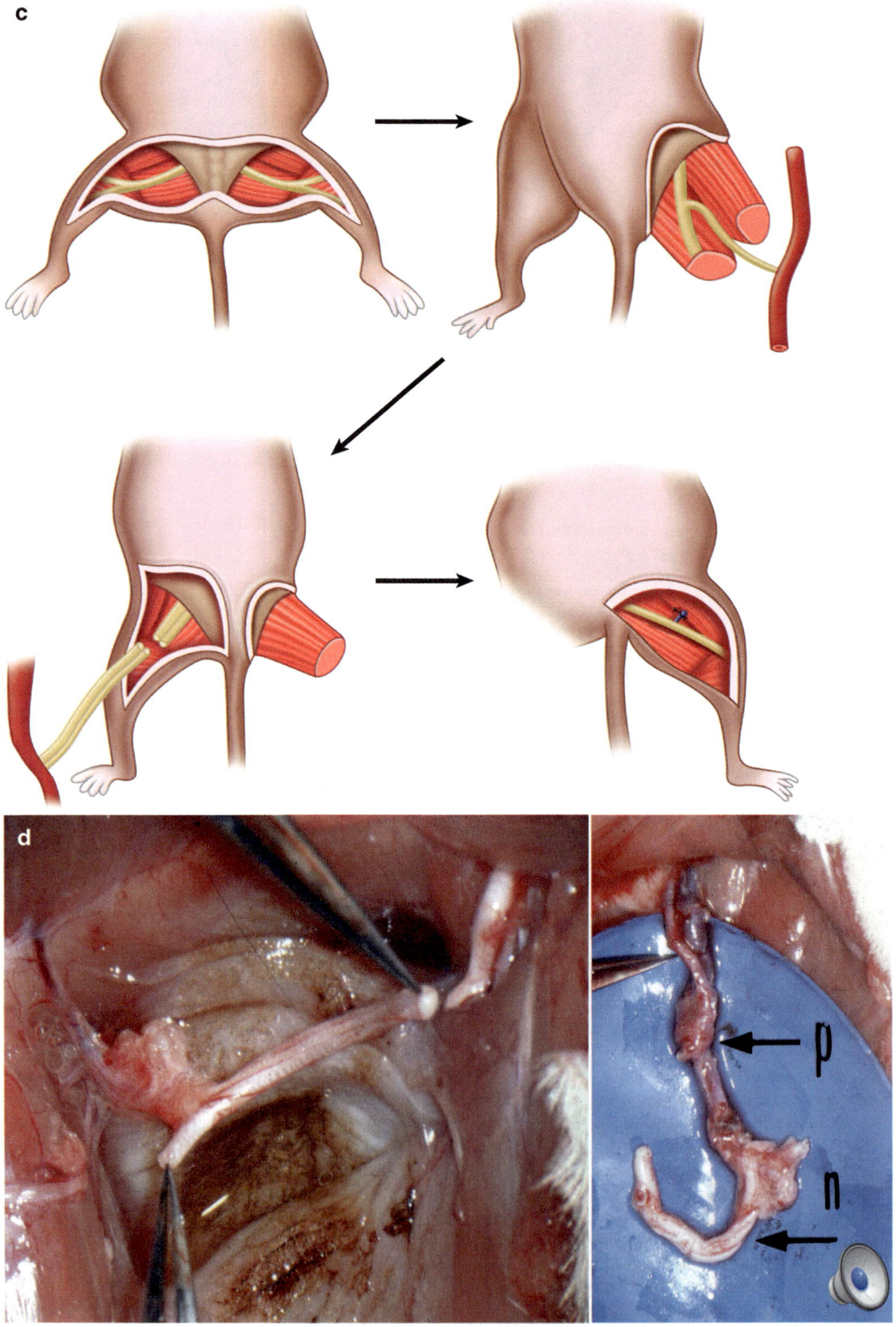

Fig. 36.6 (continued)

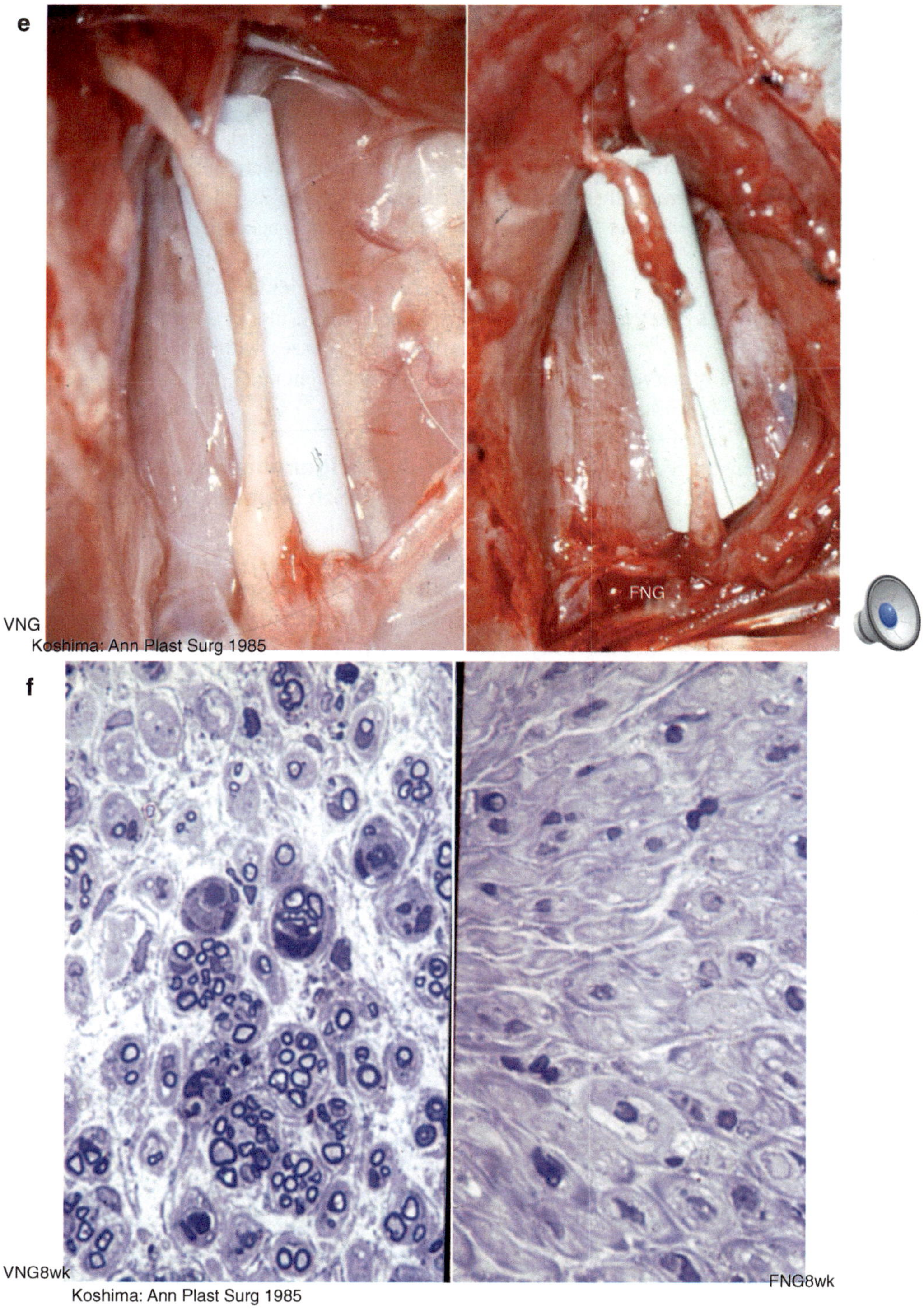

Fig. 36.6 (continued)

from the either distal or proximal stump is preferable. However, in cases with longer digital nerve gap over 20 mm in length, fascicular turnover flaps from bilateral distal and proximal stumps are preferable to join the middle portion of nerve gap. Because excellent circulation of bilateral short flaps can be expected rather than ipsilateral longer nerve flap as in Case 1 (Sect. 36.2.1.1).

36.5.3 Nerve Graft vs Nerve Flap

Regarding the selection of nerve grafting or fascicular nerve flap for digital nerve defects, our cases had not fresh but established scarred recipient beds. Excellent sensory recovery could not be expected with nonvascularized nerve grafts in poorly vascularized bed. Meanwhile, free vascularized nerve flap from distant sides might result in excellent recovery (Fig. 36.6). However, the techniques were complicated, time consuming, and resulted in some donor site morbidity. Our cases with fascicular flap showed good sensory recovery. With these results, it is assumed that the fascicular flap method is superior to other grafting or flap methods.

Regarding cases with facial nerve gaps, some methods using vascularized nerve flaps have been reported from Japanese groups including us [6, 9–11]. The fascicular turn over flap is superior to previous vascularized nerve flaps, because this simple fascicular flap method showed excellent result without any donor site morbidity. Based on our Case 2, longer nerve gap can be easily shortened with lifting up the distal musculoaponeurotic fascia. This lifting up seems to be very important to obtain early nerve sprouting in facial nerve reconstruction.

36.5.4 Advantages of Fascicular Turnover Flap

The advantages of this method are: No need for sacrificing the donor nerve, short time operation, and digital nerve gaps can be repaired under local anesthesia. Fascicular flap is a vascularized nerve flap with fast and accurate nerve sprouting rather than non-vascularized graft. Excellent nerve regeneration can be expected even in cases with longer nerve gap and scarred recipient bed (Fig. 36.6). It is simple and shorter time surgery compare to free vascularized nerve flaps. In addition, there is no functional loss resulted from sacrificed fascicle in the operated area. The disadvantage is a necessity of supermicrosurgical techniques using 50 μm needle. In conclusion, we believe fascicular turn over flap is less invasive and can results in accurate nerve regeneration even in cases with longer nerve deficit and scarred recipient bed.

36.5.5 Trigeminal Nerve Transfer with Supermicrosurgery

Based on our experimental microanatomical studies on peripheral nerves, fascicles can also maintain blood circulation even when the fascicle is separated as a pedicle flap or island flap [2, 3, 12]. This concept of fascicular flap transfer in nerve surgery is based upon the same principles as the pedicle skin flap. However, the fascicular transfer is not as simple because it requires particularly fine techniques. With the recent development of supermicrosurgical techniques appropriate for the microanatomy of peripheral nerves [2, 3, 9, 12, 13], fascicular transfers are possible. Thus it was possible to engineer a new method of intraoral "cross-face trigeminal nerve transfer," used successfully in the context of trigeminal nerve II palsy. Our cases investigating trigeminal nerve transfer show that this method is indicated for patients with long-standing trigeminal nerve palsy resulting from traumatic injuries and cancer ablation.

36.5.6 Advantages of Trigeminal Nerve Transfer

One advantage of this method is that excellent nerve regeneration is expected, even in patients who have endured prolonged periods of trigeminal palsy. In addition, the fascicular flap is a vascularized nerve flap with fast and accurate nerve sprouting in comparison to the free nerve graft. Furthermore, the method is simple and brief compared to free nerve grafts. Trigeminal nerve transfer is a less invasive surgery with an intraoral approach: an operation without visible scarring. It does not damage sensation of the donor and may be possible under local anesthesia. The patients achieve nearly normal sensation on the affected side, not contralateral donor site sensation. This is a completely different result from that obtained wit extremity sensory reconstructions with nerve transfers. Finally, postoperative cortical reeducation may further improve the results of trigeminal nerve transfer. The disadvantage of this method is the necessity of supermicrosurgical technique using a needle less than 80 μm.

In conclusion, we believe that intraoral cross-face trigeminal nerve transfer is less invasive. The method can result in accurate nerve regeneration even in cases with longer periods of facial sensory loss.

Disclosure The authors of this paper have no financial interest nor any commercial association related to the information presented in this paper. There are no conflicts of interest or any funding sources that require disclosure.

References

1. Taylor GI, Ham FJ. The free vascularized nerve graft. A further experimental and clinical application of microvascular techniques. Plast Reconstr Surg. 1976;57:413–25.
2. Koshima I, Harii K. Experimental study of vascularized nerve grafts: multifactorial analyses of axonal regeneration of nerves transplanted into an acute burn wound. J Hand Surg Am. 1985;10:64–72.
3. Koshima I, Harii K. Experimental study of vascularized nerve grafts: morphometric study of axonal regeneration of nerves transplanted into silicone tubes. Ann Plast Surg. 1985;14:235–43.
4. Rose EH, Kowalski TA. Restration of sensibility to aesthetic scarred digits with free vascularized nerve grafts from the dorsum of the foot. J Hand Surg. 1985;10A:514–21.
5. Doi K, Tamaru K, Sakai K, Kuwata N, Kurafuji Y, Kawai S. A comparison of vascularized and conventional sural nerve grafts. J Hand Surg Am. 1992;17:670–6.
6. Koshima I, Yamamoto H, Moriguchi T, Kawada S, Ono Y. Combined anteroposterior tibial perforator-based flap with a vascularized deep peroneal nerve for repair of facial defect. Ann Plast Surg. 1994;33:421–5.
7. Koshima I, Okumoto K, Umeda N, et al. Free vascularized deep peroneal nerve grafts. J Reconstr Microsurg. 1996;12:131–41.
8. Koshima I, Nanba Y, Tsutsui T, Takahashi Y, Kawai A. Vascularized femoral nerve graft with anterolateral thigh true perforator flap for massive defects after cancer ablation in the upper arm. J Reconstr Micosurg. 2003;19:299–302.
9. Koshima I, Nanba Y, Tsutsui T, Takahashi Y, Itoh S. New one-stage nerve pedicle grafting technique using the great auriclar nerve for reconstruction of facial nerve defects. J Reconstr Microsurg. 2003;19:299–302.
10. Kimata Y, Sakuraba M, Hishinuma S, Ebihara S, Hayashi R, Asakage T. Free vascularized nerve grafting for immediate facial nerve reconstruction. Laryngoscope. 2005;115:331–6.
11. Iida T, Nakagawa M, Asano T, Fukushima C, Tachi K. Free vascularized lateral femoral cutaneous nerve graft with anterolateral thigh flap for reconstruction of facial nerve defects. J Reconstr Microsurg. 2006;22:343–7.
12. Lundborg G. The intrinsic vascularization of human peripheral nerves: structural and functional aspect. J Hand Surg Am. 1979;4:34–41.
13. Koshima I, Nanba Y, Tsutsui T, Takahashi Y. Deep peroneal nerve transfer for established plantar sensory loss. J Reconstr Microsurg. 2003;19:451–4.

Facial Reanimation in Face Transplantation

37

Waleed Gibreel, Carrie E. Robertson, Marissa Suchyta, Hatem Amer, and Samir Mardini

Key Points

- The success of face transplant is largely dependent on the extent of facial reanimation and motor recovery.
- Distal coaptation of nerve branches near the donor muscle reduces aberrant nerve regeneration and decreases the time to functional muscle recovery.
- Adjuvant therapies to improve facial reanimation in the context of face transplant include hyperbaric oxygen therapy, physical therapy; immunosuppressive regimens may also contribute to improved nerve regeneration.
- Standardized outcome scoring of facial reanimation after face transplant is necessary to compare outcomes and determine best practices.

W. Gibreel · M. Suchyta · S. Mardini (✉)
Division of Plastic Surgery, Department of Surgery, Mayo Clinic, Rochester, MN, USA
e-mail: Mardini.samir@mayo.edu

C. E. Robertson
Department of Neurology, Mayo Clinic, Rochester, MN, USA

H. Amer
Department of Medicine, Center for Reconstructive Transplant Surgery, Essam and Dalal Obaid, Mayo Clinic, Rochester, MN, USA

37.1 Introduction

Face transplantation (FT) is a life-transforming surgery that allows patients with severe facial deformities to reintegrate into society. Facial transplantation can restore orofacial complex function in situations that have exhausted the conventional reconstructive armamentarium [1–30] (Fig. 37.1). To date, over 40 face transplantation procedures have been performed worldwide, [31] including one re-transplant. Success of face transplant, however depends upon the restoration of spontaneous, symmetric facial movement, smile, and emotional expression. Facial reanimation is therefore an integral goal of this life-restoring surgery [32].

37.2 Goals of Facial Reanimation in Face Transplantation

Goals of facial reanimation in face transplantation are largely similar to those of facial reanimation in facial paralysis. In full face transplantation, the general aims are to restore symmetric eyelid closure, brow elevation, competent external nasal valves, a symmetric and spontaneous smile, lower lip depression, and a competent upper and lower lip "oral sphincter" with no synkinesis. These goals vary depending on the extent of the recipient defect and transplanted tissue [11, 25, 26, 33] (Fig. 37.2). In this chapter, the word "syn-

© Springer Nature Switzerland AG 2021
C.-H. J. Tzou, A. Rodríguez-Lorenzo (eds.), *Facial Palsy*,
https://doi.org/10.1007/978-3-030-50784-8_37

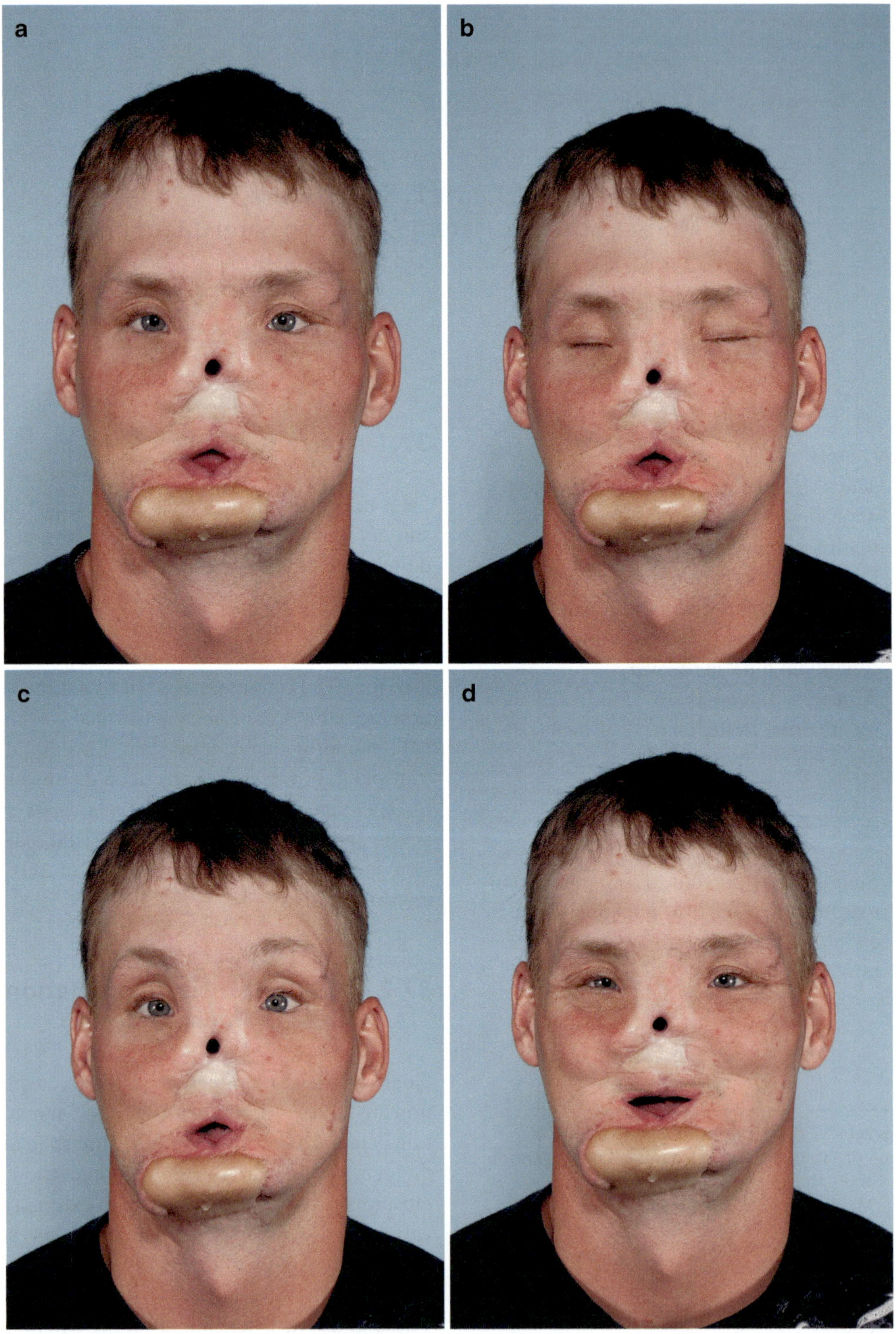

Fig. 37.1 (**a** through **d**) Preoperative photos of the patient showing him in repose (**a**), demonstrating eyelid closure and brow elevation which needed to be preserved during the transplant (**b**, **c**), and demonstrating a smile (**d**). (**e** through **i**), Postoperative views in repose (**e**), showing the preserved eyelid closure and brow elevation (**f** and **g**), demonstrating a smile (**h**) and oral sphincter closure (**i**). (Copyright retained by Mayo Clinic)

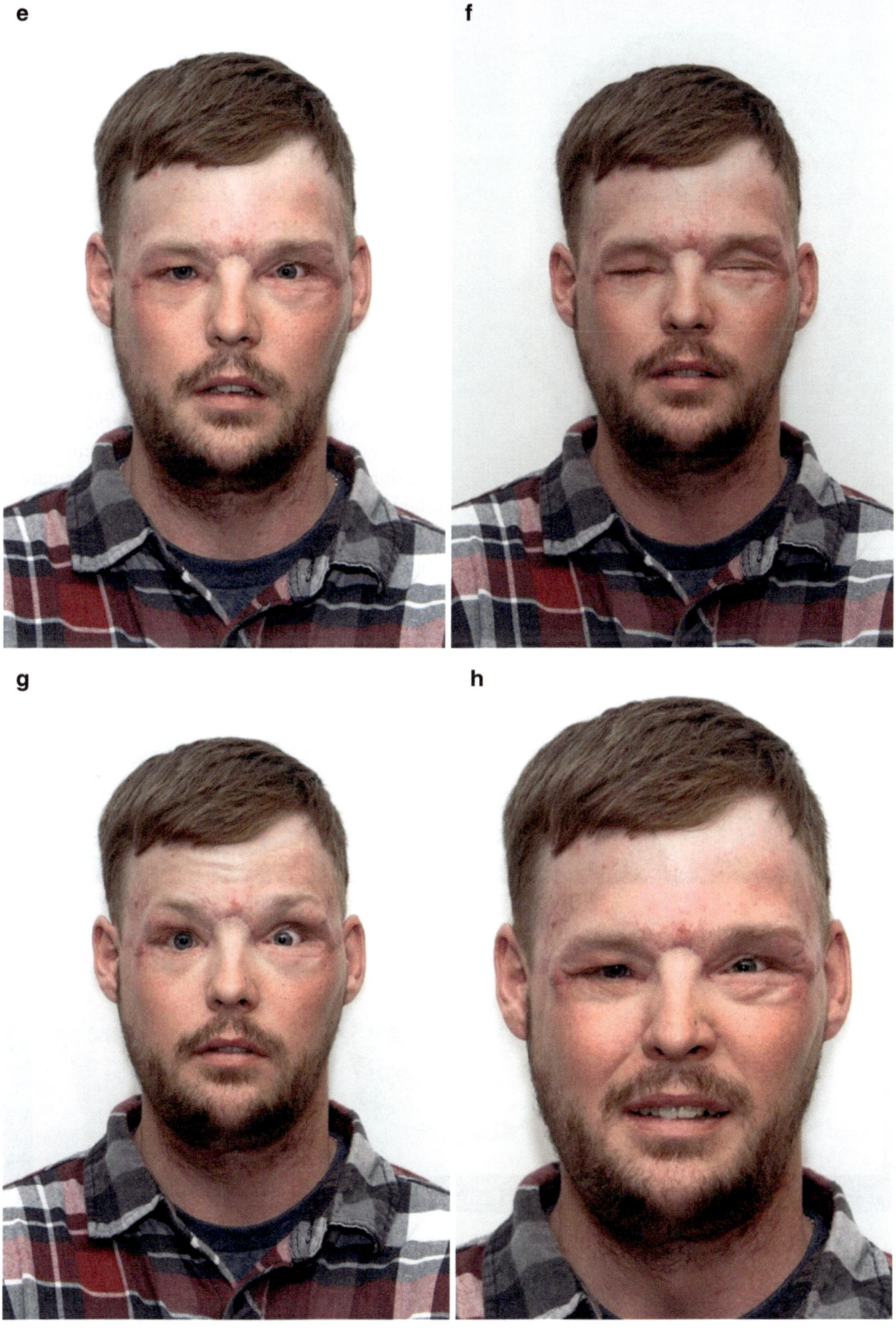

Fig. 37.1 (continued)

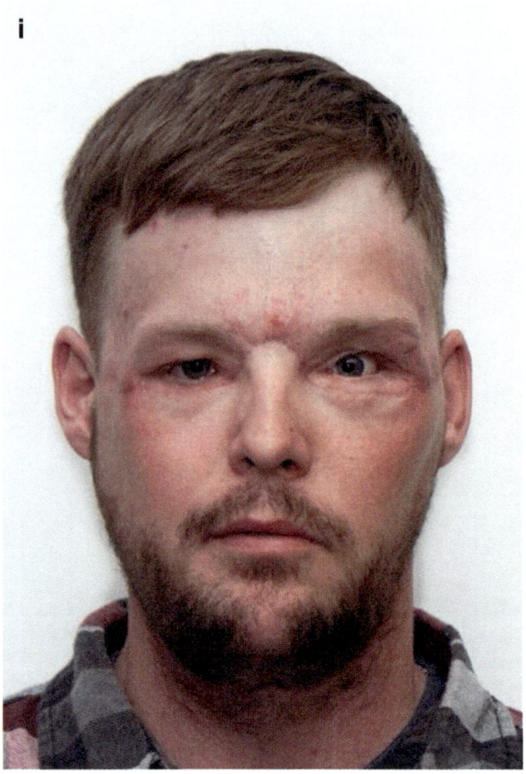

Fig. 37.1 (continued)

kinesis" is used to describe aberrant and undesired muscle reinnervation that results in contraction of muscles other than the intended target muscles; for example, involuntary eye closure with smile. Synkinesis may occur as a result of mass contractions or co-contraction.

37.3 Assessment of Facial Nerve Function in the Recipient and Donor

Assessment of the recipient's facial nerve function begins during preoperative visits. A detailed history and comprehensive physical examination with particular emphasis on facial nerve function are crucial to help understand the extent of the functional deficit of the facial nerve. Information related to prior facial nerve surgeries should be clearly outlined and documented. During preoperative visits, goals, and expectations of facial reanimation should be openly discussed. The patient's priorities should be discussed extensively and recorded. This clear communication between the surgeon and the FT candidate sets

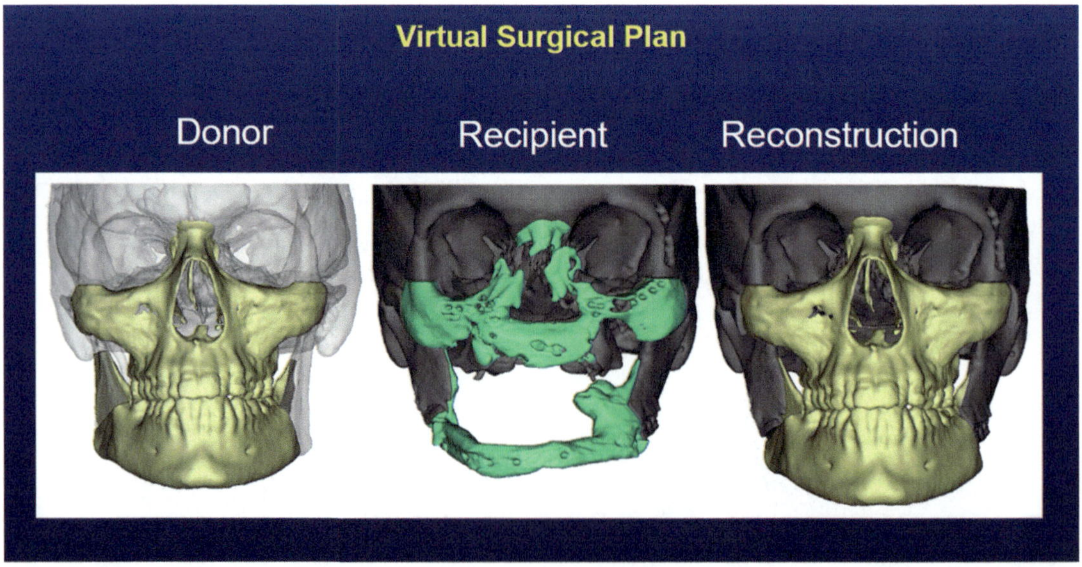

Fig. 37.2 Shows the virtual surgical plan for the donor (left), the recipient demonstrating the extent of the defect (middle) and the surgical transplant (right). (Copyright retained by Mayo Clinic)

the stage for a successful reconstruction. The transplant candidate's defect should be assessed thoroughly and carefully to evaluate the full extent of skin, subcutaneous fat, mimetic muscles, nerve, and bone deficits as each one of these has implications when deciding on the size and tissue components of the face allograft. The function of intact mimetic neuromuscular units should be assessed via a detailed exam, as information gleaned from this exam will prove useful when performing the surgery. In general, intact neuromuscular units should be preserved [21]. Preoperative function of the facial nerve should be documented by obtaining photos and videos that depict different facial expressions, as is standard for facial paralysis patients.

Since preoperative clinical assessment of the face transplant donor is not possible, information pertaining to donor facial nerve function should be obtained from the family by the organ procurement team with a particular emphasis on any history of current or prior facial injury or deformity. This may include reviewing photos and videos if they are available, and careful review of intraoperative stimulation of facial nerve branches at the time of the allograft procurement.

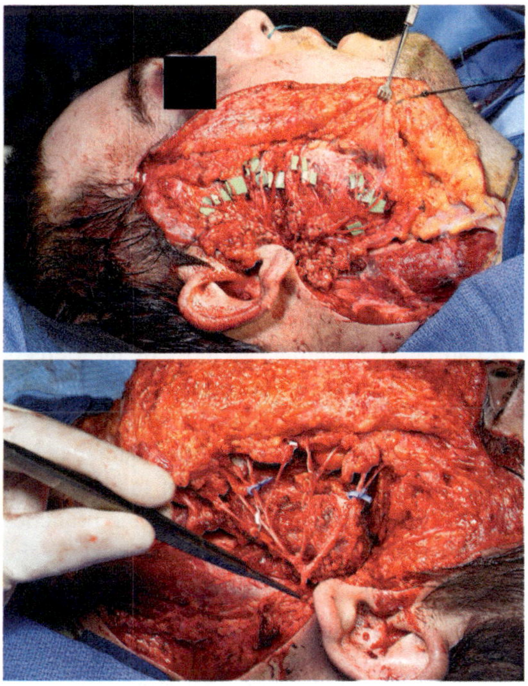

Fig. 37.3 Branches of the facial nerve are identified in the donor as they exit the parotid gland. These branches are then tagged with either vessel loops or sutures and stimulation of the branches is video recorded to review. (Copyright retained by Mayo Clinic)

37.4 Mapping Facial Nerve Branches During Allograft Procurement

FT donors are usually donors for solid organs including liver, heart, lungs, and kidneys. The sequence of organ procurement must be coordinated with solid organ transplant teams to allow the face graft to be recovered prior to cross clamping of the aorta and cessation of blood circulation. As such, the face is typically the first organ to be procured [34, 35]. The size and tissue components of the allograft are determined preoperatively based on the recipient's soft tissue and bone defects. Typically, pretragal incisions are made and dissection in the sub SMAS (superficial musculo-aponeurotic system) is performed. The facial nerve trunk is identified as it exits the stylomastoid foramen. Superficial parotidectomy allows identification of the facial nerve branches within the parotid gland and to minimize the amount of bulk of the cheek after the transplant. Branches of the facial nerve are identified as they exit the parotid gland. Our preference is to continue the dissection distally (toward the center of the midface) until all distal branches are clearly identified (Fig. 37.3). A nerve stimulator is used to functionally identify each distal branch. The function of each identified branch is recorded and the nerve is tagged to allow subsequent identification. Vessel loops or sutures of different color are used to tag different facial nerve branches. Photos and videos are obtained to show the function of each identified and stimulated nerve. The facial nerve trunk is divided as proximally as technically feasible. The decision of where to divide the facial nerve or its distal branches should be performed after completion of allograft inset and revascularization. Dividing the facial nerve distally during the procurement can result in creation of unexpected gaps during the reconstruction, when nerve coaptation is performed between the recipient's and donor's facial nerves.

37.5 Mapping the Facial Nerve Branches in the Recipient

Mapping the facial nerve branches in the recipient can be challenging, as most of the defects requiring FT involve the central portion of the face. Therefore, target mimetic muscles in the midface region are frequently damaged or absent. If some of the muscles of facial expression are still intact and functional, the branches of the facial nerve are stimulated to assess the function of individual nerve branches. Nerve branches are tagged and photos and videos are obtained in a similar fashion as in the donor (Fig. 37.4). Without functional stimulation, the surgeon is dependent solely on anatomic landmarks when deciding which branch to connect to in the recipient.

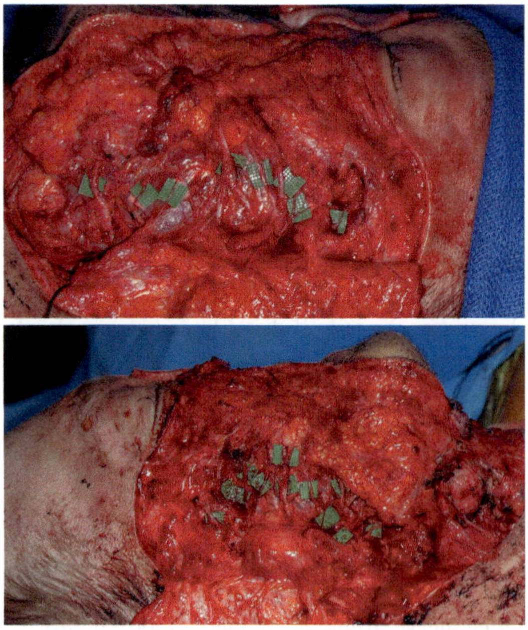

Fig. 37.4 In the recipient, nerve branches are tagged and photos and videos are obtained in a similar fashion as in the donor. Each nerve is tagged with a suture of different color. These sutures are marked on the picture along with the function that each nerve provides. (Copyright retained by Mayo Clinic)

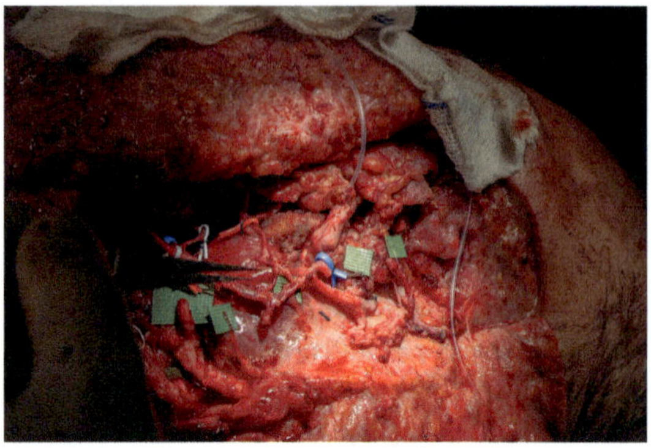

Fig. 37.5 The nerves of the donor allograft, cut as proximally as possible, are shown here overlaid over the recipient nerve branches, but as distally as possible. Video recording of facial nerve mapping in the donor and recipient is helpful when deciding on nerve coaptation of these nerves. (Copyright retained by Mayo Clinic)

Video recording of facial nerve mapping in the donor and recipient is helpful when deciding on nerve coaptation. This enables the surgeon to review the recording and formulate a nerve coaptation plan (Fig. 37.5). No paralytic agents are used to allow for nerve stimulation and observation of the effect on the target muscles. Our preference is that total intravenous anesthesia rather than inhalational anesthesia is performed throughout the donor and recipient surgery until all nerve branches have been identified and stimulated.

37.6 Principles of Motor Nerve Repair

Nerve coaptation takes place following bony fixation and allograft revascularization. When repairing the facial nerve in FTs, tension free coaptation of the donor and recipient nerves should be the goal. If for any reason, tension free primary nerve repair cannot be performed, nerve grafts can be used. The use of such grafts in facial VCA has been associated with satisfactory outcomes, and is described below [32]. Direct nerve repair as close as possible to the target muscles minimizes the risk of synkinesis and unpredictable facial movements [36]. By procuring the entire facial nerve proximally to the stylomastoid foramen during donor dissection and performing the nerve anastomoses as distally as possible in the recipient, one should be able to minimize the need for nerve grafts during face transplantation.

37.6.1 Nerve Grafts to Bridge Nerve Gaps

The use of nerve grafts has been described in facial nerve reconstruction in FTs (Sect. 37.3). Pomahac used a recipient's thoracodorsal nerve from a previous free flap as a nerve autograft to bridge multiple gaps during a full FT [32]. Siemionow has also used a donor's vagus nerve graft on one side and a recipient's hypoglossal nerve on the other side as interposition nerve grafts. These grafts were used as interposition grafts to bridge the recipient's upper trunk of the facial nerve to the main trunk of the donor's facial nerve [6]. In addition to the use of vagus and hypoglossal nerves, the ansa cervicalis has been used to bridge nerve gaps in FT recipients [37, 38]. In general, sensory nerve grafts are associated with less morbidity than motor nerve grafts, but motor nerve grafts have been associated with superior outcomes when used to bridge motor nerve gaps due to the difference in nerve architecture and the higher axonal density of motor nerves [39–42].

Dealing with nerve gaps should be an uncommon occurrence during FT and can be avoided with surgical planning and dividing the facial nerve trunk in the donor as proximal as possible. As previously stated, during the nerve procurement the surgeon should resist the temptation to divide the facial nerve distally, as this can result in creation of unexpected gaps later when nerve coaptation is performed between the recipient's and donor's facial nerves.

37.6.2 Proximal Versus Distal Coaptation

The coaptation technique of the motor branches of the facial nerves has been a subject of much debate over the last few years. Some groups advocate for proximal facial trunk coaptation to decrease operative time and simplify the coaptation technique [5, 10, 37, 43, 44] while others advocate for distal coaptations of individual facial nerve branches [32, 36]. Early reports of return of facial motor function among groups performing proximal facial nerve repair revealed higher rates of synkinesis. To avoid the risk of synkinesis, we recommend that repair of the facial nerve branches be performed distally, as close as possible to the target muscles [32, 36].

In the majority of FT patients, the defect involves the central face and the majority of the central targets muscles and their respective nerves are damaged. In these situations, proximal coaptation to the facial nerve trunk or divisions can be the only available option [4]. Coaptation to the proximal facial nerve trunk does not allow for targeted reconnection to distal nerves and relies on a single proximal nerve segment to reinnervate all muscles of facial expression. Facial movements in these situations are characterized by significant synkinesis [27]. Proximal coaptation thus has been demonstrated to lead to suboptimal results and should be attempted only when distal facial branches are not available.

In situations in which the existing facial musculature of the recipient is determined to be sufficient for adequate facial function and expression, nerve coaptation does not have to be performed [45]. This situation is a rare occurrence in FT patients and, when present, is usually confined to a small area of the face with intact mimetic musculature. Many patients with midfacial injuries have intact eyelid and brow function. Therefore preserving the nerve branches to these muscles is important during the dissection of recipient facial nerve branches.

Occasionally, the distal aspect of the muscle can be missing while the proximal aspect is still intact. In these situations, primary repair of the donor muscles to the recipient's muscles can be performed and has been reported to lead to good functional motor outcomes [2, 21].

Our preference is to perform distal nerve instead of proximal nerve coaptation for multiple reasons. We feel that the chance of aberrant reinnervation is less with distal coaptation. Moreover, the distance to the target muscles is shorter with distal coaptation, which has the potential to shorten the time needed for return of function. Delayed return of motor function can lead to atrophy of the target muscles to the point that may not be restorable with reinnervation. It is also preferable to perform the coaptation to a nerve that produces only one function. For example, if there are two nerves; one produces a smile only upon nerve stimulation and the other produces a smile and eyelid closure, it is preferable to perform the coaptation to the nerve that produces the smile only. This careful selection minimizes the chance of development of synkinesis. To date, there are no published studies comparing the outcomes of these two different coaptation methods due to the paucity of the reported cases and lack of detailed measured functional outcomes. Furthermore, the heterogenicity of defects in different patients prevents direct comparison. Studies comparing the incidence of the synkinesis and hyperkinesis between the two coaptation methods are ultimately needed to determine the method of coaptation associated with better outcomes.

37.7 Nerve Transfers and Cross-Face Nerve Grafts

In patients in whom a proximal facial nerve stump is not available or not suitable for coaptation, nerve transfer (such as nerve to the masseter or hypoglossal nerve) can be used as a donor motor nerve and coapted to the donor's facial nerve either primarily or via a nerve graft [27]. In patients with intact contralateral facial nerve function or distal facial nerve branches, cross-face nerve grafts can be performed and the distal zygomatic, buccal, or marginal mandibular branches can be used as donor nerves [27].

37.8 Recovery of the Facial Motor Function After Face Transplantation

Studies utilizing surface electromyography (sEMG) have reported evidence of detectable signals as early as 1 month following transplantation [46]. Recovery of clinically appreciable facial movement has been reported as early as 2–3 months, with an average of 6–8 months [32, 43, 47].

A period of absent facial motor function is expected following FTs which contributes to the "mask face" look of FT recipients. This period is followed by gradual return of motor function as motor nerves continue to regenerate and innervate target muscles. The speed of motor recovery depends on axonal regrowth of the recipient's nerve past the coaptation site which occurs at a rate of approximately 1 mm/day following an initial delay of about 1 month.

Hyperbaric oxygen treatment has been shown in both experimental and clinical settings to enhance peripheral nerve regeneration [48–55] by reducing the impact of ischemia reperfusion injury, promoting neovascularization, and enhancing the production of growth factors [50]. Hyperbaric oxygen treatment may enhance and accelerate axonal regeneration and could be a useful adjunct in FT patients.

37.9 The Role of Immunosuppression in Facial Nerve Regeneration

Tacrolimus (FK506) has been found in multiple experimental animal studies to accelerate nerve regeneration [56–60] even when allografts are used [27, 56, 57, 59–63]. The molecular mechanism of this enhancement is through binding to FKBP-12 and inhibition of calcineurin, which increases the phosphorylation of several substrate molecules such as growth-associated protein- 43.

This protein plays an important role in neural plasticity and is highly expressed in regenerative growth cones [64]. In addition, non-immunosuppressant derivatives of FK506 do not inhibit calcineurin, but do accelerate nerve regeneration [61]. The effects of Tacrolimus in accelerating nerve regeneration may explain the early return of facial motor function observed in some of the face transplant recipients.

37.10 Treatment of Suboptimal Recovery of Facial Motor Function

Irreversible changes to the facial neuromuscular units can occur following a prolonged period of denervation that exceeds 12 months. Therefore, early identification and intervention has the potential to restore facial motor function. Regular and frequent clinical and electromyographic evaluation of FT recipients provides invaluable information that can guide subsequent management. We recommend that these evaluations occur at intervals not exceeding three months. In cases of suboptimal return or no return of motor function at 9–12 months following FT, nerve transfer should be considered [32]. Pomahac et al. reported the first and only FT case to undergo a nerve transfer procedure to restore animation. They performed a nerve to masseter transfer using a great auricular interposition nerve graft following a unilateral lack of motor function return at 11 months in a fullface transplant recipient [32]. Regional muscle transfer, cross-face nerve grafts, and free functional muscle transfers for facial reanimation in the FT recipients have not yet been described.

37.11 Sensory Recovery, Trigeminofacial Communication, and Their Role in Motor Function Recovery

Restoration of facial sensation has not received the same attention as the recovery of motor function [65]. Among FT recipients, thermal and mechanical sensation can occur as early as 3 months after surgery [5, 14] with satisfactory sensory restoration often by 8 months (defined by recovery of heat and cold sensation, discrimination of light touch assessed by static monofilament, well localized two-point touch discrimination, and response to painful stimuli) [3, 5, 14, 43, 47].

Cutaneous branches of all three divisions of the trigeminal nerve and the great auricular nerve show plexiform connections with the terminal rami of the facial nerve. These trigeminofacial communications can occur either in the proximal (auriculotemporal, great auricular) or distal (supraorbital, infraorbital, buccinators, mental) region of the facial nerve distribution [65]. Although there is no common agreement on the function of the nerve fibers in the communicating rami, it has been suggested that the trigeminal nerve fibers in the communicating rami convey the proprioception of the mimetic muscles [66]. In addition, it has been shown that the trigeminofacial communications could also provide additional motor supply to the superficial facial musculature; some investigators hypothesize the presence of a sensory component in the facial nerve that explains the preservation of deep facial sensation after trigeminal neurectomy [65, 67].

Despite the variation in the technique (end-to-end mental and infraorbital neurorrhaphy versus simple placement of the mental and infraorbital nerves near their respective foramina) and sensory nerve repair technique among transplant centers, sensory recovery has been reported even when neurorrhaphy was not performed [47]. This recovery of sensory function when sensory neurorrhaphy was not performed has been attributed to many factors. Possible mechanisms include the presence of alternative sensory pathways such as trigeminofacial communications, somatic afferents of the facial nerve, the presence of nervi nervosum of the facial nerve, somatic afferents of the facial nerve, the adrenergic fibers around the allograft's vascular pedicle [65], or the retention of facial corpuscles within the allograft [68]. The restoration of sympathetic innervation of the skin contributes to the restoration of thermal regulation mechanisms of the graft [65].

These observations highlight the complex interplay between the trigeminal and facial nerves and the potential positive influence of normal facial sensation on optimal motor recovery among FT recipients. Further studies are needed to clearly assess the role of neurorrhaphy in affecting the rate, integrity, and topography of facial sensory innervation [47].

37.12 Synkinesis in Face Transplant Patients

Synkinesis following facial nerve reconstruction in FT has been reported with both proximal and distal coaptations, although distal coaptation closer to the target muscles is hypothesized to be associated with less synkinesis [31, 32]. Biofeedback, botulinum toxin injection, selective neurectomies, and myectomies have all been described in the management of post-facial paralysis synkinesis [69–72]. Neither the effectiveness nor the safety of these strategies has been investigated in the management of synkinesis in FT patients.

Revision surgeries, including facial nerve coaptations, have been successfully and safely performed in FT recipients while on maintenance immunosuppressive treatment [5, 28, 30]. If biofeedback is not successful in alleviating synkinesis, selective neurectomy or myectomy could be considered.

In an experimental transplantation model, botulinum toxin A was found to have properties that may increase allograft acceptance by stimulating VEGF expression, a mediator of angiogenesis. Additionally, botulinum toxin A was also demonstrated to inhibit CD4 expression, which is a surface marker of immune cells such as T helper cells, monocytes, macrophages, and dendritic cells [73]. No clinical study has evaluated the effect of botulinum toxin A or antitoxin antibodies on allograft survival, immunologic tolerance, or interaction with the other immunosuppressive regimens in FT patients. Therefore, the safety of botulinum toxin in the treatment of synkinesis in FT patients is yet to be determined.

37.13 Physical Therapy and Rehabilitation

Early initiation of a physical, biofeedback-driven exercise program, and neuromuscular rehabilitation is paramount to the success of FT [22, 32, 46, 74]. Personalized rehabilitation programs, cognitive rehabilitation, and functional electrical stimulation are beneficial in improving facial emotional expressions and restoring symmetric voluntary and spontaneous facial movements in FT patients [46]. Regular participation in rehabilitative programs also allows early identification and treatment of synkinesis via mirror feedback and muscle retraining [69]. Surface EMG has been used in FT patients to detect early development and treatment of synkinesis [46].

37.14 Reporting and Comparison of Surgical Outcomes

Accurate assessment and comparison of facial motor function among FT recipients is challenging for many reasons. Bone and soft tissue defects in FT patients are heterogeneous and each patient has a unique profile of functional and aesthetic challenges addressed by the FT. Moreover, underreporting of the return of motor function following FTs is another obstacle to accurate assessment of motor function outcomes following FT [13, 15, 16, 75]. Even among the majority of reported cases, facial nerve function is not discussed in a detailed manner that permits comprehensive assessment of subtleties of facial nerve motor function, such as synkinesis [22]. Rodriguez and colleagues have reviewed the outcomes of 28 FTs performed between 2005 and 2013 [47]. In 13 out of 28 patients, recovery of motor nerve function was not reported. Even among the remaining 15 patients in whom motor nerve recovery was reported, the report of outcomes was not clearly detailed or comprehensive. As more surgeries are performed and reported, data pertaining to facial nerve function following transplantation will become available. This additional information will hopefully enhance our understanding of the complexities of facial reanimation following face transplant.

However, to ultimately compare outcomes pertaining to facial nerve motor function, a standardized tool allowing measurement of facial nerve motor function with precision and accuracy is needed. Multiple assessment tools have been used to evaluate motor function recovery in FT recipients, including manual muscle testing [22, 32], EMG [21, 22, 43], Sunnybrook Facial Grading System (measures voluntary muscle movement, symmetry, and synkinesis) [32, 76] and Facial Disability Index (FDB) [77], in addition to others [78]. The lack of precise and standardized tool has led to the proposal of utilizing computerized video analysis software of objective, precise and reproducible analysis of facial movements and functions after FT [79]. The presence and utilization of a standardized reporting tool is needed to enhance our ability to understand challenges facing the field of FT in general and, more specifically, to evaluate facial nerve motor function and facial expression among face transplant recipients.

References

1. Siemionow M, Ozturk C. An update on facial transplantation cases performed between 2005 and 2010. Plast Reconstr Surg. 2011;128(6):707e–20e.
2. Devauchelle B, Badet L, Lengele B, Morelon E, Testelin S, Michallet M, et al. First human face allograft: early report. Lancet. 2006;368(9531):203–9.
3. Dubernard JM, Lengele B, Morelon E, Testelin S, Badet L, Moure C, et al. Outcomes 18 months after the first human partial face transplantation. N Engl J Med. 2007;357(24):2451–60.
4. Guo S, Han Y, Zhang X, Lu B, Yi C, Zhang H, et al. Human facial allotransplantation: a 2-year follow-up study. Lancet. 2008;372(9639):631–8.
5. Lantieri L, Meningaud JP, Grimbert P, Bellivier F, Lefaucheur JP, Ortonne N, et al. Repair of the lower and middle parts of the face by composite tissue allotransplantation in a patient with massive plexiform neurofibroma: a 1-year follow-up study. Lancet. 2008;372(9639):639–45.
6. Siemionow M, Papay F, Alam D, Bernard S, Djohan R, Gordon C, et al. Near-total human face transplantation for a severely disfigured patient in the USA. Lancet. 2009;374(9685):203–9.
7. Siemionow MZ, Papay F, Djohan R, Bernard S, Gordon CR, Alam D, et al. First U.S. near-total human face transplantation: a paradigm shift for massive complex injuries. Plast Reconstr Surg. 2010;125(1):111–22.
8. Barret JP, Gavalda J, Bueno J, Nuvials X, Pont T, Masnou N, et al. Full face transplant: the first case report. Ann Surg. 2011;254(2):252–6.
9. Gomez-Cia T, Sicilia-Castro D, Infante-Cossio P, Barrera-Pulido F, Gacto-Sanchez P, Lagares-Borrego A, et al. Second human facial allotransplantation to restore a severe defect following radical resection of bilateral massive plexiform neurofibromas. Plast Reconstr Surg. 2011;127(2):995–6.
10. Meningaud JP, Hivelin M, Benjoar MD, Toure G, Hermeziu O, Lantieri L. The procurement of allotransplants for ballistic trauma: a preclinical study and a report of two clinical cases. Plast Reconstr Surg. 2011;127(5):1892–900.
11. Pomahac B, Pribaz J, Eriksson E, Annino D, Caterson S, Sampson C, et al. Restoration of facial form and function after severe disfigurement from burn injury by a composite facial allograft. Am J Transplant. 2011;11(2):386–93.
12. Guntinas-Lichius O, Finkensieper M. Three patients with full facial transplantation. N Engl J Med. 2012;366(19):1841; author reply -2
13. Petruzzo P, Testelin S, Kanitakis J, Badet L, Lengele B, Girbon JP, et al. First human face transplantation: 5 years outcomes. Transplantation. 2012;93(2):236–40.
14. Pomahac B, Pribaz J, Eriksson E, Bueno EM, Diaz-Siso JR, Rybicki FJ, et al. Three patients with full facial transplantation. N Engl J Med. 2012;366(8):715–22.
15. Diaz-Siso JR, Parker M, Bueno EM, Sisk GC, Pribaz JJ, Eriksson E, et al. Facial allotransplantation: a 3-year follow-up report. J Plast Reconstr Aesthet Surg. 2013;66(11):1458–63.
16. Dubernard JM, Sirigu A, Seulin C, Morelon E, Petruzzo P. Fifteen years later: main lessons from composite tissue allografts. Clin Transpl. 2013:113–9.
17. Maciejewski A, Krakowczyk L, Szymczyk C, Wierzgon J, Grajek M, Dobrut M, et al. The first immediate face transplant in the World. Ann Surg. 2016;263(3):e36–9.
18. Sosin M, Rodriguez ED. The face transplantation update: 2016. Plast Reconstr Surg. 2016;137(6):1841–50.
19. Krakowczyk L, Maciejewski A, Szymczyk C, Oles K, Poltorak S. Face transplant in an advanced neurofibromatosis type 1 patient. Ann Transplant. 2017;22:53–7.
20. Theodorakopoulou E, Meghji S, Pafitanis G, Mason KA. A review of the world's published face transplant cases: ethical perspectives. Scars Burn Heal. 2017;3:2059513117694402.
21. Lassus P, Lindford A, Vuola J, Back L, Suominen S, Mesimaki K, et al. The Helsinki face transplantation: surgical aspects and 1-year outcome. J Plast Reconstr Aesthet Surg. 2018;71(2):132–9.
22. Lindford AJ, Makisalo H, Jalanko H, Lauronen J, Anttila VJ, Juteau S, et al. The Helsinki approach to face transplantation. J Plast Reconstr Aesthet Surg. 2019;72(2):173–80.

23. Coffman KL, Gordon C, Siemionow M. Psychological outcomes with face transplantation: overview and case report. Curr Opin Organ Transplant. 2010;15(2):236–40.
24. Pomahac B, Aflaki P, Nelson C, Balas B. Evaluation of appearance transfer and persistence in central face transplantation: a computer simulation analysis. J Plast Reconstr Aesthet Surg. 2010;63(5):733–8.
25. Caterson EJ, Diaz-Siso JR, Shetye P, Junker JP, Bueno EM, Soga S, et al. Craniofacial principles in face transplantation. J Craniofac Surg. 2012;23(5):1234–8.
26. Pomahac B, Papay F, Bueno EM, Bernard S, Diaz-Siso JR, Siemionow M. Donor facial composite allograft recovery operation: Cleveland and Boston experiences. Plast Reconstr Surg. 2012;129(3):461e–7e.
27. Pomahac B, Bueno EM, Sisk GC, Pribaz JJ. Current principles of facial allotransplantation: the Brigham and Women's Hospital Experience. Plast Reconstr Surg. 2013;131(5):1069–76.
28. Mohan R, Fisher M, Dorafshar A, Sosin M, Bojovic B, Gandhi D, et al. Principles of face transplant revision: beyond primary repair. Plast Reconstr Surg. 2014;134(6):1295–304.
29. Roche NA, Vermeersch HF, Stillaert FB, Peters KT, De Cubber J, Van Lierde K, et al. Complex facial reconstruction by vascularized composite allotransplantation: the first Belgian case. J Plast Reconstr Aesthet Surg. 2015;68(3):362–71.
30. Aycart MA, Alhefzi M, Kueckelhaus M, Krezdorn N, Bueno EM, Caterson EJ, et al. A retrospective analysis of secondary revisions after face transplantation: assessment of outcomes, safety, and feasibility. Plast Reconstr Surg. 2016;138(4):690e–701e.
31. Rifkin WJ, David JA, Plana NM, Kantar RS, Diaz-Siso JR, Gelb BE, et al. Achievements and challenges in facial transplantation. Ann Surg. 2018;268(2):260–70.
32. Aycart MA, Perry B, Alhefzi M, Bueno EM, Kueckelhaus M, Fischer S, et al. Surgical optimization of motor recovery in face transplantation. J Craniofac Surg. 2016;27(2):286–92.
33. Cavadas PC, Ibanez J, Thione A. Surgical aspects of a lower face, mandible, and tongue allotransplantation. J Reconstr Microsurg. 2012;28(1):43–7.
34. Bueno J, Barret JP, Serracanta J, Arno A, Collado JM, Valles C, et al. Logistics and strategy of multiorgan procurement involving total face allograft. Am J Transplant. 2011;11(5):1091–7.
35. Brazio PS, Barth RN, Bojovic B, Dorafshar AH, Garcia JP, Brown EN, et al. Algorithm for total face and multiorgan procurement from a brain-dead donor. Am J Transplant. 2013;13(10):2743–9.
36. Pomahac B, Pribaz JJ, Bueno EM, Sisk GC, Diaz-Siso JR, Chandawarkar A, et al. Novel surgical technique for full face transplantation. Plast Reconstr Surg. 2012;130(3):549–55.
37. Meningaud JP, Benjoar MD, Hivelin M, Hermeziu O, Toure G, Lantieri L. Procurement of total human face graft for allotransplantation: a preclinical study and the first clinical case. Plast Reconstr Surg. 2010;126(4):1181–90.
38. Dorafshar AH, Bojovic B, Christy MR, Borsuk DE, Iliff NT, Brown EN, et al. Total face, double jaw, and tongue transplantation: an evolutionary concept. Plast Reconstr Surg. 2013;131(2):241–51.
39. Ray WZ, Mackinnon SE. Management of nerve gaps: autografts, allografts, nerve transfers, and end-to-side neurorrhaphy. Exp Neurol. 2010;223(1):77–85.
40. Bassilios Habre S, Bond G, Jing XL, Kostopoulos E, Wallace RD, Konofaos P. The surgical management of nerve gaps: present and future. Ann Plast Surg. 2018;80(3):252–61.
41. Nichols CM, Brenner MJ, Fox IK, Tung TH, Hunter DA, Rickman SR, et al. Effects of motor versus sensory nerve grafts on peripheral nerve regeneration. Exp Neurol. 2004;190(2):347–55.
42. Moradzadeh A, Borschel GH, Luciano JP, Whitlock EL, Hayashi A, Hunter DA, et al. The impact of motor and sensory nerve architecture on nerve regeneration. Exp Neurol. 2008;212(2):370–6.
43. Lantieri L, Hivelin M, Audard V, Benjoar MD, Meningaud JP, Bellivier F, et al. Feasibility, reproducibility, risks and benefits of face transplantation: a prospective study of outcomes. Am J Transplant. 2011;11(2):367–78.
44. Lantieri L, Grimbert P, Ortonne N, Suberbielle C, Bories D, Gil-Vernet S, et al. Face transplant: long-term follow-up and results of a prospective open study. Lancet. 2016;388(10052):1398–407.
45. Sosin M, Ceradini DJ, Hazen A, Levine JP, Staffenberg DA, Saadeh PB, et al. Total face, eyelids, ears, scalp, and skeletal subunit transplant cadaver simulation: the culmination of aesthetic, craniofacial, and microsurgery principles. Plast Reconstr Surg. 2016;137(5):1569–81.
46. Topcu C, Uysal H, Ozkan O, Ozkan O, Polat O, Bedeloglu M, et al. Recovery of facial expressions using functional electrical stimulation after full-face transplantation. J Neuroeng Rehabil. 2018;15(1):15.
47. Khalifian S, Brazio PS, Mohan R, Shaffer C, Brandacher G, Barth RN, et al. Facial transplantation: the first 9 years. Lancet. 2014;384(9960):2153–63.
48. Bradshaw PO, Nelson AG, Fanton JW, Yates T, Kagan-Hallet KS. Effect of hyperbaric oxygenation on peripheral nerve regeneration in adult male rabbits. Undersea Hyperb Med. 1996;23(2):107–13.
49. Haapaniemi T, Nylander G, Kanje M, Dahlin L. Hyperbaric oxygen treatment enhances regeneration of the rat sciatic nerve. Exp Neurol. 1998;149(2):433–8.
50. Sanchez EC. Hyperbaric oxygenation in peripheral nerve repair and regeneration. Neurol Res. 2007;29(2):184–98.
51. Vilela DS, Lazarini PR, Da Silva CF. Effects of hyperbaric oxygen therapy on facial nerve regeneration. Acta Otolaryngol. 2008;128(9):1048–52.
52. Wei LX, Cao YT, Liu HQ. Effects of neural growth factor and hyperbaric oxygen on nerve regeneration after hypoxic ischemic brain injury in newborn mice. Zhonghua Er Ke Za Zhi. 2008;46(9):714–6.

53. Ince B, Arslan A, Dadaci M, Oltulu P, Bilgen F. The effect of different application timings of hyperbaric oxygen treatment on nerve regeneration in rats. Microsurgery. 2016;36(7):586–92.
54. Tal S, Hadanny A, Sasson E, Suzin G, Efrati S. Hyperbaric oxygen therapy can induce angiogenesis and regeneration of nerve fibers in traumatic brain injury patients. Front Hum Neurosci. 2017;11:508.
55. Tan JW, Zhang F, Liu HJ, Li Z. Hyperbaric oxygen ameliorated the lesion scope and nerve function in acute spinal cord injury patients: a retrospective study. Clin Biochem. 2018;53:1–7.
56. Konofaos P, Terzis JK. FK506 and nerve regeneration: past, present, and future. J Reconstr Microsurg. 2013;29(3):141–8.
57. Shahraki M, Mohammadi R, Najafpour A. Influence of tacrolimus (FK506) on nerve regeneration using allografts: a rat sciatic nerve model. J Oral Maxillofac Surg. 2015;73(7):1438.e1–9.
58. Yeh C, Bowers D, Hadlock TA. Effect of FK506 on functional recovery after facial nerve injury in the rat. Arch Facial Plast Surg. 2007;9(5):333–9.
59. Lyons WE, George EB, Dawson TM, Steiner JP, Snyder SH. Immunosuppressant FK506 promotes neurite outgrowth in cultures of PC12 cells and sensory ganglia. Proc Natl Acad Sci U S A. 1994;91(8):3191–5.
60. Kano Y, Hiragami F, Kawamura K, Kimata Y, Nakagiri S, Poffenberger CK, et al. Immunosuppressant FK506 induces sustained activation of MAP kinase and promotes neurite outgrowth in PC12 mutant cells incapable of differentiating. Cell Struct Funct. 2002;27(5):393–8.
61. Gold BG, Zeleny-Pooley M, Wang MS, Chaturvedi P, Armistead DM. A nonimmunosuppressant FKBP-12 ligand increases nerve regeneration. Exp Neurol. 1997;147(2):269–78.
62. Saxena K, Patro N, Patro I. FK506 protects neurons following peripheral nerve injury via immunosuppression. Cell Mol Neurobiol. 2007;27(8):1049–57.
63. Kim JP, Hundepool CA, Friedrich PF, Moran SL, Bishop AT, Shin AY. The effect of full dose composite tissue allotransplantation immunosuppression on allograft motor nerve regeneration in a rat sciatic nerve model. Microsurgery. 2018;38(1):66–75.
64. Benowitz LI, Routtenberg A. GAP-43: an intrinsic determinant of neuronal development and plasticity. Trends Neurosci. 1997;20(2):84–91.
65. Siemionow M, Gharb BB, Rampazzo A. Pathways of sensory recovery after face transplantation. Plast Reconstr Surg. 2011;127(5):1875–89.
66. Riessner D. Surgical procedure in tumors of parotid gland; preservation of facial nerve and prevention of postoperative fistulas. AMA Arch Surg. 1952;65(6):831–48.
67. Ley A, Guitart JM. Clinical observations on sensory effects of trigeminal dorsal root section. J Neurol Neurosurg Psychiatry. 1971;34(3):260–4.
68. Connor NP, Abbs JH. Orofacial proprioception: analyses of cutaneous mechanoreceptor population properties using artificial neural networks. J Commun Disord. 1998;31(6):535–42; 53
69. Terzis JK, Karypidis D. Therapeutic strategies in post-facial paralysis synkinesis in adult patients. Plast Reconstr Surg. 2012;129(6):925e–39e.
70. Azuma T, Nakamura K, Takahashi M, Ohyama S, Toda N, Iwasaki H, et al. Mirror biofeedback rehabilitation after administration of single-dose botulinum toxin for treatment of facial synkinesis. Otolaryngol Head Neck Surg. 2012;146(1):40–5.
71. Filipo R, Spahiu I, Covelli E, Nicastri M, Bertoli GA. Botulinum toxin in the treatment of facial synkinesis and hyperkinesis. Laryngoscope. 2012;122(2):266–70.
72. Azizzadeh B, Frisenda JL. Surgical management of postparalysis facial palsy and synkinesis. Otolaryngol Clin N Am. 2018;51(6):1169–78.
73. Park YJ, Lee JW, Chong Y, Park TH. Botulinum toxin A increases allograft tolerance in an experimental transplantation model: a preliminary study. Biosci Rep. 2018;38(2):BSR20171721.
74. Perry BJ, Richburg BD, Pomahac B, Bueno EM, Green JR. The effects of lip-closure exercise on lip strength and function following full facial transplantation: a case report. Am J Speech Lang Pathol. 2017;26(2S):682–6.
75. Bassiri Gharb B, Frautschi RS, Halasa BC, Doumit GD, Djohan RS, Bernard SL, et al. Watershed areas in face transplantation. Plast Reconstr Surg. 2017;139(3):711–21.
76. Ross BR, Fradet G, Nedzelski JM. Development of a sensitive clinical facial grading system. Eur Arch Otorhinolaryngol. 1994:S180–1.
77. VanSwearingen JM, Brach JS. The Facial Disability Index: reliability and validity of a disability assessment instrument for disorders of the facial neuromuscular system. Phys Ther. 1996;76(12):1288–98; discussion 98-300
78. Slade GD, Spencer AJ. Development and evaluation of the oral health impact profile. Community Dent Health. 1994;11(1):3–11.
79. Fischer S, Diehm Y, Dorante MI, Kotsougiani D, Kueckelhaus M, Alhefzi M, et al. Software-based video analysis of functional outcomes of face transplantation. Microsurgery. 2019;39(1):53–61.

38 3D, 4D, Mobile APP, VR, AR, and MR Systems in Facial Palsy

Johannes Steinbacher, Aaron Antaeus Metz, and Chieh-Han John Tzou

Key Points

- 3D facial surface imaging systems are a fast, noninvasive instrument, which provides accurate measurement of the 3D movement of facial markings and can be used as an objective system for evaluating the effectiveness of various facial reanimation procedures, as well as for preoperative consultation.
- 4D imaging allows capturing the movement of a 3D surface over time and is therefore especially suited for dynamic measurements, such as facial expressions.
- Mobile apps are a new trend, which will continue to evolve and further support the plastic surgeon. At present, the areas of application in facial surgery remain limited to supporting the patient during rehabilitation, surgical simulations, or helping with the application of clinical scores (e.g., eFace).
- The use of VR/AR offers a fast and patient-safe training to acquire surgical skills and help plastic surgeons operate faster and more accurately and therefore improve patient outcomes and reduce surgical morbidity.

The authors declare that they have not received support in any kind from companies mentioned herein, and they have no conflict of interest regarding the publication of this chapter.

J. Steinbacher
Plastic and Reconstructive Surgery, Department of Surgery, Hospital of Divine Saviour Vienna (Krankenhaus Goettlicher Heiland Wien), Vienna, Austria

A. A. Metz
TZOU MEDICAL, Vienna, Austria

C.-H. J. Tzou (✉)
Plastic and Reconstructive Surgery, Hospital of Divine Savior (Krankenhaus Goettlicher Heiland), Sigmund Freud University, TZOU MEDICAL, Vienna, Austria

Faculty of Medicine, Sigmund Freud University, Vienna, Austria
e-mail: science@tzoumedical.com

© Springer Nature Switzerland AG 2021
C.-H. J. Tzou, A. Rodríguez-Lorenzo (eds.), *Facial Palsy*, https://doi.org/10.1007/978-3-030-50784-8_38

38.1 Introduction

In plastic and reconstructive surgery, many diagnoses are based on visual examinations; therefore, imaging technologies provide essential aids to support diagnosis and therapy. Objective analysis of facial movement is essential to quantify the extent of facial paralysis. This helps to predict the postoperative course of recovery and allows comparison of postoperative outcomes. Quantifying the degrees of facial palsy and the dimensions of facial movements has long been assessed with various grading systems.

38.1.1 Subjective Diagnostic Tools

Subjective facial motion analysis tools like the House-Brackmann, Sidney, or Sunnybrook facial scoring system [1–4], and patient questionnaire, such as the Facial Clinimetric Evaluation (FaCE) Scale, are subject to evaluation by the examiner and may comprise investigator's rating [5]. The House-Brackmann scale for facial grading, introduced in 1985, is the North American standard used for evaluating facial function and classifying facial paralysis [3]. In further consequence, subsections for the diagnosis of facial synkinesia had been developed. These included the "Facial Grading System" [1], the "regional House-Brackmann facial nerve grading system" [6], the "Sydney facial grading system" [7], and patient questionnaires specifically aiming at synkinesia, such as the "Synkinesis Assessment Questionnaire" [8] and the "FaCE Scale Instrument" [5], were introduced. Subjective diagnostic tools for facial function are easy to use and inexpensive, but do not provide completely accurate facial function.

38.1.2 Objective Diagnostic Tools

Sawyer et al. highlight the importance of quantitative analysis of the healthy side in unilateral facial palsy to aid reconstruction of the paralyzed side, as well as the additional help for Mobius syndrome with bilateral facial palsy in recreating the smile [9]. Classic technologies include stereolithography, stereophotogrammetry, structured light, moiré topography, image subtraction techniques, light luminance scanning, laser scanning, and video systems [10].

Objective assessment of facial nerve function is crucial for adequate planning and evaluating therapeutic interventions in patients with facial palsy [11–13]. In particular, the three-dimensional analysis of facial function for pre- and postoperative examination, adequate surgical planning, and evaluation and research in facial surgery has become indispensable [12]. Diagnostic systems that rely on the technique of three-dimensional video analysis, like the "3D Video Analysis System" developed by Frey et al. [11, 13–15], provide both quantitative and qualitative data of facial function [16–18]. Three-dimensional analysis allows the most precise assessment of facial movement. Gross et al. found that two-dimensional analysis underestimates three-dimensional excursions by up to 43% [19].

Chuang et al. developed an objective scoring system for assessing smile excursion that is fast and easy to use. Since the mid-1990s, this has been used at Chang Gung Memorial Hospital for pre- and postoperative assessment of smile reconstruction outcomes [20].

38.1.3 Current Status

Several subjective and objective diagnostic tools have been reported for the quantification of facial nerve palsy. Multiple centers around the world have created their individual diagnostic instruments, but an international standard has not yet been created [21]. A brief summary of the subjective and objective diagnostic of a facial palsy grading system is provided in the following paragraphs. Quality assurance in facial reanimation surgery is essential and requires adequate tools to document the preoperative and postoperative status. Due to the versatile changes of the surface of three-dimensional nature of facial movements and expressions, these set challenging requirements for 3D and 4D systems [9, 10, 22–26].

This chapter introduces the technical aspects of 3D and 4D systems, mobile apps, and virtual technologies relevant for the facial palsy surgeon. Reflecting rapidly ongoing advances in optical systems and data-processing software, this chapter focuses on the typical features and strengths of each system, rather than on technical data, which tend to become outdated quickly.

38.2 Technical Aspects

Most 3D and 4D systems fall into three systems: structured light analysis, stereophotogrammetry, and optical-based analysis of images/frames of videoshots.

Laser- and optics-based technologies for surface imaging have evolved considerably over time and are increasingly used in medicine. Optics-based technologies for surface imaging include stereophotogrammetry and structured light. In the following section, the basic principles of these technologies are presented in more detail.

38.2.1 Structured Light

This technique is probably best known for the touchless 3D scanning of fingerprints. Visualization of three-dimensional surfaces utilizing structured light requires the projection of known patterns such as grids, dots, or horizontal bars onto the desired object. At least one camera from a different perspective is needed to capture the distortion of this structured light from its original pattern. The information is then processed for the geometrical reconstruction of the surface structure.

Imperceptible light, such as infrared light, can be used to avoid undesired interference of these patterns with other imaging software; however, if multiple cameras are used, pictures need to be taken in sequence to avoid pattern overlapping due to the different viewpoints. This results in a prolonged data acquisition process, which in human subjects can be disadvantageous for data accuracy [27].

38.2.2 Stereophotogrammetry

Three forms of stereophotogrammetry can be distinguished: active, passive, and hybrid.

Active stereophotogrammetry combines natural texture correspondences with random unstructured light patterns projected on the surface of the desired object. In contrast to structured light, the camera is not previously calibrated with the characteristics of the projected light pattern. The latter simply works as an additional source for two-dimensional information that can be captured by the stereo triangulation process and converted into a more detailed three-dimensional image. Active stereophotogrammetry resists the otherwise confounding effects of ambient lighting.

Passive stereophotogrammetry relies heavily on sufficient texture correspondences (e.g., skin imperfections, freckles, wrinkles) on the surface of the target object. High-resolution cameras are needed to feed the associated imaging software with high-quality two-dimensional images, which are processed into a three-dimensional geometry model by using sophisticated stereo triangulation algorithms. After the surface has been calculated, color is added by the software. Passive stereophotogrammetry requires careful management of ambient light. In contrast to active stereophotogrammetry, with this method highly directional ambient light can cause glare effects on the surface of the subject, which affects the detail of the texture. Scattered light can produce undesired reflections, potentially disturbing data processing. The detailed mathematical and optical design principles of photogrammetry for the creation of three-dimensional surface images have already been described in detail in the literature [27, 28]. Compared with older surface-imaging modalities, the coverage of up to 360° and a fast acquisition speed are particularly noteworthy.

Hybrid stereophotogrammetry integrates both active and passive techniques, to provide higher quality and accuracy in creating a three-dimensional surface image.

For evaluation of follow-up data taken with 3D stereophotogrammetry, interobserver reliability was less than intraobserver reliability; it was therefore recommended that only one observer should assess 3D stereophotogrammetry data for follow-up measurements [29].

38.2.3 Analysis of Images

For analyzing the images, the patient will usually be photographed digitally or videotaped. To access images from videotaped data, video sequences are edited and saved to image files for analysis.

38.2.3.1 Landmark-Based Approaches

The most common approach to grading facial palsies from a single RGB image is to use facial landmarks. Facial movements are measured by calculating the distance and angle between facial landmarks.

Comaniciu et al. performed tracking of landmarks marked on the face using the software After Effects® CS 5 (Adobe Inc.). A special "mean-shift tracking algorithm" was implemented for this purpose [30] (Fig. 38.1). Accuracy of about 99% was achieved. Landmarks covered by skin creases (e.g., lower eyelid rim) were recalculated with additional software programs [24].

Gaber et al. [31, 32] implemented an automatic system based on Kinect v2 real-time facial recognition software, where there is no need to place markers on the face.

Similarly, Park et al. [33] proposed a landmark-based system using a smartphone video recording (iPhone 4S and iPhone 6) without marker placing, which can distinguish facial palsy from normal subjects by analyzing three states of facial expression—resting, smiling, raising eyebrows—without interference from the recording suroundings (Fig. 38.2).

Other methods, using facial landmark assessment and asymmetrical facial features for objective quantitative assessment of facial palsy, provide promising results, which can be implemented in clinical routines [34, 35].

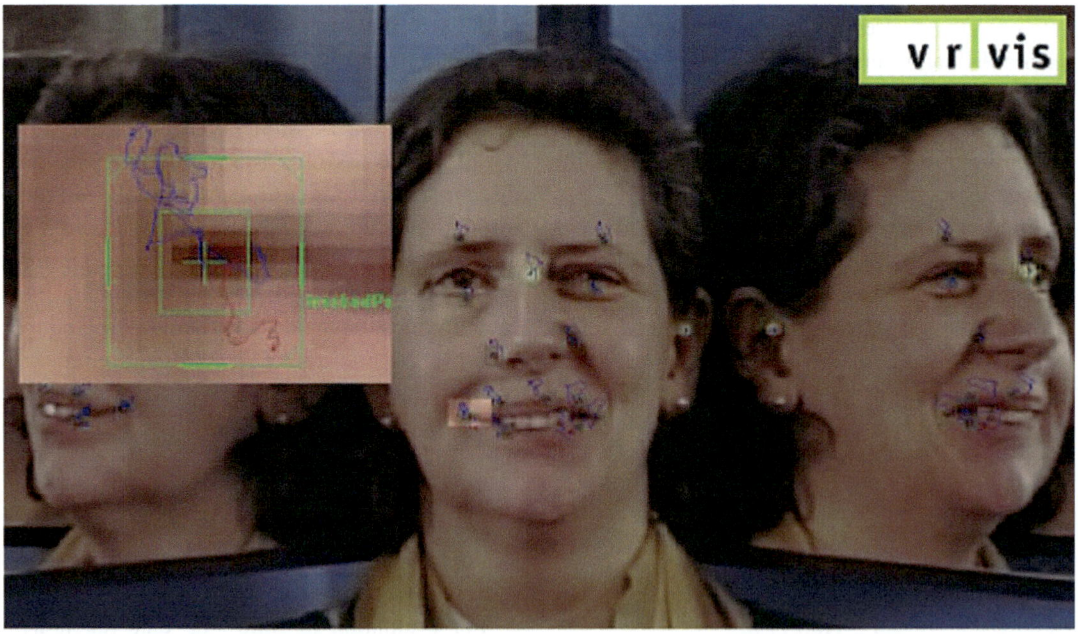

Fig. 38.1 This photograph demonstrates the function of the automatic tracking function of the software. The zoom window shows the tracking of right mouth corner during movement. The red trace visualizes the excursion already tracked, while the blue trace shows the excursion still to be tracked. (Reproduced with permission from Center for Virtual Reality and Visualization Research Ltd., Vienna, Austria, © 2010 VRVis Gmbh [24])

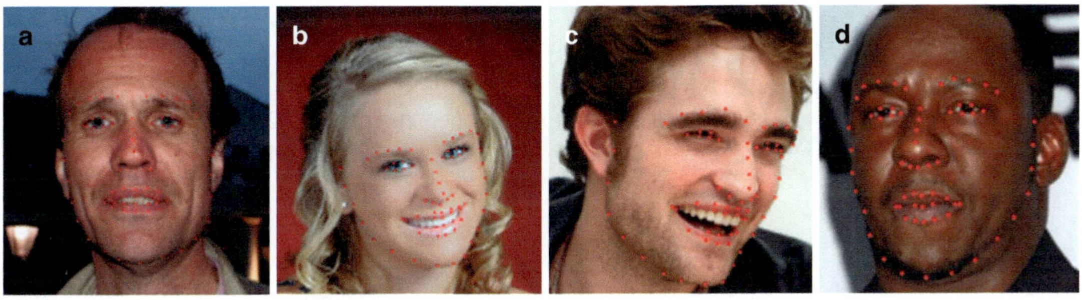

Fig. 38.2 Examples of images analyzed (**a–d**). The red dots represent 68 selected landmarks [33]. (© Figure distributed under the Creative Commons Attribution License)

38.2.3.2 Intensity-Based Approaches

Studies that recommend identifying facial motions using intensity-based features have been rare to date. In 2007, Monhar et al. proposed to use so-called optical flow-strain patterns as a simplified and appropriate method for visualizing and characterizing facial soft tissue [36] (Fig. 38.3). The proposed method has several unique characteristics. (a) Instead of using the image intensity, the strain pattern is used here for grading, as it is related to the biomechanical properties of the facial tissue that are unique to each individual. (b) The strain pattern is less sensitive to different illumination effects and face camouflage because it remains constant as long as the facial changes are reliably captured. (c) No special imaging equipment is required, as photos or videos of facial deformations can be captured with a regular video camera. In addition to generating an "identity signature," the generated facial strain pattern of an expression reveals the facial dynamics of a person [37]. Although this system was able to track almost all (99%) pixels, a 3D calculation of pixel excursion in millimeters was not yet feasible.

The optical flow-based method [38] and the multiresolution local binary pattern (MLBP) [39] showed promising results in automatic objective facial palsy grading. Guo et al. [40] proposed a Convolution Neural Network (CNN) based on GoogLeNet [41] by exploiting pattern recognition methods to perform objective facial palsy classification with a pretrained inception model. This system provided 91.25% accuracy for predicting the degree of facial palsy using the House-Brackmann scale based on a facial palsy image dataset.

Compared with landmark-based approaches by AAM technology [42], the application of a pretrained CNN [43], in combination with the Supervised Descent Method (SDM) [44], has the advantage of numerical stability during localization of landmarks, improved speed, and less sensitivity against slight nuances of facial expressions in the CNN training model (usually standard emotions using publicly available datasets) and the ability to analyze expression of facial palsy that differs from normal facial movements [45]. However, Zhuang suggested that a combination of landmarks-based and intensity-based approaches is essential to produce the most accurate results in facial palsy grading, when compared with either landmarks or intensity approaches separately [46].

38.3 Overview of 3D and 4D Surface-Imaging Software

Advances in optical systems and data processing software allowed ongoing improvements in the assessment of facial expressions. The 3D systems presented below are briefly explained in the following sections.

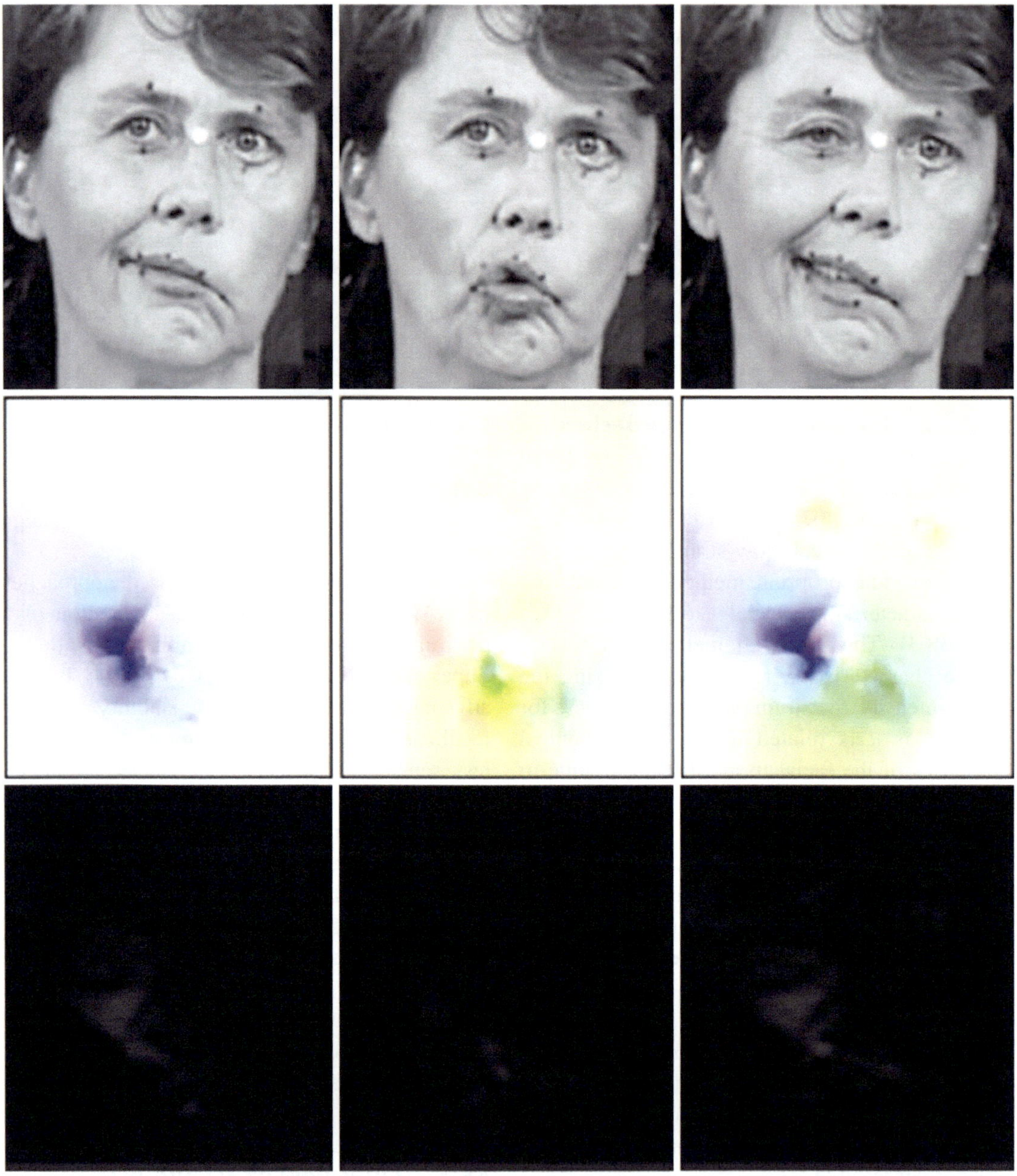

Fig. 38.3 Representation of facial expressions in the form of an "optical flow" (line 2) and as an "optical stretch" (line 3) in the example sequence. Different colors correspond to different directions of vectors; intensity of color correlates with strength of deformation. Whiter regions correspond to higher strain strength, while black regions contain no strain. (Reproduced with permission from the Department of Computer Science and Engineering, University of South Florida, Tampa, FL, © 2010 [24])

38.3.1 3D Video Analysis

The 3D video analysis system presented here consists of a system of specially arranged mirrors, a grid for calibration, and a commonly used digital video camera (Fig. 38.4). Eighteen facial anatomical landmarks were set, which are standardized and easy to reproduce. Three of

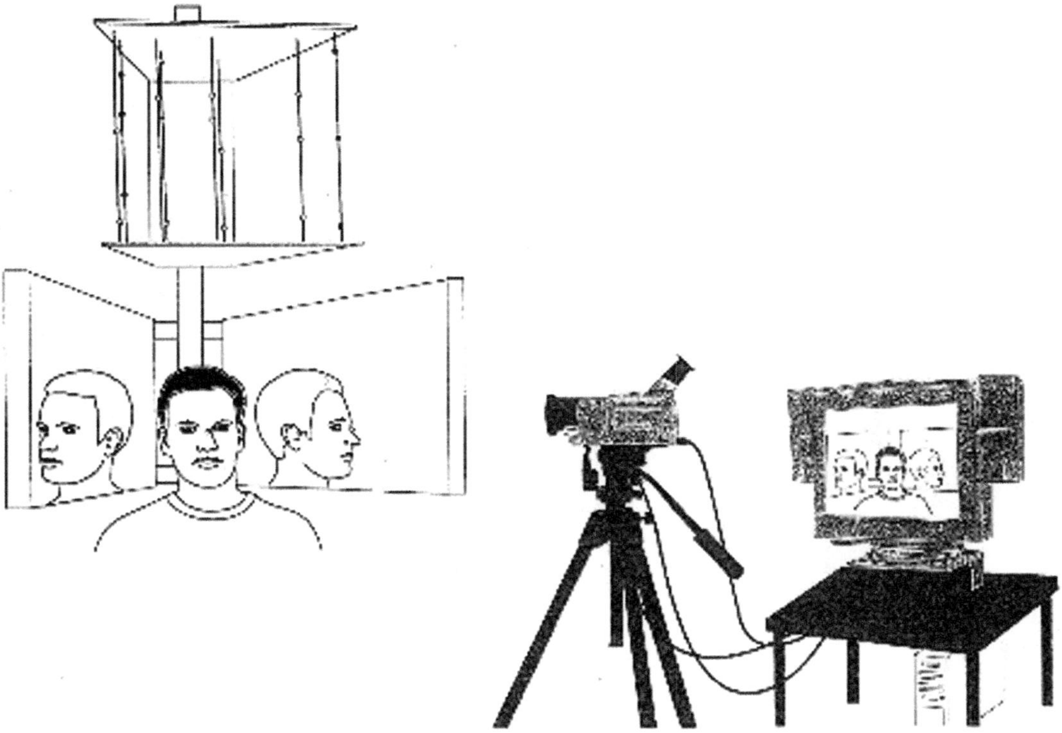

Fig. 38.4 Schematic drawing of the "3D video analysis system" setup. (Reproduced with the permission of Lippincott Williams & Wilkins [47])

them are static and 15 are dynamic. The static points are marked with 5 mm plastic light balls. Black eyeliner is used to mark the dynamic landmarks as 2 mm black dots. All markings, except for the points of the philtrum and the center of the nose, were placed on each side of the face [11]. Frey et al. performed standardized video recordings of the subjects. After selecting the most suitable video sequences, these were edited and saved as video and image files on a storage medium. Subsequently, the 3D coordinates of landmarks in the face were generated using the specially programmed software Facialis®. Visualization of the generated data was done with the FaciShow® program. Both programs were specially developed by the Laboratory of Biomechanics of the Swiss Federal Institute of Technology, Zurich, Switzerland. This allows two- and three-dimensional trajectories of each set marker in motion to be evaluated [15, 24].

38.3.2 3dMD

3dMD (www.3dmd.com), since 1999 based in London, UK, and Atlanta, GA, USA, combines modular hardware architecture with an adaptable software environment. This interchangeability of components and the ability to upgrade existing systems allow for significant efficiency. These modular units consist of industry standard cameras that work with a set of scaffolding and mounting systems. The 3dMD technology utilizes hybrid stereophotogrammetry (active and passive) with software algorithms using the texture of the skin, as well as projected random patterns, to stereo-triangulate and generate a three-dimensional surface image. For the facial plastic surgeon, the following are the most suitable: *3dMDface* (Fig. 38.5), *3dMDhead,* and *3dMDdynamic 4D systems*. The *3dMDDynamic 4D system* enables 4D video analysis (3D over time).

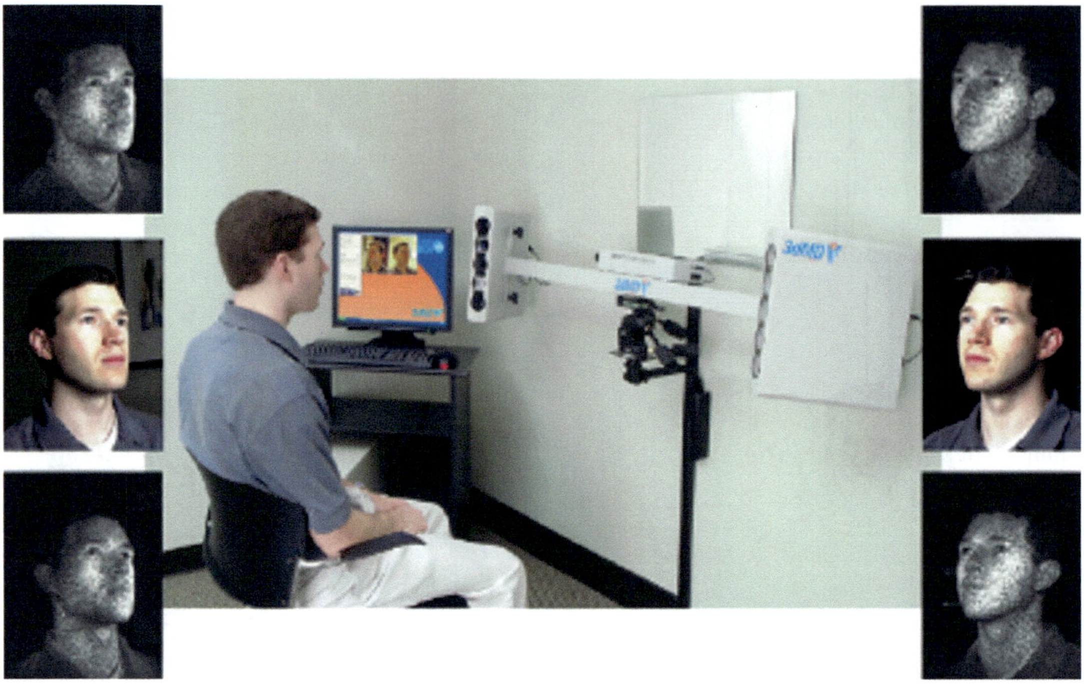

Fig. 38.5 Mounted 3dMDface System. (Reproduced with permission from 3dMD, © 2020)

3dMD provides image fusion software called 3dMDvultus that combines a 3dMD surface image with computer tomography (CT), cone-beam computed tomography (CBCT), or digitalized training models. The program offers a variety of features to help assess patient condition, plan and simulate treatments and surgeries, and evaluate results. Other features include real-time 3D volume and cross-sectional visualization. There is the option to automatically load DICOM with stored orientation transformation. Patient images can be overlaid; surface measurement (distance/angle) and sophisticated 3D landmarking can be accomplished. Of particular interest are the superimposition and thus the comparison of pre- and postoperative conditions as well as the quantitative evaluation of surface and volume changes.

The 3dMDtempus software even allows the analysis of the skin dynamics of the subject in ultra-dense resolution. Furthermore, it allows dynamic analysis of posture, functional motion as well as a visualization of soft tissue deformations in sequence or in isolation.

Several studies confirmed the high precision and reproducibility of the 3dMD Systems. By comparing the data captured with 3dMD's system and Maxilim (Medicim NV, Mechelen, Belgium), for the evaluation of outcomes in oral and maxillofacial surgery, Maal et al. found the intra- and interobserver error of the reference-based registration to be 1.2 and 1.0 mm, respectively [48]. In a comparison with anthropometric landmark coordinate data in terms of precision, error, and repeatability, Aldridge et al. attest to the high repeatability and precision of the 3dMDface System [49].

Lubbers et al. recommend the 3dMD system for evaluating and documenting the facial surface. In a measurement on mannequins, they state the reliability with a mean global error of 0.2 mm (range, 0.1–0.5 mm) [50]. Hong et al. confirmed the accuracy of all landmarks and parameters analyzed in this study with the 3dMDface system by measurements on a mannequin. The mean total errors were below 1.00 mm for both linear and surface parameter measurements [51]. De Menezes found that the 3dMd method was repeatable, and random errors were always lower than 1 mm [52]. Concordance between craniofacial measurements using the 3dMDface system compared with manual anthropometry showed a significantly greater variability in manual compared with 3D assessments ($p < 0.02$) [53].

38.3.3 Artec3D

Artec3D (https://www.artec3d.com) is an international group of companies with their headquarters in Luxembourg, where it was founded in 2007, and subsidiaries in the USA and Russia. Its products and services are used in various industries, including mechanical engineering, healthcare, media and design, and entertainment. Its scanners are structured (white) light scanners. The three-dimensional coordinates obtained in this way are used to digitally reconstruct the real object. Artec3D offers a variety of different formats of 3D scanners, from portable solutions, like the Artec Eva (Fig. 38.6), to the Artec Ray for capturing large objects, like an airplane. For plastic surgery, only the formats Artec Leo, Artec Eva, Artec Eva Lite, and Artec Space Spider are of practical and reasonable size.

Artec Studio is 3D scanning and post-processing software. It guides the user through a series of questions regarding the properties of the scanned object and offers the ability to assist

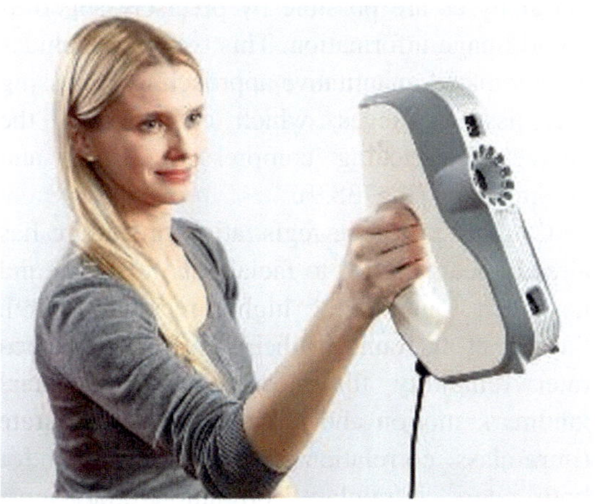

Fig. 38.6 Scanning a subject with Artec Eva. (Reproduced with permission from Artec3D, © 2020)

throughout the post-processing process. The autopilot mode automatically joins the scans within a parent coordinate system, selects post-processing algorithms, and cleans up captured data. Artec Scanning SDK is a freely distributed software development kit (SDK) that allows individual users or companies to modify existing software or develop new software to work with Artec handheld scanners. It comes with tools and libraries that allow users to develop their own scan app to control their Artec 3D scanner and edit the recorded data. It is possible to add support for the Artec scanners to existing software or create a C++ plug-in for any commercially available software.

Koban et al. compared the Artec3D scanner with a reference imaging system (Vectra XT from Canfield Scientific Inc) and demonstrated that three-dimensional surfaces captured for facial imaging by Artec Eva are similar in accuracy to those of Vectra XT reference images [54].

38.3.4 Di4D

Dimensional Imaging (Di4D, formerly Di3D, https://www.di4d.com) was founded in 2003 and is based in Glasgow, Scotland (UK), with a subsidiary in Los Angeles, California (USA). The Oscar-winning company provides systems, solutions, and services for high-resolution 3D and 4D visual field acquisition. Its systems, based on passive stereophotogrammetry, with nine synchronized 12-megapixel machine vision cameras create ultrahigh-resolution three-dimensional surface images able to cover 180° of the face using standard digital still cameras and allow the capture of fine nuances of the unique nature of facial expressions.

Di4D also offers the world's first commercial head-mounted camera system (Fig. 38.7) using passive stereophotogrammetry, remote control, and live recording at up to 60 frames per second. The data video sequence can be evaluated with DI4D optical flow tracking software.

Winder et al. analyzed the geometric accuracy and found a mean error of 0.057 mm, a repeatability error (variance) of 0.0016 mm, and a mean

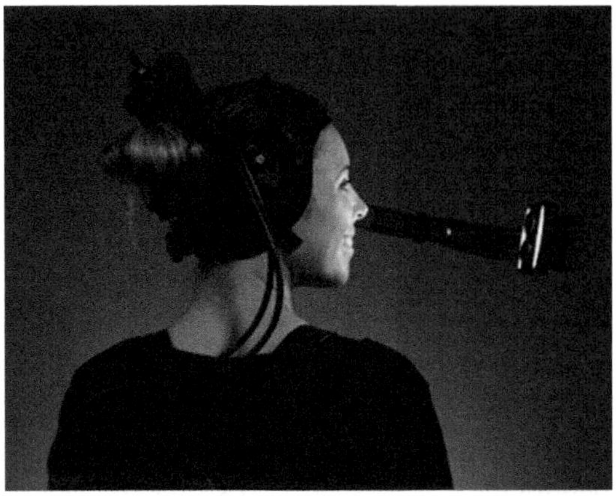

Fig. 38.7 Di4D's portable head-mounted camera. (Reproduced with permission from Dimensional Imaging Limited, © 2020)

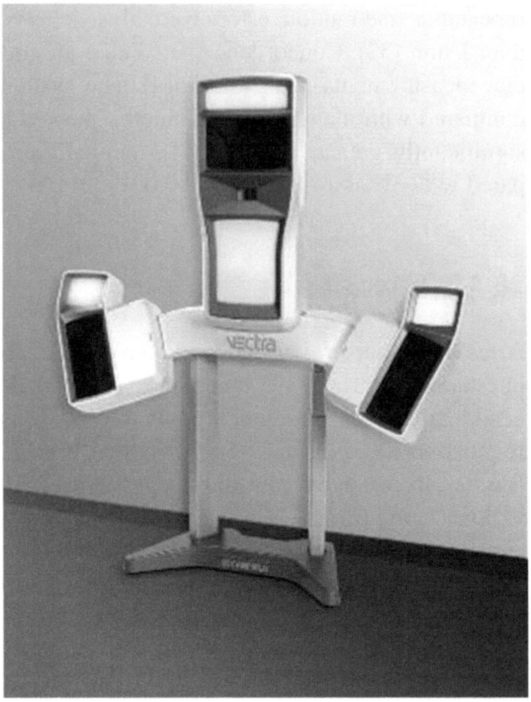

Fig. 38.8 Canfield Vectra XT system. (Courtesy of Canfield, Fairfield, New Jersey. Reproduced with permission from Canfield, © 2020)

error of 0.6 mm for linear measurements compared to manual measurements [55]. Khambay et al. evaluated the accuracy and reproducibility compared to a coordinate measuring machine and found an average system error of 0.21 mm (range 0.14–0.32 mm) [56]. Fourie et al. compared 3D stereophotogrammetry (Di3D system), laser surface scanning (Minolta Vivid 900), and CBCT (3dMD) and concluded that all are precise and reliable for use in research and clinical applications [57]. Wong et al. demonstrated that their digital measurements with the 3dMD system were reliable, precise (with a mean absolute difference across all measures lesser than 1 mm), accurate, and unbiased relative to direct anthropometry [58].

38.3.5 Canfield

Canfield Scientific Inc. (www.canfieldsci.com), located in Fairfield, NJ, USA, was founded in 1988. Canfield's 3D surface imaging systems are based on passive stereophotogrammetry. VECTRA® H1 and H2 are handheld stand-alone units that use precision optics to produce high-resolution 3D images for facial aesthetics, breast and body aesthetics, and clinical documentation. The VECTRA® XT (Fig. 38.8) creates 3D images of the face, breast, and body as 360° images and circumferential measurements.

Canfield's Mirror® imaging software is a fully integrated solution for medical image management, visual communication, and aesthetic simulation. After defining the area of interest, the software automatically calculates the root mean square (RMS) distance values between the facial halves separately for each facial third, thus providing a set of symmetry values. Biomechanical 3D analyses are possible by precisely superimposed image information. This software includes an automated quantitative approach for assessing soft tissue changes, which characterizes the degree of stretching, compression, lifting, and volumization (Fig. 38.9).

Canfield's surface registration procedure has already been applied to facial palsy patients and has been found to be highly repeatable [59]. Sawyer et al. found in their research that intra-rater reliability for measurements of facial landmark motion and angle was very accurate (intra-class correlation coefficients >0.93 for both raters; intra-class correlation coefficients >0.92 for inter-rater reliability) [9]. Oliveira-Santos et al. evaluated the accuracy of the 3D-FACE-Simulator by comparing synthetic and

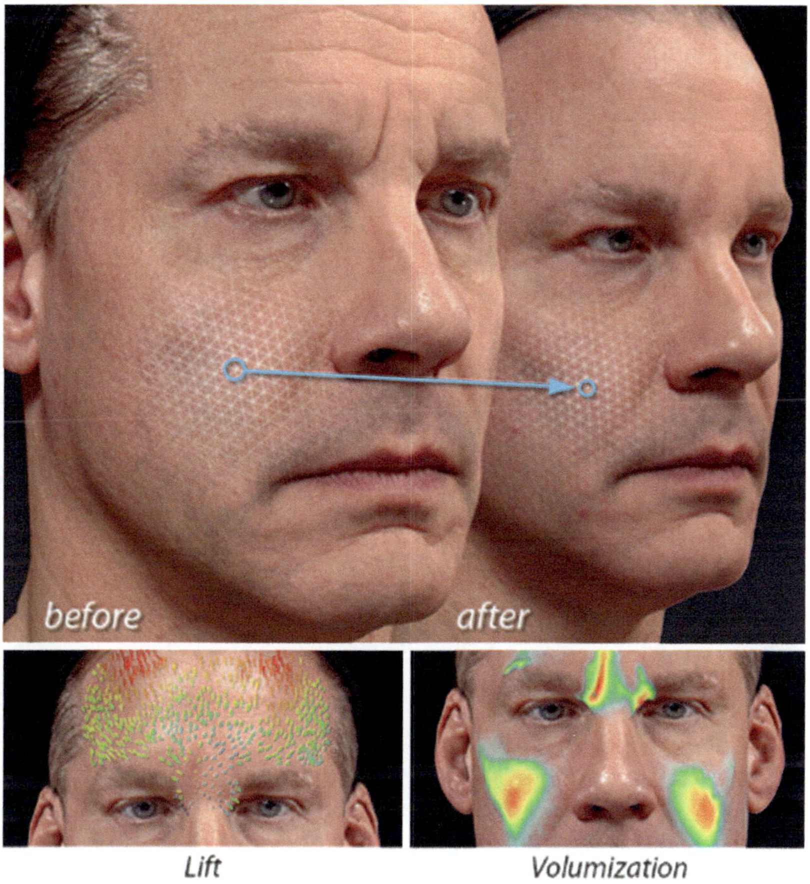

Fig. 38.9 Canfield's software assesses the degree of extension, compression, elevation, and volumization. (Reproduced with permission from Canfield, © 2020)

real faces. Their investigations revealed an average reconstruction error over the entire data set (338 faces) of less than 2 mm [60]. They conclude from their results that the simulation is sufficient for use in consulting. De Menezes et al. showed that Canfield's 3D stereophotogrammetric imaging system can assess the coordinates of facial landmarks with good precision and reproducibility and confirm that Canfield's method is fast and can obtain facial measurements with few errors [52]. In a study by Spanholtz et al., the Vectra technology reliably recorded even volume differences of less than 3 cm^3 and the values measured manually on the body and those measured by the Vectra system showed a mean deviation of only 0.55 mm [61]. Vectra H1 showed high repeatability and is suggested to be accurate and reliable enough for clinical and research applications [62].

38.3.6 Crisalix

Crisalix (http://www.crisalix.com), founded in 2009 and based in Bern, Switzerland, is a leading tech company in the field of 3D aesthetic simulation. In contrast to the other companies presented, Crisalix does not offer any hardware but is purely a web-based 3D simulator for plastic surgery and aesthetic procedures. The patient can be imaged in 3D by either uploading three standard digital photographs of the patient (front view and both profiles) or by using a portable 3D sensor ("Structure Sensor" from Occipital Inc.) connected to an iPad (Fig. 38.10). Crisalix software simulates plastic surgery procedures such as breast augmentation, nose correction, body contouring, and real-time 3D simulations via the Crisalix software. Crisalix software simulation can be

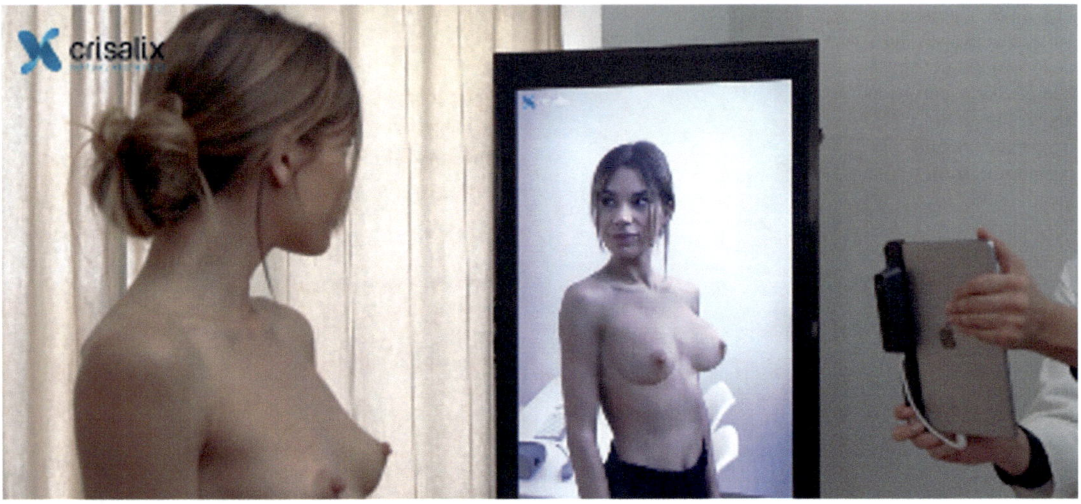

Fig. 38.10 Crisalix live simulation with 3D scanner plugged into iPad and streaming the simulation on a special mirror. (Reproduced with permission. © 2020 Crisalix S.A.)

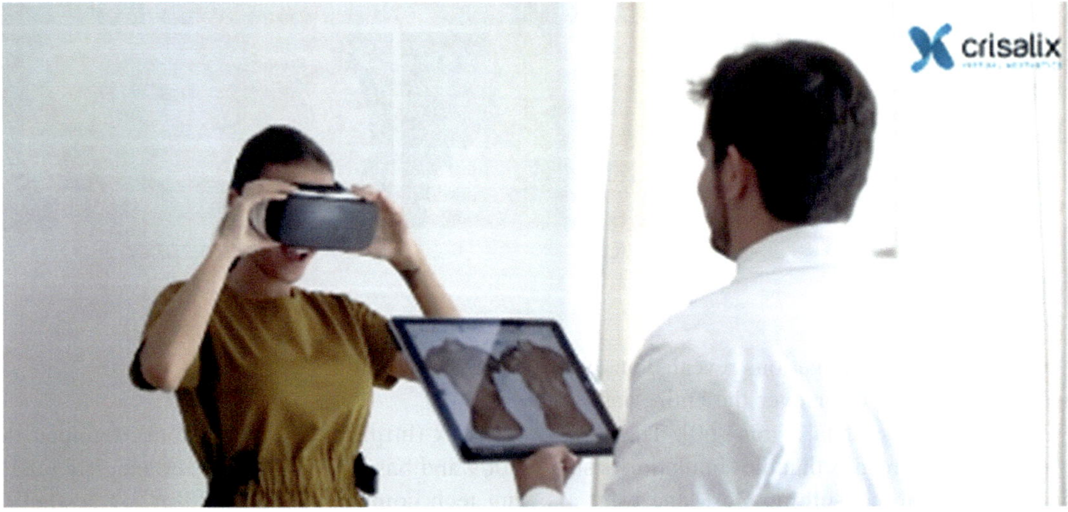

Fig. 38.11 With VR glasses, patients can access the Crisalix virtual showroom, where surgery simulations can be shown in real time. (Reproduced with permission. © 2020 Crisalix S.A.)

viewed with virtual reality goggles: Oculus (Samsung) and Google Cardboard (Google) (Fig. 38.11).

There are only limited data available for validating the Crisalix system. Oliveira-Santos et al. evaluated the accuracy of the 3D-FACE-Simulator by comparing artificial and real faces. The average reconstruction error was below 2 mm [60]. They conclude that the simulations provide sufficient precision for communication between the doctor and the patient to visualize facial treatment options.

38.3.7 Facegramm

Facegramm was first presented in 2016 by researchers in Porto, Portugal. This system is capable of quantitatively and objectively evaluating complicated three-dimensional facial move-

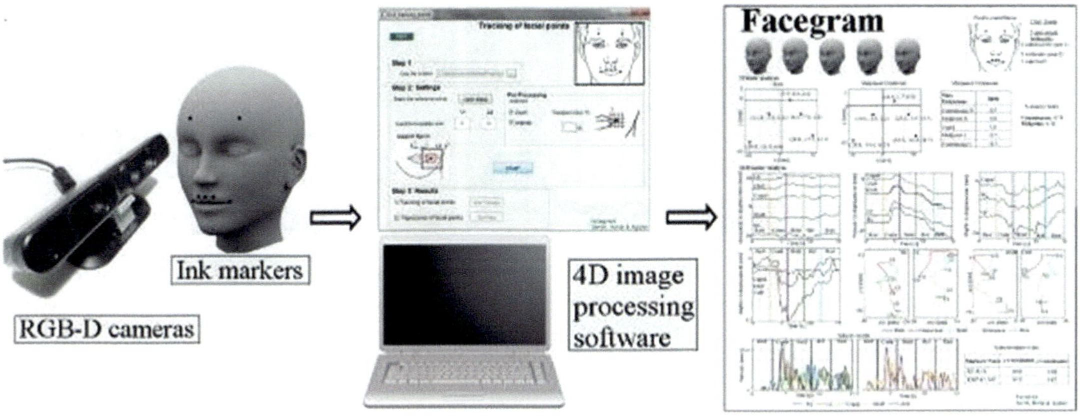

Fig. 38.12 Graphical abstract of Facegramm system [25]

ments by taking a series of static, dynamic, and morphological measurements. Color and depth images can be acquired using specific RGB-D cameras. An algorithm then tracks the location of anatomical landmarks of interest (Fig. 38.12). The system provides useful and detailed quantitative information, both static and dynamic. These characteristics make this system a suitable solution for objective quantitative evaluation of facial movements in a clinical setting [25].

This system has been used in various clinical applications to evaluate facial functions, as in postoperative radiotherapy [63], and in long-term follow-up of facial palsy patients, whose paralytic lower eyelid retraction was improved with midcheek lifts [64]. Validation of this system was performed using a 3D print in an orthogonal three-dimensional coordinate system and resulted in 100 μm accuracy in all three directions [25].

38.3.8 FACE System

Facial Assessment by Computer Evaluation (FACE) software was announced in 2012 by ENT surgeons in Boston, USA [65], designed for 2D facial analysis. This system was built on the "Scaled Measure of Improvement in Lip Excursion" (SMILE) program [66], which used a MATLAB-based image analysis software tool from Mathworks Inc. for quantifying oral commissure excursions.

It evaluates the static positions of the anatomical landmarks in the face as well as the dynamic facial movements. Photoshop (Adobe Inc) is used to scale the images to be analyzed to the iris diameter (11.8 mm) for normalization [67] before assessment. To facilitate measurements with the built-in measurement tool for the areas of interest, a horizontal line is set through the pupils and a vertical line is set to bisect the interpupillary line.

38.3.9 Kinect

Kinect (Version I and II, Microsoft, Albuquerque, United States) is based on structured light technology and time-of-flight measurement. The RMS accuracy of 3D images generated with Kinect I and Kinect II ranges between 0.84 and 2.0 mm [68]. Kinect II was used to assess facial palsy and offers assessment scores according to three widely used traditional grading systems [32, 69]. Various studies have applied Kinect system for automated classification of facial palsy [70–73], interactive oral rehabilitation system [74], and systems that can grade facial palsy to set up a suitable rehabilitation program [75].

38.3.10 RealSense

Studies were carried out in Nijmegen, The Netherlands, in 2017 and 2020 [76, 77], validating the 3D geometric (depth) accuracy of facial palsy patients analysis with RealSense Depth Systems (Intel® RealSense™ Depth Camera D415 and

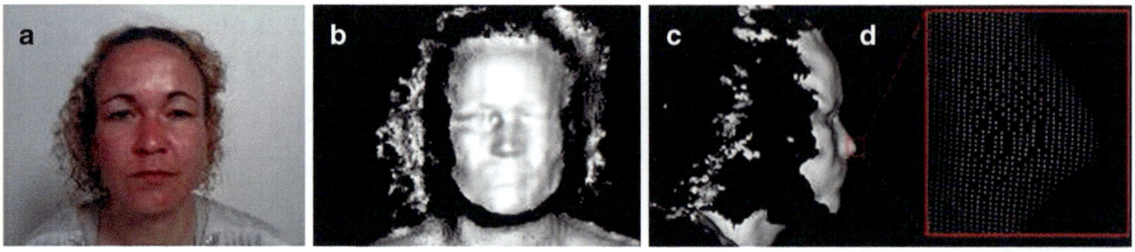

Fig. 38.13 A single frame from a RealSense data set is shown, which at the same time captures the color image (**a**) and the depth image (**b**), by the color sensor and the IR sensor, respectively. The depth data can be also shown from different angles, e.g., from a lateral view (**c**). When zooming in, the individual points of the cloud become visible (**d**) (ten Harkel et al., 2017). (© Figure distributed under the Creative Commons Attribution License)

RealSense™ Camera F200, Santa Clara, USA) by comparing these systems with a clinically validated 3dMD system. RealSense simultaneously captures both the color image and the depth image through the respective sensors (Fig. 38.13). Its measurements and 3dMD measurements expressed on average the agreement of −0.90 mm (−4.04 to 2.24) and −0.89 mm (−4.65 to 2.86) for intra- and inter-rater agreement, respectively [76]. Based on the reported reliability and agreement of the RealSense measurements, RealSense can be considered as a viable option to perform objective 3D facial palsy measurements. These studies were intended to be a foundation for implementing RealSense in a clinical or telemedicine setting, to assess facial palsy patients.

38.3.11 Smart Facial System

Scientist from Rome, Italy, proposed a video system that captures patients' facial movement with gray, circular retroreflective self-adhesive markers. The video was recorded using a commercial smartphone, within a weakly illuminated room, with the smartphone light switched on. Virtual Instrument (VI) software developed in LabVIEW (Laboratory Virtual Instrument Engineering Workbench) was used to grade the patients' facial palsy. Video recordings of patients were assessed by three blinded examiners using the House-Brackmann and Sunnybrook facial scoring systems; the third investigator, an independent technician, performed the assessment using the SMART FACIAL system. Consistency of rating between scores obtained using all three assessment methods was observed in 87% ($n = 41$ patients). Statistical analysis found a significant correlation between these three grading systems ($p < 0.0001$) [78, 79].

38.4 Mobile Apps

Mobile apps for smartphones or tablets are an emerging trend. From playful apps that allow users to apply "beauty filters" to their photos to complex programs that simulate plastic surgery operations on the face, there is a wide variety of apps for smartphones. There is even an app to support and guide patients during rehabilitation after facial paresis. A few interesting and helpful apps for the plastic facial surgeon are briefly described below. It can be assumed that the market for apps for both physicians and patients will continue to grow. VR apps can help not only during the counseling process, but also in incorporating the patient's expectations.

38.4.1 FACE2FACE® App

The Face2Face Facial-Palsy-App (Kapios Health, Toledo, USA) supports the treatment and rehabilitation of patients with facial paralysis (Fig. 38.14). The application uses the prin-

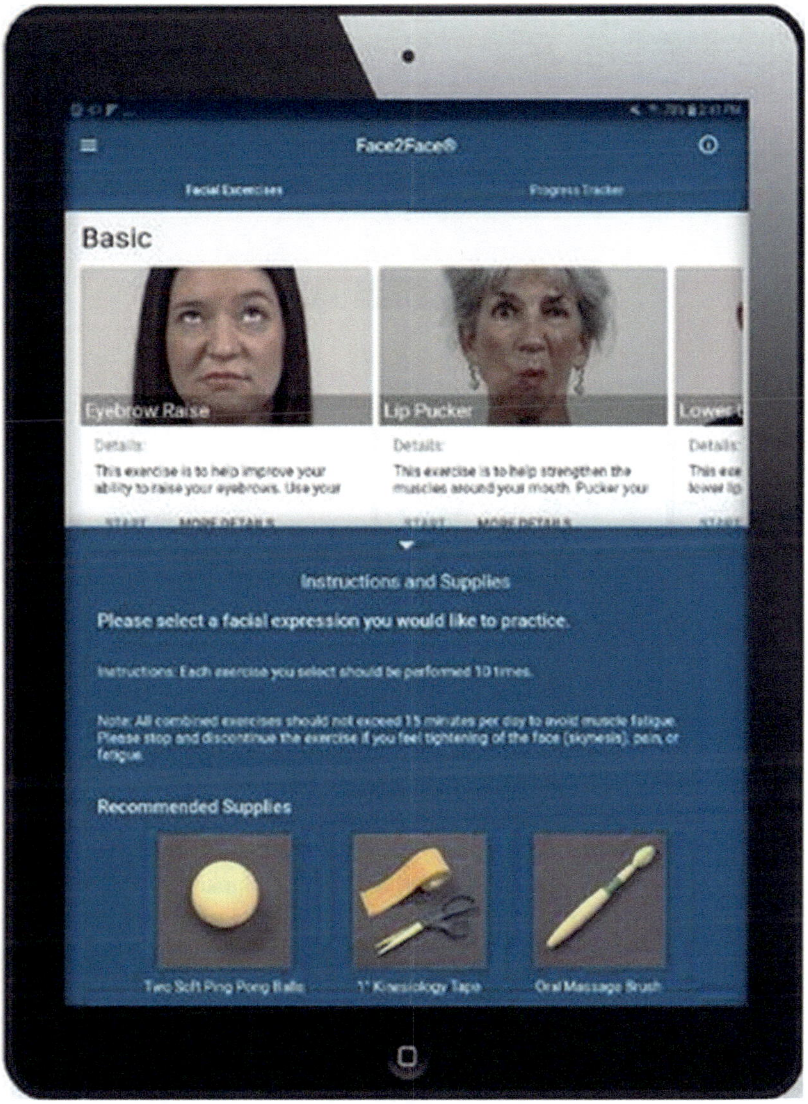

Fig. 38.14 Face2Face Facial-Palsy-App on the iPad. (Reproduced with permission from Kapioshealth.com, © 2020)

ciple of mirror biofeedback therapy, which has been associated with positive results in treating idiopathic facial paralysis [80, 81]. The program works like a double-mirrored slit mirror and projects the unaffected side onto the affected side, creating the illusion of a complete, symmetrical face. This is intended to put the patient in a positive and motivating environment while performing the exercises with sufficient repetition to bring about long-term synaptic changes [82].

38.4.2 eFace App

The eFace App is a Clinician-Graded Electronic Facial Paralysis Assessment (eFACE) by Massachusetts Eye and Ear Infirmary (Boston, USA) (Fig. 38.15). The app is available through the Apple Appstore for iOS devices. This application can be used for rapid quantitative and graphical representation of various facial function values in patients with unilateral facial paralysis using visual analog scales [83]. It evaluates resting

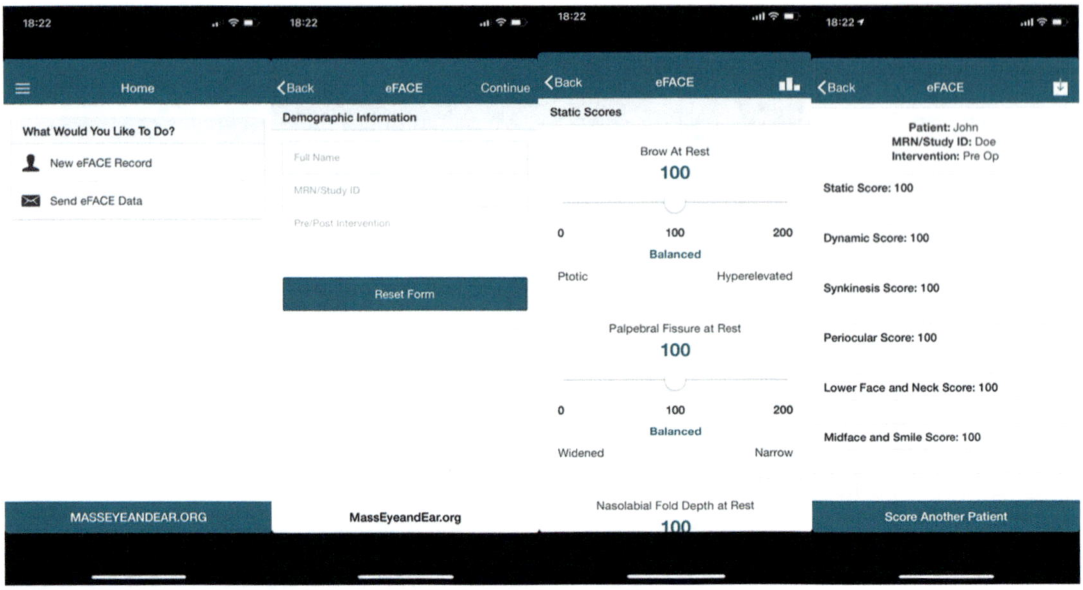

Fig. 38.15 The eFace App for mobile devices. (© Massachusetts Eye and Ear)

(static), dynamic motion, and synkinesis movements in facial palsy patients. It has a high test-retest correlation [84], validity and reliability [85].

38.5 Virtual, Augmented, and Mix Reality in Plastic Surgery

Virtual reality (VR) is the representation and simultaneous perception of reality in a real-time computer-generated interactive virtual environment. In other words, it is a fully immersive experience, where a user leaves the real-world environment behind to enter a fully digital environment via a VR headset. In contrast to this, a user in augmented reality (AR) experiences virtual objects superimposed onto the real-world environment via smartphones, tablets, and heads-up displays via AR glasses or displays. Mixed reality works with digital overlay displays that project interactive holograms into the user's field of view.

The user sees the real world while being able to modify the digital content generated by the device. Control over the imaged content is often possible through verbal commands and hand gestures [86].

These technologies provide physicians with hands-free, real-time access to internet resources, prebuilt content environments, or even electronic medical records. VR is a powerful tool, which is increasingly being used in surgical training for laparoscopic procedures [87, 88]. With AR glasses, surgeons can project details of ultrasound, X-ray, or MRI images directly in the operating area [89]. This feature benefits trainees in technically sensitive procedures by overlaying the surgical field with patient-specific clinical information (e.g., flap perfusion or depth and location of vessels) [90]—which was proven to have positive effects on the learning curve and the improvement of basic psychomotor skills in the operating room [91–95]. Radiological anatomy 3D VR trainings can be achieved by transforming 2D images into a 3D model by using thresholding and segmentation [96].

For highly specialized and complex surgery, it would be beneficial for doctors and patients to train for each specific facial palsy surgery. Region modules for each specific facial palsy surgery can be created with inputs to control the rotational and translational movement of 3D models in the virtual space. 3D models can be rendered to allow users to explore 3D models by using head tilt and controller input, visualizing essential steps and structures during each surgical procedure. These modular VR trainings will increase educational interactivity (www.facialpalsy.eu). VR provides a rich, interactive, and engaging educational context, which supports learning-by-doing and intuitive understanding of anatomic structures in 3D space. With the enhanced learning curve, it raises interest and motivation and effectively supports knowledge retention and skills acquisition [97].

The benefits of microsurgery VR simulators are endless repetitions of surgery, a safe environment for trainee and patients, a return to the training program wherever the user has left it, possible stress-free conditions for best learning, and reduced costs associated with maintaining animal-based and cadaver-based surgical training [98].

In today's society, interest in safer patient and medical staff workplaces is growing. The need for cost-effective training of personnel and the use of live data as training modules to model certain surgical scenarios are increasing. Surgical situations may involve a multiprofessional team of surgeons, anesthesians, nurses, and medical specialists, all working on one patient at the same time. However, existing simulations are focused on monoprofessional training, omitting the crucial communications and interactive collaboration between the teams. Models for multiprofessional medical team training can be developed from following emergency management education that addresses the combination of activity theory and naturalistic decision-making and recognition-primed decision models, implemented to build a basis for a pedagogical model for multiprofessional emergency management training [99].

Virtual Surgical Planning (VSP) is an evolving technology that updates reconstructive surgery with increased reconstructive accuracy, faster surgical procedures, and improved outcomes [100, 101]. AR has already been successfully used in the preoperative planning and execution of various plastic surgery procedures [101–104].

38.6 Telemedicine

Telemedicine is an upcoming technology, which facilitates the exchange of medical information to assist medical staff to diagnose and treat at a distance. Because the numbers of plastic surgery specialists are limited and because plastic surgery diagnoses are based on visual examination, this technology can extend our expertise to remote sites, beyond major medical centers [105]. Telemedical assessment of facial palsy patients with the House-Brackmann and Sunnybrook grading systems was tested and found to be as reliable as face-to-face assessment, but insufficient when synkineses needed to be evaluated [106]. Moreover, telemedicine has the potential to increase the efficiency of postoperative care for microsurgical procedures, improve care coordination and management of burn wounds, and facilitate interprofessional collaboration, thus eliminating unnecessary referrals and connecting patients located far from major medical centers with plastic surgery specialist "without impinging on—and in some cases improving—the quality or accuracy of care provided" [107]. During the COVID-19 crises, telemedicine served as an essential tool, to provide continuous personal medical service to high-risk patients and patients unable to travel long distances [108]. Furthermore, a study in the United Kingdom reported that telemedicine could improve access to the delivery of facial palsy therapy via telerehabilitation, and that "one legacy of the pandemic may be lower organizational barriers to telemedicine, especially if cost effectiveness can be demonstrated" [109]. Telemedicine potentially has far-reaching effects on healthcare delivery—locally, nationally, and internationally [110]. Since telemedicine has been used and expanded by a variety of healthcare professionals, its legal implications need to be thoroughly considered to safely integrate privacy and medico-legal issues of electronic communications into daily practice. Further research is needed to conclusively demonstrate its benefit in routine clinical care.

38.7 Conclusion

Although a lot of research has been conducted over the decades to analyze facial movements, no objective method for facial grading has yet become universally accepted. Surgical therapy results are therefore difficult or impossible to compare [12, 111]. Subjective methods for facial palsy classifications, such as the House-Brackmann scale [3] and the Sunnybrook facial grading system [1], are reliable and easy to apply. However these systems are observer-dependent subjective assessments [112] and have a pronounced intersubject and interobserver variability [21], restricting the clinical use of such subjective analysis instruments, particularly planning treatments or evaluating interventions [13, 113].

Technologies have evolved rapidly over the past few decades, leading surgeons into a new era of opportunity that will transform working as a surgeon, training, preoperative planning, comparing outcomes, and communicating with patients. Technologies used in 3D and 4D imaging systems and in virtual, augmented, and mixed reality are emerging and beginning to be applied clinically; however, more trials and evidence will be needed to define the practicability of these systems in routine work.

References

1. Ross B, Fradet G, Nedzelski J. Development of a sensitive clinical facial grading system. Otolaryngol Head Neck Surg. 1996;114:380–6.
2. Terzis JK, Noah ME. Analysis of 100 cases of free-muscle transplantation for facial paralysis. Plast Reconstr Surg. 1997;99:1905–21.
3. House JW, Brackmann DE. Facial nerve grading system. Otolaryngol Head Neck Surg. 1985;93:146–7.
4. Coulson SE, O'Dwyer NJ, Adams RD, Croxson GR. Expression of emotion and quality of life after facial nerve paralysis. Otol Neurotol. 2004;25:1014–9.
5. Kahn J, et al. Validation of a patient-graded instrument for facial nerve paralysis: the FaCE scale. Laryngoscope. 2001;111:387–98.
6. Yen T, Driscoll C, Lalwani A. Significance of House-Brackmann facial nerve grading global score in the setting of differential facial nerve function. Otol Neurotol. 2003;24:118–22.
7. Coulson S, Croxson G, Adams R, O'Dwyer N. Reliability of the "Sydney," "Sunnybrook," and "House Brackmann" facial grading systems to assess voluntary movement and synkinesis after facial nerve paralysis. Otolaryngol Head Neck Surg. 2005;132:543–9.
8. Mehta R, WernickRobinson M, Hadlock T. Validation of the synkinesis assessment questionnaire. Laryngoscope. 2007;117:923–6.
9. Sawyer AR, See M, Nduka C. Quantitative analysis of normal smile with 3D stereophotogrammetry—an aid to facial reanimation. J Plast Reconstr Aesthet Surg. 2010;63:65–72.
10. Tzou CHJ, Frey M. Evolution of 3D surface imaging systems in facial plastic surgery. Facial Plast Surg Clin North Am. 2011;19:591–602.
11. Frey M, Giovanoli P, Gerber H, Slameczka M, Stüssi E. Three-dimensional video analysis of facial movements: a new method to assess the quantity and quality of the smile. Plast Reconstr Surg. 1999;104:2032–9.
12. Frey M, Jenny A, Giovanoli P, Stussi E. Development of a new documentation system for facial movements as a basis for the international registry for neuromuscular reconstruction in the face. Plast Reconstr Surg. 1994;93:1334–49.
13. Giovanoli P, Tzou C-H, Ploner M, Frey M. Three-dimensional video-analysis of facial movements in healthy volunteers. Br J Plast Surg. 2003;56:644–52.
14. Stussi E, Handschin S, Frey M. [Quantifying facial asymmetry. A method for objective assessment of impairments of facial motoricity; a pilot study]. Biomed Tech (Berl). 1992;37:14–9.
15. Tzou C, Giovanoli P, Ploner M, Frey M. Are there ethnic differences of facial movements between Europeans and Asians? Br J Plast Surg. 2005;58:183–95.
16. Mehta R, Zhang S, Hadlock T. Novel 3-D video for quantification of facial movement. Otolaryngol Head Neck Surg. 2008;138:468–72.
17. Nakata S, et al. Quantification of facial motion for objective evaluation using a high-speed three-dimensional face measurement system—a pilot study. Otol Neurotol. 2006;27:1023–9.
18. Rogers C, et al. Automated facial image analysis: detecting improvement in abnormal facial movement after treatment with botulinum toxin A. Ann Plast Surg. 2007;58:39–47.
19. Gross M, Trotman C, Moffatt K. A comparison of three-dimensional and two-dimensional analyses of facial motion. Angle Orthod. 1996;66:189–94.
20. Tzou CH, Chuang DC, Chen HH. Facial paralysis grading system: a new and simple smile excursion score for evaluating facial reanimation surgery. Ann Plast Surg. 2015;74:210–3.
21. Linstrom CJ. Objective facial motion analysis in patients with facial nerve dysfunction. Laryngoscope. 2002;112:1129–47.
22. Alagha MA, Ju X, Morley S, Ayoub A. Reproducibility of the dynamics of facial expressions in unilateral facial palsy. Int J Oral Maxillofac Surg. 2018;47:268–75.

23. Sigaux N, Ganry L, Mojallal A, Breton P, Bouletreau P. Stereophotogrammetry and facial surgery: principles, applications and prospects. Ann Chir Plast Esthet. 2018;63:62–8.
24. Tzou CHJ, et al. Evolution of the 3-dimensional video system for facial motion analysis: ten years' experiences and recent developments. Ann Plast Surg. 2012;69:173–85.
25. Gerós A, Horta R, Aguiar P. Facegram—objective quantitative analysis in facial reconstructive surgery. J Biomed Inform. 2016;61:1–9.
26. Zhao Y, et al. Prognostic value of a three-dimensional dynamic quantitative analysis system to measure facial motion in acute facial paralysis patients. Head Face Med. 2020;16:15.
27. Lane C, Harrell W. Completing the 3-dimensional picture. Am J Orthod Dentofac Orthop. 2008;133:612–20.
28. Velkley DE, Oliver GD. Stereo-photogrammetry for the determination of patient surface geometry. Med Phys. 1979;6:100–4.
29. van Veen MM, ten Berge JHA, Werker PMN, Dijkstra PU. Three-dimensional stereophotogrammetry assessment of facial asymmetry in facial palsy. J Craniofac Surg. 2020;31:893–7.
30. Comaniciu D, Ramesh V, Meer P. Real-time tracking of non-rigid objects using mean shift. In: IEEE conference on computer vision and pattern recognition, vol. 2. Hilton Head Island, SC: IEEE Computer Society Press; 2000. p. 142–9.
31. Gaber A, Taher MF, Wahed MA. Quantifying facial paralysis using the Kinect v2. In: 2015 37th annual international conference of the IEEE engineering in medicine and biology society (EMBC); 2015. p. 2497–501.
32. Gaber A, Faher MF, Waned MA. Automated grading of facial paralysis using the Kinect v2: a proof of concept study. In: 2015 International conference on virtual rehabilitation (ICVR); 2015. p. 258–64.
33. Kim HS, Kim SY, Kim YH, Park KS. A smartphone-based automatic diagnosis system for facial nerve palsy. Sensors. 2015;15:26756–68.
34. Anping S, et al. Assessment for facial nerve paralysis based on facial asymmetry. Australas Phys Eng Sci Med. 2017;40:851–60.
35. Guo Z, et al. An unobtrusive computerized assessment framework for unilateral peripheral facial paralysis. IEEE J Biomed Health Inform. 2018;22:835–41.
36. Manohar V, Goldgof D, Sarkar S, Zhang Y. Facial strain pattern as a soft forensic evidence. In: 2007 IEEE workshop on applications of computer vision (WACV'07). IEEE; 2007. p. 42.
37. Manohar V, Shreve M, Goldgof D, Sarkar S. Modeling facial skin motion properties in video and its application to matching faces across expressions. In: 20th International conference pattern recognition (ICPR). Washington, DC: IEEE Computer Society; 2010. p. 2122–5.
38. He S, Soraghan J, O'Reilly B. Biomedical image sequence analysis with application to automatic quantitative assessment of facial paralysis. EURASIP J Image Video Process. 2007;2007:1–11.
39. He S, Soraghan JJ, Reilly BFO, Xing D. Quantitative analysis of facial paralysis using local binary patterns in biomedical videos. IEEE Trans Biomed Eng. 2009;56:1864–70.
40. Guo Z, et al. Deep assessment process: objective assessment process for unilateral peripheral facial paralysis via deep convolutional neural network. In: 2017 IEEE 14th international symposium on biomedical imaging (ISBI 2017); 2017. p. 135–8.
41. Szegedy C, et al. Going deeper with convolutions. In: 2015 IEEE conference on computer vision and pattern recognition (CVPR); 2015. p. 1–9.
42. Modersohn L, Denzler J. Facial paresis index prediction by exploiting active appearance models for compact discriminative features. In: VISIGRAPP (4: VISAPP); 2016. p. 271–8.
43. Donahue J, et al. DeCAF: a deep convolutional activation feature for generic visual recognition. In: Eric PX, Tony J, editors. Proceedings of the 31st international conference on machine learning. PMLR, proceedings of machine learning research, vol. 32; 2014. p. 647–55.
44. Xiong X, Torre FDL. Supervised descent method and its applications to face alignment. In: 2013 IEEE conference on computer vision and pattern recognition; 2013. p. 532–9.
45. Mothes O, et al. Automated objective and marker-free facial grading using photographs of patients with facial palsy. Eur Arch Otorhinolaryngol. 2019;276:3335–43.
46. Zhuang Y, et al. Facial weakness analysis and quantification of static images. IEEE J Biomed Health Inform. 2020;24:2260–7.
47. Frey M, et al. 3D video analysis of facial movements. Facial Plast Surg Clin N Am. 2011;19:639–46., viii.
48. Maal TJJ, et al. Registration of 3-dimensional facial photographs for clinical use. J Oral Maxillofac Surg. 2010;68:2391–401.
49. Aldridge K, Boyadjiev SA, Capone GT, DeLeon VB, Richtsmeier JT. Precision and error of three-dimensional phenotypic measures acquired from 3dMD photogrammetric images. Am J Med Genet A. 2005;138A:247–53.
50. Lübbers HT, Medinger L, Kruse A, Grätz KW, Matthews F. Precision and accuracy of the 3dMD photogrammetric system in craniomaxillofacial application. J Craniofac Surg. 2010;21:763–7.
51. Hong C, et al. Evaluation of the 3dMDface system as a tool for soft tissue analysis. Orthod Craniofacial Res. 2017;20:119–24.
52. De Menezes M, Rosati R, Ferrario VF, Sforza C. Accuracy and reproducibility of a 3-dimensional stereophotogrammetric imaging system. J Oral Maxillofac Surg. 2010;68:2129–35.
53. Naini FB, et al. Validation of a new three-dimensional imaging system using comparative craniofacial anthropometry. Maxillofac Plast Reconstruct Surg. 2017;39:23.

54. Koban KC, et al. Validation of two handheld devices against a non-portable three-dimensional surface scanner and assessment of potential use for intraoperative facial imaging. J Plast Reconstruct Aesthet Surg. 2020;73:141–8.
55. Winder RJ, Darvann TA, McKnight W, Magee JDM, Ramsay-Baggs P. Technical validation of the Di3D stereophotogrammetry surface imaging system. Br J Oral Maxillofac Surg. 2008;46:33–7.
56. Khambay B, et al. Validation and reproducibility of a high-resolution three-dimensional facial imaging system. Br J Oral Maxillofac Surg. 2008;46:27–32.
57. Fourie Z, Damstra J, Gerrits PO, Ren Y. Evaluation of anthropometric accuracy and reliability using different three-dimensional scanning systems. Forensic Sci Int. 2011;207:127–34.
58. Wong JY, et al. Validity and reliability of craniofacial anthropometric measurement of 3D digital photogrammetric images. Cleft Palate Craniofac J. 2008;45:232–9.
59. Gibelli D, et al. Three-dimensional assessment of restored smiling mobility after reanimation of unilateral facial palsy by triple innervation technique. Int J Oral Maxillofac Surg. 2020;49:536–42.
60. Oliveira-Santos T, et al. 3D face reconstruction from 2D pictures: first results of a web-based computer aided system for aesthetic procedures. Ann Biomed Eng. 2013;41:952–66.
61. Spanholtz TA, et al. 3-dimensionale Bilderfassung: Erste Erfahrungen in der Planung und Dokumentation plastisch-chirurgischer Operationen. Handchirurgie Mikrochirurgie Plastische Chirurgie. 2012;44:234–9.
62. Camison L, et al. Validation of the Vectra H1 portable three-dimensional photogrammetry system for facial imaging. Int J Oral Maxillofac Surg. 2018;47:403–10.
63. Yi CR, Oh TM, Jeong WS, Choi JW, Oh TS. Quantitative analysis of the impact of radiotherapy on facial nerve repair with sural nerve grafting after parotid gland surgery. J Craniomaxillofac Surg. 2020;48:724–32.
64. Min K, Lee JH, Kim SC, Choi JW, Oh TS. Quantitative analysis of paralyzed lower eyelid elevation technique: suspension sling versus supporting midcheek lift. Plast Reconstr Surg. 2019;143:829e–39e.
65. Hadlock TA, Urban LS. Toward a universal, automated facial measurement tool in facial reanimation. Arch Facial Plast Surg. 2012;14:277–82.
66. Bray D, Henstrom DK, Cheney ML, Hadlock TA. Assessing outcomes in facial reanimation: evaluation and validation of the SMILE system for measuring lip excursion during smiling. Arch Facial Plast Surg. 2010;12:352–4.
67. Spörri S, Simmen D, Briner HR, Jones N. Objective assessment of tip projection and the nasolabial angle in rhinoplasty. Arch Facial Plast Surg. 2004;6:295–8. ; discussion 299–300.
68. Pöhlmann STL, Harkness EF, Taylor CJ, Astley SM. Evaluation of Kinect 3D sensor for healthcare imaging. J Med Biol Eng. 2016;36:857–70.
69. Gaber A, Taher MF, Wahed MA. Quantifying facial paralysis using the Kinect v2. Conf Proc IEEE Eng Med Biol Soc. 2015;2015:2497–501.
70. Mattila R. Automatic rating system for unilateral facial palsy. 2019.
71. Carro R, Huerta E, Caporal R, Hernandez J, Cruz F. Facial expression analysis with kinect for the diagnosis of paralysis using Nottingham grading system. IEEE Lat Am Trans. 2016;14:3418–26.
72. Guanoluisa GM, Pilatasig JA, Flores LA, Andaluz VH. GY MEDIC v2: quantification of facial asymmetry in patients with automated Bell's palsy by AI. In: International conference on augmented reality, virtual reality and computer graphics. New York: Springer; 2019. p. 351–61.
73. Guntinas-Lichius O, Denzler J. Automatic and objective facial palsy grading index prediction using deep feature regression. In: Medical image understanding and analysis: 24th annual conference, MIUA 2020, Oxford, UK, July 15–17, 2020, proceedings. Cham: Springer; 2020. p. 253.
74. Pan T-Y, Wong Y-X, Lee T-C, Hu M-C. A Kinect-based oral rehabilitation system. In: 2015 International conference on orange technologies (ICOT). IEEE; 2015. p. 71–4.
75. Guanoluisa GM, Pilatasig JA, Andaluz VH. GY MEDIC: analysis and rehabilitation system for patients with facial paralysis. In: International symposium on integrated uncertainty in knowledge modelling and decision making. Springer; 2019. p. 63–75.
76. Harkel TCT, et al. Reliability and agreement of 3D anthropometric measurements in facial palsy patients using a low-cost 4D imaging system. IEEE Trans Neural Syst Rehabil Eng. 2020;28:1817–24.
77. ten Harkel TC, et al. Depth accuracy of the RealSense F200: low-cost 4D facial imaging. Sci Rep. 2017;7:16263.
78. Monini S, et al. Validation of the objective assessment of facial movement with a new software-based system. Acta Otolaryngol. 2019;139:456–60.
79. Monini S, et al. Proposal of a video-recording system for the assessment of Bell's palsy: methodology and preliminary results. Otol Neurotol. 2017;38:1178–85.
80. Beurskens CHG, Heymans PG. Mime therapy improves facial symmetry in people with long-term facial nerve paresis: a randomised controlled trial. Aust J Physiother. 2006;52:177–83.
81. Lindsay RW, Robinson M, Hadlock TA. Comprehensive facial rehabilitation improves function in people with facial paralysis: a 5-year experience at the Massachusetts Eye and Ear Infirmary. Phys Ther. 2010;90:391–7.
82. Dorion J. Facial neuromuscular retraining. Perspect Swallow Swallow Disord (Dysphagia). 2005;14:18–23.
83. Banks CA, Bhama PK, Park J, Hadlock CR, Hadlock TA. Clinician-graded electronic facial paralysis assessment: the eFACE. Plast Reconstruct Surg. 2015;136:223e–30e.
84. Banks CA, Jowett N, Hadlock TA. Test-retest reliability and agreement between in-person and

video assessment of facial mimetic function using the eFACE facial grading system. JAMA Facial Plast Surg. 2017;19:206–11.
85. Chong LSH, et al. Validation of the clinician-graded electronic facial paralysis assessment. Plast Reconstr Surg. 2017;140:159–67.
86. Verhey JT, Haglin JM, Verhey EM, Hartigan DE. Virtual, augmented, and mixed reality applications in orthopedic surgery. Int J Med Robot Comput Assist Surg. 2020;16:e2067.
87. Schijven M, Jakimowicz J. Virtual reality surgical laparoscopic simulators. Surg Endosc Other Interv Tech. 2003;17:1943–50.
88. Okrainec MM. Validation of three virtual reality fundamentals of laparoscopic surgery (FLS) modules. Med Meets Virtual Real 19: NextMed. 2012;173:349.
89. Tepper OM, et al. Mixed reality with HoloLens: where virtual reality meets augmented reality in the operating room. Plast Reconstr Surg. 2017;140:1066–70.
90. Sayadi LR, et al. The new frontier: a review of augmented reality and virtual reality in plastic surgery. Aesthet Surg J. 2019;39:1007–16.
91. Clevin L, Grantcharov TP. Does box model training improve surgical dexterity and economy of movement during virtual reality laparoscopy? A randomised trial. Acta Obstet Gynecol Scand. 2008;87:99–103.
92. Larsen CR, et al. Effect of virtual reality training on laparoscopic surgery: randomised controlled trial. BMJ. 2009;338:1253.
93. Palter VN, Grantcharov TP. Individualized deliberate practice on a virtual reality simulator improves technical performance of surgical novices in the operating room. J Am Coll Surg. 2011;213:S126.
94. Palter VN, Grantcharov TP. Development and validation of a comprehensive curriculum to teach an advanced minimally invasive procedure: a randomized controlled trial. Ann Surg. 2012;256:25–32.
95. Seymour NE. VR to OR: a review of the evidence that virtual reality simulation improves operating room performance. World J Surg. 2008;32:182–8.
96. Ammanuel S, Brown I, Uribe J, Rehani B. Creating 3D models from radiologic images for virtual reality medical education modules. J Med Syst. 2019;43:166.
97. Sultan L, et al. An experimental study on usefulness of virtual reality 360° in undergraduate medical education. Adv Med Educ Pract. 2019;10:907–16.
98. Erel E, Aiyenibe B, Butler PEM. Microsurgery simulators in virtual reality: review. Microsurgery. 2003;23:147–52.
99. Prasolova-Førland E, Molka-Danielsen J, Fominykh M, Lamb K. Active learning modules for multi-professional emergency management training in virtual reality. In: 2017 IEEE 6th international conference on teaching, assessment, and learning for engineering (TALE); 2017. p. 461–8.
100. Rodby KA, et al. Advances in oncologic head and neck reconstruction: systematic review and future considerations of virtual surgical planning and computer aided design/computer aided modeling. J Plast Reconstruct Aesthet Surg. 2014;67:1171–85.
101. Vles MD, Terng NCO, Zijlstra K, Mureau MAM, Corten EML. Virtual and augmented reality for preoperative planning in plastic surgical procedures: a systematic review. J Plast Reconstruct Aesthet Surg. 2020;73(11):1951–9.
102. Avraham T, et al. Functional outcomes of virtually planned free fibula flap reconstruction of the mandible. Plast Reconstruct Surg. 2014;134:628e–34e.
103. Chang EI, Jenkins MP, Patel SA, Topham NS. Long-term operative outcomes of preoperative computed tomography-guided virtual surgical planning for osteocutaneous free flap mandible reconstruction. Plast Reconstr Surg. 2016;137:619–23.
104. Weitz J, et al. Accuracy of mandibular reconstruction by three-dimensional guided vascularised fibular free flap after segmental mandibulectomy. Br J Oral Maxillofac Surg. 2016;54:506–10.
105. Gardiner S, Hartzell TL. Telemedicine and plastic surgery: a review of its applications, limitations and legal pitfalls. J Plast Reconstr Aesthet Surg. 2012;65:e47–53.
106. Tan JR, Coulson S, Keep M. Face-to-face versus video assessment of facial paralysis: implications for telemedicine. J Med Internet Res. 2019;21:e11109.
107. Vyas KS, et al. A systematic review of the use of telemedicine in plastic and reconstructive surgery and dermatology. Ann Plast Surg. 2017;78:736–68.
108. Kramser A. Ambulanz per Videochat. (Clinic consultation via videochat). Telemedizine. In: Vinzenz Magazin, vol. 2. Vienna: Vinzenz Group Austria; 2020.
109. Szczepura A, et al. Raising the digital profile of facial palsy: national surveys of patients' and clinicians' experiences of changing UK treatment pathways and views on future role of digital technology. J Med Internet Res. 2020;22(10):e20406.
110. Pap SA, Lach E, Upton J. Telemedicine in plastic surgery: E-consult the attending surgeon. Plast Reconstr Surg. 2002;110:452–6.
111. Hontanilla B, Aubá C. Automatic three-dimensional quantitative analysis for evaluation of facial movement. J Plast Reconstr Aesthet Surg. 2008;61:18–30.
112. Hontanilla B, Marré D. Comparison of hemihypoglossal nerve versus masseteric nerve transpositions in the rehabilitation of short-term facial paralysis using the facial clima evaluating system. Plast Reconstruct Surg. 2012;130:662e–72e.
113. Frey M, Jenny A, Giovanoli P, Stüssi E. Development of a new documentation system for facial movements as a basis for the international registry for neuromuscular reconstruction in the face. Plast Reconstr Surg. 1994;93:1334–49.

Index

© Springer Nature Switzerland AG 2021
C.-H. J. Tzou, A. Rodríguez-Lorenzo (eds.), *Facial Palsy*,
https://doi.org/10.1007/978-3-030-50784-8

GPSR Compliance

The European Union's (EU) General Product Safety Regulation (GPSR) is a set of rules that requires consumer products to be safe and our obligations to ensure this.

If you have any concerns about our products, you can contact us on ProductSafety@springernature.com

In case Publisher is established outside the EU, the EU authorized representative is:

Springer Nature Customer Service Center GmbH
Europaplatz 3
69115 Heidelberg, Germany

Batch number: 10732799

Printed by Printforce, the Netherlands